MW00837148

Nutrients, Stress, and Medical Disorders

NUTRITION ◊ AND ◊ HEALTH

Adrianne Bendich, Series Editor

Nutrients, Stress, and Medical Disorders, edited by **Shlomo Yehuda and David I. Mostofsky**, 2006

Calcium in Human Health, edited by **Connie M. Weaver and Robert P. Heaney,** 2006

***Preventive Nutrition:** The Comprehensive Guide for Health Professionals, Third Edition,* edited by **Adrianne Bendich and Richard J. Deckelbaum,** 2005

***The Management of Eating Disorders and Obesity,** Second Edition,* edited by **David J. Goldstein,** 2005

Nutrition and Oral Medicine, edited by **Riva Touger-Decker, David A. Sirois, and Connie C. Mobley,** 2005

IGF and Nutrition in Health and Disease, edited by **M. Sue Houston, Jeffrey M. P. Holly, and Eva L. Feldman,** 2005

Epilepsy and the Ketogenic Diet, edited by **Carl E. Stafstrom and Jong M. Rho,** 2004

Handbook of Drug–Nutrient Interactions, edited by **Joseph I. Boullata and Vincent T. Armenti,** 2004

Nutrition and Bone Health, edited by **Michael F. Holick and Bess Dawson-Hughes,** 2004

Diet and Human Immune Function, edited by **David A. Hughes, L. Gail Darlington, and Adrianne Bendich,** 2004

Beverages in Nutrition and Health, edited by **Ted Wilson and Norman J. Temple,** 2004

Handbook of Clinical Nutrition and Aging, edited by **Connie Watkins Bales and Christine Seel Ritchie,** 2004

***Fatty Acids:** Physiological and Behavioral Functions,* edited by **David I. Mostofsky, Shlomo Yehuda, and Norman Salem, Jr.,** 2001

Nutrition and Health in Developing Countries, edited by **Richard D. Semba and Martin W. Bloem,** 2001

***Preventive Nutrition:** The Comprehensive Guide for Health Professionals, Second Edition,* edited by **Adrianne Bendich and Richard J. Deckelbaum,** 2001

***Nutritional Health:** Strategies for Disease Prevention,* edited by **Ted Wilson and Norman J. Temple**, 2001

***Clinical Nutrition of the Essential Trace Elements and Minerals:** The Guide for Health Professionals,* edited by **John D. Bogden and Leslie M. Klevey**, 2000

Primary and Secondary Preventive Nutrition, edited by **Adrianne Bendich and Richard J. Deckelbaum**, 2000

The Management of Eating Disorders and Obesity, edited by **David J. Goldstein,** 1999

***Vitamin D:** Physiology, Molecular Biology, and Clinical Applications,* edited by **Michael F. Holick,** 1999

***Preventive Nutrition:** The Comprehensive Guide for Health Professionals,* edited by **Adrianne Bendich and Richard J. Deckelbaum**, 1997

NUTRIENTS, STRESS, AND MEDICAL DISORDERS

Edited by

SHLOMO YEHUDA, PhD

Psychopharmacology Laboratory, Department of Psychology, and The Gonda Research Center, Bar Ilan University, Ramat Gan, Israel

and

DAVID I. MOSTOFSKY, PhD

Department of Psychology, Boston University, Boston, MA

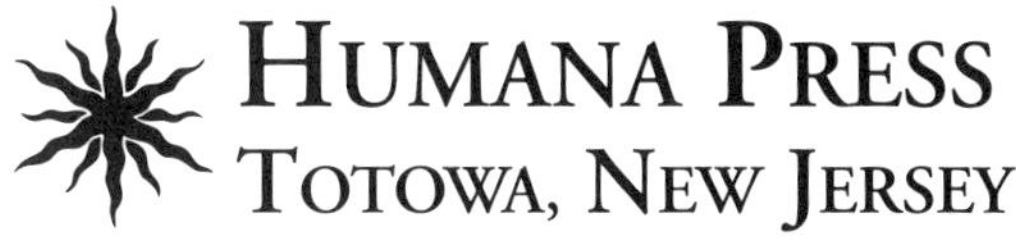

HUMANA PRESS
TOTOWA, NEW JERSEY

999 Riverview Drive, Suite 208
Totowa, New Jersey 07512

www.humanapr.com

Cover design by Patricia F. Cleary

Production Editor: Melissa Caravella

For additional copies, pricing for bulk purchases, and/or information about other Humana titles, contact Humana at the above address or at any of the following numbers: Tel.: 973-256-1699; Fax: 973-256-8341; E-mail: orders@humanapr.com; or visit our website at www.humanapress.com

This publication is printed on acid-free paper. ∞
ANSI Z39.48-1984 (American National Standards Institute) Permanence of Paper for Printed Library Materials.

Printed in the United States of America. 10 9 8 7 6 5 4 3 2 1

eISBN 1-59259-952-4

Library of Congress Cataloging-in-Publication Data

I. Mostofsky.

p. cm. — (Nutrition and health)

Includes bibliographical references and index.

ISBN 1-58829-432-3 (alk. paper) — ISBN 1-59259-952-4 (e-isbn)

1. Stress (Physiology) 2. Stress (Physiology)—Nutritional aspects. 3. Chronic diseases—Nutritional aspects. 4. Inflammation—Nutritional aspects. I. Yehuda, Shlomo. II. Mostofsky, David I. III. Series: Nutrition and health (Totowa, N.J.)

QP82.2.S8N88 2005

616.9'8—dc22

2005003216

Series Editor's Introduction

The *Nutrition and Health Series* of books have had great success because each volume has the consistent overriding mission of providing health professionals with texts that are essential because each includes (1) a synthesis of the state of the science; (2) timely, in-depth reviews by the leading researchers in their respective fields; (3) extensive, up-to-date fully annotated reference lists; (4) a detailed index; (5) relevant tables and figures; (6) identification of paradigm shifts and the consequences; (7) virtually no overlap of information between chapters, but targeted, interchapter referrals; (8) suggestions of areas for future research; and (9) balanced, data-driven answers to patient/health professionals' questions that are based on the totality of evidence rather than the findings of any single study.

The series volumes are not the outcome of a symposium. Rather, each editor has the potential to examine a chosen area with a broad perspective, both in subject matter as well as in the choice of chapter authors. The international perspective, especially with regard to public health initiatives, is emphasized where appropriate. The editors, whose trainings are both research- and practice-oriented, have the opportunity to develop a primary objective for their book, define the scope and focus, and then invite the leading authorities from around the world to be part of their initiative. The authors are encouraged to provide an overview of the field, discuss their own research, and relate the research findings to potential human health consequences. Because each book is developed *de novo*, the chapters are coordinated so that the resulting volume imparts greater knowledge than the sum of the information contained in the individual chapters.

Nutrients, Stress, and Medical Disorders, edited by Shlomo Yehuda and David I. Mostofsky, is a critical addition to the *Nutrition and Health Series* and fully exemplifies the goals of the series. Stress, health, and illness are well accepted as intimately linked. However, the critical influence of nutritional status (and/or specific dietary components that can affect the brain) on mental functions affected by stress has often been a neglected area of research focus. This volume has been developed to examine the current clinical findings and put these into historic perspective as well as point the way to future research opportunities. Both editors are internationally recognized leaders in the field of nutrition and neurological function. Both are excellent communicators and they have worked tirelessly to develop a book that is destined to be the benchmark in the field because of its extensive, in-depth chapters covering the most important aspects of the complex interactions between diet and its nutrient components, mental health, stress, and its impact on disease states. The introductory chapters provide readers with the basics so that the more clinically related chapters can be easily understood. The editors have chosen 40 of the most well-recognized and respected authors from around the world to contribute the 25 informative chapters in the volume.

The chapters of *Nutrients, Stress, and Medical Disorders* are logically organized to provide the reader with a basic understanding as well as an appreciation of the development of the field of stress research, its relationship to brain function, and the potential for nutrients to affect these variables. The first section reviews the history, methodologies, and basic scientific information that is essential to understanding the following sections. In Chapter 1, the reader is introduced to the leading investigators who developed the area of clinical stress research. Three scientific disciplines are compared: biology—exemplified by the work of Walter B. Cannon and Hans Selye; psychology—Kurt Lewin and Richard Lazarus; and psychobiology—John W. Mason and coworkers. In every experimental field of research, the animal models used have been crucial in understanding the complexities of the disease states as well as the development of drugs to treat the disease. Equally important is the understanding of the potential for nutrients to affect responses to stress and/or its treatment. Chapter 2 provides an in-depth look at the animal models used in stress research, effects of food and its deprivation, and also critiques the model's value in predicting human responses. Chapter 3 introduces the reader to the complexities of the physiological responses to stress in the brain, nervous, and endocrine systems, and also includes detailed information about the differences in responses between males and females. Chapter 4 begins the integration of nutrition, stress, and disease. The chapter includes a summary of the extensive literature that is finding a strong association between diets containing fruits and vegetables that are rich in polyphenolic compounds with antioxidant functions and reduced risks of diseases often associated with aging that affect the brain such as Alzheimer's and Parkinson's diseases. The importance of the blood–brain barrier and its role in stressful situations is discussed in-depth in Chapter 5. This chapter also includes an analysis of the roles of neuroactive amino acids and their interactions with the blood–brain barrier.

The second section of the volume includes chapters addressing the interactions between specific nutrients, effects of food, and stress. The editors and their colleagues have included an extensive chapter on the effects of fatty acids on stress responses. Both editors of this volume and Dr. Norman Salem have collaborated on another book in this series, *Fatty Acids*, and consequently, these dietary components are of special interest to the chapter authors. Chapter 6 provides relevant information on the mechanisms of actions of the major polyunsaturated long-chain fatty acids, their availability in the food supply, and their actions on the nervous system, with emphasis on their effects during stress. Chapter 7 examines the interactions between stress, glucocorticoids, and the brain. This chapter spans the research from the cellular to the behavioral levels, as well as providing information on genetic influences on stress responses that are organized in a comprehensive table. Herbal product use has increased dramatically over the last decade and in the United States, these products are classified as dietary supplements. The chapter on herbal products, stress, and the mind critically reviews the clinical literature and provides guidance to health professionals concerning the efficacy and safety of St. John's Wort, Kavakava, valerian, ginkgo and several other plant products associated with stress reduction. Chapter 9 compares and contrasts the stress reactions to drug cravings vs food cravings. Chapter 10 specifically examines the effects of alcohol and alcoholism on stress to the individual, family members, the fetus, and the neonate. Of interest are the interactions between environmental influences other than diet and the effects on stress and central nervous system (CNS) functions. These influences include the effects of temporal (rise in obesity incidence, increase in the number of women in the workforce) and space (neighborhood, city, state, and the medical benefits available) on the interactions between diet and stress.

The chapters in the third section of *Nutrients, Stress, and Medical Disorders* examine the health, mental health, and cognitive functions influenced by stress. Beginning with the discussion of the developing fetus in Chapter 12, there is an extensive review of the literature that points to the critical effects of maternal nutritional status as well as stress level on fetal physical and mental development. Certain components of the diet have specific function in the CNS and are critical for mental health. Chapter 13 examines the role of lipids in the development and treatment of depression. The exciting preliminary data indicate that eicosapentaenoic acid has beneficial effects in depressive patients as well as having virtually none of the serious side effects seen with current drug therapies. To further examine depression, Chapter 14 reviews the role of nicotine in depression as well as sleep. Chapter 15 looks at the clinical data that point to a role of fish oils, rather than any specific long-chain fatty acid, on neurological responses that may lead to the development of aggressive behaviors. Another area given a great deal of public interest is obesity. The next chapter reviews the studies that have looked at the consequences of obesity on stress and the development of eating disorders. This chapter examines the effects of eating on reducing anxiety and its potential to further increase the obesity epidemic.

The fourth and final section of *Nutrients, Stress, and Medical Disorders* reviews the effects of stress on chronic disorders and the influence of inflammation on diet, dietary components, neurological functions, disease incidence, and cognitive functions. Several of these chapters review novel findings, such as those seen in Chapter 17, which examines the adverse effects of hypercholesteremia on immune cells and their functions. To assure that readers understand the effects of high- circulating cholesterol levels on disease, there is an extensive review of the role of cholesterol in immune cell membranes and cytokines. Huntington's disease is an inherited neurodegenerative disease that progresses fairly rapidly, leaving the patient with many physical as well as behavioral abnormalities. Until fairly recently, there were no treatments available; however, as described in the Chapter 18, it appears that there are preliminary findings that eicosapentaenoic acid may slow the progression of this disease. Another critical area that has been included in this unique volume is the effects of and major causes of stress in women. The major diseases that affect women at significantly higher rates than men include several autoimmune diseases, depression, and osteoporosis. All of these medical conditions are discussed in detail in Chapter 19. Also included in this chapter are discussions of stressors associated with menstruation, including polycystic ovarian syndrome and premenstrual syndrome. Type 2 diabetes is a major chronic disease and is preceded by a syndrome that is linked to insulin resistance, syndrome X. The next chapter looks at the role of fatty acids in the development of insulin resistance as well as syndrome X and the stress this metabolic syndrome places on the individual. Another chapter with novel findings deals with the roles of specific amino acids on mental functions. Chapter 21 reviews the effects of amino acids on sleep, mood, and responses to stress. Cardiac function is acutely as well as chronically affected by stress. Less well known is the importance of certain nutrients (such as carnitine, coenzyme Q, and thiamine) on cardiac muscle and nerve responses. The new data on the nutritional requirements that may be increased in the injured or stressed heart are described in Chapter 21. Chapter 22 describes how brain functions are also often adversely affected by stress and the resulting inflammation of brain cells. Long-chain fatty acids are abundant in brain tissue and their dietary intake level has been associated with modulating complex inflammatory responses of specific cytokines in distinct areas in the brain. The next chapter continues to examine the effects of inflammation in the brain and its effects on memory functions. This chapter describes the development of memory, distinct areas of the brain and cytokines that are associated with memory, and the balance between the importance of inflammatory molecules for the development of some memories and the adverse effects of certain inflammatory mediators on memory, especially with stress and aging. The final chapter examines the complex interactions between inflammation and diet throughout the life cycle. This full-circle analysis of the major consequences of stress, dietary deficiencies, and genetic predisposition reminds us of the critical role of nutrition in modulating responses to stress-induced inflammation.

Hallmarks of all of the chapters include complete definitions of terms with the abbreviations fully defined for the reader and consistent use of terms between chapters. There are more than 20 relevant tables, and 55 useful figures, as well as more than 2000 up-to-date references; all chapters begin with a Key Points section, and close with a conclusion that provides the highlights of major findings. The volume contains a highly annotated index and within chapters, readers are referred to relevant information in other chapters.

This important reference text provides practical, data-driven integrated resources based on the totality of the evidence to help the reader evaluate the critical role of nutrition, especially in at-risk populations, in optimizing health and preventing stress-related chronic illnesses. The overarching goal of the editors is to provide fully referenced information to health professionals so they may have a balanced perspective on the value of foods and nutrients that are routinely consumed and how these help to maintain mental as well as physical health.

In conclusion, *Nutrients, Stress, and Medical Disorders*, edited by Drs. Yehuda and Mostofsky, provides health professionals in many areas of research and practice with the most up-to-date, well-referenced, and easy-to-understand volume on the importance of nutrition in reducing stress-related chronic diseases and optimizing health. This volume will serve the reader as the benchmark in this complex area of interrelationships between diet, specific nutrients, CNS function, immune responses, and mental health. The editors are applauded for their efforts to develop the most authoritative resource in the field to date and this excellent text is a very welcome addition to the *Nutrition and Health* Series.

***Adrianne Bendich,* PhD, FACN**
Series Editor

Preface

The entry of the 21st century has been accompanied by a continuing surge of interest in brain science that began with the "Decade of the Brain" initiative. The laboratory research and clinical practice that followed have contributed to a realignment of perspectives, an integration of theory and thought, and the establishment of numerous multidisciplinary collaborations. Nutrition has begun to be recognized for its pharmacological relevance and stress phenomena are no longer viewed simply as mental health constructs. The study and treatment of health and illness has become the province of a broad segment of scientists and clinicians that includes psychologists, immunologists, biochemists, and public health professionals along with physician specialists from medicine. Even a cursory scanning of the published literature reveals the vast terrain that such enterprises represent. Journals, edited volumes, and monograph publications from almost all related disciplines can be expected to report on developments that cross the once familiar disciplinary boundaries. Investigations of nutrition, behavior, and health—in all their combinations—are now more the rule than the exception. For whatever reasons this has come to be, it has taken hold. The implications for research direction inherent in such activities, and especially the potential for interventions and treatments of many serious health conditions, are profound and are attracting the attention of the entire community of health science and delivery.

In *Nutrients, Stress, and Medical Disorders* we have assembled a sampling of the issues and findings that are representative of much of the current theoretical and laboratory activity. The volume is addressed to professionals and graduate students from diverse areas, for whom the need to become better informed about concepts and methodologies from neighboring disciplines is not readily solved by the specialized scientific literature. We have attempted to provide a wide-ranging collection of chapters by established experts that will provide a useful introduction to the literature of each of the areas of stress, nutrition, and medical disorders. In doing so, we have left it to the individual reader to attempt the global integration of the various messages that are presented, and to extract the salient features that will allow extensions for future scientific investigations or clinical applications. We are most appreciative of the valuable support of Humana Press in bringing this work to publication. We are especially grateful to Paul Dolgert, Editorial Director and to Andrianne Bendich, Series Editor for their expertise and patience in working with us on this project, as well as the earlier volumes that we have prepared. Although we were not able to include all of the relevant topics nor include chapters by all of the available experts, it is our hope that the efforts of the respective authors will merit a favorable reception by the audience of those who are advancing our knowledge in each of these areas—nutrition, stress, and health—so that our boundaries of scientific knowledge will be extended and that the quality of human life will be improved.

Shlomo Yehuda, PhD
David I. Mostofsky, PhD

Contents

Contributors

RINAT ARMONY-SIVAN • *Department of Pediatrics, Shaare Zedek Medical Center, Jerusalem, Israel*
WILLIAM A. BANKS • *Department of Internal Medicine, St. Louis University School of Medicine and Geriatric Research, St. Louis, MO*
ADRIANNE BENDICH • *GlaxoSmithKline Consumer Healthcare, Parsippany, NJ*
ELLIOT M. BERRY • *Department of Human Nutrition and Metabolism, Braun School of Public Health, The Hebrew University, Hadassah Medical School, Jerusalem, Israel*
G. CASADESUS • *Institute of Pathology, Case Western Reserve University, Cleveland, OH*
ROBERT DANTZER • *Laboratoire de Neurobiologie Integrative, INRA 1244 CNRS 2723, Bordeaux, France*
UNDURTI N. DAS • *UND Life Sciences, Walpole, MA*
E. R. DE KLOET • *Division of Medical Pharmacology, Leiden/Amsterdam Center for Drug Research, Leiden University, Leiden, The Netherlands*
ROEL H. DERIJK • *Division of Medical Pharmacology, Leiden/Amsterdam Center for Drug Research, Leiden University, Leiden, The Netherlands*
RENÉ DRUCKER-COLÍN • *Departamento de Neurociencias, Instituto de Fisiología Celular, Universidad Nacional Autónoma de México, Mexico City, México*
GAL DUBNOV • *Department of Human Nutrition and Metabolism, Braun School of Public Health, The Hebrew University, Hadassah Medical School, Jerusalem, Israel*
ARTHUR I. EIDELMAN • *Department of Pediatrics, Shaare Zedek Medical Center, Hebrew University School of Medicine, Jerusalem, Israel; The Faculty of Health Sciences, Ben Gurion University of the Negev, Beer Sheva, Israel*
MARTHA M. FARADAY • *Department of Medical and Clinical Psychology, Uniformed Services University of the Health Sciences, Bethesda, MD*
MICHAEL R. FOY • *Department of Psychology, Loyola Marymount University, Los Angeles, CA*
CARLA GAMBARANA • *Department of Neuroscience, University of Siena, Siena, Italy*
MARIA M. GLAVAS • *Department of Cellular and Physiological Sciences, University of British Columbia, Vancouver, BC, Canada*
ROBERT F. GRIMBLE • *Institute of Human Nutrition, University of Southampton, Southampton, UK*
TOMOHITO HAMAZAKI • *Department of Clinical Sciences, Institute of Natural Medicine, Toyama Medical and Pharmaceutical University, Toyama, Japan*
J. A. JOSEPH • *USDA Human Nutrition Research Center on Aging, Tufts University, Boston, MA*
ICHIRO KAWACHI • *Department of Society, Human Development, and Health, Harvard School of Public Health, Boston, MA*
DANIEL KIM • *Department of Society, Human Development, and Health, Harvard School of Public Health, Boston, MA*

JEANSOK J. KIM • *Department of Psychology, University of Washington, Seattle, WA*
SOPHIE LAYÉ • *Laboratoire de Neurobiologie Integrative, INRA 1244 CNRS 2723, Bordeaux, France*
ROGER M. LORIA • *Department of Microbiology and Immunology, Virginia Commonwealth University, Richmond, VA*
DAVID I. MOSTOFSKY • *Department of Psychology, Boston University, Boston, MA*
BASANT K. PURI • *Lipid Neuroscience Group, MRI Unit, MRC Clinical Sciences Centre, Imperial College London, University of London, London, UK*
SHARON RABINOVITZ • *Department of Criminology and Psychopharmacology Laboratory, The Gonda Research Center, Bar Ilan University, Ramat Gan, Israel*
TRACEY J. SHORS • *Department of Psychology, Rutgers University, Piscataway, NJ*
B. SHUKITT-HALE • *USDA Human Nutrition Research Center on Aging, Tufts University, Boston, MA*
MIRO SMRIGA • *Ajinomoto Europe SAS, Paris, France*
MICHAEL J. SOLE • *Heart and Stroke Richard Lewar Centre of Excellence, University Health Network and University of Toronto, Toronto, Canada*
LISA A. TEATHER • *Department of Psychology, Wilfrid Laurier University, Waterloo, Ontario, Canada; Department of Brain and Cognitive Sciences, Massachusetts Institute of Technology, Cambridge, MA*
RICHARD F. THOMPSON • *Neuroscience Program, University of Southern California, Los Angeles, CA*
KUNIO TORII • *Institute of Life Sciences, Ajinomoto Co. Inc., Tokyo, Japan*
AKIHIKO URAYAMA • *Department of Internal Medicine, St. Louis University School of Medicine and Geriatric Research, St. Louis, MO*
JAVIER VELÁZQUEZ-MOCTEZUMA • *Area de Neurociencias, Universidad Autónoma Metropolitana-Iztapalapa, Mexico City, México*
JOANNE WEINBERG • *Department of Cellular and Physiological Sciences, University of British Columbia, Vancouver, BC, Canada*
DAVID WHEATLEY • *Psychopharmacology Research Group, Kingston-on-Thames, UK*
SHLOMO YEHUDA • *Department of Psychology, Psychopharmacology Laboratory, and The Gonda Research Center, Bar Ilan University, Ramat Gan, Israel*
RONIT ZILBERBOIM • *Lonza Loce, Allendale, NJ*

I

History, Methodology, and Basic Science

1 Stress Revisited

A Methodological and Conceptual History

Martha M. Faraday

KEY POINTS

- The modern concept of stress developed over the last 150 yr in two separate branches of science: biology and psychology.
- Because biology and psychology historically are informed by different philosophical traditions with regard to the purpose of science, the concepts of stress that emerged from these two streams are quite different.
- The philosophical differences between biology and psychology dictate the methodological and statistical tools employed by each group of scientists—and therefore shape how questions are asked and answered.
- In the late 20th century, scientists with a psychobiological orientation have attempted to bridge these gaps, drawing on the strengths of both disciplines.
- Better understanding of the relationship between stress, health, and disease and of factors that protect or make the individual vulnerable require integrated conceptual and methodological approaches.

1. INTRODUCTION

Threats or challenges to self precipitate a cascade of responses. The threat or challenge may be physical, environmental, social, or psychological. It may be anticipated, presently occurring, remembered, or imagined. It may be tangibly dangerous, symbolically threatening, or demanding of personal growth. Responses to threats and challenges also take on many forms, including psychological and biological reactions. Emotional life may be overcast by anxiety, and the presence of others sought for reassurance and reevaluation of the threat. Decisions about coping strategies are sifted, weighed, and implemented. The individual's body and brain are steeped in powerful biochemicals. This process, in which internal or external events—stressors—threaten or challenge an organism's existence and well-being and stress responses occur that are directed toward reducing the event's impact, is stress (Baum, Gatchel, & Krantz, 1997; Baum, Grunberg, & Singer, 1982; Baum, Singer, & Baum, 1981).

From: *Nutrients, Stress, and Medical Disorders*
Edited by: S. Yehuda and D. I. Mostofsky © Humana Press Inc., Totowa, NJ

This concept of stress captures the work of many different kinds of stress investigators, including those who regard organisms as primarily biological entities, those who regard organisms as primarily psychological entities, and, less commonly, those who regard organisms as psychobiological entities. These different theoretical orientations have resulted necessarily in different methodological approaches to understand stress, health, and disease. This divergence in approach is rooted in the historical emergence of stress research in which the biological and psychological streams developed largely in isolation from one another. These historical traditions are sufficiently powerful that the remarkable insights of early investigators as well as their errors of omission continue to be perpetuated methodologically and conceptually in today's work. The hybrid psychobiological tradition is beginning to bridge this gap by conceptualizing health and disease as holistic states, recognizing that the subjective psychological world exists inseparable from the biological activities of the body and brain.

This historical and present-day methodological and conceptual divergence in the stress field also reflects a broader, more fundamental difference in point of view about the purpose of science and the tension between two apparently conflicting goals: the need to discover the laws that govern systems and the need to understand individual differences. This critical difference influences the formulation of scientific questions, how experiments are designed, and how data are collected and interpreted and has been described by Kurt Lewin as a conflict between the Aristotelian and Galilean modes of thought (Lewin, 1935).

Lewin notes that the Aristotelian approach assigned paramount importance to an object's membership in a given class because the class itself defined the essence of the object (Lewin, 1935). Classes were dichotomous, mutually exclusive, and defined as the total of characteristics that the group of objects had in common. The laws of science consisted of events or behaviors that occurred frequently and without exception (Lewin, 1935). Importantly, in the Aristotelian conceptualization lawful events were distinct from chance events; chance events were not subject to scientific laws. Because Aristotelian lawfulness can only be demonstrated by frequency, laws implicitly have a statistical, probabilistic nature, and the individual *per se* not only disappears but is not susceptible to lawful explanation (Lewin, 1935).

In contrast, Galilean physics assumed that the entire physical world was comprehensibly lawful, that "[t]he same law govern[ed] the courses of the stars, the falling of stones, and the flight of birds" (Lewin, 1935, p. 10). Membership in a conceptual class as a criterion for understanding an object was irrelevant because the outward appearance of an object did not define its behavior. Mutually exclusive, antithetical categories also lacked meaning and were replaced with the concepts of gradations and series. The fact that an object behaved in a particular way frequently or only once also became irrelevant because laws describing the physical world applied regardless of observed frequency. The distinction between lawful events and chance events disappeared—both common and uncommon events were subject to laws.

The psychologist, generally speaking, is an Aristotelian. Phenomena must be manifested frequently and in groups of organisms in order to be studied meaningfully. Differences in how organisms respond to a manipulation constitute within-group error—the noise of individual differences. Organisms that respond in an extreme way to the manipulation may be considered outliers that bias the group mean. An experiment is successful when probabilistic functions indicate that a group mean is unlikely to have occurred by chance if this group indeed belongs to a population that the control group is assumed to represent. For the psychologist, lawfulness and, by extension, truth, are frequency.

The biologist pursues truth as a Galilean. According to the Galilean point of view, all phenomena are governed by "strict exceptionless lawfulness" (Lewin, 1935, p. 23). The law and, by extension, the truth of a phenomenon can be demonstrated by the responses of one subject. Whether this subject's responses are similar to other subjects' responses makes no difference to the validity of the law. A consequence of this point of view is that there is no need to express subjects' responses as a mean and apply statistical techniques. Each subject's data stand validly alone as expression of particular laws; parametric manipulations blur the underlying laws and their interrelationships. For the biologist, truth is embodied in all observations.

This chapter differs from traditional reviews of the stress literature in several ways. First, in addition to describing the concepts of stress that emerged from each tradition, this review highlights conceptual omissions. Conceptual omissions are important because lines of research are driven by the perception of what is known and what is not known but would be worthwhile to know. Second, methodological inclusions and omissions also are identified. These inclusions and omissions are important because how experiments are designed, what is measured, who is measured, whether and how measurements are manipulated (e.g., statistical analyses), how measurements are interpreted, and how error is conceptualized together determine the nature of the truth that is discovered. The two streams of stress research historically have found different remedies to issues of design, measurement, interpretation, and error that flow from the Aristotelian vs Galilean distinction. These remedies persist today in ongoing work; each has limitations and advantages.

2. THE BIOLOGISTS

Walter B. Cannon's classic work on the fight-or-flight response and Hans Selye's influential conceptualization of stress in terms of the general adaptation syndrome (GAS) are the essence of the biological approach to stress. These investigators were central to carly the definition of the stress concept as it related to health and illness, and their influence can be seen clearly today in the focus on the sympathetic nervous system (SNS) and the hypothalamic–pituitary–adrenal (HPA) axis. To understand the context in which the biological tradition of stress research developed, however, one must first consider the methodological and conceptual approach of 19th-century physiologists. It is against this backdrop that the early 20th-century Cannon proposed that stress is an interaction between external or internal events and homeostatic capacities and the mid-20th-century Selye promulgated the concept that the stress response is nonspecific and occurs in the three stages of the GAS.

Two individuals are relevant. The methodological approach in which Cannon and Selye were trained was epitomized by the work of revered American physiologist William Beaumont. The rationale for this methodological approach was articulated by the great French physiologist Claude Bernard (1813–1866). Bernard's theoretical approach and discoveries also laid the conceptual groundwork for Cannon's contributions to the modern understanding of stress.

2.1. Biological Methodology: Inclusions and Omissions

The methodological hallmarks of the biological approach to the study of stress are: simple experimental designs that often are not fully factorial, one or two independent variables, and multiple control groups; use of small numbers of subjects; careful observation and description and meticulous quantitation of observations; and measurement of biological variables directly related to the question under study. Omissions include the lack of statistical description or analysis; complex experimental designs in which interactions as well as simple main effects can be examined; use of dependent variables such as behaviors that may indicate whether a biological change has behavioral relevance; explicit consideration of the possible role of individual differences such as subjects' sex; and, generally, controls for psychological variables present in the experimental situation that may alter biological responses.

During the 19th century, physiologists were concerned about two kinds of error: error of measurement and error produced by individual differences among subjects. The error associated with individual differences might occur as a result of within-species biologically based differences but also might occur as a result of varying subject–environment interactions. These interactions included factors such as whether an animal was acclimated to the laboratory and its procedures. Because the measurement devices available to early investigators required reference to the whole animal or human as a check on their validity, factors affecting the whole subject were considered important sources of potential error. This 19th-century methodological approach is epitomized in William Beaumont's work.

Beaumont, an Army physician stationed at Fort Crawford in the wilderness of early 19th-century Prairie du Chien, Wisconsin, cared for the French hunter Alexis St. Martin after a penetrating injury to the abdomen. As a result of the wound, St. Martin developed a permanent fistula through which the stomach lining and secretions could be observed (Beaumont, 1833). Beaumont worked with improvised equipment and without journals or colleagues. Nevertheless, he recorded many fundamental principles of digestive physiology. His discoveries included a stress-related fact well known today: extreme emotional states such as anger inhibit digestive activities. Beaumont's work was proof that a single scientist working with meticulous care could reveal the laws of a phenomenon by observations made on one subject.

In contrast, by the late 20th century, biologists generally recognized only error of measurement. In part, this development is a consequence of biology's ever-growing capacity for measurement. It is possible to measure the activity of a single cell, the opening and closing of a single receptor, the activation of chemical cascades linked to G protein receptors, the contents of one vesicle as it empties into a synapse, and particles down to the femptomole concentration. The measured responses cannot be observed directly; they are inferred from instruments and techniques. It is ironic that a scientific tradition grounded in the power of observation to reveal truth now uses instrumentation as a surrogate for observation. One consequence of measurement at a level remote from the whole organism is that the relevance of the whole organism and its environment has tended to disappear. As a result, although over 100 yr of investigations have revealed that subject–environment interactions can alter responses of biological systems, variables such as age, sex, housing conditions, and familiarity with being handled are not generally considered sources of potential error in modern biology.

Classically, statistical methods were also absent. Claude Bernard addressed the biologist's aversion for statistics in his classic 1865 work *An Introduction to the Study of Experimental Medicine.* Bernard objected to the use of data analytical techniques for three reasons: their probabilistic nature obscured the individual, the use of statistics was inappropriate once a cause was defined, and mathematical manipulations that depended on probabilistic functions could never establish causality (Bernard, 1957). Bernard noted that disease outcomes depended on the age, sex, and temperament of the patient as well as on the disease process itself. The use of averages to express outcomes, therefore, could never inform the clinician about the future welfare of a particular patient, although mean outcomes might well describe the general phenomenon:

> The results of statistics, even statistics of large numbers, seem indeed to show that some compensation in the variations of phenomena leads to a law; but as this compensation is indefinite, even the mathematicians confess that it can never teach us anything about any particular case; for they admit that if the red ball comes out fifty times in succession, that is no reason why a white ball would be more likely to come out the fifty-first time. (Bernard, 1957, p. 138)

According to Bernard, different experimental results, once measurement error had been controlled, were the result of variables in the experiment of which the investigator might not be aware. Determining why experiments thought to be similar produced different findings was, in Bernard's view, the window of opportunity for making great discoveries about fundamental principles of biological systems.

2.2. The Biological Conceptualization of Stress: Inclusions and Omissions

Bernard's influence also can be discerned in the biologic conceptualization of stress. He wrote about the instructive value of nonreplicating experiments to communicate a theoretical perspective about the underlying truths of biology: that processes that constituted and sustained life were no different from processes that accounted for changes in inanimate objects (Bernard, 1957). Both consist of chemical reactions that follow measurable laws. In framing physiological investigations this way, Bernard explicitly countered an older scientific tradition that, when confronted with individual differences in susceptibility to disease, assigned causality to differences in "vitality" in order to account for the discrepancies (Bernard, 1957). By putting physiology in a lawful context, Bernard also made clear that all processes operating in normal or diseased states were susceptible to scientific, biological explanation.

Bernard's great contribution to the study of stress was his insight that an organism's ability to move freely in the external environment depended on the capacity of its internal environment (*le milieu interne*) to buffer external influences. The more complex and stable the internal environment, the freer the organism was from fluctuations in the external world. A one-celled organism with a permeable membrane is at the mercy of environmental change. A plant can withstand environmental changes within limits but cannot remove itself from a hostile environment. Amphibians can remove themselves from a hostile environment but still are vulnerable to the temperature of their surroundings. Mammals, however, have developed to the point that they are largely free of the external environment, and humans have perfected this freedom. Because of the complexity and stability of the human internal environment, humans are largely liberated from fluctuations in the external world. In Cannon's words,

> [t]hough the world outside us may be distressingly cold, though the heat and acid which arise from our own strenuous exertions may tend to become an overwhelming menace, we are not greatly disturbed, for our living parts touch only the body fluids which are maintained in an even and steady state. So long as this personal, individual sack of salty water, in which each one of us lives and moves and has his being, is protected from change, we are freed from serious peril. Because that protection is afforded by special physiologic agencies, I have suggested that the stable state of the fluid matrix be given the name *homeostasis*. (Cannon, 1935, p. 2)

2.2.1. Walter B. Cannon

Bernard laid the groundwork for Cannon's remarkable contributions to the study of stress. These contributions include that activity of the SNS could be provoked by internal manipulations or by external physical, environmental, or psychological events; that these homeostatic responses had evolutionary, adaptive, self-preserving significance; that the primary function of the SNS was to preserve homeostasis; and that stress could be conceptualized as an interaction between an organism and an external or internal event mediated by the processes of homeostasis.

Following in the tradition of Beaumont, Cannon's early work focused on digestion using the then newly discovered X-ray technology to follow the course of food treated with bismuth (an X-ray-opaque substance) through the digestive tract. In experiments aimed at determining the purpose of stomach wall movements, Cannon observed that some animal subjects did not exhibit the characteristic waves. After reviewing the experimental methodology for errors in preparation and technique, the frustrated Cannon realized that the waves were absent only in animals that appeared distressed by the experimental procedure (Cannon, 1898, 1945). This observation led to a series of studies on other bodily changes provoked by strong emotions such as rage and fear and the capacity of the sympathetic nerves and adrenal medulla to enact these changes via adrenalin release (e.g., Cannon, 1914, 1928; Cannon & de la Paz, 1911).

At first these adrenalin-provoked changes appeared to be chaotic and disconnected responses of multiple body systems: blood sugar increased to the point of glycosuria; circulation was shunted preferentially to the heart, lungs, brain, and large muscles and markedly diminished to the other viscera; the digestive tract essentially ceased activity; clotting speed increased; and thresholds for muscular exhaustion increased. Cannon, however, was well acquainted with Darwin's *The Origin of Species*. If one assumed that all of the changes had adaptive utility, then the apparent chaos resolved itself into a beautifully orchestrated response geared to the organism's survival. In Cannon's words,

> [t]he changes are, each one of them, *directly serviceable in making the organism more efficient in the struggle which fear or rage or pain may involve*; for fear and rage are aspects of organic preparations for action, and pain attends conditions which naturally evoke supreme exertion. And the organism which with the aid of increased adrenal secretion can best muster its energies, best call forth sugar to supply the laboring muscles, best lessen fatigue, and best send blood to the parts essential in the run or the fight for life, is most likely to survive. (Cannon, 1914, p. 270)

Further studies highlighted the importance of the sympathetic system in maintaining the various necessary steady states of the body (e.g., Cannon, 1929, 1932, 1933, 1935). The sympathetic system's role was to keep the various bodily systems within narrow homeostatic boundaries in the face of challenges. When this process reached a point where the homeostatic system could no longer compensate, then homeostatic resistance was broken, the stress process became a "breaking strain," and the organism was likely to suffer permanent injury, illness, or death (Cannon, 1935). Further, responses that were adaptive when the organism was confronted with a threat that may be physically fought or fled may well be destructive when the threat is not one that can be countered by physical action.

> If the emotion is transformed into action, then the preparation is useful, and the body by anticipation is protected against a low blood sugar, an excessive heat, and a limiting shift in the direction of the acidity of the blood. If no action succeeds the excitement, however, and the emotional stress—even worry or anxiety—persists, then the bodily changes due to the stress are not a preparatory safeguard against disturbance of the fluid matrix but may be in themselves profoundly upsetting to the organism as a whole. (Cannon, 1933, p. 84)

What factors did Cannon omit? Other aspects of the stress concept that became the center of the psychological approach to stress (e.g., perception and appraisal) were also recorded in Cannon's writings but were not examined systematically. Cannon clearly understood the importance of psychological influences, but his goal was the elucidation of the mechanisms by which physiological systems maintained the living organism. The idea that subjective processes influence the stress experience was not revisited experimentally for almost 50 yr, when John W. Mason emphasized the role of appraisal in the 1960s and 1970s, and Richard Lazarus made appraisal his theoretical centerpiece.

2.2.2. Hans Selye

Selye's theory of stress is not only conceptually distinct from Cannon's "fight-or-flight" response but specifically excludes homeostatic adjustments as stress responses. Selye's influence on the field has been enormous. He was a proselytizer of stress, lecturing and writing extensively on his theory during a lengthy career, with more than 1500 scientific publications at his death. He also wrote several popular books on stress that were widely read.

Many different stimuli can raise heart rate—bounding up the stairs, worrying about finances, experiencing rage, joy, hope, or fear. To the extent that the heart rate increases regardless of the specific nature of the stimulus, the individual is experiencing stress according to Selye. Stress is the nonspecific response of the body to demands for adaptation—a deceptively simple concept that often has been misinterpreted to mean that responses to stressors are necessarily and by definition nonspecific. To grasp Selye's conceptual structure, it is important to remember that he was trained as a physician.

In 1925, as a second-year medical student at the University of Prague, Selye observed that the process of diagnosing specific illnesses was complicated by the fact that many different diseases presented similarly (Selye, 1956/1976). Regardless of whether the sufferer endured scarlet fever or influenza, the patient was likely to report loss of appetite, diffuse pains in the joints, and fever and manifest an enlarged spleen or liver. So similar were diverse disease manifestations that the art of the physician, Selye realized, depended on learning to discern subtle, specific, identifying symptoms against the broader nonspecific background of "the syndrome of just being sick" (Selye, 1956/1976). Ten years later, as a research assistant at McGill University, Selye thought he was on the trail of a new and important sex hormone. He attempted to identify the substance with a crude bioassay—injecting ovarian and placental extracts into rats and examining their organs for changes that were not known to be the result of identified sex hormones. His initial experiments yielded striking findings. Animals displayed a triad of symptoms: enlargement of the adrenal cortex; atrophy of the thymus, spleen, and lymph nodes; and deep, bleeding ulcers in the stomach lining (Selye, 1936). As the extracts were purified, however, their effects diminished. Selye realized that the triad was a response to the toxicity of the initial preparations. To test this hypothesis, he treated rats with formalin and other known irritating, toxic agents, and again the same triad was manifested (Selye, 1956/1976).

Selye reported that at this point he remembered the nonspecific "syndrome of just being sick" he had observed as a medical student (Selye, 1956/1976). He believed that this nonspecific syndrome was the key to understanding and treating commonalities among disease processes (Selye, 1956/1976). Continued experimentation revealed that the triad could be produced by multitudinous "stressors"—by injecting other biological substances and also by the use of physical agents such as cold, heat, X-rays, trauma, hemorrhage, pain, or forced exercise.

Further work was interpreted to indicate that this syndrome was manifested in three phases that Selye labeled the GAS: alarm, resistance, and exhaustion (Selye, 1936, 1946, 1956/1976). Initial exposure to the stressor—the alarm stage—resulted in production of adrenocorticotropic hormone (ACTH) by the pituitary which stimulated the adrenal cortices to produce corticoids. Later this model was modified to include the role of the hypothalamus and corticotropin-releasing factor (CRF) as instigators of the pituitary response (Selye, 1956/1976). The influence of the corticoids, Selye believed, produced the other distinguishing features of the triad—thymic involution and stomach ulcers. Other manifestations of the alarm stage included weight loss, hemoconcentration, and general tissue catabolism. If the stressor overwhelmed the body during this stage, the organism died. If the stressor did not overwhelm the body during this initial stage, then a period of adaptation to the presence of the stressor ensued—the resistance stage. In the resistance stage, production of corticoids dropped to only slightly above normal as the organism adapted to the stressor and body weight returned to normal. If the stressor continued long enough, however, the organism's capacity for adaptation was overwhelmed and the stage of exhaustion ensued, in which corticoid production again rose and multiple "diseases of adaptation," related to the destructive effects of continued excess corticoid production, might occur.

Over the next 40 yr, Selye's original formulation of the concept of stress and the GAS evolved but remained consistent with his early ideas of a nonspecific syndrome in response to a specific stressor that also had specific, nonstress effects. In its most extensive articulation by Selye, stress is the *nonspecific* response of the body to any demand (pleasant or unpleasant) for adaptation (Selye, 1956, 1973). Stressors are *specific* stimuli that produce the nonspecific syndrome of stress (Selye, 1973). Stressor effects depend on the intensity of the demand made on the adaptive capacity of the body. Stress explicitly is *not* tension, the discharge of hormones from the adrenal medulla, necessarily the result of damage, or any deviation from homeostasis. Further, stress is distinct from the stressor and also distinct from the GAS. Stress is "the state manifested by a specific syndrome which consists of all the nonspecifically induced changes within a biologic system" (Selye, 1956, p. 54). It is a construct whose existence can be inferred by the presence of specific indices.

Selye's contention that stress is indexed by a nonspecific syndrome and occurs according to the GAS has been challenged by a number of investigators, including Mason (*see* Section 4). Criticisms of the nonspecificity tenet include that the same stressor does not produce the same syndrome across individuals. Selye counters in two ways. First, Selye noted that "conditioning" factors—internal (e.g., genetic predispositions, age, gender, past experience) or external (e.g., drug treatments, dietary factors, climate)—can enhance or inhibit the GAS, rendering individuals differentially susceptible to stress (Selye, 1975). Stimuli that demand adaptation have two kinds of action: stressor (nonspecific) effects (by definition the effects that produce stress) and specific effects. Specific effects are variable and characteristic of the individual agent. The organism's response depends on both kinds of effects as well as on the organism's reactivity.

Although best known for his emphasis on the corticosteroids, Selye's model of stress effects as early as 1956 incorporated multiple organ systems. In addition to the HPA axis, it included the hypothalamic–pituitary–thyroid axis; the liver and its multiple metabolic functions; the kidneys, blood vessels, and connective tissues, and the immune system. Selye's insight that stress potentially affected every bodily system was an important contribution to understanding how stress and disease states might be related.

What were Selye's conceptual omissions? His model included every tissue in the body except for the brain. He speculated that corticoids might influence cognitive processes (Selye, 1976), but did not pursue this line of work. For Selye, the brain was primarily the anatomical locale for the hypothalamus and pituitary. In addition, despite his inclusion of individual differences in his model in the form of conditioning factors that mediate stress responses, his experimental work did not reflect a systematic attempt to model and manipulate conditioning factors. Further, although he knew that psychological stimuli were sufficient to evoke stress responses, he concentrated on physical and pharmacological stressors almost exclusively. Ironically, Selye's parenthetical observation that psychological stimuli (which Selye considered mild in comparison to physical stressors) were sufficient to elicit such responses was one of the reasons Mason focused on psychological stress (Mason, 1971).

3. THE PSYCHOLOGISTS

Whereas biologists sought to understand the mechanisms by which the body responded to external or internal challenges, psychologists focused on the psychological apparatus through which events are sifted and experienced. The conceptual exemplar for the predominantly psychological approach to stress is Richard S. Lazarus, who emphasized appraisal, coping responses, and the process nature of the stress experience.

The methodological approach of experimental psychologists has a long and complex history in which the contributions of many individuals are relevant. Conceptually, the idea that the subjective psychological world constitutes the overwhelming reality for the individual and therefore can explain behavior was classically articulated by Kurt Lewin.

3.1. Psychological Methodology: Inclusions and Omissions

Experimental psychology and psychological field and epidemiological studies are predicated on the assumptions of Aristotelian science described by Lewin. For psychologists, truth is a probabilistic phenomenon, the validity of which is indicated by frequency of occurrence and the manifestation of which is assumed to follow a normal distribution. This probabilistic emphasis necessitates the use of groups of subjects, descriptive as well as inferential data analytical techniques, and, in theory, allows statements about a phenomenon only in terms of quantified uncertainty. The use of data analytical techniques allows complex multivariate (multiple independent variables as well as multiple dependent variables) experimental designs. With the tools of multivariate analysis and design, complex interrelationships among variables can be examined. The methodological hallmarks of the psychological approach to the study of stress also include measurement of psychological variables directly related to the phenomenon under investigation by self-report and, occasionally, measurement of behaviors and physiological responses. Error is assumed to be normally distributed, and random or quasi-random subject assignment is intended to optimize the probability that error is spread equally across treatment groups, allowing the treatment effect to stand out against the background of error.

Like early biologists, early experimental psychologists were aware of two kinds of error: error associated with measurements and individual difference error. As in biology, it is the treatment of individual difference error that has changed. Modern experimental psychology has largely overlooked the fact that statistical examination of individuals or very small groups is possible when subjects are measured repeatedly. As a result of the focus on group means as the unit of analysis, differences among subjects in the same group (within-group variance) are considered noise.

The general methodological approach of psychology is based on the work of many individuals from the 18th–20th centuries. That multicausal phenomena—ranging from reaction times to record a star's movement across a stationary line in the eyepiece of a telescope to marriage, birth, and death rates in a country's population—were more accurately described with many measurements rather than with a few was well-known in the 18th and 19th centuries. The work of Pierre S. Laplace (1749–1827) and Carl F. Gauss (1777–1855) in particular demonstrated that error is decreased when observations are combined and that patterns of error as well as patterns of data can be described with normal curves (Stigler, 1986). Many workers in the social sciences speculated that the curve also might have inferential utility. Adolphe Quetelet (1796–1874) struggled to use the curve as an inferential tool. In Quetelet's words, "*The greater the number of individuals observed, the more do individual peculiarities, whether physical or moral, become effaced, and allow the general facts to predominate, by which society exists and is preserved*" (Quetelet, 1842, p. 6). One incontrovertible fact thwarted Quetelet: human behaviors were the complex outcome of multitudinous causes. Quetelet did not succeed in developing inferential statistical tools for the social sciences, but his work contributed to the insights of those who ultimately developed such tools: Sir Francis Galton, Francis Y. Edgeworth, Karl Pearson, and Ronald A. Fisher (Stigler, 1986).

As social scientists struggled with the complexity of large data sets, the psychophysicists found a way around the problem of multicausality in the context of experimental psychology. The powerful tool of the factorial design, a mainstay of modern experimental psychology, emerged from Fechner's work on the differential perceptual sensitivity of individuals. Like the social scientists of the time, Fechner knew that any given measurement was affected by a multitude of factors. From Gauss and Laplace he borrowed the assumption that patterns of error were normally distributed and applied the principle to the responses of a single subject. Fechner realized that these factors could be systematically manipulated and controlled by conducting experiments with many different conditions (Fechner, 1860). Herman Ebbinghaus took the next step in his studies of a more complex, multicausal phenomenon—memory—by using the normal distribution as a test for the validity of a set of data and casting departures from the central tendency in terms of their probable error. Modern statisticians have gone well beyond these insights, but the pychophysicists' contributions of the factorial design to dissect causality and the applicability of the normal curve to inference were crucial to these later advances.

Methodologically, what was lost? Despite the fact that experimental psychology adopted the powerful tool of the factorial design that originated in psychophysics, the concept of the individual as a unit of study disappeared. Because early work focused on perceptual and cognitive properties of humans or on epidemiological and sociological outcomes, the use of animal models to study human conditions was not explored. Although Fechner in particular was aware that perceptual abilities were affected by factors such as whether the subject had recently eaten (Fechner, 1860), the idea that human behavior was a consequence of biological as well as psychological forces was not considered.

3.2. The Psychological Conceptualization of Stress: Inclusions and Omissions

Kurt Lewin focused on the role of the subjective psychological world in human experience—the cornerstone of appraisal, coping, predictability, and controllability. Lewin's work has been chosen as the conceptual prelude to Richard S. Lazarus's work because of Lazarus's theme of subjective experience as crucial to understanding stress.

3.2.1. Kurt Lewin

In 1917, while serving in the German army during World War I, Lewin wrote a paper called "The War Landscape" in which he described how the soldier's "life-space" is dramatically different from that of the civilian's. A civilian might consider a secluded place as ideal for a picnic, whereas a soldier might consider the same place as likely to harbor an ambush (Hothersall, 1990). After the war Lewin continued to develop this theme into what became his theory of topological psychology, most extensively described in *Principles of Topological Psychology* (1936).

Lewin's theory is centered on the concept of the life-space. The life-space constitutes the subjective psychological world of the individual. Within the life-space is a constantly changing complex of needs (innate states that involve tension, e.g., hunger) and quasi-needs (states that involve learned tensions, e.g., social acceptance or achievement). These tensions give rise to forces that are given direction (e.g., vectors) depending on the valence of particular goal regions. Any behavior could be explained, Lewin believed, by understanding the interrelationships among all of the operating vectors and goal regions in the "psychological field *at that time*" (Lewin, 1943, p. 294).

Lewin's relevance to stress research is that the objective existence of an event in the external world is experienced by the individual within the subjective world of the life-space. Human reality is psychological, cognitive, subjective, and fluid. Whether the event is a threat or challenge depends on how the event is perceived to impinge on the life-space. The subjective nature of the person–environment interaction is the essence of Lazarus's work.

3.2.2. Richard S. Lazarus

"Psychological stress is a particular relationship between the person and the environment that is appraised by the person as taxing or exceeding his or her resources and endangering his or her well-being" (Lazarus & Folkman, 1984, p. 19). For Lazarus the subjective psychological experience of stress is a function of the psychological factors that the person brings to the transaction—past experiences, memories, biases, early childhood influences—and of the stimuli that the environment presents to the person. The implication of this definition is that individuals vary in the degree to which they experience stress in a particular situation and that objectively defined properties of the environmental stimulus are insufficient to explain the stress process.

According to Lazarus, two processes mediate the person–environment relationship: cognitive appraisal and coping. Appraisal is a process of evaluation in which it is determined to what extent a particular transaction or series of transactions between the person and the environment is stressful. Coping is the process through which the person–environment relationship demands and the emotions they generate are managed (Lazarus & Folkman, 1984).

Primary appraisal refers to the evaluation of a person–environment transaction as irrelevant, benign-positive, or stressful. The judgment that a transaction is irrelevant implies that nothing is to be lost or gained. A benign-positive transaction is one construed to enhance or potentially enhance well-being. The evaluation of a transaction as stressful indicates the possibility of harm/loss, threat, or challenge. When harm or loss is anticipated but has not yet occurred, the appraisal is one of threat and the resulting emotions are negative—fear, anxiety, or anger. The appraisal of challenge occurs when the transaction holds the potential for growth. The emotional responses to the challenge appraisal are positive—eagerness, excitement, and exhilaration (Lazarus & Folkman, 1984). Secondary appraisal involves assessing which coping options are available, how likely those options are to successfully address the problem, and to what extent the individual is able to carry out those options effectively.

The processes of appraisal are themselves modified by other factors within the person: commitments and beliefs. These variables exert influence on the appraisal process in three ways: (a) by determining what is salient for well-being in a given encounter, (b) by shaping the person's understanding of the event and the resulting emotions and coping behaviors, and (c) by providing the basis for evaluating outcomes (Lazarus & Folkman, 1984). Situational factors also influence the stress experience. Lazarus and Folkman (1984) distinguish between uncertainty—the person not knowing what the event might mean—and ambiguity—lack of information about the situation itself. In ambiguous situations, factors about the person become the most important determinants of responses, and these factors also determine whether the ambiguity makes the experience more or less stressful. The processes of appraisal continue as the stressful transaction continues. This process is called reappraisal and reflects the essential process nature of the stress experience.

Coping is the "constantly changing cognitive and behavioral efforts to manage specific external and/or internal demands that are appraised as taxing or exceeding the resources of the person" (Lazarus & Folkman, 1984, p. 141). Coping responses can be divided into two categories: responses aimed at the problem itself—problem-focused coping—and responses aimed at managing emotional responses to the problem—emotion-focused coping (Folkman & Lazarus, 1980). Problem-focused coping is more likely to occur when the situation is perceived to be susceptible to action, and emotion-focused coping is more likely when appraisal indicates that nothing can be done about the event. Problem-focused coping includes strategies such as defining the problem, looking for alternative solutions, weighing the costs and benefits of various alternatives, choosing among the solutions, and acting on the decision. Emotion-focused coping includes cognitive processes such as distancing, minimization, avoidance, and selective attention. These strategies may lead to reappraisal of the situation as less harmful than originally believed even though the situation remains objectively the same. Emotion-focused coping also consists of behaviors that may lead to reappraisals such as exercising in order to distract oneself from a problem, venting anger or fear, drinking alcohol, and seeking social support.

Omitted from the psychological model is the idea that humans also are complex biological organisms and that biological activity may affect psychological processes. Lazarus' work is driven by a one-way, top-down assumption—that cognition drives the stress experience including biological stress responses, and that biological responses, if they are relevant, are trivial compared to psychological processes. As a consequence, possible biological contributions to the subjective nature of the stress experience are not considered. It is possible, however, that appraisal and coping depend to some extent on the individual's biological responses during a given person–environment interaction. Lazarus left unexamined the possibility that people's cognitions are a coping response for their idiosyncratic physiological responses. In addition, because the subjective, psychological world is conceived of as a peculiarly human one, the possible role of animal models is not explored.

4. THE PSYCHOBIOLOGISTS

The psychobiologists' conceptual contributions to the understanding of stress integrate psychology and biology. John W. Mason is the prototypical stress psychobiologist. Mason's investigations are organized around two themes: that psychological stress is a potent inducer of stress responses and that the biological consequences of stress are homeostatic and depend on psychological factors. Biology's capacity for sensitive and accurate measurement of biological processes, its potential to illuminate underlying mechanisms governing diverse bodily systems, and its emphasis on the presence of lawful phenomena as revealed in the individual coupled with psychology's awareness of the power of environment and the subjective psychological world to influence behavior and the appropriate use of inferential statistics are united in Mason's 40 yr of investigations. The result is an approach to stress research that attempts to integrate the activity of multiple endocrine systems, cognitive variables such as appraisal, personality factors, and environmental or situational variables.

4.1. Psychobiological Methodology: Inclusions and Omissions

Methodologically, Mason's work blends the biological and psychological traditions. In part, his work reflects the methodological emphases of the early physiologists—meticulous and repeated measurement of biological responses, small numbers of subjects and appreciation for the individual, and a disinclination to consider extreme responses as aberrant. He also draws from the psychological tradition, using field studies of soldiers during war to study human stress responses and creating animal models of psychological stress with classical and operant conditioning paradigms. Noting that means obscured individual differences in highly variable hormonal responses, he also used nonparametric tests and presented the data of individual human and animal subjects to demonstrate reported variability. He emphasized the need when examining hormonal responses to have repeated sampling and concurrent measurements of psychological states in order to interpret biological data (e.g., Mason, 1968c).

What did Mason omit methodologically? Missing from the human and animal work is measurement of behavior not directly related to the question under examination. In the animal work, this omission was partly a consequence of using conditioning paradigms in which the only behavior that could be measured in the experimental situation was lever-pressing. He also generally used only male subjects. Further, the stressors employed (e.g., exposure to war, 3-d avoidance task interfering with feeding and sleeping) were extreme.

4.2. The Psychobiological Conceptualization of Stress: Inclusions and Omissions

Mason conceptualizes stress as an interaction between psychological, environmental, and biological variables. The individual's experience of stress and manifestation of stress responses depends on appraisal of a situation or stimulus, personality factors, situational or environmental influences, and an integrated multihormonal response. He focused on endocrinological responses as evolutionarily functional reactions associated with extreme psychological stress in normal humans and animals. From Bernard and Cannon he took the assumption that biological responses to disruption are homeostatic, prepare the organism for exertion, and are aimed at preserving the organism. Mason adds that psychoendocrine responses are essentially anticipatory in nature (Mason, 1968b).

In general, human studies conducted by Mason and coworkers (Bourne, Rose, & Mason, 1967, 1968; Mason, Giller, Kosten, & Harkness, 1988; Mason, Kosten, Southwick, & Giller, 1990; Poe, Rose, & Mason, 1970; Rose, Poe, & Mason, 1968) demonstrated that the magnitude of corticosteroid responses

> did not correspond to objective measures of the significance of the threat, particularly in terms of the extent to which it was life-threatening. This suggested that for any individual the significance of any event in the environment could only be interpreted as a function of the interaction of his ego defenses, and the manner in which he perceived the environment. (Bourne et al., 1967, p. 104)

Studies in men under the extreme stressor of combat or threat of combat also revealed the power of psychological forces to influence HPA axis activity. In helicopter ambulance medics corticosteroid levels not only were lower than in a noncombat control group but remained low regardless of whether the individual was in combat (Bourne et al., 1967). The authors attributed stable low corticosteroid levels to the use of complex psychological defenses that enabled subjects to perceive reality in a way that minimized danger and led to feelings of invincibility and invulnerability. These defenses included feelings of job gratification, prestige accorded by other troops, expressions of gratitude by evacuated casualties, religious beliefs, ritualistic behaviors, and calculations of the probability of being injured or killed.

From these studies and an extensive series of animal studies, Mason and colleagues concluded that (a) responses to psychological stressors were profound, often not linked closely in time with the actual experience, persisted for days or weeks after the stressor ceased, and exhibited marked individual differences; (b) acute hormonal responses are sensitive to subtle differences in the psychological parameters of the stressor (i.e., presence or absence of ambiguity) (Mason, 1968a, 1975, Mason, Mangan, Brady, Conrad, & Rioch, 1961; Mason, Hartley, Mougey, Ricketts, & Jones, 1973); (c) hormonal responses to psychological stress are provoked by *anticipated* metabolic needs and are aimed at meeting those needs and restoring homeostasis (Mason, 1968a); and (d) the responses of individual hormones during and after stress must be evaluated in a multihormonal context because individual hormones have multiple and sometimes opposing effects on metabolic processes and hormones interact with one another in a complex, mutually regulatory manner at any given time-point as well as over time (Mason, 1968b).

Mason also counters Selye's nonspecificity concept. He notes that endocrinological responses to physical stressors such as heat, cold, blood loss, and hyperinsulinemia counter the challenge in specific homeostatic ways rather than in nonspecific ways (Mason, 1971, 1975). Second, Mason points out that physical stressors such as fasting, exercise, cold, and heat have inherent psychological stress components. Mason argues that the effects of physical stressors have historically been confounded with effects of psychological stress and demonstrated empirically that when psychological components are reduced or eliminated, adrenocorticol responses are also reduced or eliminated (Mason, Jones, Ricketts, Brady, & Tolliver, 1968; Mason, Wool, Mougey, Wherry, Collins, & Taylor, 1968). The major disadvantage of Mason's psychobiological stress model is the failure to entertain the possibility that psychological and biologic responses may interact in a bidirectional manner. Like Lazarus, Mason's theoretical approach assumes a top-down process in which psychological factors affect biological processes, but not *vice versa*.

5. CONCLUSIONS

Theory as a guide for empirical work is essential to making progress in a field. In Lewin's words, "it is an illusion to believe that it is possible to develop on a purely empirical basis any science which deals with questions of interdependence and causation" (Lewin, 1938, p. 12). How stress, health, and illness are defined, therefore, guides the choice of question under investigation, the design of experiments, the interpretation of data, and the choice of future directions. Given the retrospective clarity that historical consideration offers, it is clear that better understanding of the relationship between stress and disease requires viewing the individual as a psychobiological entity. Psychological forces are the perceptible core of human existence: awareness of self, the relevance of the threat or challenge to self, and cognitive and behavioral responses aimed at preserving self. Biological forces operate largely beneath the level of psychological awareness, are evolutionarily old, and follow their own mute teleology of homeostasis—another form of self-preservation.

The challenge for stress researchers in the 21st century is to discover the mechanisms by which individual differences that are the product of culture, gender, environment, personal history, personality, genotype, physiology, and neurochemistry make the individual vulnerable or resistant to stress-induced physical and psychological disease. Approaches to this challenge that incorporate awareness of humans as psychobiological entities and that comprise a variety of methodological tools are the most likely to make important contributions to the field.

REFERENCES

Baum, A., Gatchel, R. J., & Krantz, D. S. (1997). *An introduction to health psychology*, 3rd ed. New York: McGraw-Hill.

Baum, A., Grunberg, N. E., & Singer, J. E. (1982). The use of psychological and neuroendocrinological measurements in the study of stress. *Health Psychology, 1*(3), 217–236.

Baum, A., Singer, J. E., & Baum, C. S. (1981). Stress and the environment. *Journal of Social Issues, 37*(1), 4–35.

Beaumont, W. (1833). *Experiments and observations on the gastric juice and the physiology of digestion.* Plattsburgh, NY: F. P. Allen.

Bernard, C. (1957). *An introduction to the study of experimental medicine.* New York: Dover.

Bourne, P. G., Rose, R. M., & Mason, J. W. (1967). Urinary 17-OHCS levels: Data on seven helicopter ambulance medics in combat. *Archives of General Psychiatry, 17*, 104–110.

Bourne, P. G., Rose, R. M., & Mason, J. W. (1968). 17-OHCS levels in combat. *Archives of General Psychiatry, 19*, 135–140.

Cannon, W. B. (1898). The movements of the stomach studied by means of the roentgen rays. *American Journal of Physiology, I*, 359–382.

Cannon, W. B. (1914). The interrelations of emotions as suggested by recent physiological researches. *American Journal of Psychology, XXV*, 256–282.

Cannon, W. B. (1928). The mechanism of emotional disturbance of bodily functions. *The New England Journal of Medicine, 198*(17), 877–884.

Cannon, W.B. (1929). Organization for physiological homeostasis. *Physiological Reviews, IX*(3), 399–431.

Cannon, W. B. (1932). *The wisdom of the body.* New York: W.W. Norton.

Cannon, W. B. (1933). *Some modern extensions of Beaumont's studies on Alexis St. Martin.* Reprinted from the *Journal of the Michigan State Medical Society*, March-May, 1933.

Cannon, W. B. (1935). Stresses and strains of homeostasis. *The American Journal of the Medical Sciences, 189*(1), 1–14.

Cannon, W. B. (1945). *The way of an investigator.* New York: W.W. Norton.

Cannon, W. B., & de la Paz, D. (1911). Emotional stimulation of adrenal secretion. *American Journal of Physiology, 28*, 64–70.

Fechner, G. T. (1860). *Elements of psychophysics* (H. E. Adler, D. H. Howes, & E. G. Boring, Eds. and Trans.). New York: Holt, Rinehart & Winston.

Folkman, S., & Lazarus, R. S. (1980). An analysis of coping in a middle-aged community sample. *Journal of Health and Social Behavior, 21*, 219–239.

Hothersall, D. (1990). *History of psychology.* New York: McGraw-Hill.

Lazarus, R. S., & Folkman, S. (1984). *Stress, appraisal, and coping.* New York: Springer.

Lewin, K. (1935). *A dynamic theory of personality: Selected papers.* New York: McGraw-Hill.

Lewin, K. (1936). *Principles of topological psychology* (F. Heider & G. Heider, Trans.). New York: McGraw-Hill.

Lewin, K. (1938). *The conceptual representation and the measurement of psychological forces.* Durham, NC: Duke University Press.

Lewin, K. (1943). Defining the "field at a given time." *Psychological Review, 50*, 292–310.

Mason, J.W. (1968a). Organization of the multiple endocrine response to avoidance in the monkey. *Psychosomatic Medicine, 30*(5, Part II), 774–790.

Mason, J.W. (1968b). "Over-all" hormonal balance as a key to endocrine organization. *Psychosomatic Medicine, 30*(5, Part II), 791–808.

Mason, J.W. (1968c). A review of psychoendocrine research on the pituitary-thyroid system. *Psychosomatic Medicine, 30*(5, Part II), 666–681.

Mason, J.W. (1971). A re-evaluation of the concept of "non-specificity" in stress theory. *Journal of Psychiatric Research, 8*, 323–333.

Mason, J. W. (1975, June). A historical view of the stress field. *Journal of Human Stress*, 22–36.

Mason, J. W., Giller, E. L., Kosten, T. R., & Harkness, L. (1988). Elevation of urinary norepinephrine/cortisol ratio in posttraumatic stress disorder. *The Journal of Nervous and Mental Disease, 176*(8), 498–502.

Mason, J. W., Hartley, L. H., Mougey, E. H., Ricketts, P., & Jones, L. G. (1973). Plasma cortisol and norepinephrine responses in anticipation of muscular exercise. *Psychosomatic Medicine, 35*, 406–414.

Mason, J. W., Jones, J. A., Ricketts, P. T., Brady, J. V., & Tolliver, G. A. (1968). Urinary aldosterone and urine volume responses to 72-hr avoidance sessions in the monkey. *Psychosomatic Medicine, 30*(5, Part II), 733–745.

Mason, J. W., Kosten, T. R., Southwick, S. M., & Giller, E. L. (1990). The use of psychoendocrine strategies in post-traumatic stress disorder. *Journal of Applied Social Psychology, 20*(21), 1822–1846.

Mason, J. W., Mangan, G. F., Brady, J. V., Conrad, D., & Rioch, D. (1961). Concurrent plasma epinephrine, norepinephrine and 17-hydroxycorticosteroid levels during conditioned emotional disturbances in monkeys. *Psychosomatic Medicine, 23*, 344.

Mason, J. W., Wool, M. S., Mougey, E. H., Wherry, F. E., Collins, D. R., & Taylor, E. D. (1968). Psychological vs. nutritional factors in the effects of "fasting" on hormonal balance. *Psychosomatic Medicine, 30*, 554–575.

Poe, R. O., Rose, R. M., & Mason, J. W. (1970). Multiple determinants of 17-hydroxycorticosteroid excretion in recruits during basic training. *Psychosomatic Medicine, 32*(4), 369–378.

Quetelet, A. (1842). *A treatise on man and the development of his faculties*. Edinburgh: Chambers.

Rose, R. M., Poe, R. O., & Mason, J. W. (1968). Psychological state and body size as determinants of 17-OHCS excretion. *Archives of Internal Medicine, 121*, 406–413.

Selye, H. (1936). A syndrome produced by diverse nocuous agents. *Nature, 138*, 32.

Selye, H. (1946). The general adaptation syndrome and the diseases of adaptation. *Journal of Clinical Endocrinology, 6*, 117–230.

Selye, H. (1973). The evolution of the stress concept. *American Scientist, 61*, 692–699.

Selye, H. (1975). Confusion and controversy in the stress field. *Journal of Human Stress*, 37–44.

Selye, H. (1976). *The stress of life*. New York: McGraw-Hill. (Original work published 1956)

Selye, H., & Heuser, G. (1954). *Fourth annual report on stress—1954*. Montreal, Canada: Acta Medical Publications.

Stigler, S. M. (1986). *The history of statistics: The measurement of uncertainty before 1900*. Cambridge, MA: Belknap Press of Harvard University Press.

2 Experimental Protocols for the Study of Stress in Animals and Humans

Carla Gambarana

KEY POINTS

- Stress is the response of an organism to a stressor of physical, chemical, or emotional nature.
- Exposure to stressors induces behavioral and neuroendocrine consequences in experimental animals as well as in humans, and this complex response can be adaptive or maladaptive.
- Experimentally, the exposure to different stressors is used in order to study the evoked responses and the mechanisms underlying them or to modify the behavior of animals in an attempt to reproduce reliable models of psychiatric symptoms with a stress-related component in humans.
- In animals of the same species, strain, sex, and age maintained in controlled environmental conditions, we can expect reproducible behavioral and neuroendocrine responses to stressful protocols, which are proportional to the intensity of the stressor and the duration of the exposure. The reproducibility of the response is crucially bound to the controlled experimental conditions used.
- In human experiments, the main difficulties in controlling experimental conditions are not related to the stressor (intensity and duration of exposure ethically acceptable), but are mainly related to the large interindividual variability in sensitivity to any kind of traumatic stimulus or event, which can sometimes be explained on the basis of genetic variables or particular personal histories.

1. INTRODUCTION

The term "stress" has several meanings; in behavioral research it is used in the sense of "a physical, chemical, or emotional factor (as trauma, histamine, or fear) to which an individual fails to make a satisfactory adaptation" or "the state or condition of strain (Webster's dictionary, 1971)." Selye used "stress" to indicate the response of an organism to a "stressor" and made a distinction between adaptive and maladaptive responses (Selye, 1950, 1974). Emotional stimuli such as novelty, withholding of reward, and anticipation of punishment (rather than punishment itself) are the most frequent stressors and among the most efficacious activators of the neuroendocrine systems that play a role

From: *Nutrients, Stress, and Medical Disorders*
Edited by: S. Yehuda and D. I. Mostofsky © Humana Press Inc., Totowa, NJ

in stress responses (Mason, 1968, 1975). A more comprehensive definition of stress given by Goldstein (1987) is a condition when expectations, whether genetically programmed or established by a prior learning, do not match the current or anticipated perceptions of internal or external environment. This discrepancy causes a complex range of adaptive responses, whose pattern is dependent upon the type and duration of the provoking event (Chrousos, 1998; Pacak & Palkovits, 2001).

1.1. Modeling of Stress in Animals

Exposure to stressors induces behavioral and neuroendocrine sequelae that are often used to experimentally mimic in animals the symptoms that characterize specific human psychiatric disorders (Willner, 1995). This is possible because animals of the same species, strain, sex, and age maintained in controlled environmental conditions show a sufficiently homogeneous response to stressful conditions that is proportional to the intensity of the stressor and the duration of the exposure. Thus, a stress protocol can be calibrated and standardized in order to obtain reproducible behavioral and neuroendocrine modifications. These stress procedures should never exceed the rigid limits imposed by the international ethical committees, and their reproducibility is crucially bound to the controlled experimental conditions used. Within these limits we can design stressful procedures that may result in either adaptive or maladaptive reactions by acting more on the degree of control allowed to the animal on the stressor than on the stressor intensity.

1.2. Modeling of Stress in Humans

Exposure to comparable levels of stressful situations and controlled conditions is not possible in experiments on human beings, as common sense and stringent ethical rules absolutely limit the use of aversive stimuli. On the other hand, solving a simple arithmetical problem or participating in an easy game in front of one or more examiners may elicit an emotional reaction similar to that of a student undergoing examination, and different tests have been devised and validated in healthy voluntary subjects that induce psychological stress and measurable neuroendocrine responses. The main difficulties in controlling experimental conditions in human experiments are not primarily related to the stressor, but to the vast interindividual variability in sensitivity to any kind of traumatic stimulus or event (Kroll, 2003). This point seems to contradict the *Diagnostic and Statistical Manual of Mental Disorders*, which, when defining the causes of posttraumatic stress disorder (PTSD), states that "[the] severity, duration, and proximity of an individual exposure to the traumatic event are the most important factors affecting the likelihood of developing this disorder" (American Psychiatric Association [APA], 2000). There is no doubt that trauma is the necessary disease agent, but it is never a sufficient predictor of PTSD development. Other factors, both genetic (Bouchard, Lykken, McGue, Segal, & Tellegen, 1990) and acquired, such as previously experienced traumatic events (Breslau, Chilcoat, Kessler, & Davis, 1999) or strong cultural traditions (Welsaeth, 2002), may exert strong control over the individual acute reactivity to stressful events and the long-term consequences.

1.3. Uses of Stress Models

To minimize confusion we will use the terms "stressor" to define a stimulus or event that perturbs the equilibrium in an organism and "stress" to define the response of the organism to such a stimulus or event. Experimentally, the effects of different stressors are useful to study the evoked responses and the mechanisms underlying them or to modify the behavior of animals in an attempt to reproduce reliable models of psychiatric symptoms that may have a stress-related component in humans. The two approaches differ only in the final aim, as both require very strictly controlled experimental conditions. An experimental model of a psychiatric disease must fulfill three basic requirements: face validity, as the behavioral modification should mimic a psychiatric symptom; predictive validity, as the behavioral modification should be reverted by the psychotropic drugs that control the spontaneous symptom; and construct validity, as the mechanisms underpinning the behavioral modification should be similar to those considered responsible, or associated with, the psychiatric symptom (Willner, 1995). These requirements are used to validate a model independently of the modality (pharmacological, genetic, or environmental) used to obtain it.

2. STRESSOR EXPOSURE AS A MODEL OF PSYCHIATRIC SYMPTOMS

2.1. Depression

We have devised two models for studying depression based on animal exposure to unavoidable stressors (Gambarana, Scheggi, Tagliamonte, Tolu, & De Montis, 2001). Rats exposed to a noxious avoidable stimulus quickly learn to avoid it; thus, when administered a sequence of threshold electric tail-shocks, a naive animal escapes from an average of 26 out of 30 shocks. This escape competence can be disrupted by previous exposure to an unavoidable stressor; in this condition, when tested for escape, the animal escapes from an average of 3–5 out of 30 consecutive tail-shocks (Gambarana et al., 2001). This escape deficit, which is a modification of the classical learned helplessness syndrome (Overmier & Seligman, 1967; Sherman, Sacquitine, & Petty, 1982), implies an *N*-methyl-D-aspartate (NMDA)-dependent neuronal plasticity process, since the acute administration of 0.1 mg/kg of dizocilpine, an NMDA receptor antagonist, 30 min before unavoidable stressor exposure completely prevents the development of escape deficit (Gambarana et al., 2001). The unavoidable stressor has been standardized (Maier, 1986) and consists of a series of 48 tail-shocks administered in 50 min in a condition of complete immobilization. It appears that the stressed rat "learns" that any effort to avoid the noxious stimulus is ineffective. This form of aversive memory is short-lived: it is maximal 24 h after unavoidable stressor exposure, and it rapidly declines within 48–72 h (Gambarana et al., 2001). This decline is dependent on μ-opioid receptor functionality, since the subcutaneous infusion of naloxone by osmotic minipump (1 mg/kg/24 h) postpones recovery as long as naloxone is infused (Fig. 1). The development of acute escape deficit is prevented by previous repeated administration of classical antidepressants. That is, imipramine, fluoxetine, clomipramine, phenelzine, mirtazapine, and reboxetine administered acutely before an unavoidable stressor show no protective effect; however, when they are administered for 14–21 d, depending on the compound, a preventive, protective effect is consistently observed (Gambarana et al., 1995; Raugg, et al., 2005). The experimental conditions must be strictly controlled, as adjunctive stressors may easily alter animals' performance. For instance, experiments are always carried out on rats fed *ad libitum*, since the condition of fasting may completely protect them from the behavioral sequelae of unavoidable stressor exposure (Fig. 2).

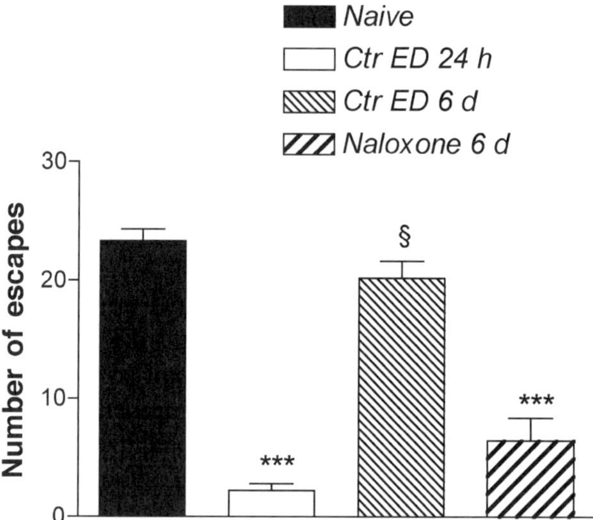

Fig. 1. Critical role of μ-opioid receptors in the extinction of unavoidable stressor-induced escape deficit. Twenty-four hours after exposure to unavoidable shocks, rats showed a clear-cut escape deficit (*Ctr ED 24 h*) compared to the performance of stress-naive rats (*Naive*). This behavioral deficit rapidly declined within 48–72 h, and by d 6 rats had completely recovered (*Ctr ED 6 d*). Rats infused with naloxone subcutaneously by osmotic minipumps (1 mg/kg/24 h), exposed to unavoidable shocks under naloxone infusion and 6 d later to escape test (*Naloxone 6 d*), did not recover a normal escape response. Values represent mean 6 SEM of number of escapes ($n = 8$ in each group). $^{***}p < 0.001$ compared to the number of escapes of the *Naive* group, $^{§}p < 0.001$ compared to the number of escapes of the *Ctr ED 24 h* group (one-way ANOVA followed by Bonferroni's test).

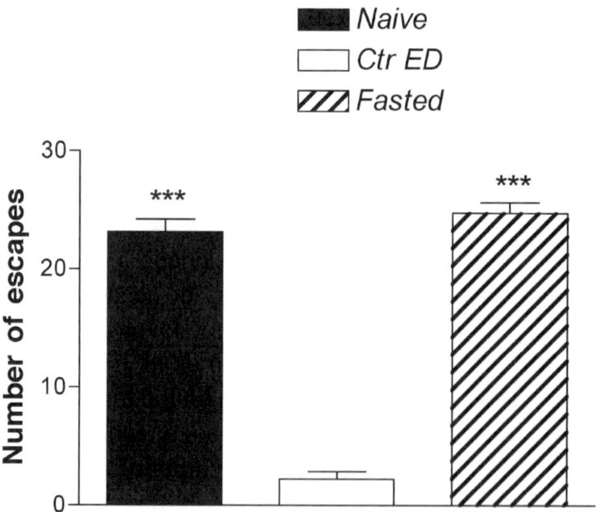

Fig. 2. Protective effect of a 24-h fast period on the development of escape deficit (*ED*). Rats were fasted for 24 h and then exposed to unavoidable shocks. Eight hours after stressor exposure, rats had unlimited access to food and they underwent the escape test 24 h after the unavoidable shocks. Values represent mean 6 SEM of number of escapes ($n = 9$ in each group). $^{***}p < 0.001$ compared to the number of escapes of the *Ctr ED* group (one-way ANOVA followed by Bonferroni's test).

The stressor-induced models of depression most often used in rats or mice are the forced swim test and the tail suspension test. The forced swim test, also known as the Porsolt test, involves placing the animal in a tank filled with tepid water, where both rats and mice will struggle in the attempt to jump out, and measuring the latency for the animal to become immobile (Porsolt, LePichon, & Jalfre, 1977). Acute or short-term (3–4 administrations within 24 h) treatment with most antidepressants prolongs this latency and decreases the duration of immobility. A skilled experimenter can distinguish the class of antidepressant used from the pattern of movements of the animals; thus, norepinephrine reuptake blockers may increase climbing behavior, whereas selective serotonin reuptake inhibitors (SSRIs) increase swimming (Detke, Rickels, & Lucki, 1995). An interpretation of the test as a model of depression is that immobility time is a symptom of reduced reactivity to an aversive environment, and the fact that the administration of an antidepressant prolongs the struggling or swimming time should give predictive validity to the model. A main criticism o f this interpretation is that a very short-term treatment is sufficient for shortening immobility time, and this fact conflicts with the delay necessary for an antidepressant compound to develop its therapeutic activity. This discrepancy limits the validity of Porsolt's test as a model of depression, but does not reduce its utility as a relatively rapid testing protocol for detecting agents with antidepressant-like activity. The tail suspension test, a variant of the forced swim test, is used in mice (Steru, Chermat, Thierry, & Simon, 1985; Steru et al., 1987). The mouse is suspended by its tail and the time it takes to become immobile (i.e., to hang passively upside down) is measured. Acute administration of most antidepressants decreases immobility. Thus, this model presents the same limits as the forced swim test, but the same adaptability as a quick screening tool.

False positives in the three described acute tests include drugs that are stimulants (and hence decrease immobility) but not antidepressants. In the acute escape deficit model, central stimulants increase the number of escapes when administered before the escape test but show no protective activity when given before the unavoidable stressor (Gambarana, Ghiglieri, Taddei, Tagliamonte, & De Montis, 1995).

2.2. Anxiety

The spontaneous capacity of animals to avoid aversive stimuli is often used to model anxiety. Both mice and rats prefer a protected to an open environment, and when placed in an elevated-plus maze (i.e., a maze with two closed arms and two open arms elevated above the floor level) they explore it but spend most of the time in the arms of the maze protected by walls. Since the acute administration of benzodiazepines or other anxiolytic drugs at a dose that does not modify spontaneous motility prolongs the time spent by animals in the open arms, the elevated-plus maze is used as a model of anxiety (Lister, 1987; Pellow, Chopin, File, & Briley, 1985). A mild physical stressor such as a continuous electric current in the metal tip of a water bottle does not completely prevent rats from drinking, but it reduces water consumption. Again, acute benzodiazepine administration reinstates basal water consumption, and this behavioral paradigm is used as a model of anxiety (Vogel, Beer, & Clody, 1971).

2.3. Chronic Models

The models so far described allow almost exclusively the study of the preventive effects of drugs on experimentally modified behaviors. When exposure to unavoidable stressors is repeated, the condition of reduced reactivity to environmental stimuli may be prolonged, and it may outlast by several days the end of stressor exposure. Different kinds of stressors, such as immobilization, repeated electric shocks, etc., have been used. Repeated episodes of immobilization are frequently used to study the neuroendocrinological and metabolic stress responses, rather than to induce reliable behavioral modifications. One of the most elegant long-term models of depression is the chronic mild stress (CMS) procedure devised by Willner (Papp, Moryl, & Willner, 1996; Papp, Willner, & Muscat, 1991). In the CMS model, chronic sequential exposure of rats to a variety of mild stressors has been shown to decrease the drinking of a sweetened solution, a condition that could be reversed by the chronic administration of classical antidepressant drugs as well as dopaminergic agonists (Muscat, Papp, & Willner, 1992a, 1992b; Muscat, Sampson, & Willner, 1990; Papp et al., 1996). Exposure to chronic mild stress also impairs the acquisition of place preference conditioning, in parallel with sucrose consumption (Papp et al., 1991). All of these deficits are reversed by chronic treatment with clinically effective antidepressant drugs (Moreau, Jenck, Martin, Mortas, & Haefely, 1992; Muscat et al., 1990, 1992b; Papp et al., 1991, 1996; Willner, Towell, Sampson, Sophokleous, & Muscat, 1987).

The condition of escape deficit induced by a single exposure to unavoidable shocks can be maintained indefinitely by exposing rats that have developed the deficit to a sequence of milder stressors on alternate days, such as a brief immobilization period, a few tail-shocks, or exposure to the room in which shocks were previously administered (Gambarana et al., 2001). Moreover, 14 d after the last stressor exposure, chronically stressed rats still present a clear-cut escape deficit (Mangiavacchi et al., 2001). No significant differences in the amount of daily food and water consumption or in the curve of body weight increase is observed between control rats and rats exposed to this procedure for 3 wk (Mangiavacchi et al., 2001). Daily administration of a classical antidepressant, beginning 24 h after initial exposure to unavoidable shocks and continuing during chronic stressor exposure, results in reversal of the escape deficit after ≥3 wk of treatment (Gambarana et al., 2001). Thus, repeated administration of antidepressant compounds not only prevents the development of escape deficit, but also reverts it once established. This is strong proof of predictive validity in favor of the escape deficit as a model of depression.

After a 3-wk exposure to chronic stressors, rats show a decreased output of dopamine (DA) and serotonin (5-HT) in the medial prefrontal cortex (mPFC) and in the shell of the nucleus accumbens (NAcS), as detected by microdialysis procedure, which may last for days after the last stressor exposure (Mangiavacchi et al., 2001). Moreover, these rats also show a steady increase in plasma corticosterone levels and a decrease in glucocorticoid receptors in discrete brain areas such as the hippocampus and mPFC (De Montis, Rauggi, Scheggi, & Tagliamonte, 2004). These intense, long-lasting monoaminergic deficits, associated with a condition of increased hypothalamic–pituitary–adrenal (HPA) axis activity, are reminiscent of the serotonergic and catecholaminergic theories of depression and of the enhanced HPA axis activity observed in depressed patients (Halbreich, Asnis, Schindledecker, Zurnoff, & Nathan, 1985; Meltzer & Lowy, 1987; Schildkraut, 1965; Willner, 1983). Thus, altogether they constitute a strong neurobiological and endocrinological construct validity proof for defining chronic escape deficit as a model of depression.

Exposure to chronic stressful procedures also reduces spontaneous reactivity to rewarding stimuli in rats, as already mentioned for the CMS model. Rats are very fond of vanilla sugar (VS), and they still consume it when fed *ad libitum* on a standard diet. Indeed, VS maintains its reinforcing property in satiated rats that consistently learn to choose between the two divergent arms of a Y-maze, the one contingently baited with VS (Ghiglieri et al., 1997). The disruption of the VS-sustained appetitive behavior (VAB) by chronic exposure to unavoidable stressors was developed as a model of anhedonia, which is a core symptom of depression, since rats exposed to the chronic stressor procedure during the training phase show reduced interest in the bait and never acquire the appetitive behavior (Ghiglieri et al., 1997). Interestingly, both the escape deficit and the impairment of VAB learning in the Y-maze are reversed by a chronic treatment with antidepressant drugs such as imipramine or fluoxetine. These findings further strengthen the face validity of the chronic stressor procedure, which is able to induce a reduced reactivity to both aversive and pleasurable stimuli. In addition, they also strengthen its predictive validity, as the administration of classical antidepressants antagonizes both its behavioral and neurochemical effects (Ghiglieri et al., 1997).

The effect of chronic exposure to an unavoidable stressor on VAB acquisition was crucial for clarifying the mechanism that underlies the chronic stress-reduced enticement toward palatable food. In fact, we observed that the dopaminergic response to VS consumption in satiated rats presented with VS for the first time is predictive of VS-reinforcing activity (Gambarana et al., 2003). Only rats that show a consistent increase in dopamine release in the mPFC and NAcS in response to VS consumption are able to learn VAB (Gambarana et al., 2003). Accordingly, rats that underwent CMS also showed a decreased DA response to palatable food consumption in the mesolimbic areas (Di Chiara & Tanda, 1997).

The administration of antidepressant drugs antagonizes the disrupting effect of chronic stressors on VAB acquisition to the limited extent that the treatment is initiated long before stress exposure (Gambarana et al., 2001). When rats begin imipramine or fluoxetine treatment soon after exposure to unavoidable shocks and escape test and they begin Y-maze training after a 7-d exposure to chronic stressors and antidepressant treatment, they never acquire VAB (Gambarana et al., unpublished results). Interestingly, VS consumption at the end of the first week of combined stressor exposure and antidepressant treatment does not induce a dopaminergic response in the NAcS (Table 1). Rats exposed to this experimental protocol began Y-maze training in a condition of decreased or absent competence to perceive VS as a palatable food, and they probably perceived Y-maze training as an adjunctive stressor. Accordingly, after 3 wk of daily antidepressant treatment, the escape deficit was reverted, but they had not learned the appetitive behavior. Thus, while imipramine and fluoxetine can reverse a state of stressor-induced escape deficit, they seem to have no effect on stressor-induced devaluation of food palatability.

2.4. Models of Adaptive Stress

We try, experimentally, to calibrate stressor intensity and length of exposure on the basis of the stress response of an organism, since it is impossible to predict *a priori* the limit between an adaptive and a maladaptive stress. The experimental protocols described so far are designed to induce a maladaptive stress response in the organism, and thus mimic some of the core symptoms of psychiatric diseases. A very common stressor used to induce adaptive stress is food restriction of different degrees; fasted animals show a very low response threshold to different environmental stimuli and appear to be in a latent state

Table 1

Dopamine Accumulation in Response to Palatable Food Consumption in the Nucleus Accumbens Shell of Rats Fed *Ad Libitum*

Group	*Maximum (pg/10 μL) increase in DA levels*
Ctr	37.3 ± 1.1
Stress	5.4 ± 3.3***
Stress + IMI	3.3 ± 2.3***
Stress + FLX	4.6 ± 2.2***

Rats were exposed to unavoidable shocks and escape test, then to chronic stressor protocol for 7 d. Imipramine (IMI) (5 mg/kg i p, twice a day) and fluoxetine (FLX) treatments (5 mg/kg/day, ip) began soon after the escape test. Twenty-four hours after the last stressor exposure and drug treatment, rats were implanted with microdialysis probes in the nucleus accumbens shell, and microdialysis was performed the following day. When consistent baseline dopamine (DA) levels were attained (≥10% between sample variation), rats were presented with five vanilla sugar (VS) pellets. Rats in the *Ctr* group ate all the pellets in less than 5 min; only 5 rats out of 12 in the *Stress* group, 6 out 12 in the *Stress + IMI* group, and 5 out of 11 in the *Stress + FLX* group ate the VS pellets. Values represent the mean ± SEM of maximum increases in extraneuronal DA levels after VS consumption minus baseline levels in each rat (n = 10 in the *Ctr* group, 5 in the *Stress* and *Stress + FLX* group, 6 in the *Stress + IMI* group). $^{***}p < 0.001$ compared to the maximum increase in the *Ctr* group (one-way ANOVA followed by Bonferroni's test).

of alert. Basal glucose consumption in the brain is significantly higher than that in any other organ, and this consumption further increases in a condition of stress. Thus, the stress response includes a cascade of metabolic events aimed at decreasing glucose consumption by peripheral organs in order to spare it for brain function (Peters et al., 2004). Exposure to a condition of caloric restriction is considered to be the easiest method of causing stress in animals, because eating is entirely instinctive, natural, and the most desirable behavior for animals, particularly for fasting animals (Martin & Seneviratne, 1997; Rodeck, 1969). A condition of partial, well-controlled food restriction produces gastric stress ulcers in rats (Yi & Stephan, 1998) and it is a widely used model of stressor. Moreover, chronic food restriction enhances sensitivity to the rewarding and motor-activating effects of amphetamine, cocaine, and other drugs of abuse (Bell, Stewart, Thompson, & Meisch, 1997; Cabeza de Vaca & Carr, 1998; Cabib, Orsini, Le Moal, & Piazza, 2000; Carr, Kim, & Cabeza de Vaca, 2000; Carroll & Meisch, 1984; Deroche et al., 1995), as many other stressors do (Antelman, Eichler, Black, & Kocan, 1980; Bozarth, Murray, & Wise, 1989; Deminihre et al., 1992; Deroche et al., 1992; Deroche, Piazza, Le Moal, & Simon, 1994; Pacchioni, Gioino, Assis, & Cancela, 2002).

Chronic food restriction activates complex endocrine and autonomic mechanisms that control food intake and energy metabolism (Berthoud, 2002). These mechanisms may lead to the initiation of ingestion, or they may simply lead to an adjustment in autonomic and/or endocrine outflow. In experimental chronic food restriction, the ingestive response is by definition partial, and the resulting changes in energy balance are orchestrated by a central neural network centered in the hypothalamus that receives and integrates neural, metabolic, and endocrine signals and organizes appropriate responses of energy resources allocation and expenditure (Peters et al., 2004). The neocortex and the limbic–hypothalamus–pituitary–adrenal system control both energy resource allocation and intake. Brain neurons utilize glucose almost exclusively, and ATP-sensitive potassium channels are considered the detectors of glucose concentration in neurons of the neocortex that control the HPA axis and the autonomic sympathetic system (Peters et al., 2004). HPA axis and sympathetic system activation results in reduced glucose utilization in skeletal muscles and increased brain glucose availability, among other effects. High-affinity mineralocorticoid and low-affinity glucocorticoid receptors, located in the neurons of limbic areas such as the hippocampus and hypothalamus, determine the setpoint of the HPA system (Herman et al., 2003; Jacobson & Sapolsky, 1991). This setpoint can be modified by exposure to a chronic stressor, such as partial food restriction or decreased environmental temperature, and it can reach a new functional equilibrium characterized by increased reactivity to stressful stimuli. On the other hand, it can be permanently and pathologically disrupted by extreme chronic metabolic, psychological, and physical stressors such as starvation, infectious diseases, hormones, drugs, substances of abuse, or chemicals disrupting the endocrine system.

In this context, we may define the response to chronic food restriction as adaptive stress and the response to the chronic escape deficit procedure as maladaptive stress. Accordingly, diet-restricted rats and mice have improved cardiovascular stress responses (Wan, Camandola, & Mattson, 2003) and increased resistance to high temperature (Hall et al., 2000) and to a number of different toxins (Bruce-Keller, Umberger, McFall, & Mattson, 1999; Duan & Mattson, 1999), as well as to unavoidable stressor exposure (Fig. 2). Conversely, exposure to the chronic stress procedure results in a condition of chronic escape deficit and anhedonia that is used to model mental depression.

2.5. Models of Stress in Humans

Dietary restriction in humans can increase life span and reduce the incidence of age-related diseases including cancer, diabetes, and kidney disease (Weindruch & Sohal, 1997), and it is the basis for the treatment of several metabolic and cardiovascular disorders. Dietary restriction, particularly in overweight subjects, is a stressful experience, and compliance with a rigid diet can be as poor as spontaneous abstinence is in drug abusers. On the other hand, dieting is just one of the many stressful tools employed in treating patients.

Returning to experimental stress, the use of stressors on humans is limited to the evaluation of the emotional threshold in healthy subjects and in well-defined forms of psychopathology. The stressors used are light physical stimuli, such as a brief foot immersion in cold water (Oshima et al., 2001), or a protocol of simple tasks to be solved, such as the Trier Social Stress Test (TSST) (Kirschbaum, Pirke, & Hellhammer, 1993), which induces a psychological stress. TSST consists mainly of a free speech and a mental arithmetic task in front of an audience. Including introduction to the free speech and a preparation phase, the total procedure takes approx 15 min. The most frequently measured variables are plasma or salivary cortisol, plasma adrenocorticotropic hormone (ACTH), and cardiovascular parameters such as heart rate and blood pressure. Salivary cortisol has been shown to be a reliable, noninvasive method of assessing plasma cortisol levels (Kirschbaum & Hellhammer, 1989; Reid, Intrieri, Susman, & Beard, 1992) and has the further advantage of measuring plasma free cortisol levels, hypothesized to be the more biologically active form of plasma cortisol (Elkins, 1990). Salivary cortisol provides a measure of non-protein-bound, "free" cortisol levels. Salivary "free" cortisol levels track closely with plasma levels, showing a 1- to 2-min lag, and have been previously used to monitor cortisol activity in both ambulatory and laboratory challenge paradigms (Kirschbaum and Hellhammer, 1994).

The great number of studies conducted in healthy volunteers aimed at defining gender differences in cardiovascular and HPA axis responses to psychological stress in healthy men and women of different ages did not reach consistent results (Gaab et al., 2003; Kirschbaum, Klauer, Filipp, & Hellhammer, 1995; Kudielka, Buske-Kirschbaum, Hellhammer, & Kirschbaum, 2004; Kudielka et al., 1998; Kudielka, Schmidt-Reinwald, Hellhammer, Schurmeyer, & Kirschbaum, 2000; Seeman, Singer, Wilkinson, & McEwen, 2001; Watamura, Donzella, Alwin, & Gunnar, 2003; Wolf, Schommer, Hellhammer, McEwen, & Kirschbaum, 2001).

Besides the different experimental conditions used, the main reason for the discrepancies among studies is the immense interindividual variability (Berger et al., 1987), which can sometimes be explained on the basis of genetic variables (Wust et al., 2004) or particular personal histories (Brody, 2002).

Controlled studies aimed at the assessment of psychological and physiological reactions to psychological stress provocation are less frequently carried out in psychiatric patients. This may be due to the complex interactions among the various factors that modulate the stress response and the dynamics of the disease under investigation. Thus, in different forms of psychiatric disorders the basal activity of the HPA axis is studied, rather than the susceptibility to standardized stressors. The better assessed alteration in the HPA axis is the decreased response to the dexamethasone suppression test (DST) in major depression (Carroll et al., 1981), a psychiatric disorder characterized by high plasma cortisol levels. A vast number of studies have established that the sensitivity of DST in major depression is no more than 40–50% (Arana, Baldessarini, & Ornsteen, 1985). In this context, Holsboer, von Bardeleben, Wiedemann, Müller, and Stalla (1987) serially performed corticotropin-releasing hormone (CRH) challenge on major depressive episode cases after pretreatment with dexamethasone (DEX) and found that the hyperresponses of ACTH and cortisol during the episode were normalized with recovery. This phenomenon was confirmed in a large-scale study by Holsboer-Trachsler, Stohler, and Hatzinger (1991). Heuser, Yassouridis, and Holsboer (1994) concluded that the sensitivity of this combined DEX/CRH test in major depression is >80%, which far exceeds that of the standard DST. The DEX/CRH test has also been proposed as a predictor of medium-term outcome in patients with remitted depression (Zobel et al., 2001). On the other hand, a decreased response to the DST is not specific for major depression since it has also been observed in schizophrenic patients (Tandon et al., 1991).

Cortisol, ACTH plasma levels, and cortisol salivary concentration are all reliable markers of HPA axis activity in humans, but modifications of these parameters elicited by mild stressor exposure are bound to a number of variables that render any findings or conclusions impossible. Thus, experimental models based on stressor exposure have several useful applications in animal research but are still of limited clinical value in human research.

3. CONCLUSIONS

Exposure to stressors induces a complex behavioral and neuroendocrine response—stress—in experimental animals as well as in humans. This response can be adaptive or maladaptive.

In animals maintained under controlled experimental conditions, stress is reproducible and proportional to the intensity of the stressor and the duration of the exposure. This notion allows the study of the mechanisms underlying the responses to stressors and the use of stress-induced behavioral modifications as models of psychiatric symptoms.

The experimental study of stress is still of limited clinical value in human research because of ethical problems. However, it is the large interindividual variability in the sensitivity to any kind of traumatic stimulus or event that largely accounts for the low concordance in the conclusions of the existing studies.

REFERENCES

American Psychiatric Association. (2000). *Diagnostic and statistical manual of mental disorders*, (4th ed., Rev.). Washington, DC: American Psychiatric Association.

Antelman, S. M., Eichler, A. J., Black, C. A., & Kocan, D. (1980). Interchangeability of stress and amphetamine sensitization. *Science, 207*, 329–331.

Arana, G. W., Baldessarini, R. J., & Ornsteen, M. (1985). The dexamethasone suppression test for diagnosis and prognosis in psychiatry—commentary and review. *Archives of General Psychiatry, 42*, 1193–1204.

Bell, S. M., Stewart, R. B., Thompson, S. C., and Meisch, R. A. (1997). Food-deprivation increases cocaine-induced conditioned place preference and locomotor activity in rats. *Psychopharmacology, 131*, 1–8.

Berger, M., Bossert, S., Krieg, J. C., Dirlich, G., Ettmeier, W., Schreiber, W., and von Zerssen, D. (1987). Interindividual differences in the susceptibility of the cortisol system: An important factor for the degree of hypercortisolism in stress situations? *Biological Psychiatry, 22*, 1327–1339.

Berthoud, H.-R. (2002). Multiple neural systems controlling food intake and body weight. *Neuroscience and Biobehavioral Reviews, 26*, 393–428.

Bouchard, T. J., Jr., Lykken, D. T., McGue, M., Segal, N. L., and Tellegen, A. (1990). Sources of human psychological differences: the Minnesota study of twins reared apart. *Science, 250*, 223–228.

Bozarth, M. A., Murray, A., and Wise, R. A. (1989). Influence of housing conditions on the acquisition of intravenous heroin and cocaine self-administration in rats. *Pharmacology Biochemistry and Behavior, 33*, 903–907.

Breslau, N., Chilcoat, H. D., Kessler, R. C., and Davis, G. C. (1999). Previous exposure to trauma and PTSD effects of subsequent trauma: Results from the Detroit area survey of trauma. *American Journal of Psychiatry, 156*, 902–907.

Brody, S. (2002). Age at first intercourse is inversely related to female cortisol stress reactivity. *Psychoneuroendocrinology, 27*, 933–943.

Bruce-Keller, A. J., Umberger, G., McFall, R., and Mattson, M. P. (1999). Food restriction reduces brain damage and improves behavioral outcome following excitotoxic and metabolic insults. *Annals of Neurology, 45*, 8–15.

Cabeza de Vaca, S., and Carr, K. D. (1998). Food restriction enhances the central rewarding effect of abused drugs. *Journal of Neuroscience, 18*, 7502–7510.

Cabib, S., Orsini, C., Le Moal, M., and Piazza, P. V. (2000). Abolition and reversal of strain differences in behavioral responses to drugs of abuse after a brief experience. *Proceedings of the National Academy of Sciences of the United States of America, 289*, 463–465.

Carr, K. D., Kim, G.-Y., and Cabeza de Vaca, S. (2000). Chronic food restriction augments the central rewarding effect of cocaine and the δ-1 opioid agonist, DPDPE, but not the δ-2 agonist, deltorphin-II. *Psychopharmacology, 152*, 200–207.

Carroll, B. J., Feinberg, M., Greden, J. F., Tarika, J., Albala, A. A., Haskett, R. F., James, N. M., Kronfol, Z., Lohr, N., Steiner, M., de Vigne, J. P., and Young, E. (1981). A specific laboratory test for the diagnosis of melancholia—standardization, validation, and clinical utility. *Archives of General Psychiatry, 38*, 15–22.

Carroll, M. E., and Meisch, R. A. (1984). Increased drug-reinforced behavior due to food deprivation. *Advances in Behavioral Pharmacology, 4*, 47–88.

Chrousos, G. P. (1998). Stressors, stress, and neuroendocrine integration of the adaptive response. The 1997 Hans Selye Memorial Lecture. *Annals of the New York Academy of Sciences, 851*, 311–335.

Deminihre, J. M., Piazza P. V., Guegan, G., Abrous, N., Maccari, S., Le Moal, M., and Simon, H. (1992). Increased locomotor response to novelty and propensity to intravenous amphetamine self-administration in adult offspring of stressed mothers. *Brain Research, 586*, 135–139.

De Montis, M. G., Rauggi, R., Scheggi, S., and Tagliamonte, A. (2004). Effect of chronic unavoidable stress exposure on glucocorticoid receptor levels in different areas of rat brain. *FENS Abstracts, 2*, A011.5.

Deroche, V., Marinelli, M., Maccari, S., Le Moal, M., Simon, H., and Piazza, P. V. (1995). Stress-induced sensitization and glucocorticoids: I. Sensitization of dopamine-dependent locomotor effects of amphetamine and morphine depends on stress-induced corticosterone secretion. *Journal of Neuroscience, 15*, 7181–7188.

Deroche, V., Piazza, P. V., Casolini, P., Maccari, S., Le Moal, M., and Simon, H. (1992). Stress-induced sensitization to amphetamine and morphine psychomotor effects depend on stress-induced corticosterone secretion. *Brain Research, 598*, 343–348.

Deroche, V., Piazza, P. V., Le Moal, M., and Simon, H. (1994). Social isolation-induced enhancement of the psychomotor effects of morphine depends on corticosterone secretion. *Brain Research, 640*, 136–139.

Detke, M. J., Rickels, M., and Lucki I. (1995). Active behaviors in the rat forced swimming test differentially produced by serotonergic and noradrenergic antidepressants. *Psychopharmacology, 12*, 66–72.

Di Chiara, G., and Tanda, G. (1997). Blunting of reactivity of dopamine transmission to palatable food: A biochemical marker of anhedonia in the CMS model? *Psychopharmacology, 134*, 351–353.

Duan, W., and Mattson, M. P. (1999). Dietary restriction and 2-deoxyglucose administration improve behavioral outcome and reduce degeneration dopaminergic neurons in models of Parkinson's disease. *Journal of Neuroscience Research, 57*, 195–206.

Elkins, R. (1990). Measurement of free hormones in blood. *Endocrine Reviews, 11*, 5–46.

Gaab, J., Blattler, N., Menzi, T., Pabst, B., Stoyer, S., and Ehlert, U. (2003). Randomized controlled evaluation of the effects of cognitive-behavioral stress management on cortisol responses to acute stress in healthy subjects. *Psychoneuroendocrinology, 28*, 767–779.

Gambarana, C., Ghiglieri, O., & De Montis, M. G. (1995). Desensitization of the D_1(pg/10 μL) dopamine receptors in rats reproduces a model of escape deficit reverted by imipramine, fluoxetine and clomipramine. *Progress Neuro-Psychopharmacology and Biological Psychiatry, 19*, 741–755.

Gambarana, C., Ghiglieri, O., Taddei, I., Tagliamonte, A., and De Montis M. G. (1995). Imipramine and fluoxetine prevent the stress-induced escape deficits in rats through a distinct mechanism of action. *Behavioural Pharmacology, 6*, 66–73.

Gambarana, C., Scheggi, S., Tagliamonte, A., Tolu, P., and De Montis, M. G. (2001). Animal models for the study of antidepressant activity. *Brain Research Protocols, 7*, 11–20.

Gambarana, C., Masi, F., Leggio, B., Grappi, S., Nanni, G., Scheggi, S., De Montis, M. G., and Tagliamonte, A. (2003). Acquisition of a palatable-food-sustained appetitive behavior in satiated rats is dependent on the dopaminergic response to this food in limbic areas. *Neuroscience, 121*, 179–187.

Ghiglieri, O., Gambarana, C., Scheggi, S., Tagliamonte, A., Willner, P., and De Montis, M. G. (1997). Palatable food induces an appetitive behaviour in satiated rats which can be inhibited by chronic stress. *Behavioural Pharmacology, 8*, 619–628.

Goldstein, D. S. (1987). Stress-induced activation of the sympathetic nervous system. *Bailliere's Clinical Endocrinology and Metabolism, 1*, 253–278.

Grappi, S., Nanni, G., Leggio, B., Rauggi, R., Scheggi, S., Masi, F., and Gambarana, C. (2003). The efficacy of reboxetine in preventing and reverting a condition of escape deficit in rats. *Biological Psychiatry, 53*, 890–898.

Halbreich, U., Asnis, G. M., Schindledecker, R., Zurnoff, B., and Nathan, R. S. (1985). Cortisol secretion in endogenous depression. I. Basal plasma levels. *Archives of General Psychiatry, 2*, 909–914.

Hall, D. M., Oberley, T. D., Moseley, P. M., Buettner, G. R., Oberley, L. W., Weindruch, R., and Kregel, K. C. (2000). Caloric restriction improves thermotolerance and reduces hyperthermia-induced cellular damage in old rats. *FASEB Journal, 14*, 78–86.

Herman, J. P., Figueiredo, H., Mueller, N. K., Ulrich-Lai, Y., Ostrander, M. M., Choi, D. C., and Cullinan, W. E. (2003). Central mechanisms of stress integration: Hierarchical circuitry controlling hypothalamo-pituitary-adrenocortical responsiveness. *Frontiers in Neuroendocrinology, 24*, 151–180.

Heuser, I., Yassouridis, A., and Holsboer, F. (1994). The combined dexamethasone/CRH test: A refined laboratory test for psychiatric disorders. *Journal of Psychiatric Research, 28*, 341–356.

Holsboer, F., von Bardeleben, U., Wiedemann, K., Müller, O. A., and Stalla, G. K. (1987). Serial assessment of corticotropin-releasing hormone response after dexamethasone in depression—implications for pathophysiology of DST nonsuppression. *Biological Psychiatry, 22*, 228–234.

Holsboer-Trachsler, E., Stohler, R., and Hatzinger, M. (1991). Repeated administration of the combined dexamethasone-human corticotropin releasing hormone stimulation test during treatment of depression. *Psychiatric Research, 38*, 163–171.

Jacobson, L., and Sapolsky, R. (1991). The role of the hippocampus in feedback regulation of the hypothalamic–pituitary–adrenocortical axis. *Endocrine Reviews, 12*, 118–134.

Kirschbaum, C., and Hellhammer, D. H. (1989). Salivary cortisol in psychobiological research: An overview. *Neuropsychobiology, 22*, 150–169.

Kirschbaum, C., and Hellhammer, D. H. (1994). Salivary cortisol in psychoneuroendocrine research: Recent developments and applications. *Psychoneuroendocrinology, 19*, 313–333.

Kirschbaum, C., Klauer, T., Filipp, S. H, and Hellhammer, D. H. (1995). Sex-specific effects of social support on cortisol and subjective responses to acute psychological stress. *Psychosomatic Medicine, 57*, 23–31.

Kirschbaum, C., Pirke, K. M., and Hellhammer, D. H. (1993). The "Trier Social Stress Test"—a tool for investigating psychobiological stress responses in a laboratory setting. *Neuropsychobiology, 28*, 76–81.

Kroll, J. (2003). Posttraumatic symptoms and the complexity of responses to trauma. *Journal of the American Medical Association, 290*, 667–670.

Kudielka, B. M., Buske-Kirschbaum, A., Hellhammer, D. H., and Kirschbaum, C. (2004). HPA axis responses to laboratory psychosocial stress in healthy elderly adults, younger adults, and children: impact of age and gender. *Psychoneuroendocrinology, 29*, 83–98.

Kudielka, B. M., Hellhammer, J., Hellhammer, D. H., Wolf, O. T., Pirke, K. M., Varadi, E., Pilz, J., and Kirschbaum, C. (1998). Sex differences in endocrine and psychological responses to psychosocial stress in healthy elderly subjects and the impact of a 2-week dehydroepiandrosterone treatment. *Journal of Clinical Endocrinology and Metabolism, 83*, 1756–1761.

Kudielka, B. M., Schmidt-Reinwald, A. K., Hellhammer, D. H., Schurmeyer, T., and Kirschbaum, C. (2000). Psychosocial stress and HPA functioning: no evidence for a reduced resilience in healthy elderly men. *Stress, 3*, 229–240.

Lister, R. G. (1987). The use of a plus-maze to measure anxiety in the mouse. *Psychopharmacology, 92*, 180–185.

Maier, S. F. (1986). Stressor controllability and stress-induced analgesia. *Annals of the New York Academy of Sciences, 46*, 55–72.

Mangiavacchi, S., Masi, F., Scheggi, S., Leggio, B., De Montis, M. G., and Gambarana, C. (2001). Long-term behavioral and neurochemical effects of chronic stress exposure in rats. *Journal of Neurochemistry, 79*, 1113–1121.

Martin, P. R., and Seneviratne, H. M. (1997). Effects of food deprivation and a stressor on head pain. *Health Psychology, 16*, 310–318.

Mason, J. W. (1968). A review of psychoendocrine research on the pituitary-adrenal cortical system. *Psychosomatic Medicine, 30*, 576–607.

Mason, J. W. (1975). A historical view of the stress field. *Journal of Human Stress*, 1, 6–12.

Meltzer, H. W., and Lowy M. T. (1987). The serotonin hypothesis of depression. In H. W. Meltzer (Ed.), *Psychopharmacology: The third generation of progress* (pp. 513–526). New York: Raven.

Moreau, J. L., Jenck, F., Martin, J. R., Mortas, P., and Haefely, W. E. (1992). Antidepressant treatment prevents chronic unpredictable mild stress-induced anhedonia as assessed by ventral tegmentum self-stimulation behavior in rats. *European Neuropsychopharmacology* , *2*, 43–49.

Muscat, R., Papp, M., and Willner, P. (1992a). Antidepressant-like effects of dopamine agonists in an animal model of depression. *Biological Psychiatry, 31*, 937–946.

Muscat, R., Papp, M., and Willner, P. (1992b). Reversal of stress-induced anhedonia by the atypical antidepressants, fluoxetine and maprotiline. *Psychopharmacology, 109*, 433–438.

Muscat, R., Sampson, D., and Willner, P. (1990). Dopaminergic mechanism of imipramine action in an animal model of depression. *Biological Psychiatry, 28*, 223–230.

Oshima, A., Miyano, H., Yamashita, S., Owashi, T., Suzuki, S-, Sakano, Y., and Higuchi, T. (2001). Psychological, autonomic and neuroendocrine responses to acute stressors in the combined dexamethasone/CRH test: A study in healthy subjects. *Journal of Psychiatric Research, 35*, 95–104.

Overmier, J. B., and Seligman, M. E. P. (1967). Effects of inescapable shock upon subsequent escape and avoidance learning. *Journal of Comparative Physiology and Psychology, 63*, 23–33.

Pacak, K. and Palkovits, M. (2001). Stressor specificity of central neuroendocrine responses: implications for stress-related disorders. *Endocrine Reviews, 22*, 502–548.

Pacchioni, A. M., Gioino, G., Assis, A., and Cancela, L. M. (2002). A single exposure to restraint stress induces behavioral and neurochemical sensitization to stimulating effects of amphetamine. Involvement of NMDA receptors. *Annals of the New York Academy of Sciences, 965*, 233–246.

Papp, M., Moryl, E., and Willner, P. (1996). Pharmacological validation of the chronic mild stress model of depression. *European Journal of Pharmacology, 296*, 129–136.

Papp, M., Willner, P., and Muscat, R. (1991). An animal model of anhedonia: Attenuation of sucrose consumption and place preference conditioning by chronic unpredictable mild stress. *Psychopharmacology, 104*, 255–259.

Pellow, S., Chopin, P., File, S. E., and Briley, M. (1985). Validation of open:closed arm entries in an elevated plus-maze as a measure of anxiety in the rat. *Journal of Neuroscience Methods, 14*, 149–167.

Peters, A., Schweiger, U., Pellerin, L., Hubold, C., Oltmanns, K. M., Conrad, M., Schultes, B., Born J., and Fehm, H. L. (2004). The selfish brain: competition for energy resources. *Neuroscience and Biobehavioral Reviews, 28*, 143–180.

Porsolt, R. D., LePichon, R., and Jalfre, R. (1977). Depression: a new animal model sensitive to antidepressant treatments. *Nature, 266*, 730–732.

Rauggi, R., Cassanelli, A., Raone, A., Tagliamonte, A., & Gambarana, C. (2005). Study of mirtazapine antidepressant effects in rats. *International Journal of Neuropsychopharmacology, 15*, 1–11.

Reid, J. D., Intrieri, R .C., Susman, E. J., and Beard, J. L. (1992). The relationship of serum and salivary cortisol in a sample of healthy elderly. *Journal of Gerontology: Psychological Sciences, 47*, 176–179.

Rodeck, H. (1969). Animal experimental studies on the influence of hunger on the development of the neurosecretory hypothalamo-neurohypophyseal system. *Journal of Neuro-Visceral Relations, 31*, 136–160.

Schildkraut, J. J. (1965). The catecholamine hypothesis of affective disorders: A review of supporting evidence. *American Journal of Psychiatry, 122*, 509–522.

Seeman, T. E., Singer, B., Wilkinson, C. W., and McEwen, B. (2001). Gender differences in age-related changes in HPA axis reactivity. *Psychoneuroendocrinology, 26*, 225–240.

Selye, H. (1950). *Stress*. Montreal: Acta Inc.

Selye, H. (1974). *Stress without distress*. Toronto: McClelland and Stewart Ltd.

Sherman, A. D., Sacquitine, J. L., and Petty, F. (1982). Specificity of the learned helplessness model of depression. *Pharmacology Biochemistry and Behavior, 16*, 449–454.

Steru, L., Chermat, R., Thierry, B., and Simon, P. (1985). The tail suspension test: A new method for screening antidepressants in mice. *Psychopharmacology, 85*, 367–370.

Steru, L., Chermat, R., Thierry, B., Mico, J. A., Lenegre, A., Steru, M., Simon, P., and Porsolt, R. D. (1987). The automated tail suspension test: A computerized device which differentiates psychotropic drugs. *Progress in Neuro-Psychopharmacology and Biological Psychiatry, 11*, 659–671.

Tandon, R., Mazzara, C., DeQuardo, J., Craig, K. A., Meador-Woodruff, J. H., Goldman, R., and Greden, J. F. (1991). Dexamethasone suppression test in schizophrenia: Relationship to symptomatology, ventricular enlargement and outcome. *Biological Psychiatry, 29*, 953–964.

Vogel, J. R., Beer, B., and Clody, D. E. (1971). A simple and reliable conflict procedure for testing anti-anxiety agents. *Psychopharmacologia, 21*, 1–7.

Wan, R., Camandola, S., and Mattson, M. P. (2003). Intermittent food deprivation improves cardiovascular and neuroendocrine responses to stress in rats. *Journal of Nutrition, 133*, 1921–1929.

Watamura, S. E., Donzella, B., Alwin, J., and Gunnar, M. R. (2003). Morning-to-afternoon increases in cortisol concentrations for infants and toddlers at child care: Age differences and behavioral correlates. *Child Development, 74*, 1006–1020.

Webster's Third New International Dictionary. (1971). Springfield, MA: Merriam Webster.

Weindruch, R., and Sohal, R. S. (1997). Seminars in medicine of the Beth Israel Deaconess Medical Center: caloric intake and aging. *New England Journal of Medicine, 337*, 986–994.

Welsaeth, L. (2002). The European history of psychotraumatology. *Journal of Traumatic Stress, 15*, 443–452.
Willner, P. (1983). Dopamine and depression: a review of recent evidence. I. Empirical studies. *Brain Research, 287*, 211–224.
Willner, P. (1995). Animal models of depression: validity and applications. *Advances in Biochemistry and Psychopharmacology, 49*, 19–41.
Willner, P., Towell, A., Sampson, D., Sophokleous, S., and Muscat, R. (1987). Reduction of sucrose preference by chronic unpredictable mild stress and its restoration by a tricyclic antidepressant. *Psychopharmacology, 93*, 358–364.
Wolf, O. T., Schommer, N. C., Hellhammer, D. H., McEwen, B. S., and Kirschbaum, C. (2001). The relationship between stress induced cortisol levels and memory differs between men and women. *Psychoneuroendocrinology, 26*, 711–720.
Wust, S., Van Rossum, E. F., Federenko, I. S., Koper, J. W., Kumsta, R., and Hellhammer, D. H. (2004). Common polymorphisms in the glucocorticoid receptor gene are associated with adrenocortical responses to psychosocial stress. *Journal of Clinical Endocrinology and Metabolism, 89*, 565–573.
Yi, I., and Stephan, F. K. (1998). The effects of food deprivation, nutritive and non-nutritive feeding and wheel running on gastric stress ulcers in rats. *Physiology and Behavior, 63*, 219–225.
Zobel, A. W., Nickel, T., Sonntag, A., Uhr, M., Holsboer, F., and Ising, M. (2001). Cortisol response in the combined dexamethasone/CRH test as predictor of relapse in patients with remitted depression: A prospective study. *Journal of Psychiatric Research, 35*, 83–94.

3 Neurobiological Foundations of Stress

Michael R. Foy, Jeansok J. Kim, Tracey J. Shors, and Richard F. Thompson

KEY POINTS

- The body produces a common, integrated set of responses in an attempt to adapt to many different types of stress.
- Physical or psychological stressors increase the activity of the body's autonomic system, ultimately resulting in the release of endogenous substances, including epinephrine, norepinephrine, and cortisol into the bloodstream.
- Acute stress can activate specific brain regions to enhance or impair memory consolidation, and chronic stress can alter nervous system structure and function and cause memory dysfunction.
- Deleterious effects of cortisol on brain tissue occur in the hippocampus and amygdala, limbic system structures rich in glucocorticoid receptors and important for the consolidation of memory.
- Hippocampal long-term potentiation, a mechanism of memory storage, is impaired by behavioral stress, but can be reversed by the administration of the female hormone estrogen.
- Detrimental effects of stress on learning in females is dependent on the stage of estrous during which the learning occurs and is enhanced during periods when low or no (via ovariectomy) estrogen levels occur, with detrimental effects being minimized during periods when elevated estrogen levels occur.
- Male and female reactivity to stress is quite different and most likely due to variations of circulating levels of sex hormones in the bloodstream and their influence on nervous system structures responsive to stress.

1. NEUROBIOLOGICAL FOUNDATIONS OF STRESS

Modern understanding of stress stems from classic work in the 1930s by Hans Selye, who developed the notion of the general adaptation syndrome (Selye, 1936). Selye posited that the body shows a common, integrated set of responses in an attempt to adapt to many different kinds of stress. Until his work, many scientists viewed different kinds of stress as having different effects on the body; for example, the effect of exposure to severe cold was thought to be very different from the effect of blood loss. Indeed, each particular

From: *Nutrients, Stress, and Medical Disorders*
Edited by: S. Yehuda and D. I. Mostofsky © Humana Press Inc., Totowa, NJ

type of stressor does have unique effects. However, Selye showed that different severe stressors also have common features. He identified three stages. First is the shock (or alarm) phase, involving decreased blood pressure, body temperature, and muscle tone (the reader has no doubt experienced at least some degree of shock following a minor or not so minor injury, particularly if blood loss occurred). Selye termed the second phase of the adaptation response the stage of resistance, when the body fights back. If the stress is severe and continues for a long period, the body defenses break down and the third stage, exhaustion, ensues. Among other things, this stage includes a marked impairment of the immune system.

Selye focused on physical stressors. Blood loss is a simple and common example—even donating blood can activate the general adaptation syndrome. Extensive blood loss causes an immediate drop in blood pressure and body temperature and feeling faint—the shock stage. Shock triggers in the hypothalamus the release of corticotropin-releasing hormone (CRH), causing the pituitary to release adrenocorticotropic hormone (ACTH), which acts on the cortex of the adrenal gland to release glucocorticoids (cortisol). A wide range of actions on body tissues prepares the body to deal with stress (Fig. 1) (i.e., resistance). All of these effects may occur the first time you donate blood.

The release of cortisol acts at multiple levels to redirect bodily energy resources, including an increase in blood glucose level for energy mobilization. It causes suppression of the immune system, inhibition of tissue growth processes, vasoconstriction via potentiation of the sympathetic nervous system, increased metabolism of proteins and fats, and suppression of reproductive functions.

All the actions of cortisol are meant to prepare the organism to deal with trauma and stress by restoring normal physiological conditions. Increased glucose can replenish lost energy stores, inhibiting T-cell proliferation will control the inflammatory response, and so on. These processes, helpful in the short-term response to stress, are catabolic in nature and have very damaging long-term effects. Indeed, hypersecretion of cortisol is thought to be a major factor in the aging process (Landfield, Waymire, & Lynch, 1978) and in many disease states (McEwen & Stellar, 1993). Fortunately, there are built-in controls that regulate the production of cortisol. In particular, increased blood levels of cortisol inhibit the release of CRH from the hypothalamus and ACTH from the pituitary (Fig. 1).

The second time you donate blood these stress effects will probably not occur. There is, of course, much more to stress than physical trauma. Blood loss is a clear physical stress—you donate the same amount of blood each time. But psychological factors are also critically important in causing stress; this is true in all mammals, not just humans. In recent years the focus on stress has shifted from physical trauma *per se* to psychological or, more accurately, psychobiological factors. Many types of stress, particularly chronic stress, do not produce the initial shock phase, but they do cause to varying degrees, the resistance phase and even, in extreme cases, the exhaustion phase.

2. THE ADRENAL GLAND

The adrenal gland is the major gland in mammals for coping with stress. It consists of two almost completely independent glands, a central part called the adrenal medulla and an outer covering called the adrenal cortex (Fig. 1). The adrenal medulla functions in the same way as the sympathetic ganglia. It is controlled by the axons of autonomic motor neurons from the spinal cord. However, there are no postganglionic neurons in the adre-

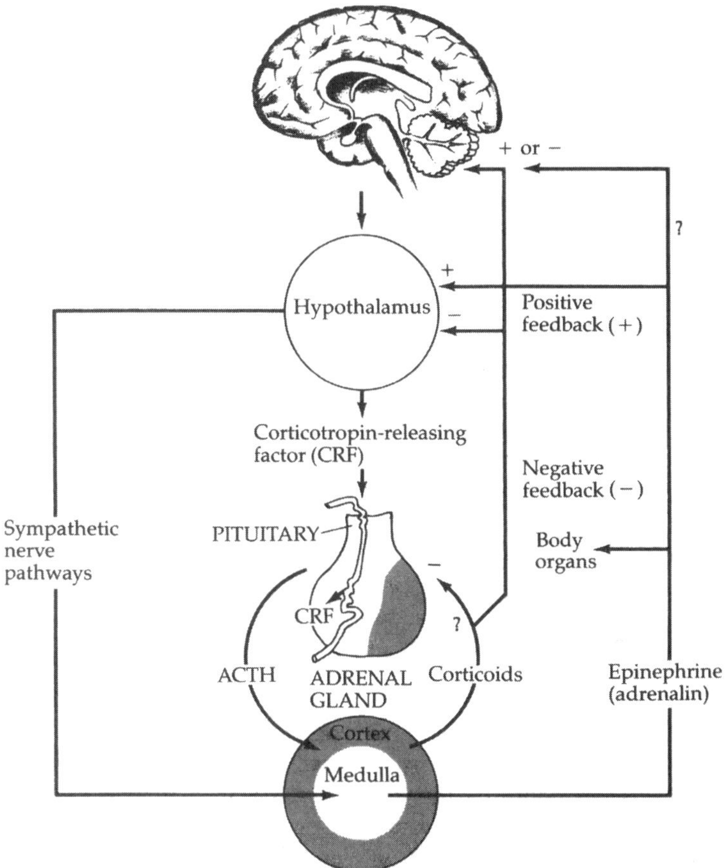

Fig. 1. Schematic representation of interrelations of the pituitary gland and the adrenal gland—the pituitary–adrenal axis or system. The adrenal medulla releases epinephrine (adrenaline), which acts on body organs and back on the hypothalamus (and perhaps other brain regions) to facilitate the activity of the autonomic nervous system. The adrenal cortex releases corticoids, which act on body organs and act back on the pituitary gland, the hypothalamus, and other brain regions. The highest density of corticoid receptors in the brain is actually in the hippocampus.

nal medulla. Instead, the motor axon terminals synapse with gland cells in the medulla called chromaffin cells. When chromaffin cells are activated by the motor neurons (release of acetylcholine [ACh]), they release norepinephrine (NE) and epinephrine (E) directly into the bloodstream. In humans, mostly E is released, but a small amount of NE is released as well. Endogenous opioids are also released.

Almost any type of sudden stress, either physical or psychological, will cause the sympathetic part of the autonomic nervous system (ANS), the emergency system, to increase its activity. This in turn causes the adrenal medulla to increase its secretion of E and NE into the blood. This is felt very rapidly: the heart immediately begins to pound. Other actions of E and NE include elevation of blood pressure, dry mouth, sweating from the palms of the hands and under the arms, and several metabolic changes that ensure an immediate supply of energy. Most of these effects are also produced by direct actions of the sympathetic nervous system on target organs. Release of E and NE by the adrenal medulla reinforces these effects. The adrenal medulla is really a part of the sympathetic division of the ANS, although it behaves in some ways as an endocrine gland.

The adrenal cortex is composed of glandular tissue and surrounds the adrenal medulla. It is the part of the adrenal gland that is a typical endocrine gland. Under certain conditions, neurons in a region of the hypothalamus release CRH into the portal circulation. It is carried by the local blood supply directly to the anterior pituitary gland, where it causes the release of ACTH into the general circulation. When ACTH reaches the adrenal cortex, endocrine gland cells release cortisol and a small amount of aldosterone. Aldosterone regulates the levels of sodium, potassium, and chloride ions by controlling the extent to which they are reabsorbed by the kidneys. The release of aldosterone by the adrenal cortex is primarily controlled by blood potassium concentration and extracellular fluid volume. Consequently, it plays an important role in thirst and drinking.

As of this writing, nine hormones have been identified as being released by the adrenal cortex, including androgens and progesterones (*see* Hierholzer & Buhler, 1996, for a detailed overview). We focus here on cortisol; the major action of ACTH is to cause the adrenal cortex to release cortisol (the only way cortisol can be released). Cortisol exerts powerful effects on all body tissues. As noted, it increases blood glucose levels and stimulates the breakdown of proteins into amino acids, inhibits the uptake of glucose by body tissues but not by the brain, and regulates the response of the cardiovascular system to persisting high blood pressure (hypertension). All of these actions help an animal deal with stress. An animal faced with a threat must usually forgo eating but needs energy in the form of glucose in the blood. The brain, in particular, needs a good supply of glucose. The increased blood levels of amino acids help repair possible tissue damage. Increased vascular tone is also of great importance. For unknown reasons, an immediate effect of stress is that certain arteries dilate, which reduces blood pressure. Cortisol counteracts this and maintains the correct blood pressure. The increased release of cortisol in response to stress is normal and very adaptive. However, long-term increases in cortisol level can result in damage and loss of neurons in the hippocampus (McEwen, 1996; Sapolsky, 1990).

3. HYPOTHALAMIC CONTROL OF THE STRESS RESPONSE

The hypothalamic nucleus directly concerned with stress is the periventricular nucleus (PVN) (Fig. 2). It is only about half a square millimeter of tissue and contains roughly 10,000 neurons in humans. There are two groups of endocrine neurons in the PVN: large neurons that convey oxytocin and vasopressin to the posterior pituitary for release (not directly involved in the stress response) and smaller neurons that release CRH into the portal circulation to activate secreting cells in the anterior pituitary to release ACTH into the general blood circulation. As we saw earlier, ACTH triggers release of cortisol from the adrenal cortex.

In addition to endocrine neurons, other neurons in the PVN make axonal connections with neurons in the reticular formation, brainstem, and spinal cord. Most of these neurons terminate on motor neurons for the ANS.

Interestingly, the PVN does not appear to contain any interneurons—neurons that interconnect within the nucleus. Hence, activity of the nucleus is under the direct control of the input projections to the nucleus—dozens of such inputs have been described. We note here four major input systems. First is an autonomic input, primarily from the vagus

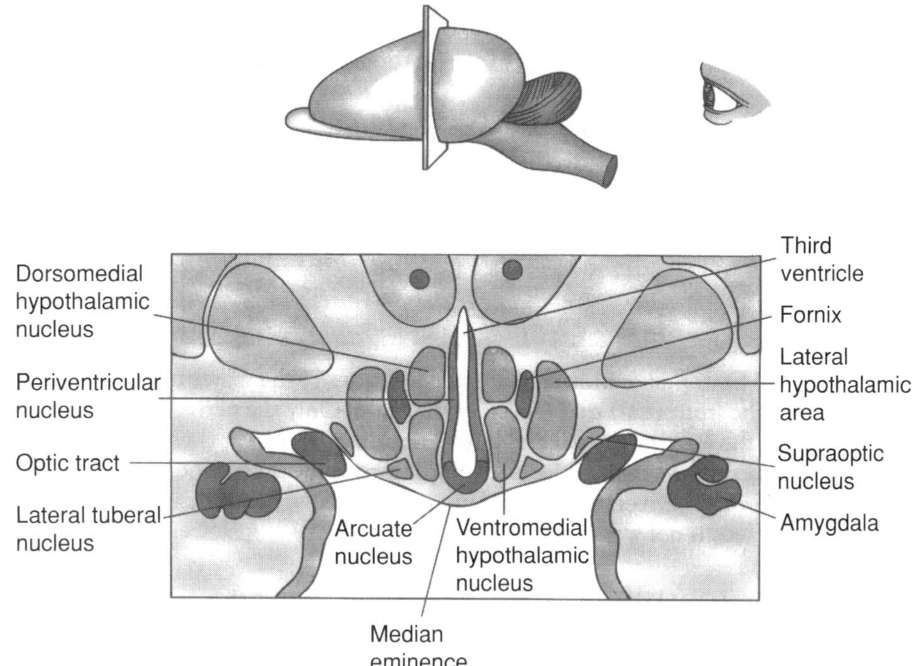

Fig. 2. Cross-section of the brain showing some of the hypothalamic nuclei. The schematic showing the plane of section is a rat brain; the actual section is of a human brain. The nuclei discussed in the text include the paraventricular nuclei (PVN), dorsomedial nuclei, and the amygdala. The fornix is a fiber bundle connecting the hippocampal system (limbic forebrain) to the hypothalamus, and the amygdala is another major structure of the limbic forebrain with strong connections to the hypothalamus.

nerve (containing sensory as well as motor fibers), that projects to autonomic nuclei in the brainstem and from there to the PVN. This system presumably conveys information about the state of the internal organs. The second input system comes from the subfornical organ, a small structure on the outside of the blood–brain barrier that has no such barrier itself. It detects levels of certain neurochemicals and hormones in the blood. The third class of input is relayed from the forebrain limbic system, particularly the hippocampus, amygdala, and prefrontal cerebral cortex. Finally, there are many projections to the PVN from other hypothalamic nuclei (Akil et al., 1999).

A schematic of some of these inputs is shown in Fig. 3. All of these can be grouped into two general categories, which Herman et al. (2003) have classed as reactive responses vs anticipatory responses (*see* Table 1). In a rough sense, these correspond to the older distinction between physiological and psychobiological sources of stress.

Reactive stressors invoke direct input pathways to the PVN; induction of these systems occurs the first time the stimulus is presented, and damage to these systems markedly impairs the cortisol response. Anticipatory responses involve forebrain structures, particularly cerebral cortex, hippocampus, and amygdala. These in turn act on the PVN polysynaptically and relay through structures that also mediate reactive responses, for example, the nucleus of the solitary tract, the parabrachial nucleus, the dorsomedial hypothalamus, the preoptic area, and the surround area of the PVN (*see* Fig. 3).

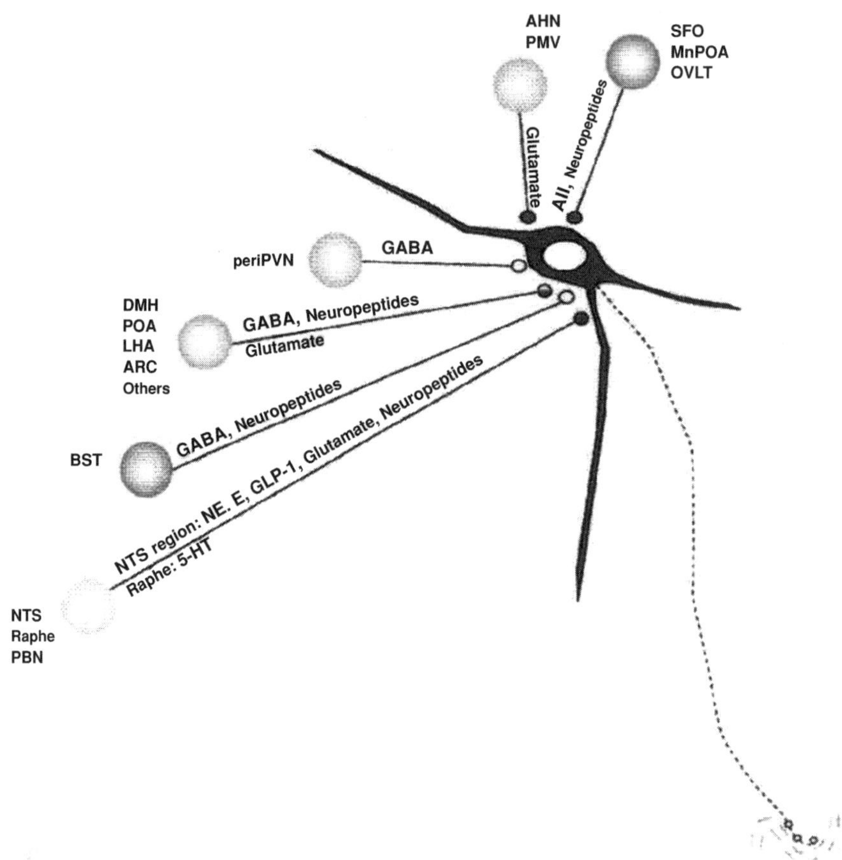

Fig. 3. Major direct projections to a prototypical medial parvocellular PVN neuron. The PVN receives direct innervation from several extrahypothalamic pathways regulating homeostatic functions, including: (1) the subfornical organ (SFO)-median preoptic nucleus (MnPOA)-organum vasculosum of the lamine terminalis (OVLT), regulating fluid and electrolyte balance; (2) norepinephrine (NE), epinephrine (E), glucagon-like peptide 1 (GLP-1), and other neuropeptidergic neurons in the nucleus of the solitary tract (NTS) and parabrachial nucleus (PBN), subserving relay of autonomic and immune system afferents; and (3) hypothalamic nuclei subserving autonomic/metabolic/immune/arousal signals, including the dorsomedial hypothalamus (DMH), medial preoptic area (POA), lateral hypothalamic area (LHA), arcuate nucleus (ARC), peri-PVN zone, anterior hypothalamic nucleus (AHN) and ventral premammillary nucleus (PMV), among others. Some of these projections are largely GABAergic (○), some are predominantly glutamatergic (●), whereas others contain mixed populations of cells. The bed nucleus of the stria terminalis (BST) is predominantly GABAergic, suggesting a largely inhibitory influence on the PVN. (From Herman et al., 2003.)

4. THE BIOCHEMICAL SWITCHING HYPOTHESIS

Many neurons in the brain have more than one neuropeptide that can function as a neurotransmitter or modulator substance. This principle seems to be carried to the extreme in the hypothalamus. The CRH-containing neurons in the PVN may contain as many as eight different neuroactive substances, including CRH, dynorphin, dopamine, and angiotensin. Swanson and colleagues at the University of Southern California have

Table 1
Stimuli Triggering Reactive vs Anticipatory HPA Stress Responses

Reactive responses	*Anticipatory responses*
Pain	Innate programs
Visceral	Predators
Somatic	Unfamiliar environments/situations
Neuronal homeostatic signals	Social challenges
Chemoreceptor stimulation	Species-specific threats (e.g., illuminated spaces for rodents, dark spaces for humans)
Baroreceptor stimulation	Memory programs
Osmoreceptor stimulation	Classically conditioned stimuli
Humoral homeostatic signals	Contextually conditioned stimuli
Glucose	Negative reinforcement/frustration
Leptin	
Insulin	
Renin–angiotensin	
Atrial natriuretic peptide	
Others	
Humoral inflammatory signals	
IL-1	
IL-6	
TNF-α	
Others	

IL, interleukin; TNF, tumor necrosis factor; HPA, hypothalamic–pituitary–adrenal.
Source: Herman et al., 2003.

developed clear evidence that a given neuron will express more or less several of these neuroactive substances, depending on the kind of stress involved (Swanson, 1991). Remember that these substances are expressed from the genes, the DNA in the cell nucleus, manufactured via the RNA, and conveyed to the terminals of the secreting PVN neurons. For example, increased blood cortisol level causes an increase in CRH but no change in vasopressin in one type of PVN neuron but a decrease in both types of peptide in another type of neuron. Other aspects of stress can produce different changes in the peptides expressed in PVN neurons.

Swanson suggests that different kinds of stress could produce differential genetic expression and production of different peptide hormones and neurotransmitters in the neurons, which could result in fine-tuning of the most adaptive type of response to the particular stress involved. The biochemical switching hypothesis is illustrated in Fig. 4. This hypothesis proposes that an anatomically fixed circuit can change its functions by altering the gene expression of peptides in the neurons. This provides an intriguing example of biochemical plasticity without anatomical plasticity.

5. THE PSYCHOBIOLOGICAL NATURE OF STRESS

The rate of cortisol secretion is extremely sensitive to psychological factors. A seemingly mild experience, such as a rat being placed in a new environment, can cause a massive increase in the release of corticosterone (the rat analog of human cortisol). When

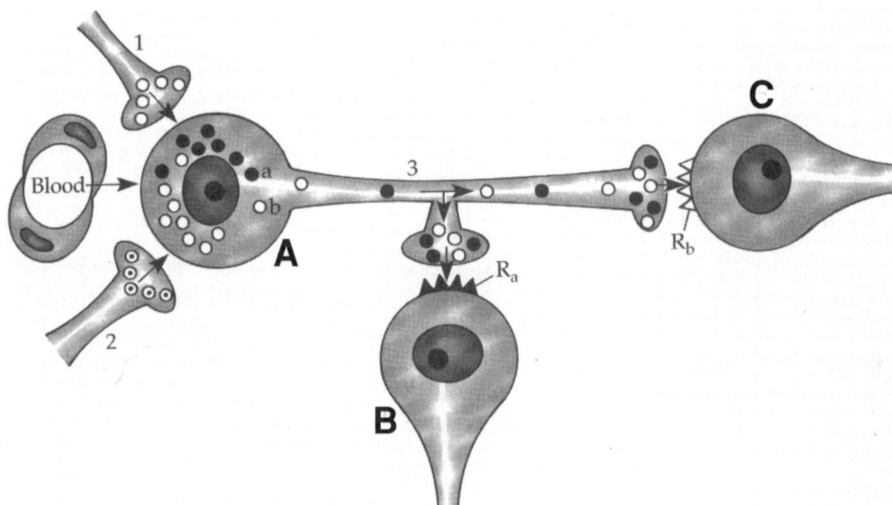

Fig. 4. Biochemical switching in a neuroanatomically fixed circuit may be implemented by changes in the ratio of neuropeptides a and b within a particular neuron (A) if the neuron innervates two different cell types (B,C), each of which expresses receptors (R_a, R_b) for one neuropeptide or the other. The a/b ratio may be altered by substances released from neural inputs 1 and 2 or by steroid hormones entering from nearby capillaries.

a person boards an airplane, there is often a massive increase in cortisol release. Cortisol release means that CRH has been released from the hypothalamus and ACTH from the pituitary. As cortisol is released, it causes the hypothalamus–pituitary to inhibit the release of CRH and ACTH, as noted above. As ACTH release decreases, release of cortisol by the adrenal cortex decreases. The release of these substances appears to be much more finely tuned and sensitive to environmental and psychological factors than the increased activity of the sympathetic nervous system in response to a sudden stress or an emergency.

It has long been known for many years that performance on various learning and skill tasks has an inverted-U relation to degree of arousal in both humans and other mammals. At the extreme low end of arousal, sleep, there is no performance. If you are exhausted and very sleepy, your performance will be poor. If you are alert, full of energy, and aroused, your performance will be optimal. However, if you are extremely aroused and under a great deal of stress, your performance will deteriorate. In general, stress impairs performance in proportion to the severity of stress—the right side of the inverted U (Hennessey & Levine, 1979).

It is now clear that stress cannot be identified simply with physical trauma. The extent to which situations are stressful is determined by how the individual understands, interprets, sees, and feels about a situation. It is fundamentally a "cognitive" phenomenon depending more on how the individual construes the situation than on the nature of the situation itself. The key aspects are uncertainty and control: the less knowledge the individual has about a potentially harmful situation and the less control he or she feels can be exerted, the more stressful the situation is. Conversely, the more understanding and certainty the individual has about a situation, the more he or she feels in control and the less stressful it is. We and other mammals appear to be driven by nature toward certainty.

This may in fact be the basis for the existence of various belief systems. A person firmly committed to a belief system does in fact "understand" the world and the nature of the controls that operate, even though this understanding may be quite wrong.

There are many examples from both the human and animal literatures. A classic study was conducted on humans in parachute training (Ursin, Baade, & Levine, 1978). In that study, the hormonal and behavioral responses of a group of Norwegian paratroop trainees were examined after repeated jumps off a 10-m tower on a guidewire. After the first jump there was a dramatic elevation of cortisol in the blood, but after the second jump there was a significant drop to basal levels; basal levels persisted on subsequent jumps. It is also important to note that the fear ratings changed dramatically following the first and second jumps: very little fear was expressed after the second jump, even though there had been a very high rating of fear prior to the first jump.

To take a simple example from the animal literature (Dess, Linwick, Patterson, Overmier, & Levine, 1983), dogs were subjected to a series of electric shocks that were either unpredictable or predictable. The predictable condition involved presenting the animal with a tone prior to the onset of shock. In the unpredictable condition, no such tone was presented. The adrenocortical response observed on subsequent testing of these animals clearly indicated the importance of reducing uncertainty by predictability. Animals that did not have the signal preceding the shock showed an adrenocortical response that was two to three times that observed in animals with previous predictable shock experiences.

It should be noted that the procedures used in this experiment are typical of those used in experiments examining learned helplessness (Seligman, 1975). Learned helplessness refers to the protracted effects of prolonged exposure to unpredictable and uncontrollable stimuli of an aversive nature. It has been observed that organisms exposed to this type of experimental regimen show long-term deficits in their ability to perform appropriately under subsequent testing conditions. Furthermore, these animals show a much greater increase in adrenocortical activity when exposed to novel stimuli than do control animals (Levine, Madden, Conner, Moskal, & Anderson, 1973). Thus, an organism exposed to an uncontrollable and unpredictable set of aversive stimuli shows not only a dramatic increase in adrenocortical activity while exposed to these conditions but also long-term deficits in other, unrelated test conditions.

The key element in these examples and in virtually all recent work on stress is uncertainty (*see*, e.g., Druckman & Swets, 1988, pp. 115–132). This applies also to positive or rewarding events. In animal studies, frustration, with the attendant elevation of serum corticosterone, can be induced by changing the conditions of reward so that previously learned expectancies no longer hold.

6. STRESS AND MEMORY

Since the time of Selye's pioneering research on stress more than 60 yr ago, it has been known that people subjected to highly stressful situations in their lives show evidence of poor health. Many subsequent descriptive studies have examined the negative impact of stress on health in people, including concentration camp survivors of World War II, air traffic controllers who work at busy airports, and drivers of subway trains that injure or kill people (Cobb & Rose, 1973; Cohen, 1953; Theorell et al., 1992). Much of our current understanding of the adverse effects of stress on health has come from experimental human and animal studies. Many of these studies show that severe stress can alter nervous system structure and function and, as a consequence, cause memory problems. Other studies show that lower amounts of acute stress may, in fact, activate specific brain regions that enhance memory consolidation, the process by which memories become strengthened. Because hormones released during stress influence memory, we can now begin to understand why stress or emotional arousal have such powerful effects on how well we remember certain information during these events. A basic understanding of how hormones and brain systems become activated during stress will be examined by reviewing human and animal studies that focus in large part on their influence on the brain and memory formation.

The role of stress and emotional memory has been studied extensively by James McGaugh and colleagues. In one of McGaugh's experiments, two groups of healthy adult human subjects were shown the same series of slides but were told different stories to accompany them (Cahill & McGaugh, 1995). The neutral story was emotionally innocuous, with the other story being similar, except that an emotionally arousing description occurred in the middle of the story. After 2 wk, the subjects were asked to state what they remembered of the slides. The group that heard the neutral story remembered the slides from all parts of the story equally well (or poorly). No differences were found in these subjects as they recalled the slides from the beginning, middle, or end of the neutral story. The group that heard the emotionally arousing story, however, had a significantly enhanced recall of the slides in the middle of the story, the ones they were looking at when they heard the emotionally arousing description. This was one of the first experimental studies in humans to support the idea that emotional arousal can influence long-term memory in healthy human subjects.

In humans, emotional arousal activates a variety of stress hormones, including adrenaline. Since adrenaline binds to adrenergic receptors in the brain, it would be possible to pharmacologically block these receptors via β-adrenergic blockers (β-blockers) and observe what impact this blocking effect has on subsequent recall of information stored following an emotional event. In an experiment subsequent to the one described above from McGaugh's laboratory, a similar study was done on healthy adult human volunteers, except that half of the subjects were given the β-blocker propranolol before the experiment started (Cahill, Prins, Weber, & McGaugh, 1994). For the group that heard the neutral story, propranolol made no difference in their recall of the slides they were shown. However, for the group that heard the emotionally arousing story, propranolol completely blocked the arousing effects of emotion on memory, preventing them from recalling details of the emotionally arousing component of the story. The different results from the two groups of experimental subjects provides strong evidence that adrenaline enables the formation of memories of emotionally arousing events.

In a recent clinical study, emergency room patients who had just experienced a traumatic event, such as an automobile accident, were administered propranolol to prevent them from developing strong emotional memories of the accident that might lead them to develop posttraumatic stress disorder (PTSD) symptoms (Pitman et al., 2002). Subjects were studied up to 3 mo following the traumatic event, and those who were given propranolol were found to have a reduction in PTSD symptoms compared to emergency room patients who were given a placebo instead of propranolol. This study suggests that acute posttrauma propranolol administration may prevent PTSD symptoms and that adrenaline may play a major role in remembering under emotion-laden, stressful conditions.

Under more chronic or long-lasting stress, the adrenal cortex produces and releases cortisol, a glucocorticoid hormone that increases glucose metabolism in the blood to help supply more energy to the body, and activates other processes that stimulate behavioral responsiveness. While cortisol levels in the blood normally fluctuate over the course of a 24-h period, the levels become extremely high when a person is confronted with a stressful situation. Sustained levels of stress or exposure to cortisol can have a variety of severe effects on both body and function. In another of McGaugh's experiments, healthy adult human subjects administered cortisone pills performed poorly on a cognitive task in which the subjects needed to remember a list of words compared to control subjects who were administered placebo pills (de Quervain, Roozendaal, Nitsch, McGaugh, & Hock, 2000). Cortisone is a compound that is quickly absorbed in the body and converted into hydrocortisone (cortisol). In sum, these studies suggest that acute levels of stress may enhance certain types of memory, whereas chronic levels of stress impair them.

7. STRESS AND THE HIPPOCAMPUS

Some of the most deleterious effects of cortisol on brain tissue occur in the hippocampus, a structure rich in glucocorticoid receptors and important for the consolidation of memory. The discovery that the hippocampus has a highly concentrated population of glucocorticoid receptors has resulted in much research on the effects of stress on hippocampal structure and function (McEwen, 2000). Sapolsky found that exposing young rats to high levels of corticosterone (cortisol) or stress adversely affects the organism by reducing the number of hippocampal neurons and making it more difficult for the organism to survive the effects of seizures and ischemia, which involves the blockage of oxygen to the brain associated with stroke (Sapolsky, Krey, & McEwen, 1985). The stress-induced hippocampal damage that Sapolsky first identified was not specific to rats. The stress associated with being a subordinate in a social group of vervet monkeys caused damage to the hippocampi of some male members of the group (Uno et al., 1989) (Fig. 5). Although female monkeys had also undergone similar degrees of social subordination and developed several physical symptoms associated with chronic stress, such as stomach ulcers and immune suppression, there was no evidence of hippocampal damage in this population. This may be a result of the neurotrophic or neuroprotective properties of the female hormone estrogen, which will be discussed later. Nonetheless, the adverse effects of prolonged and severe stress that Sapolsky found in the male vervet monkey hippocampus are sufficient enough to damage the brain and cause deleterious behavioral consequences.

In patients with Cushing's syndrome, noncancerous tumors in the pituitary gland give rise to an excessive overproduction and release of glucocorticoids that lead to hypertension, diabetes, immune system problems, and memory impairment (Starkman, Gebarski, Berent, & Schteingart, 1992). Magnetic resonance imaging scans of Cushing's syndrome patients showed that the amount of glucocorticoid secretion is correlated with the extent of hippocampal atrophy and the extent of impairment in hippocampal-dependent cognition (Sapolsky, 1996). These studies suggest a strong relationship between sustained stress or glucocorticoid secretion and damage to the hippocampus, ultimately resulting in various pathologies and memory impairment.

Excitatory synaptic transmission in the hippocampus is mediated by glutamate, the most common excitatory neurotransmitter in the brain. Several types of receptors bind

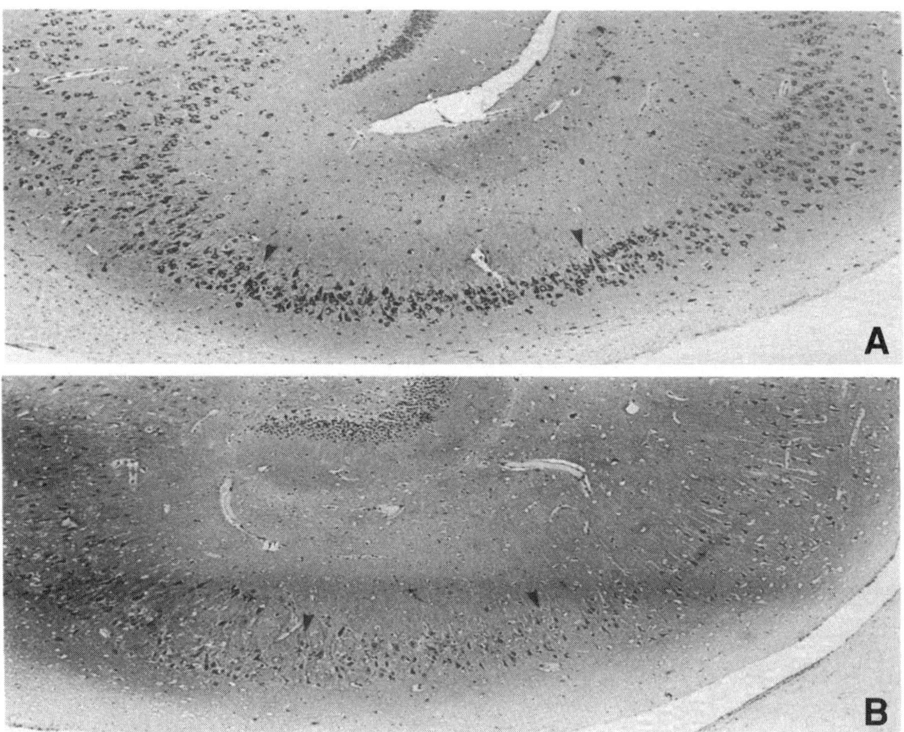

Fig. 5. Photomicrographs showing brain damage caused by stress: (a) section through the hippocampus of a normal vervet monkey: (b) section through the hippocampus of a vervet monkey of low social status subjected to stress. Compare the regions between the arrowheads, normally filled with large pyramidal cells. (From Uno et al., 1989.)

glutamate, including *N*-methyl-D-aspartate (NMDA) and AMPA receptors. When glutamate binds to these receptors, the neuron becomes excited. Activation of these receptors in the hippocampus is thought to be responsible, in part, for normal learning and memory processing. However, when glutamate is present in very high doses, it becomes toxic to the cells to which it binds. Brain damage in the hippocampus of rats exposed to high levels of glucocorticoids might, in fact, be owing to a disruption in the regulation of glutamate, ultimately resulting in high concentrations of glutamate causing damage to these neurons (Sapolsky, Krey, & McEwen, 1986b). The hippocampus may regulate the hormonal stress response, sending inhibitory messages to the hypothalamus, where the hormonal stress response is first controlled. During stress, rats and monkeys with damage to the hippocampus take longer to turn off their stress response, resulting in higher levels of glucocorticoids. As noted above from McGaugh's research, these stress hormones, presumably by acting on the hippocampus, can enhance the storage of important experiences in long-term memory. However, excessive or chronically elevated levels of these same hormones can damage the very part of the brain that regulates them. Consequently, increased secretion of glucocorticoids further damages portions of the hippocampus, resulting in deficits in learning and memory.

As we have seen, the hippocampus has special relevance to human and animal cognitive processes. Stress studies have made it clear that important stress hormones can significantly impact hippocampal structure and function. McEwen has studied the effects of stress on age-related brain degeneration that causes cognitive deficits in humans and animals. In studies of elderly humans, individual differences in human brain aging were correlated with cortisol levels in otherwise healthy individuals followed over a number of years. Elderly subjects who showed a significant and progressive increase in basal cortisol levels during yearly exams spanning 4 yr performed more poorly on tasks measuring explicit memory than those of age-matched controls who did not show progressive cortisol increases (Lupien et al., 1998). Furthermore, brain scans revealed that the hippocampi of the impaired group were 14% smaller than those of the control group. This research highlights the vulnerability of the brain—and the hippocampus, in particular—to factors associated with chronic stress and the human aging process.

Experimental animal studies suggest a mechanism whereby stress and aging interact. In young rats, repeated exposure to stress causes a decrease in the number of glucocorticoid receptors in the brain. In this case, high levels of cortisol actually are less effective because cortisol now binds to fewer receptors. However, with increasing age, the rats' glucocorticoid receptors do not decrease, allowing more of the receptors to be present when there really should be fewer (Sapolsky, Krey, & McEwen, 1986a). In aged rats, stress-generated cortisol has a much broader target area to which it can bind, thereby disrupting the normal balance of glucocorticoid receptors and presumably increasing the risk of hippocampal damage. These studies provide strong support for an association between cognitive impairment and aging that might be related to cortisol and glucocorticoid receptor dysregulation in the hippocampus. A clearer understanding of the mechanisms underlying the effect of these hormones on cognition and memory may help in providing therapeutic approaches for people needing them.

8. STRESS AND SYNAPTIC PLASTICITY

A number of hormones secreted from the pituitary–adrenal system during stress affect learning and memory processes. The phenomenon of hippocampal long-term potentiation (LTP), characterized by an increase in synaptic efficacy, is viewed by many as a putative mechanism of memory storage and has proven to be a most valuable model for the study of neuronal plasticity at the cellular level. An uncontrollable acute stress experience in rats (30 min body restraint + 1 s tail-shock/min) was found to markedly impair the subsequent ability of a region within the hippocampus to develop LTP (Foy, Stanton, Levine, & Thompson, 1987). This was the first demonstration of an acute behavioral stressor to impair the induction and maintenance of a form of synaptic plasticity within the brain (Fig. 6). In a further study, LTP was much less impaired in rats that could control the shock stress than in rats that could not exert control, even though both groups of rats received identical physical stress (Shors, Seib, Levine, & Thompson, 1989).

Although it is unknown whether behavioral stress impairs LTP specifically or plasticity in general, other forms of hippocampal plasticity, such as the more recently discovered hippocampal homosynaptic long-term depression (LTD), may also be modified by stress. LTD, contrary to LTP, is characterized by a decrease in synaptic efficacy and is considered as a mechanism of memory storage (Bear & Malenka, 1994). Behavioral stress, similar to that administered in the LTP experiments, facilitated hippocampal LTD in rats (Kim, Foy, & Thompson, 1996). In contrast, hippocampal recordings from unstressed controls failed to display LTD.

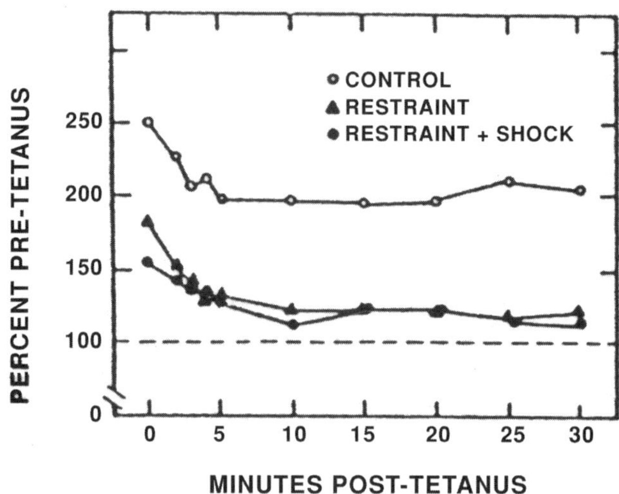

Fig. 6. Long-term potentiation differences in hippocampus from rats exposed to behavioral stress. Means of extracellular hippocampal waveforms after stimulation designed to induce long-term potentiation from nonstressed (○) vs stressed (body restraint + tail-shocks) rats (●). (From Foy et al., 1987.)

The failure to obtain LTD in control animals requires an explanation. It appears that while LTD occurs in the hippocampus of very young rats (e.g., ~12–15 d old), it seems to occur less reliably in adult rats (e.g., ~3–5 mo old). Adult rats were used in both the original LTP and LTD experiments. Also, it has been discovered that hippocampal LTD is most prominent in aged rats (e.g., ~18–24 mo old) (Norris, Korol, & Foster, 1996). In normal aging, the hippocampus undergoes a number of changes in morphology and physiology that may contribute to age-related differences in functioning and behavior (Geinisman, de Toledo-Morrell, Morrell, & Heller, 1995); these changes may be responsible for the effects of stress on synaptic plasticity in the aged animals. In the study by Kim et al. (1996) mentioned above, it was also found that the behavioral stress enhancement of LTD and the stress impairment of LTP in rats required activation of NMDA receptors, because the stress effect on both forms of hippocampal synaptic plasticity was blocked by NMDA receptor antagonists. Such modifications in hippocampal plasticity may contribute to learning and memory impairments associated with stress.

9. STRESS AND ESTROGEN

After more than three decades of research, it has been well established that estrogen influences nervous system activity. Decreased hippocampal seizure thresholds were found in animals primed with estrogen and also during proestrus, the stage of the estrous cycle when estrogen levels are at their highest (Terasawa & Timiras, 1969). Since then, many studies have confirmed the powerful electrophysiological effects of estrogen, including excitatory and inhibitory influences on hippocampal excitability, plasticity, and anatomy (Foy, 2001; Foy et al., 1999; Teyler, Vardaris, Lewis, & Rawitch, 1980; Wong & Moss, 1991, 1992; Woolley, Weiland, McEwen, & Schwartzkroin, 1997). For example, hippocampal neurons from young adult male rats exposed to moderate concen-

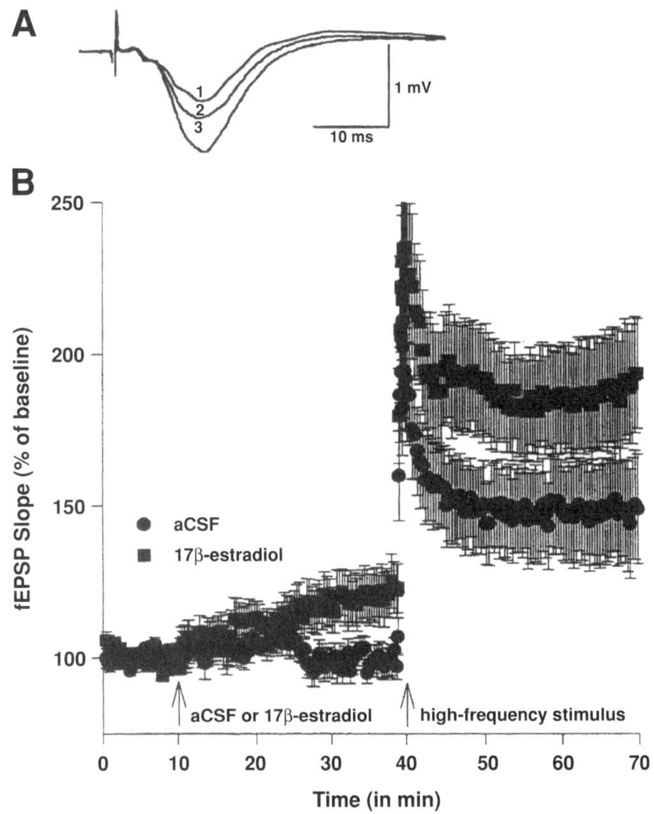

Fig. 7. Waveform recordings from hippocampal tissues exposed to control artificial cerebrospinal fluid (aCSF) or 17β-estradiol. (A1) Waveform recordings at the end of 10 min of aCSF perfusion (control). (A2) Waveform recordings at the end of 30 min of 17β-estradiol perfusion. (A3) Waveform recordings at end of 30 min of 17β-estradiol perfusion with high-frequency stimulation designed to produce LTP. (B) Averaged waveform data points from control (aCSF) and experimental (17β-estradiol) hippocampal tissues throughout entire 70-min experiment. (From Foy et al., 1999.)

trations of 17β-estradiol, the most potent of the biologically relevant estrogens, exhibit an increase in synaptic transmission occurring within several minutes of administration. Following high-frequency stimulation designed to induce LTP, 17β-estradiol induces a pronounced, persisting, and significant enhancement of LTP of extracellular hippocampal waveforms compared to control conditions (Foy et al., 1999) (Fig. 7). In females, circulating estrogen levels appear to produce a tonic activation of hippocampal synaptic plasticity because the magnitude of LTP in intact female rats recorded during proestrus is greatest, compared to a decreased magnitude of LTP recorded during the female rat's diestrus (low estrogen level) stage of the estrous cycle (Bi, Foy, Vouimba, Thompson, & Baudry, 2001).

Estrogen's influence on hippocampal synaptic plasticity has been under intensive study due, in part, to clinical evidence indicating that estrogen hormone replacement therapy may delay the progression of Alzheimer's disease and reduce the memory decline observed during normal aging and menopause (Kawas et al., 1997; Paganini-Hill &

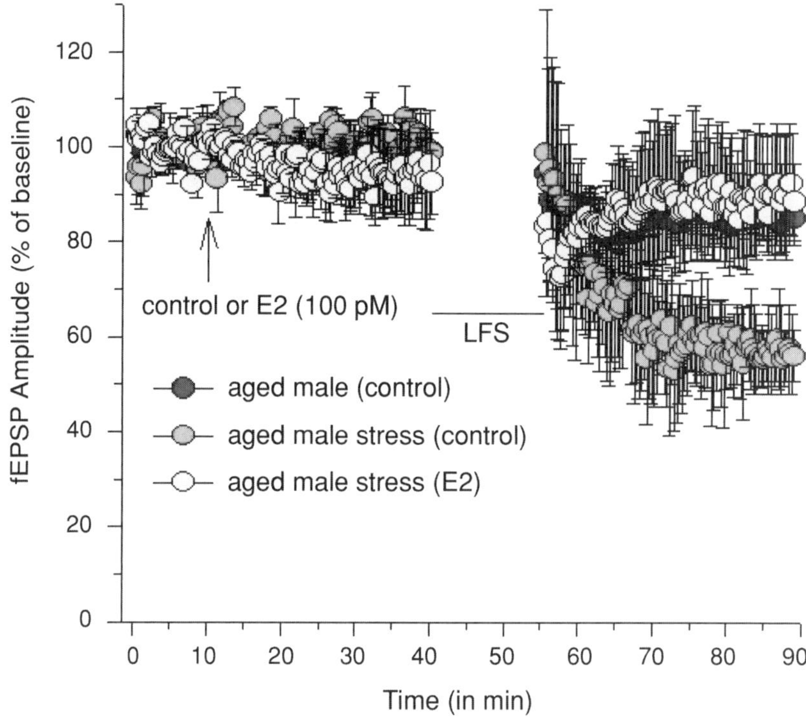

Fig. 8. Long-term depression differences in hippocampus from aged rats exposed to behavioral stress. Means of extracellular hippocampal waveforms (field excitatory postsynaptic potentials) before and after stimulation designed to induce long-term depression from nonstressed (dark gray circles), stressed (medium gray circles), and stressed + estrogen-treated (E2) (light gray circles) aged rats. (From Tran et al., 2003.)

Henderson, 1996; Tang et al., 1996). However, evidence also suggests that treatment with estrogen once the disease is clearly established has no beneficial effect (Mulnard et al., 2000) or that estrogen may even be detrimental to nervous system functioning (for review, *see* Brinton, 2004).

As already discussed, hippocampal LTD is enhanced in aged rats compared to young adult rats. This age enhancement of hippocampal LTD is suppressed by treatment with 17β-estradiol (Vouimba, Foy, Foy, & Thompson, 2000). From the research mentioned above, it is known that stress has a marked effect in enhancing hippocampal LTD in both adult and aged rats, with aged animals showing a more marked effect. Estrogen reverses the stress enhancement of hippocampal LTD in adult and aged rats, such that the amount of hippocampal LTD recorded from the rats treated with estrogen is similar to that recorded from nonstressed, young adult controls (Tran, Foy, & Thompson, 2003) (Fig. 8). The results from these animal studies examining the effects of estrogen on synaptic plasticity suggest that estrogen may act to improve memory storage by suppressing forgetfulness via a synaptic mechanism, such as hippocampal LTD. Furthermore, estrogen may be protective against the effects of acute behavioral stress on learning and memory function and may also reverse learning and memory deficits associated with age.

In summary, the hippocampus is critical for key aspects of memory formation. The current most widely accepted putative mechanisms of memory storage in the hippocampus are LTP and LTD. There are stress- and age-related alterations in hippocampal LTP and LTD that correlate with stress and age impairments in hippocampal-dependent memory tasks. Recent evidence in humans suggests that estrogenic hormones appear to ameliorate the early effects of Alzheimer's disease on memory in women. Studies on rats indicate that estrogen can modulate synaptic transmission in the hippocampus of both stressed and aged animals by enhancing LTP and by blocking or suppressing LTD. Detailed studies examining the mechanisms of action of estrogen on hippocampal plasticity and the role of estrogen in stress and aging may help us to better understand how each of these components influences memory processes in humans.

10. STRESS AND THE AMYGDALA

There is a growing literature indicating that the amygdala is critically involved in mediating stress-related behaviors and in modulating hippocampal mnemonic functioning. For example, lesions and pharmacological inactivation of the amygdala prevent stress-induced gastric erosion (Henke, 1981) and analgesia (Adamec, Burton, Shallow, & Budgell, 1999). McGaugh and colleagues have shown that various drug manipulations (specifically agonists and antagonists affecting opioid, GABAergic, noradrenergic, and cholinergic neurotransmission) in the amygdala can modulate (strengthen or weaken) memory formation in the hippocampus (McGaugh, 2000; Roozendaal, Griffith, Buranday, de Quervain, & McGaugh, 2003). Amygdalar lesions also prevent stress-induced increases in catecholamine turnover in the prefrontal cortex, which is thought to impair working memory function (Goldstein, Rasmusson, Bunney, & Roth, 1996).

The amygdala is also implicated in the development of LTP in the hippocampus. Abe and colleagues have shown that lesions to the basolateral nucleus of the amygdala (BLA) significantly attenuated perforant path-dentate gyrus LTP in vivo (Ikegaya, Saito, & Abe, 1994), whereas lesions to the central nucleus of the amygdala did not. Conversely, high-frequency stimulation of the BLA amplified the magnitude of LTP in the dentate gyrus (Ikegaya, Saito, & Abe, 1996). Targeted infusions of the NMDA receptor antagonist APV (DL-2-amino-5-phosphonovaleric acid) into the BLA reduced the magnitude of LTP in the dentate gyrus (without affecting the baseline f-EPSP), a finding that suggests that amygdalar NMDA receptors are involved in regulating hippocampal LTP (Ikegaya, Saito, & Abe, 1995). Recently, stimulation of the amygdala and exposing rats to stress (forced exposure to a brightly lit chamber) have been found to produce similar time-dependent biphasic (an immediate excitatory and a longer-lasting inhibitory) effects on hippocampal LTP (Akirav & Richter-Levin, 1999).

Anatomically, the amygdala is connected both directly (amygdalo-hippocampal bundles arise from the magnocellular and parvicellular divisions of the basolateral amygdala and terminate at CA1 and the subiculum) and indirectly (via the entorhinal cortex) to several hippocampal regions (Pikkarainen, Ronkko, Savander, Insausti, & Pitkanen, 1999). Via these routes, the amygdala may exert influences on the hippocampus, such as stress effects on hippocampal LTP and memory.

Consistent with the aforementioned findings, a recent study demonstrated that amygdalar lesions effectively block stress effects on hippocampal LTP and hippocampal-dependent spatial memory (Kim, Lee, Han, & Packard, 2001). Specifically, hippocampal slices obtained from control (sham-lesioned) animals exposed to stress exhibited LTP impairments in the CA1 area, whereas slices from control animals not exposed to stress demonstrated robust LTP, replicating earlier in vitro and in vivo findings of stress-

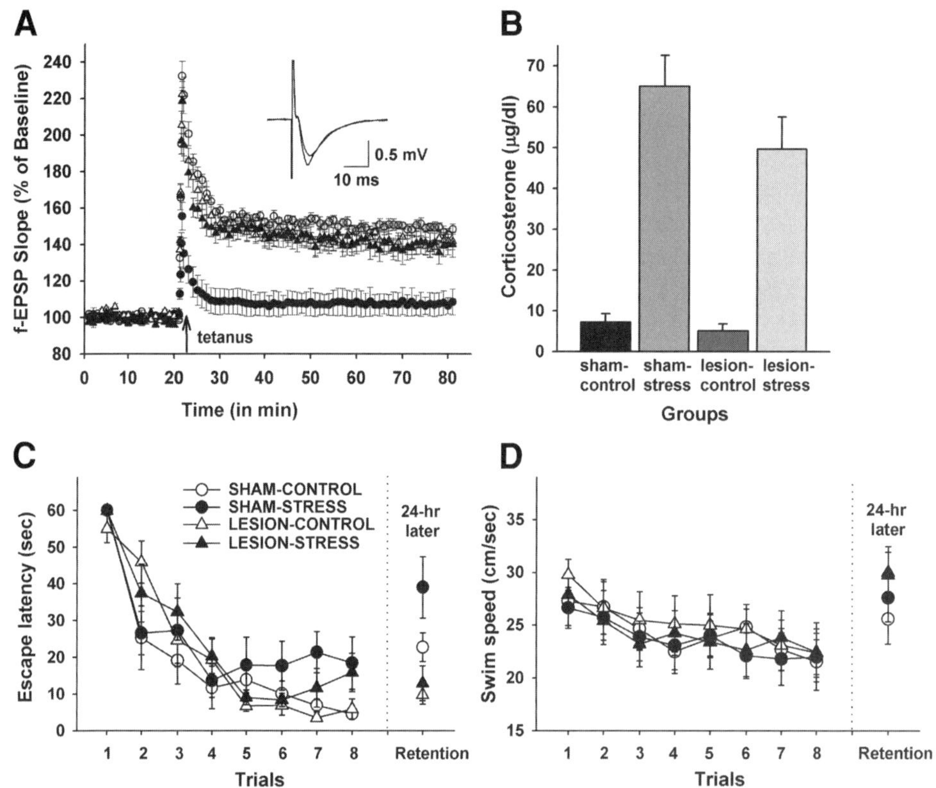

Fig. 9. (A) Amygdalar lesions block stress-induced impairments in Schaffer collateral/commissural-CA1 LTP (SHAM-CONTROL, ○; SHAM-STRESS, ●; LESION-CONTROL, △; LESION-STRESS, ▲), (B) but do not interfere with stress-induced corticosterone secretion (I^{125} radioimmunoassay). (C) Behaviorally, amygdalar lesions prevent stress-induced impairments in spatial memory, (D) without affecting swim speed. (Data from Kim & Diamond, 2002.)

induced impairments of LTP (Diamond & Rose, 1994; Foy et al., 1987; Kim et al., 1996; Shors et al., 1989; Xu, Anwyl, & Rowan, 1997). In contrast, LTP was observed reliably in hippocampal slices prepared from amygdala lesioned animals, regardless of whether or not they experienced stress (Fig. 9). Behaviorally, amygdalar lesions blocked stress-induced impairments in spatial memory when rats were tested in a hippocampal-dependent hidden platform water maze task. Stress effects on hippocampal LTP and spatial memory were also blocked by micro-infusing the $GABA_A$ receptor agonist muscimol into the amygdala prior to stress (Kim et al., 2001). Interestingly, immediate post-stress infusions of muscimol into the amygdala failed to prevent stress effects on LTP and memory, indicating that amygdalar activities during stress, but not after stress, are critical for the emergence of stress effects on hippocampus. Shors and Mathew's (1998) finding that intra-amygdalar infusions of APV block stress-induced facilitation of eyeblink conditioning suggests that NMDA receptors in the amygdala are likely to be important in mediating stress effects on hippocampal LTP and memory as well. These electrophysiological and behavioral findings that the amygdala is critically involved in mediating stress effects on the hippocampus are consistent with the view that one function of the amygdala is to modulate memory processes in other brain structures, such as the hippocampus (Cahill & McGaugh, 1998; Gallagher & Kapp, 1978; Ikegaya et al., 1994; McGaugh, 2000; Roozendaal et al., 2003).

Interestingly, although amygdalar lesions block stress effects on CA1 LTP in vitro, the lesions themselves did not affect the magnitude of LTP in unstressed animals. This finding contrasts with LTP observed in the dentate gyrus (Ikegaya et al., 1994), where the amygdalar lesion *per se* significantly impaired LTP. It appears then the amygdala differentially influences synaptic plasticity in different regions of the hippocampus.

As mentioned previously, stress is known to activate an ensemble of neurochemical responses (such as secretions of glucocorticoids, catecholamines, and opiates) from the hypothalamic–pituitary–adrenal (HPA) axis and in the ANS (Kim & Yoon, 1998; McEwen & Sapolsky, 1995). There is strong support for the notion that corticosterone is the main neuromodulator of stress effects on LTP and memory. However, the corticosterone effects on hippocampal LTP are complex, in that there is a biphasic relationship between the level of corticosterone and the magnitude of LTP: both low (through adrenalectomy) and high (produced by stress or exogenous administration) levels of corticosterone are associated with LTP impairments, with maximal LTP occurring at an intermediate level of corticosterone (Diamond, Bennett, Fleshner, & Rose, 1992). Subsequent studies indicate that low-to-intermediate levels of corticosterone enhance hippocampal LTP by preferentially stimulating the high-affinity Type I mineralocorticoid receptors (MRs), whereas high levels of corticosterone (reflecting a heightened stress state) produce greater activation of the low-affinity Type II glucocorticoid receptors (GRs), which results in an inhibitory effect on hippocampal LTP (Conrad, Lupien, & McEwen, 1999). The relatively greater importance of GRs, compared with MRs, in mediating the adverse effects of corticosterone on the hippocampus is also supported by findings that GR agonists and MR antagonists can impair spatial memory (de Kloet, Oitzl, & Joels, 1999) and that a point mutation in the mouse GR gene blocks the exogenous effects of corticosterone on spatial memory (Oitzl, Reichardt, Joels, & de Kloet, 2001).

Corticosterone can also influence the intrinsic properties of hippocampal neurons. Bath application of corticosterone has been shown to prolong the afterhyperpolarization (AHP) of CA1 pyramidal neurons by increasing the level of internal Ca^{2+} and thereby activating Ca^{2+}-gated K^+ channels (Joels, 2001; Kerr, Campbell, Hao, & Landfield, 1989). Correspondingly, corticosterone also promotes the expression of genes that encode channels that enhance Ca^{2+} influx (Nair et al., 1998). Recent work has shown that stress levels of corticosterone initially enhance MR-mediated hippocampal cellular excitability, which is then overtaken by a GR-mediated suppression of cellular activity (Joels, 2001), which could impede the development of LTP.

However, an increase in the corticosterone concentration *per se* does not seem to be sufficient to affect hippocampal LTP. This conclusion is based on findings that LTP can still be inhibited by stress in rats that have been depleted of corticosterone as a result of adrenalectomy (Shors, Levine, & Thompson, 1990). Moreover, in normal rats administered dexamethasone (a synthetic glucocorticoid that blocks the release of corticosterone), stress impairments of LTP still transpired (Foy, Foy, Levine, & Thompson, 1990). More recent work has provided three different conditions in which there was dissociation between the level of corticosterone and hippocampal functioning.

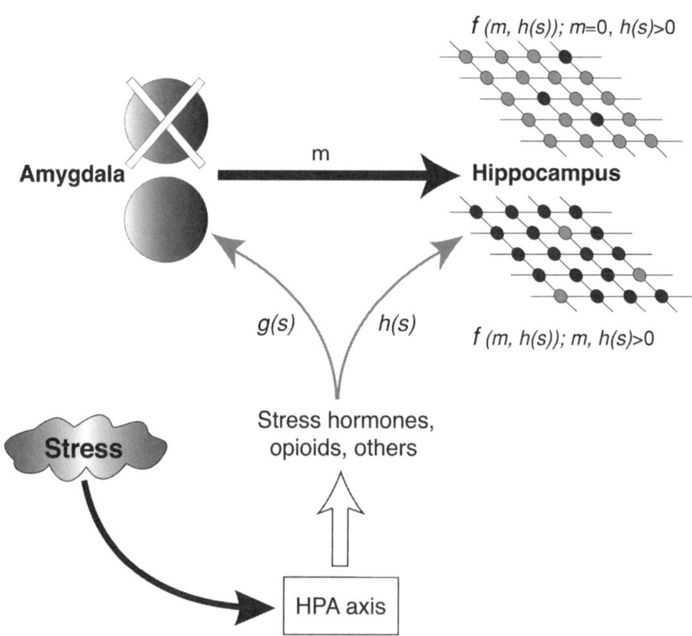

Fig.10. A hypothetical model of how neuromodulator–amygdala interactions mediate stress effects on hippocampal plasticity. Stress-induced elevations in neuromodulators (glucocorticoids, catecholamines, enkephalins) can directly affect the hippocampus [denoted by *h(s)*] and amygdala [denoted by *g(s)*]. The output from the amygdala (variable *m*) is a crucial component of the stress-induced modulation of hippocampal plasticity. The interaction between influences from the amygdala (*m*) and stress neuromodulators directly on the hippocampus (*h(s)*) is a function of both *m* and *h(s)* and is denoted by *f[m,h(s)]*. The model thus illustrates that when there is a reduction of amygdala input to the hippocampus (e.g., owing to amygdalar lesions or inactivation, $m = 0$), plasticity in the hippocampus is intact under stress conditions (top matrix). Conversely, with intact amygdalar input in response to stress, plasticity in the hippocampus is disturbed (i.e., impaired long-term potentiation [LTP]; bottom matrix). The light gray circles on the matrices represent synapses with normal capacity to generate plasticity (e.g., normal LTP), thereby accommodating normal hippocampal-dependent memory. The dark gray circles represent synapses following stress with altered plasticity property (e.g., impaired LTP), which impairs subsequent hippocampal-dependent memory. (Adapted from Kim & Diamond, 2002.)

First, rats with lesions of the amygdala did not develop stress impairments of LTP, despite the fact that the lesioned rats had significantly elevated corticosterone levels (Kim et al., 2001). Second, the exogenous administration of stress levels of corticosterone, under nonstress conditions, did not produce impairments in hippocampal-dependent spatial memory in rats (Woodson, Macintosh, Fleshner, & Diamond, 2003). Third, male rats given access to a sexually receptive female had elevations of serum corticosterone, but no spatial memory deficit (Woodson et al., 2003). Thus, the elevated corticosterone in the absence of an intact amygdala (or amygdalar-based activity such as fear) is not sufficient to produce deficits in hippocampal LTP and memory. Collectively, multiple factors—glucocorticoids and other neuromodulators in conjunction with amygdalar activities—are likely to be involved in mediating stress effects on hippocampal functioning (Fig. 10).

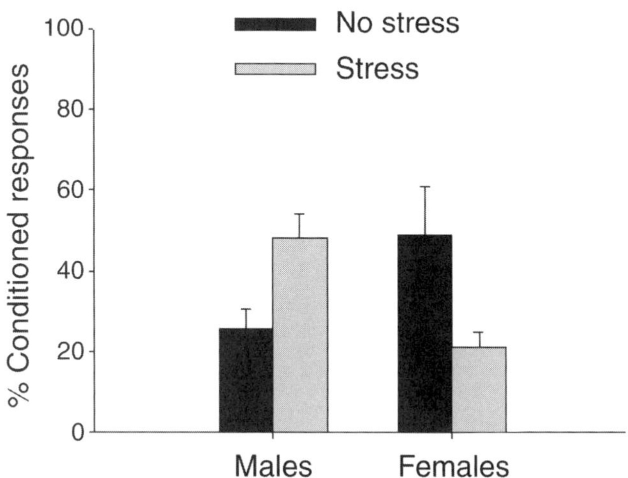

Fig. 11. The bar graph depicts the percentage of conditioned responses in males and females 24 h after being exposed to an acute stressor of brief intermittent tail-shocks relative to the percentage of conditioned responses in unstressed controls.

11. SEX-SPECIFIC RESPONSES TO STRESS

Males and females can respond to stressful experience in very different ways. The most robust sex difference occurs with endogenous levels of glucocorticoids. In many species, glucocorticoid levels are higher in females than in males (Viau & Meaney, 1991). This sex difference is apparent under unstressed and stressed conditions, and in rats, glucocorticoid levels are elevated in females during proestrus relative to other stages of estrous. Stressful experience can also elicit very different behavioral responses in males vs females, particularly in procedural memory tasks. For example, female rats exposed to an acute stressful event are severely handicapped in their ability to learn the classically conditioned eyeblink response (Wood & Shors, 1998). Oddly enough, males exhibit enhanced performance after exposure to the same stressful event (Shors, 2001; Shors, Weiss, & Thompson, 1992) (Fig. 11). The stressful event consists of either brief exposure to intermittent tail-shocks or brief swim stress (20 min), both of which are common methods for inducing behavioral depression in laboratory animals.

If these effects of uncontrollable stressful experience on learning in rats are relevant to the human condition, they should possess some characteristics of mental illness, particularly those associated with stressful experience such as PTSD. After experiencing a traumatic stressful event, some humans develop a series of behaviors that are maladaptive and cause distress and dysfunction, such as avoidance, reduced responsiveness, increased arousal, and anxiety. Often, they reexperience frightening aspects of the traumatic event, particularly if presented with cues associated with the event. To determine whether the effects of stress on learning in rats were sensitive to these factors, rats were exposed to cues associated with the stressful event days after it had ceased and at a time when the effects of stress would not be reduced or no longer evident. Indeed, days after the stressor, males reintroduced to the stress context were further enhanced in their performance, whereas females were further impaired (Shors & Servatius, 1997; Wood, Beylin, & Shors, 2001). Minimally, these results suggest that the effects of acute stress on learning

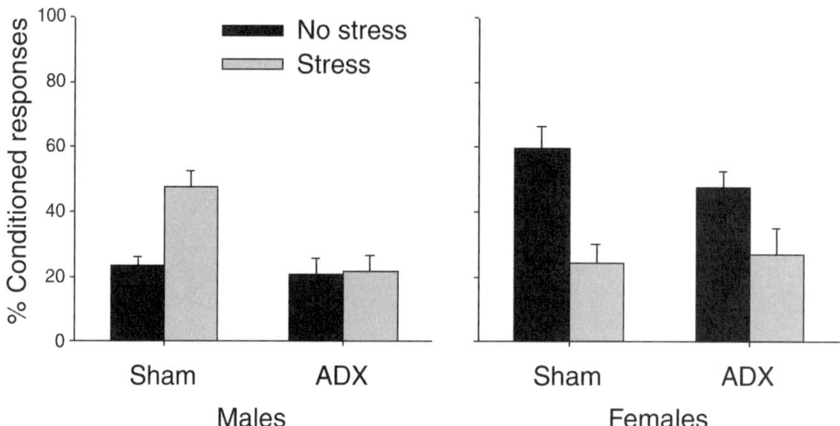

Fig. 12. The graph depicts the percentage of conditioned responses in males and females 24 h after being exposed to an acute stressor of brief intermittent tail-shocks relative to the percentage of conditioned responses in unstressed controls. Groups of animals either had their adrenal glands removed (ADX) or were exposed to a sham surgery.

are not entirely dependent on sensory stimulation, but rather can be stimulated by associations established with the stressful environment. More generally, they suggest that the effects of acute stress on later learning in rats may model some aspects of posttraumatic experience in humans.

12. STRESS HORMONES AND STRESS EFFECTS ON MEMORY FORMATION

Given its importance in the stress response, it seems logical that corticosterone would be involved in modulating learning processes after stress. Indeed, removal of endogenous glucocorticoids via adrenalectomy prevents the enhanced eyeblink conditioning in males after stress. Somewhat surprisingly, however, adrenalectomy did not alter the female response to stress (Wood & Shors, 1998) (Fig. 12). Thus, exposure to the acute stressful event not only has opposite effects on this measure of performance in males and females, but these effects are mediated by different hormonal systems.

Obviously, there are many different types of stressors, and their effects on learning are varied depending on the task, training conditions, and sex. Despite the variety of responses, many are assumed to occur via glucocorticoid activation and most often by activity within the hippocampal formation. The hippocampus has an abundance of GRs, particularly the Type I, or MR, and has been implicated in feedback of the HPA axis. Thus, the results regarding the male response to stress is generally consistent with much of the literature. That the female response is not dependent on the presence of glucocorticoids may be an aberration or simply reflect the fact that so few studies have been conducted in females.

Although glucocorticoids are not critically involved in the stress effect in females, ovarian hormones are. Their removal via ovariectomy prevents the stress effect on eyeblink conditioning, suggesting that their presence is necessary for inducing a learning impairment after stress. Of the two primary ovarian hormones, estrogen seems most

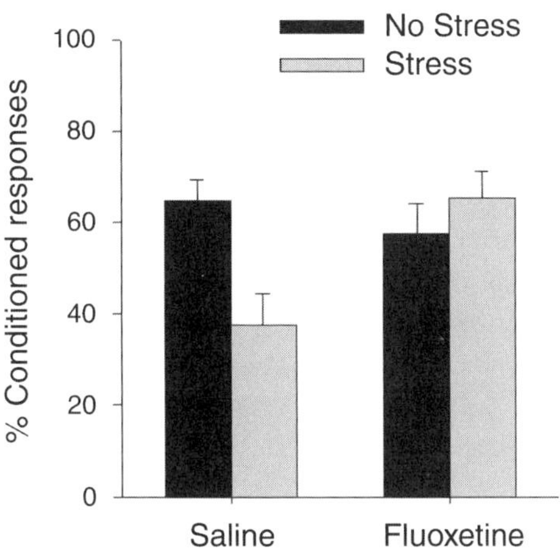

Fig. 13. The percentage of conditioned responses in females 24 h after being exposed to an acute stressor of brief intermittent tail-shocks relative to the percentage of conditioned responses in unstressed controls. Groups of females were either treated for approx 14 d with the antidepressant fluoxetine (Prozac) or injected with the vehicle.

critical since treatment with the estrogen antagonist tamoxifen also prevents the stress effect on conditioning (Wood & Shors, 1998). Together, these data suggest that estrogen is critically involved in the stress effect on conditioning in females. It is also noted that the detrimental effect of stress on learning is dependent on the stage of estrous in which the learning occurs. Of the stages of estrous, females trained during proestrus (stressed 24 h earlier in diestrus) are most impaired by stressor exposure (Shors, Lewczyk, Paczynski, Mathew, & Pickett, 1998). Since this stage is associated with elevated levels of estrogen, estrogen is again implicated in the stress effects on conditioning. Interestingly, as noted above, an enhanced amount of hippocampal LTP was recorded from female rats during the proestrus stage of their cycle (Bi et al., 2001). Also, results from both the human and animal literature now show the powerful influence of estrogen on enhancing procedural (e.g., Wood & Shors, 1998) and declarative memories (e.g., Sherwin & Tulandi, 1996). How these different systems are studied may advance our understanding of the mechanisms responsible for the effects of estrogen on NMDA receptor-mediated responses and on synaptic connectivity within the hippocampus related to stress.

13. THE ROLE OF SEROTONIN IN THE FEMALE RESPONSE TO STRESS

There has been much interest in the neural mechanisms that underlie antidepressants, especially the newer generation compounds such as fluoxetine (Prozac). Not only do these affect neural plasticity, especially in the hippocampus, but they also interact with estrogen (Malberg, Eisch, Nestler, & Duman, 2000; Shors & Leuner, 2003). Based on these connections, one might wonder whether the stress effect on learning in females could be ameliorated by chronic treatment with Prozac. In one study, female rats were injected daily with 5 mg/kg for at least 2 wk. As shown in Fig. 13, chronic treatment with the antidepressant prevents the negative effect of stress on learning (Leuner, Mendolia,

Falduto, & Shors, 2002). The effects of stress and Prozac on anxiety behavior were also measured by time spent in the open exposed arms of the plus maze. As might be expected, exposure to the stressful event enhanced anxiety behavior. Treatment with antidepressants also enhanced anxiety, but there was no interaction between the effects of stress and Prozac on anxiety behavior. These results suggest that the amelioration of the stress effect on learning by Prozac is distinct from its known anxiogenic effects during the first few weeks of treatment (Silva & Brandao, 2000). Moreover, they indicate that the females treated with Prozac did experience the stressor and that it had persistent effects on some behaviors—just not on learning itself.

Prozac's effectiveness in treating human mental disorders emerges only after weeks. Consistent with this, treatment with Prozac only on the day of training did not lessen the impact of stress on learning (Leuner et al., 2002) (Fig. 13). These data are consistent with the efficacy of such antidepressants. Overall, these data implicate serotonergic mechanisms in the stress-induced impairment of learning in the female rat.

This brief review of sex differences in the stress response presents only a small sample of those that have been reported to exist, and likely a much smaller fraction of those that do exist. They certainly illustrate that the male stress response is not the same as the female stress response. Moreover, they indicate that laboratory findings about stress in males would not necessarily model what occurs in women after they have experienced stressful events in their lives.

14. CONCLUSIONS

The contemporary view of the neurobiological foundations of stress originates from a wealth of research undertaken during the past 70 yr, focused primarily on activation of the HPA axis. The HPA axis regulates the primary endocrine response to stress, which in turn regulates major metabolic and neural processes. Stress, either physical injury or perception of stress, results in activation of the hypothalamus to release corticotropin-releasing hormone, which acts on the anterior pituitary gland to release ACTH into the bloodstream. ACTH acts on the cortex of the adrenal gland to release cortisol, the stress hormone, which mobilizes the body to deal with the stress. In stress, the hypothalamus also acts directly on the ANS to prepare the body for emergencies and via forebrain structures to prepare the organism for "fight or flight." The sympathetic adrenomedullary system of the ANS releases directly into the bloodstream E and other catecholamines, which act on target organs to adapt to or deal with the stressful situation.

While the increased release of cortisol in response to stress is normal and adaptive, a long-term increase in cortisol levels can result in damage and loss to neurons in the hippocampus, a limbic system structure rich in GRs and important for the consolidation of memory. Sustained stress or glucocorticoid secretion and damage to the hippocampus may ultimately result in various pathologies and memory impairment, presumably through excessive binding of the excitatory synaptic transmitter glutamate to its receptors. Hippocampal LTP, a putative mechanism of memory storage involving synaptic plasticity, has been found to be impaired in animals exposed to uncontrollable, acute stress. Interestingly, LTP was impaired much less in animals that could control the stress than in rats that could not, suggesting the importance of "control" in stressful situations. More recent studies have reported that the effects of stress on hippocampal plasticity are dramatically influenced by sex (male vs female), hormone (estrogen vs testosterone), age (young vs adult), and structural (e.g., amygdala) variables that appear to correlate with sex, hormone, and age impairments in hippocampal-dependent memory tasks.

The relationship between stress and neurobiology is quite complex and indirect. While stress involves a number of physical and psychological factors, uncertainty and lack of control in potentially harmful situations appears to be the major cause of its detrimental effects. The ability to control such situations appears to provide the most successful coping strategy. All stress-inducing stimuli, both physical and psychological, exert their initial effects on the central nervous system. A contemporary perspective of the neurobiological foundations of stress has evolved from Selye's original concept of a single, stereotypical response resulting from any stress placed upon the body to one that reflects different patterns of biochemical, physiological, and behavioral responses of varying degrees to particular stressors. A more detailed understanding of these important factors should provide us with an awareness of potential and better coping strategies designed to lessen the impact of stress on the brain and body.

ACKNOWLEDGMENTS

Supported by grants from NIA (14751) (RFT, MRF); LMU Faculty Research Grant (MRF); Whitehall Foundation, NIA (P60AG10469), NIMH (MH64457) (JJK); NIMH (59970), NSF (IBN0217403) (TJS).

REFERENCES

Adamec, R. E., Burton, P., Shallow, T., & Budgell, J. (1999). Unilateral block of NMDA receptors in the amygdala prevents predator stress-induced lasting increases in anxiety-like behavior and unconditioned startle—effective hemisphere depends on the behavior. *Physiology and Behavior, 65*, 739–751.

Akil, H., Campeau, S., Cullinan, W. E., Lechan, R. M., Toni, R., Watson, S. J., & Moore, R. Y. (1999). Neuroendocrine systems I: Overview—Thyroid and adrenal axes. In M. J. Zigmond, F. E. Bloom, & S. C. Landis (Eds.), *Fundamental neuroscience* (pp. 1127–1150). San Diego: Academic.

Akirav, I., & Richter-Levin, G. (1999). Biphasic modulation of hippocampal plasticity by behavioral stress and basolateral amygdala stimulation in the rat. *Journal of Neuroscience, 19*, 10,530–10,535.

Bear, M. F., & Malenka, R. C. (1994). Synaptic plasticity: LTP and LTD. *Current Opinion in Neurobiology, 4*, 389–399.

Bi, R., Foy, M. R., Vouimba, R. M., Thompson, R. F., & Baudry, M. (2001). Cyclic changes in estrogen regulate synaptic plasticity through the MAP kinase pathway. *Proceedings of the National Academy of Sciences (USA), 98*, 13,391–13,395.

Brinton, R. D. (2004). Impact of estrogen therapy on Alzheimer's disease: A fork in the road? *CNS Drugs, 18*, 405–422.

Cahill, L., & McGaugh, J. L. (1995). A novel demonstration of enhanced memory associated with emotional arousal. *Consciousness and Cognition, 4*, 410–421.

Cahill, L., & McGaugh, J. L. (1998). Mechanisms of emotional arousal and lasting declarative memory. *Trends in Neuroscience, 21*, 294–299.

Cahill, L., Prins, B., Weber, M., & McGaugh, J. L. (1994). Beta-adrenergic activation and memory for emotional events. *Nature, 371*, 702–704.

Cobb, S., & Rose, R. M. (1973). Hypertension, peptic ulcer, and diabetes in air traffic controllers. *Journal of the American Medical Association, 224*, 489–492.

Cohen, E. A. (1953). *Human behavior in the concentration camp*. New York: W.W. Norton.

Conrad, C. D., Lupien, S. J., & McEwen, B. S. (1999). Support for a bimodal role for type II adrenal steroid receptors in spatial memory. *Neurobiology of Learning and Memory, 72*, 39–46.

de Kloet, E. R., Oitzl, M. S., & Joels, M. (1999). Stress and cognition: Are corticosteroids good or bad guys? *Trends in Neuroscience, 22*, 422–426.

de Quervain, D., Roozendaal, B., Nitsch, R., McGaugh, J., & Hock, C. (2000). Acute cortisone administration impairs retrieval of long-term declarative memory in humans. *Nature Neuroscience, 3*, 313–317.

Dess, N. K., Linwick, D., Patterson, J., Overmier, J. B., & Levine, S. (1983). Immediate and proactive effects of controllability and predictability on plasma cortisol responses to shocks in dogs. *Behavioral Neuroscience, 97*, 1005–1016.

Diamond, D. M., Bennett, M. C., Fleshner, M., & Rose, G. M. (1992). Inverted-U relationship between the level of peripheral corticosterone and magnitude of hippocampal primed burst potentiation. *Hippocampus, 2*, 421–430.

Diamond, D. M., & Rose, G. M. (1994). Stress impairs LTP and hippocampal-dependent memory. *Annals of the New York Academy of Sciences, 746*, 411–414.

Druckman, D., & Swets, J. A. (1988). *Enhancing human performance: Issues, theories, and techniques.* Washington, DC: National Academy Press.

Foy, M. R. (2001). 17ß-Estradiol: Effect on CA1 hippocampal synaptic plasticity. *Neurobiology of Learning and Memory, 76*, 239–252.

Foy, M. R., Foy, J. G., Levine, S., & Thompson, R. F. (1990). Manipulation of pituitary-adrenal activity affects neural plasticity in rodent hippocampus. *Psychological Science, 3*, 201–204.

Foy, M. R., Stanton, M. E., Levine, S., & Thompson, R. F. (1987). Behavioral stress impairs long-term potentiation in rodent hippocampus. *Behavioral and Neural Biology, 48*, 138–149.

Foy, M. R., Xu, J., Xie, X., Brinton, R. D., Thompson, R. F., & Berger, T. W. (1999). 17β-Estradiol enhances NMDA receptor-mediated EPSPs and long-term potentiation. *Journal of Neurophysiology, 81*, 925–929.

Gallagher, M., & Kapp, B. S. (1978). Manipulation of opiate activity in the amygdala alters memory processes. *Life Sciences, 23*, 1973–1978.

Geinisman, Y., de Toledo-Morrell, L., Morrell, F., & Heller, T. E. (1995). Hippocampal markers of age-related memory dysfunction: Behavioral, electrophysiological and morphological perspectives. *Progress in Neurobiology, 45*, 223–252.

Goldstein, L. E., Rasmusson, A. M., Bunney, B. S., & Roth, E. H. (1996). Role of the amygdala in the coordination of behavioral, neuroendocrine, and prefrontal cortical monoamine responses to psychological stress in the rat. *Journal of Neuroscience, 16*, 4787–4798.

Helmstetter, F. J. (1992). The amygdala is essential for the expression of conditional hypoalgesia. *Behavioral Neuroscience, 106*, 518–528.

Henke, P. G. (1981). Attenuation of shock-induced ulcers after lesion in the medial amygdala. *Physiology and Behavior, 27*, 143–146.

Hennessey, J. W., & Levine, S. (1979). Stress, arousal, and the pituitary-adrenal system: A psychoendocrine hypothesis. In J. M. Sprague & A. N. Epstein (Eds.), *Progress in psychobiology and physiological psychology* (Vol. 8, pp. 133–178). San Diego: Academic.

Herman, J. P., Figueiredo, H., Mueller, N. K., Ulrich-Lai, Y., Ostrander, M. M., Choi, D. C., & Cullinan, W. E. (2003). Central mechanisms of stress integration: Hierarchical circuitry controlling hypothalamo-pituitary-adrenocortical responsiveness. *Frontiers in Neuroendocrinology, 24*, 151–180.

Hierholzer, K., & Buhler, H. (1996). Metabolism of cortical steroid hormones and their general mode of action. In G. R. Winhorst (Ed.), *Comprehensive human physiology: From cellular mechanisms to integration* (Vol. 1, pp. 403–429). New York: Springer.

Ikegaya, Y., Saito, H., & Abe, K. (1994). Attenuated hippocampal long-term potentiation in basolateral amygdala-lesioned rats. *Brain Research, 656*, 157–164.

Ikegaya, Y., Saito, H., & Abe, K. (1995). Amygdala N-methyl-D-aspartate receptors participate in the induction of long-term potentiation in the dentate gyrus in vivo. *Neuroscience Letters, 192*, 193–196.

Ikegaya, Y., Saito, H., & Abe, K. (1996). The basomedial and basolateral amygdaloid nuclei contribute to the induction of long-term potentiation in the dentate gyrus in vivo. *European Journal of Neuroscience, 8*, 1833–1839.

Joels, M. (2001). Corticosteroid actions in the hippocampus. *Journal of Neuroendocrinology, 13*, 657–669.

Kawas, C., Resnick, S., Morrison, A., Brookmeyer, R., Corrada, M., Zonderman, A., et al. (1997). A prospective study of estrogen replacement therapy and the risk of developing Alzheimer's disease: The Baltimore longitudinal study of aging. *Neurology, 48*, 1517–1521.

Kerr, D. S., Campbell, L. W., Hao, S. Y., & Landfield, P. W. (1989). Corticosteroid modulation of hippocampal potentials: Increased effect with aging. *Science, 245*, 1505–1509.

Kim, J. J., & Diamond, D. M. (2002). The stressed hippocampus, synaptic plasticity and lost memories. *Nature Reviews Neuroscience, 3*, 453–462.

Kim, J. J., Foy, M. R., & Thompson, R. F. (1996). Behavioral stress modifies hippocampal plasticity through N-methyl-d-aspartate receptor activation. *Proceedings of the National Academy of Sciences, 93*, 4750–4753.

Kim, J. J., Lee, H. J., Han, J.-S., & Packard, M. G. (2001). Amygdala is critical for stress-induced modulation of hippocampal LTP and learning. *Journal of Neuroscience, 21*, 5222–5228.

Kim, J. J., & Yoon, K. S. (1998). Stress: Metaplastic effects in the hippocampus. *Trends in Neuroscience, 21*, 505–509.

Landfield, P. W., Waymire, J. C., & Lynch, G. (1978). Hippocampal aging and adrenocorticoids: Quantitative correlations. *Science, 202*, 1098–1102.

Leuner, B., Mendolia, S., Falduto, J., & Shors, T. J. (2002). Antidepressant treatment protects against the adverse effects of stress on learning in females. *Society for Neuroscience Abstracts, Program No. 380.1.*

Levine, S., Madden, J. I., Conner, R. L., Moskal, J. R., & Anderson, D. C. (1973). Physiological and behavioral effects of prior aversive stimulation (preshock) in the rat. *Physiology and Behavior, 10*, 467–471.

Lupien, S. J., de Leon, M., de Santi, S., Convit, A., Tarshish, C., Nair, N. P., Thakur, M., McEwen, B. S., Hauger, R. L., & Meaney, M. J. (1998). Cortisol levels during human aging predict hippocampal atrophy and memory deficits. *Nature Neuroscience, 1*, 69–73.

Malberg, J. E., Eisch, A. J., Nestler, E. J., & Duman, R. S. (2000). Chronic antidepressant treatment increases neurogenesis in adult rat hippocampus. *Journal of Neuroscience, 20*, 9104–9110.

McEwen, B. S. (1996). Hormones modulate environmental control of a changing brain. In G. R. Windhorst (Ed.), *Comprehensive human physiology: From cellular mechanisms to integration* (Vol. 1, pp. 473–493). New York: Springer.

McEwen, B. S. (2000). The neurobiology of stress: From serendipity to clinical relevance. *Brain Research, 886*, 172–189.

McEwen, B. S., & Sapolsky, R. M. (1995). Stress and cognitive function. *Current Opinion in Neurobiology, 5*, 205–216.

McEwen, B. S., & Stellar, E. (1993). Stress and the individual. Mechanisms leading to disease. *Archives of Internal Medicine, 153*, 2093–2101.

McGaugh, J. L. (2000). Memory: A century of consolidation. *Science, 287*, 248–251.

Mulnard, R. A., Cotman, C. W., Kawas, C., van Dyck, C. H., Sano, M., Doody, R., Koss, E., Pheiffer, E., Jin, S., Gamst, A., Grundman, M., Thomas, R., & Thal L. J. (2000). Estrogen replacement therapy for treatment of mild to moderate Alzheimer's disease: A randomized controlled trial. *Journal of the American Medical Association, 283*, 1007–1015.

Nair, S. M., Werkman, T. R., Craig, J., Finnell, R., Joels, M., & Eberwine, J. H. (1998). Corticosteroid regulation of ion channel conductances and mRNA levels in individual hippocampal CA1 neurons. *Journal of Neuroscience, 18*, 2685–2696.

Norris, C. M., Korol, D. L., & Foster, T. C. (1996). Increased susceptibility to induction of long-term depression and long-term potentiation reversal during aging. *Journal of Neuroscience, 16*, 1–11.

Oitzl, M. S., Reichardt, H. M., Joels, M., & de Kloet, E. R. (2001). Point mutation in the mouse glucocorticoid receptor preventing DNA binding impairs spatial memory. *Proceedings of the National Academy of Sciences, 98*, 12,790–12,795.

Paganini-Hill, A., & Henderson, V. W. (1996). Estrogen replacement therapy and risk of Alzheimer's disease. *Archives of Internal Medicine, 156*, 2213–2217.

Pikkarainen, M., Ronkko, S., Savander, V., Insausti, R., & Pitkanen, A. (1999). Projections from the lateral, basal, and accessory basal nuclei of the amygdala to the hippocampal formation in rat. *Journal of Comparative Neurology, 403*, 229–260.

Pitman, R. K., Sanders, K. M., Zusman, R. M., Healy, A. R., Cheema, F., Lasko, N. B., et al. (2002). Pilot study of secondary prevention of posttraumatic stress disorder with propranolol. *Biological Psychiatry, 51*, 189–192.

Roozendaal, B., Griffith, Q., Buranday, J., de Quervain, D., & McGaugh, J. (2003). The hippocampus mediates glucocorticoid-induced impairment of spatial memory retrieval: Dependence upon the basolateral amygdala. *Proceedings of the National Academy of Sciences, 100*, 1328–1330.

Sapolsky, R. (1990). Glucocorticoids, hippocampal damage and the glutamatergic synapse. *Progress in Brain Research, 86*, 13–23.

Sapolsky, R. M. (1996). Why stress is bad for your brain. *Science, 273*, 749–750.

Sapolsky, R. M., Krey, L., & McEwen, B. S. (1985). Prolonged glucocorticoid exposure reduces hippocampal neuron number: Implications for aging. *Journal of Neuroscience, 5*, 1221.

Sapolsky, R. M., Krey, L. C., & McEwen, B. S. (1986a). The adrenocortical axis in the aged rat: Impaired sensitivity to both fast and delayed feedback inhibition. *Neurobiology of Aging, 7*, 331–335.

Sapolsky, R. M., Krey, L. C., & McEwen, B. S. (1986b). The neuroendocrinology of stress and aging: The glucocorticoid cascade hypothesis. *Endocrine Reviews, 7*, 284–301.

Seligman, M. E. P. (1975). *Learned helplessness: On depression, development and death.* San Francisco: W.H. Freeman.

Selye, H. (1936). A syndrome produced by diverse nocuous agents. *Nature, 138*, 32.

Sherwin, B. B., & Tulandi, T. (1996). "Add-back" estrogen reverses cognitive deficits induced by a gonadotropin-releasing hormone agonist in women with leiomyomata uteri. *Journal of Clinical Endocrinology and Metabolism, 81*, 2545–2549.

Shors, T. J. (2001). Learning during stressful times. *Learning and Memory, 11*, 137–144.

Shors, T. J., & Leuner, B. (2003). Estrogen-mediated effects on depression and memory formation in females. *Journal of Affective Disorders, 74*, 85–96.

Shors, T. J., Levine, S., & Thompson, R. F. (1990). Effect of adrenalectomy and demedullation on the stress-induced impairment of long-term potentiation. *Neuroendocrinology, 51*, 70–75.

Shors, T. J., Lewczyk, C., Paczynski, M., Mathew, P. R., & Pickett, J. (1998). Stages of estrous mediate the stress-induced impairment of associative learning in the female rat. *Neuroreport, 9*, 419–423.

Shors, T. J., & Mathew, P. R. (1998). NMDA receptor antagonism in the lateral/basolateral but not central nucleus of the amygdala prevents the induction of facilitated learning in response to stress. *Learning and Memory, 5*, 220–230.

Shors, T. J., Seib, T. B., Levine, S., & Thompson, R. F. (1989). Inescapable versus escapable shock modulates long-term potentiation in the rat hippocampus. *Science, 244*, 224–226.

Shors, T. J., & Servatius, R. J. (1997). The contribution of stressor intensity, duration, and context to the stress-induced facilitation of associative learning. *Neurobiology of Learning and Memory, 67*, 92–96.

Shors, T. J., Weiss, C., & Thompson, R. F. (1992). Stress-induced facilitation of classical conditioning. *Science, 257*, 537–539.

Silva, R. C., & Brandao, M. L. (2000). Acute and chronic effects of gepirone and fluoxetine in rats tested in the elevated plus-maze: An ethological approach. *Pharmacology, Biochemistry and Behavior, 65*, 209–216.

Starkman, M., Gebarski, S., Berent, S., & Schteingart, D. (1992). Hippocampal formation volume, memory dysfunction, and cortisol levels in patients with Cushing's syndrome. *Biological Psychiatry, 32*, 756–765.

Swanson, L. W. (1991). Biochemical switching in hypothalamic circuits mediating responses to stress. *Progress in Brain Research, 87*, 181–200.

Tang, M. X., Jacobs, D., Stern, Y., Marder, K., Schofield, P., Gurland, B., Andrews, H., & Mayeux, R. (1996). Effect of oestrogen during menopause on risk and age at onset of Alzheimer's disease. *Lancet, 348*, 429–432.

Terasawa, E., & Timiras, P. S. (1969). Electrical activity during the estrous cycle of the rat: Cyclic changes in limbic structures. *Endocrinology, 83*, 207–216.

Teyler, T. J., Vardaris, R. M., Lewis, D., & Rawitch, A. B. (1980). Gonadal steroids: Effect on excitability of hippocampal pyramidal cells. *Science, 209*, 1017–1019.

Theorell, T., Leymann, H., Jodko, M., Konarski, K., Norbeck, H. E., & Eneroth, P. (1992). "Person under train" incidents: Medical consequences for subway drivers. *Psychosomatic Medicine, 54*, 480–488.

Tran, B., Foy, M. R., & Thompson, R. F. (2003). 17ß-Estradiol reverses stress-induced inhibition of LTP and stress-induced facilitation of LTD in aged rats. *Society for Neuroscience Abstracts, Program No. 255.1.*

Uno, H., Tarara, R., Ross, T., Else, J., Suleman, M., & Sapolsky, R. (1989). Hippocampal damage associated with prolonged and fatal stress in primates. *Journal of Neuroscience, 9*, 1709–1711.

Ursin, H., Baade, E., & Levine, S. (1978). *Psychobiology of stress: A study of coping men.* New York: Academic.

Viau, V., & Meaney, M. J. (1991). Variations in the hypothalamic-pituitary-adrenal response to stress during the estrous cycle in the rat. *Endocrinology, 129*, 2503–2511.

Vouimba, R., Foy, M. R., Foy, J. G., & Thompson, R. F. (2000). 17ß-Estradiol suppresses facilitation of long-term depression in aged rats. *Brain Research Bulletin, 53*, 783–787.

Wong, M., & Moss, R. L. (1991). Electrophysiological evidence for a rapid membrane action of the gonadal steroid, 17ß-Estradiol, on CA1 pyramidal neurons of the rat hippocampus. *Brain Research Bulletin, 543*, 148–152.

Wong, M., & Moss, R. L. (1992). Long-term and short-term electrophysiological effects of estrogen on the synaptic properties of hippocampal CA1 neurons. *Journal of Neuroscience, 12*, 3217–3225.

Wood, G. E., Beylin, A. V., & Shors, T. J. (2001). The contribution of adrenal and reproductive hormones to the opposing effects of stress on trace conditioning in males versus females. *Behavioral Neuroscience, 115*, 175–187.

Wood, G. E., & Shors, T. J. (1998). Stress facilitates classical conditioning in males but impairs conditioning in females through activational influences of ovarian hormones. *Proceedings of the National Academy of Sciences, 95*, 4066–4071.

Woodson, J. C., Macintosh, D., Fleshner, M., & Diamond, D. M. (2003). Emotion-induced amnesia in rats: Working memory-specific impairment, corticosterone-memory correlation, and fear versus arousal effects on memory. *Learning and Memory, 10*, 326–336.

Woolley, C. S., Weiland, N. G., McEwen, B. S., & Schwartzkroin, P. A. (1997). Estradiol increases the sensitivity of hippocampal CA1 pyramidal cells to NMDA receptor-mediated synaptic input: Correlation with dendritic spine density. *Journal of Neuroscience, 17*, 1848–1859.

Xu, J., Anwyl, R., & Rowan, M. J. (1997). Behavioural stress facilitates the induction of long-term depression in the hippocampus. *Nature, 387*, 497–500.

4 The Beneficial Effects of Fruit and Vegetable Supplementation on Neuronal Signaling and Behavior in Aging

Beyond Antioxidants

J. A. Joseph, B. Shukitt-Hale, and G. Casadesus

KEY POINTS

- The vulnerability to oxidative stress and inflammation increases in the aging brain. This increased vulnerability predisposes the aged brain to additional genetic insults that could lead to diseases such as Alzheimer's disease and certain forms of Parkinson's disease. It appears from our research and that of others that diets containing antioxidants and anti-inflammatories may retard the onset of these diseases and may actually reverse the cognitive and motor deficits seen in aging.
- Data indicate that the polyphenolic compounds from fruits such as blueberries may actually increase neuronal communication by enhancing signaling and neurogenesis. There appear to be multiple effects of the polyphenolic compounds found in fruits and possibly vegetables that could act to reduce the deleterious effects of aging.

1. INTRODUCTION

In this chapter we will describe the motor and cognitive deficits in behavior that occur in aging and show how these deficits are related to increased vulnerability to oxidative stress (OS) and inflammation, as well as deficits in signal transduction. In addition, we will describe the possible role of fruit polyphenolics, such as anthocyanins, in reversing or forestalling these deficits. From the research discussed in this chapter we will suggest that the aged brain, in combination with genetic changes, may provide a sensitive environment for the development of such devastating neurodegenerative changes of the nervous system such as Alzheimer's disease (AD) or certain forms of Parkinson's disease, resulting in even more severe deficits in memory and/or motor function. Therefore, it is critical to find methods to alter this fertile environment and perhaps reduce these enormous healthcare costs. One of these methods involves nutritional intervention.

From: *Nutrients, Stress, and Medical Disorders*
Edited by: S. Yehuda and D. I. Mostofsky

2. BEHAVIORAL CHANGES IN AGING

A great deal of research indicates the occurrence of numerous behavioral deficits that include both cognitive (Bartus, 1990) and motor (Joseph et al., 1983; Kluger et al., 1997) behaviors during "normal" aging. Numerous studies have shown that the deficits in motor function may include decreases in balance, muscle strength, and coordination (Joseph et al., 1983), while memory deficits are seen on cognitive tasks that require the use of spatial learning and memory (Bartus, 1990; Ingram, Jucker, & Spangler, 1994; Muir, 1997; Shukitt-Hale, Mouzakis, & Joseph, 1998; West, 1996).

Age-related deficits in motor performance are thought to be the result of alterations in the striatal dopamine (DA) system, as the striatum shows marked neurodegenerative changes with age (Joseph, 1992), or in the cerebellum, which also shows age-related alterations (Bickford, 1993; Bickford, Heron, Young, Gerhardt, & De La Garza, 1992). Memory alterations appear to occur primarily in secondary memory systems and are reflected in the storage of newly acquired information (Bartus, Dean, Beer, & Lippa, 1982; Joseph, 1992). It is thought that the hippocampus mediates place learning and that the prefrontal cortex is critical to acquiring the rules that govern performance in particular tasks (i.e., procedural knowledge), while the dorsomedial striatum mediates egocentric response and cue learning (Devan, Goad, & Petri, 1996; McDonald & White, 1994; Oliveira, Bueno, Pomarico, & Gugliano, 1997; Zyzak, Otto, Eichenbaum, & Gallagher, 1995). As will be discussed in subsequent sections, it appears that OS (Shukitt-Hale, 1999) and inflammation (Hauss-Wegrzyniak, Vannucchi, & Wenk, 2000; Hauss-Wegrzyniak, Vraniak, & Wenk, 1999) are contributing factors to the behavioral decrements seen in aging.

3. DYSREGULATION IN AGING

Aging can be defined as a condition where stressors are not counteracted by protective functions, leading to a dysregulation in development. In neuroscience, aging is characterized by losses in neuronal function, accompanied by behavioral declines (decreases in motor and cognitive performance) in both humans and animals. These stressors, as pointed out above, include OS and inflammation.

3.1. Oxidative Stress

Numerous studies in the literature suggest that one of the most important factors involved in the deleterious effects of aging on behavioral and neuronal function is OS (*see* Floyd, 1999, for review). Indications of increased OS have been found in studies in the brain showing that there are increases in bcl-2 (Sadoul, 1998), an endogenous antioxidant, and reductions in redox active iron (Gilissen, Jacobs, & Allman, 1999; Savory, Rao, Huang, Letada, & Herman, 1999), as well as significant lipofuscin accumulation (Gilissen et al.), increases in membrane lipid peroxidation (Yu, 1994), and alterations in membrane lipids (Denisova, Erat, Kelly, & Roth, 1998). Research has also shown that besides these alterations (e.g., reductions in glutathione levels [Olanow, 1992]), OS vulnerability in aging may be the result of additional factors including changes in the microvasculature (Floyd & Hensley, 2002) and increases in oxidized proteins and lipids (Floyd & Hensley, 2002). It also appears that the effectiveness of endogenous antioxidants may be reduced by (a) alterations in the membrane microenvironment and structure (Joseph, Denisova,

Fisher, Bickford, et al., 1998; Joseph et al., 2001) (b) alterations in calcium buffering ability, and (c) differential vulnerability of neurotransmitter receptors to OS.

For example, in the case of muscarinic receptors, our research has shown that COS-7 cells transfected with one of the five muscarinic acetylcholine receptors (MAChRs) and exposed to dopamine (Joseph, Fisher, & Strain, 2002) showed differences in OS sensitivity expressed as a function of Ca^{2+} buffering (i.e., the ability to extrude or sequester Ca^{2+} following oxotremorine-induced depolarization). The loss of calcium buffering in these experiments is similar to that reported in many studies with respect to aging (*see* Toescu & Verkhratsky, 2000; Herman, Chen, Booze, & Landfield, 1998), and such losses can have a profound effect on the functioning and viability of the cell (Lynch & Dawson, 1994; Mattson, 2000; Vannucci, Brucklacher, & Vannucci, 2001), further increasing OS (De Sarno et al., 2003) and leading ultimately to decrements in motor and memory function in senescent rats (Huidobro et al., 1993; Shukitt-Hale, Mouzakis, et al., 1998) (*see* below).

It also appears that a receptor domain in an "OS-sensitive" (M1) and "non-sensitive" (M3) subtype may be responsible for the differential vulnerability to OS between receptor subtypes. Comparison of the amino acid sequences of the two receptors has shown the third cytoplasmic loop (i3 loop) to be the domain with the most variability between M1 and M3. A recent experiment (Joseph, Fisher, Carey, & Szprengiel, 2004) has shown that deletions of the entire i3 loop increased DA sensitivity (a lower percentage of cells showing recovery following depolarization) in both the M1 and M3 subtypes. Chimerics of M1 where the i3 loop of the M3AChR was switched with the i3 loop of the M1AChR (M1M3i3) showed that DA sensitivity was reduced (percentage of cells showing increase in calcium clearance) following depolarization. In the M3 chimerics containing M1i3 (M3M1i3), the i3 loop offered no protection against DA-induced decrements in calcium buffering. These findings suggest that this loop may be critical in determining the sensitivity of muscarinic receptors to OS.

It is also important to note that there are significant differences in the rates of aging among various brain regions, with areas such as the hippocampus (Kaufmann, Bickford, & Taglialatela, 2001; Nyakas et al., 1997), cerebellum (Kaufmann et al., 2001), and striatum (Joseph et al., 1996; Kaasinen et al., 2000) showing profound alterations in aging. Given the importance of MAChRs in mediating such factors as amyloid precursor protein (for review, *see* Fisher et al., 2003), as well as motor and cognitive behaviors (Bartus et al., 1982), it is clear that their loss of function and responsiveness to agonist stimulation would have important implications in neuronal and behavioral aging.

In addition to these factors, it appears that there may be critical declines in endogenous antioxidant protection that include alterations in the ratio of oxidized to total glutathione (Olanow, 1992) and reduced glutamine synthetase (Carney, Smith, Carney, & Butterfield, 1994). Findings suggest that there are age-related changes in the neuronal plasma membrane molecular structure, and physical properties (e.g., increased rigidity) may increase vulnerability to OS and inflammation (Joseph, Denisova, Fisher, Bickford, et al., 1998; Joseph et al., 2001). Unfortunately, research also indicates that not only is the central nervous system (CNS) particularly vulnerable to OS, but this vulnerability increases during aging (see Joseph, Denisova, Fisher, Bickford, et al., 1998; Joseph, Denisova, Fisher, Shukitt-Hale, et al., 1998 for review) and may also enhance central vulnerability to inflammation (Joseph, Denisova, Fisher, Bickford, et al., 1998; Joseph et al., 2001).

3.2. Inflammation

Recent evidence also suggests that CNS inflammatory events may have an important role in affecting the neuronal and behavioral deficits in aging. Increased glial fibrillary acid protein expression is observed by middle age (Rozovsky, Finch, & Morgan, 1998) and, in the elderly, occurs in the absence of a defined stimulus (McGeer & McGeer, 1995). Increases in tumor necrosis factor (TNF)-α have also been reported (Chang et al., 1996) as a function of age as well as associated inhibition of glia (Chang et al., 2001). Similarly, research in both aged mice and humans (Chang et al., 1996; Spaulding, Walford, & Effros, 1997; Volpato et al., 2001) have found increases in both TNF-α and interleukin (IL)-6. Upregulation of C-reactive protein, an important marker of inflammation, may be an important factor in biological aging (Kushner, 2001).

In addition, important interactions of reactive oxygen species (ROS)-generating agents and cytokines have been observed. Paralleling the results seen with respect to OS are increases in sensitivity to inflammatory mediators with aging. For example, Manev and Uz (1999) showed that old rats were more sensitive to kainate-induced excitotoxic brain injuries and enhanced 5-lipoxygenase (5-LOX) expression in limbic structures. As is well known, lipoxygenases are enzymes that in the form of cyclooxygenases (COX) provide oxygen to an arachidonic molecule and induce the synthesis of inflammatory mediators such as eicosanoids and leukotrienes. It has been shown that 5-LOX is expressed in CNS neurons and may be involved in neurodegenerative processes. Data (reviewed in Manev, Uz, Sugaya, & Qu, 2000) suggest that 5-LOX may exert its actions through tyrosine kinase receptors and cytoskeletal proteins. Both 5-LOX gene expression and activity are increased in aging. Additionally, it has been shown that the expression of one form of COX, COX-2, appears to be associated with amyloid β deposition in the hippocampus (Hoozemans et al., 2002; Ho et al., 1999). Moreover, research has suggested that inflammatory prostaglandins (PG) such as PGE increase with aging, especially in such areas as the hippocampus (Casolini, Catalani, Zuena, & Angelucci, 2002). In this respect, the PG synthesis pathway appears to be a major source of ROS in several organ systems, including the brain (Baek et al., 2001).

Increases in inflammatory reactions in several pathways involving factors such as cytokines, COX, PGs, etc., may result in extracellular signals that act in concert to generate additional ROS to induce decrements in neuronal function or glial neuronal interactions (Rosenman, Shirkant, Dubb, Benveniste, & Ransohoff, 1995; Schipper, 1996; Steffen, Breier, Butcher, Schulz, & Engelhardt, 1996; Stella et al., 1997; Woodroofe, 1995). Increase in sensitivity to both OS and inflammation may be ultimately involved in inducing the deficits in behavior observed in aging. Some support for this contention is provided by studies showing that heavy particle irradiation, which acts to increase oxidative and/or inflammatory stressors, may produce behavioral deficits paralleling those observed in aging (Joseph, Erat, & Rabin, 1998; Joseph, Shukitt-Hale, McEwen, & Rabin, 2000; Shukitt-Hale, Casadesus, McEwen, Rabin, & Joseph, 2000), as discussed below. Furthermore, central administration of the inflammatory stressor lipopolysaccharide (LPS) into the brain of young rats increases several markers of inflammation and produces degeneration of hippocampal pyramidal neurons, as well as impairments in working memory (Bickford, 1993; Hauss-Wegrzyniak, Dobrzanski, Stoehr, & Wenk, 1998; Hauss-Wegrzyniak, Willard, Del Soldato, Pepeu, & Wenk, 1999; West, 1996; Yamada et al., 1999), as discussed in the following section.

4. OXIDATIVE AND INFLAMMATORY INDUCED COGNITIVE AND MOTOR DEFICITS

As reviewed in the previous sections of this chapter, there are numerous changes in both cognitive and motor behavior as a function of age, and young animals exposed to oxidative or inflammatory stressors exhibit similar neuronal and behavioral changes to those seen in aging. In this respect, we have shown that exposing young rats to particles of high energy and charge (HZE particles) disrupts the functioning of the dopaminergic system and dopamine-mediated behaviors in a manner similar to that observed in behavioral and neuronal function in aged animals (Joseph, Erat, et al., 1998; Joseph et al., 2000). Similarly, data indicate that whole-body exposure of rats to HZE particles, primarily 600 MeV or 1 GeV ^{56}Fe, impairs motor behavior (Joseph, Hunt, Rabin, & Dalton, 1992), spatial learning and memory behavior (Shukitt-Hale et al., 2000), and amphetamine-induced conditioned taste aversion (Rabin, Joseph, & Erat, 1998). Associated with these findings were deficits in oxotremorine enhancement of K^+-evoked DA release and carbachol-stimulated GTPase activity that paralleled those seen in aging (Joseph et al., 2000). These parameters are dependent upon the integrity of the central dopaminergic system (Rabin, Joseph, Shukitt-Hale, & McEwen, 2000). Therefore, the deficits induced by radiation are similar to those that occur during aging, are associated with free-radical damage, and support the hypothesis that these changes may share a common chemical/biological mechanism (Joseph et al., 1992).

Another model used to produce ROS and subsequent OS involves exposing young rats to a normobaric hyperoxia environment of 100% oxygen (O_2) at 760 mmHg (sea level pressure). We have shown that motor function, as measured by accelerating rotarod, wire suspension, small rod walk, and large rod walk, is impaired following 48 h of 100% O_2 (Shukitt-Hale, 1999), as is cerebellar β-adrenergic and striatal muscarinic receptor functioning (Bickford et al., 1999). Again, these effects are similar to those seen in aging. An additional treatment involved the induction of OS by altering the balance between ROS and antioxidant activity by reducing the levels of the endogenous antioxidant glutathione with buthionine sulfoximine (BSO) and then increasing ROS production with an injection of DA. BSO given prior to DA administration selectively impaired psychomotor (rod walking, wire suspension, and plank walking) (Shukitt-Hale, Denisova, Strain, & Joseph, 1997) and cognitive performance (spatial learning and memory measured by the Morris water maze) (Shukitt-Hale, Erat, & Joseph, 1998); however, in the reverse condition (DA + BSO), no decrements in performance were observed relative to vehicle administration. Additionally, neither BSO alone nor DA alone had detrimental effects on behavior. Therefore, reducing glutathione with BSO and then increasing ROS production with DA injections induced behavioral deficits similar to those seen in aging.

Increases in inflammatory mediators (e.g., cytokines) known to be involved in the activation of glial cells and perivascular/parenchymal macrophages, as well as increased mobilization and infiltration of peripheral inflammatory cells into the brain, have been shown to produce deficits in behavior similar to those observed during aging (Hauss-Wegrzyniak et al., 2000). Previous studies (Hauss-Wegrzyniak et al., 1998, 2000; Hauss-Wegrzyniak, Vraniak, et al., 1999; Hauss-Wegrzyniak, Willard, et al., 1999; Yamada et al., 1999) have shown that chronic (28–37 d) infusion of LPS into the ventricle of young rats can reproduce many of the behavioral, inflammatory, neurochemical, and neuropathological changes seen in the brains of AD patients in some similar regions (e.g., cingulate cortex), as well as produce changes in spatial learning and memory behavior (Hauss-Wegrzyniak et al., 1998, 2000; Hauss-Wegrzyniak, Vraniak, et al. 1999; Yamada et al. 1999). These changes include, but are not limited to, increased activated astrocytes, increased number and density of activated microglia, particularly within the hippocampus, cingulate cortex, and basal forebrain, increased levels of cytokines, degeneration of hippocampal pyramidal neurons, and an impairment in working memory (Hauss-Wegrzyniak et al., 1998, 2000; Hauss-Wegrzyniak, Vraniak, et al. 1999; Hauss-Wegrzyniak, Willard, et al. 1999; Yamada et al. 1999). Use of a chronic injection directly into the brain restricts the inflammation-induced changes to the CNS; the rats do not develop fever and plasma cytokine levels are not elevated (Hauss-Wegrzyniak, Vraniak et al. 1999). It has been shown that nonsteroidal anti-inflammatory drugs (NSAIDs) can attenuate the neuro-inflammatory reaction and reduce the inflammation-induced memory deficit associated with this model. However, it was also shown that the effects of NSAIDs are age dependent, i.e., daily peripheral administration of a NSAID significantly attenuated the memory deficit produced by chronic LPS in young (3 mo) rats and decreased the degree of inflammation in both young and adult (9 mo) rats, but did not improve water maze performance in either adult or old (23 mo) rats (Hauss-Wegrzyniak, Vraniak et al. 1999).

5. SIGNALING CHANGES

In addition to alterations in vulnerability to ROS and inflammation seen in aging, which could contribute to the behavioral deficits reported in many studies, alterations in age- and calcium-sensitive signaling molecules are associated with memory, especially the conversion of short- to long-term memory. These signaling cascades are complex and numerous, and many of the pathways remain to be discerned. A complete discussion of these cascades is beyond the scope of this chapter. However, with respect to learning and memory, one that has received a great deal of study is the MAP kinase (MAPK) cascade.

A great deal of work has shown the importance of the MAPK cascade in proliferation and differentiation (Graves, Campbell, & Krebs, 1995). In addition, MAPK has been shown to be critical in long-term memory formation through the activation of cyclic AMP response element-binding protein (CREB). More specifically, it appears that various MAPKs are involved not only in hippocampal memory formation, but also in memory modulation in other brain structures (Sgambato, Pages, Rogard, Besson, & Caboche, 1998). Recent studies have indicated that the activation of these molecules is OS sensitive (Zhang & Jope, 1999) and that they may serve as biochemical signal integrators and/or molecular coincidence detectors for modulating coordinated responses to extracellular signals in neurons (Sweatt, 2001).

Calcium-dependent protein kinase C (PKC) is important in this pathway. Studies have shown that PKC activity is important in the formation of memory, particularly spatial memory (e.g., see Leahy, Luo, Kent, Meiri, & Vallano, 1993; Micheau & Riedel, 1999, for review), and that treatment with PKC inhibitors impairs memory formation (Serrano et al., 1994). It appears that training induces calcium-induced translocation (Colombo, Wetsel, & Gallagher, 1997) of PKC from the soluble to the particulate subcellular fraction (Van der Zee, Compaan, Bohus, & Luiten, 1995). However, in aging, there appear to be alterations in this translocation (Battaini et al., 1995), which are correlated with decrements in spatial memory (Fordyce & Wehner, 1993). It has been shown that young rats with the best performance in spatial memory also had the highest levels of PKCγ in the particulate (i.e., membrane) fraction of the hippocampus and PKCβ_2 in the soluble (i.e., cytosolic) fraction (Colombo et al. 1997).

PKC does not operate in a vacuum, and there is a great amount of cross talk with other signaling molecules, such as protein kinase A (PKA) and protein tyrosine kinase (PTK), in the initiation of memory formation and the conversion of short- to long-term memory. Evidence indicates that both PKA (Rosenzweig, Bennett, Colombo, Lee, & Serrano, 1993) and PTK (for review, *see* Micheau & Riedel, 1999) may also be involved in this conversion. In the case of PTK this may be done through direct modulation of brain-derived nerve growth factor (BDNF) (Boxall & Lancaster, 1998), whereas in aging, studies indicate that BDNF expression was reduced in several brain areas (Boxall & Lancaster, 1998). PKA appears to mediate long-term memory formation by participating in CREB activation through initiation of the MAPK cascade. Particularly important in this regard are the extracellular signal-regulated kinases (ERK) 1 and 2. Studies have demonstrated the role of ERK signaling cascades in several types of learning and memory, including taste aversion (Berman, Hazvi, Rosenblum, Seger, & Dudai, 1998), novel taste learning (Swank & Sweatt, 2001), spatial learning (Selcher, Atkins, Trzaskos, Paylor, & Sweatt, 1999), and inhibitory avoidance (Schafe, Nadel, Sullivan, Harris, & Le Doux, 1999).

In the case of aging, studies indicate that ERK activities were reduced in cortical brain slices of senescent rats (24 mo) without decline in the corresponding proteins (Zhen, Uryu, Cai, Johnson, & Friedman, 1999). An additional study showed that exposure of hippocampal slices from senescent mice expressing amyloid β 1-42 produced a downregulation of hippocampal ERK activity.

Finally, there is a great deal of evidence to suggest that the downstream activation of CREB by the kinases cited above is involved in the formation of memory and regulates the transcription of immediate early genes that, in turn, activate late response genes, which ultimately initiate long-term memory formation (*see* Lamprecht, 1999; Mazzucchelli & Brambilla, 2000). As cited in Lamprecht (1999), research indicates that CREB affects the growth of new synapses and synaptic transmission, while Bourtchuladze et al. (1994) showed that CREB knockout mice were impaired in Morris water maze performance. CREB activity has also been shown to decline with age (Matsumoto, 2000). Conversely, Josselyn et al. (2001) showed that overexpression of CREB enhances the formation of long-term memory after massed training.

6. EFFECTS OF FRUIT AND VEGETABLE SUPPLEMENTATION ON BEHAVIORAL AND NEURONAL DEFICITS IN AGING

In previous sections of this chapter we outlined the changes in neuronal signaling and associated increases in the vulnerability to OS and inflammation in aging that lead, ultimately, to motor and behavioral deficits. As stated in the introduction, the problem is reducing the vulnerability of the brain to insults and preventing or reversing the deficits in behavior, possibly through nutrition. Although there are numerous studies suggesting that various antioxidant supplements (for review, *see* Casadesus, Shukitt-Hale, & Joseph, 2002) may be effective in this regard, our research suggests that the combinations of antioxidant/anti-inflammatory polyphenolics found in fruits and vegetables may show efficacy in aging. All plants, including fruit- or vegetable-bearing plants, synthesize a vast array of chemical compounds that are not necessarily involved in the plant's metabolism. These secondary compounds instead serve a variety of functions that serve to enhance the plant's survivability. These compounds may be responsible for the putative multitude of beneficial effects of fruits and vegetables on health-related issues, among the most important of which may be their antioxidant and anti-inflammatory properties.

Anthocyanins are plant polyphenols that have potent antioxidant and anti-inflammatory activities. They are natural pigments responsible for the orange, red, and blue colors of fruits, flowers, vegetables, and other storage tissues in plants (Seeram, Bourquin, & Nair, 2001; Seeram, Momin, Bourquin, & Nair, 2001; Wang et al., 1999). Anthocyanins have been reported to affect many of the parameters discussed above by inhibiting lipid peroxidation and the activity of COX-1 and COX-2 enzymes (Seeram, Cichewicz, Chandra, & Nair, 2003; Seeram, Schutzki, Chandra, & Nair, 2002).

The chemistry of anthocyanins can be reduced to six major anthocyanidins: delphinidin, cyanidin, pelargonidin, petunidin, peonidin, and malvidin. Among berry fruits, blueberries contain high levels of a wide variety of anthocyanins, including glycosides of four of the six major anthocyanidins: malvidin, petunidin, peonidin, and cyanidin (Kalt, Forney, Martin, & Prior, 1999).

Anthocyanins are a subset of a larger class of polyphenols known as flavonoids. More than 4000 flavonoids have been identified in plants. They are also abundant in seeds, fruits, and plant-derived oils such as olive oils, as well as tea and red wine. Thus, they are part of the human diet, and plants and spices containing them have been used for many years in eastern medicine. As might be expected from the above discussion of anthocyanins, flavonoids have been reported to inhibit lipid peroxidation in several biological systems, including mitochondria and microsomes (Bindoli, Cavallini, & Siliprandi, 1977; Cavallini, Bindoli, & Siliprandi, 1978) as well as erythrocytes (Maridonneau-Parini, Braquet, & Garay, 1986; Sorata, Takahama, & Kimura, 1984) and liver (Kimura et al., 1984). They appear to be potent inhibitors of both NADPH and CCl_4-induced lipid peroxidation (Afanas'ev, Dorozhko, Brodskii, Kostyuk, & Potapovich, 1989). It appears that the iron-chelating ability of the flavonoids may be very important in mediating their potent inhibitory effects on 5-LOX (Hoult, Moroney, & Paya, 1994), while CO inhibition appears to involve other mechanisms.

The antioxidant effects of flavonoids may be derived in part from their ability to upregulate antioxidant enzymes (e.g., glutathione) or enzymes related to glutathione synthesis. One mechanism that may be operational in these beneficial effects is the direct enhancement of transcription factors that enhance antioxidant enzymes or their signaling cascades. It is known, for example, that the enzymes for glutathione (reviewed in Schroeter et al., 2002; Zippe & Mulcahy, 2000) or heme oxygenase (Chen & Maines, 2000) synthesis exhibit ERK 1/2 dependency in the regulation of their expression, whereas Cu/ZnSOD is regulated by ELK-1 (Chang, Yoo, & Rho, 1999), and MnSOD expression contains binding sites for Sp1, AP-1, and CREB (Chang et al., 1999; Das, Lewis-Molok, & White, 1995), which are ERK 1/2 (Chang & Karin, 2001; Sgambato et al., 1998) regulated. Finally, it also appears that flavonoids regulating ERK 1/2 may influence iNOS activity. Thus, there is a great deal of evidence to suggest that a possible link exists between the antioxidant activity of flavonoids and their putative MAPKs, altering activity.

Because MAPKs are involved in numerous biological activities, the findings that flavonoids may influence such signaling suggests that their potential benefits may involve properties other than those involving antioxidant or anti-inflammatory effects. For example, delphinidin inhibits endothelial cell proliferation and cell cycle progression by ERK 1/2 activation (Martin, Favot, Matz, Lugnier, & Andriantsitohaina, 2003), while grapeseed proanthocyanidin can reduce ischemia reperfusion-induced activation of JNK-1 and C-Jun and reduce cardiomyocyte apoptosis (Sato, Bagchi, Tosaki, & Das, 2001). Additional research indicates that phytochemicals can regulate MAPK and other signaling pathways at the level of transcription (Frigo et al., 2002).

These findings, coupled with a plethora of studies showing the involvement of ERK in diverse forms of memory, such as contextual fear conditioning (English & Sweatt, 1996), long-term potentiation (English & Sweatt, 1997), striatal-dependent learning and memory (Mazzucchelli & Brambilla, 2000), hippocampal-dependent spatial memory (Selcher et al., 1999), and inhibitory avoidance (Schafe et al., 1999), suggest that interventions that influence MAPK signaling may have beneficial effects on cognition. Given the findings reviewed above showing alterations in signaling as a function of age, the putative signal-modifying properties of flavonoids may prove to be invaluable in altering the neuronal and behavioral effects of aging.

We believed that given the multiple properties of fruits and vegetables, they might show considerable efficacy in reducing the deleterious effects of aging on neuronal function and behavior. Therefore, we utilized fruits and vegetables that were high in antioxidant activity (via the oxygen radical absorbance capacity assay [ORAC]) (Cao, Sofic, & Prior, 1996; Prior, et al., 1998; Wang, Cao, & Prior, 1996) and showed that long-term (6- to 15-mo old F344 rats) feeding with a supplemented AIN-93 diet (strawberry extract or spinach extract [1–2% of the diet] or vitamin E [500 IU]), retarded age-related decrements in cognitive or neuronal function. Results indicated that the supplemented diets prevented the onset of age-related deficits in several indices (e.g., cognitive behavior, Morris water maze performance) (Joseph, Shukitt-Hale, et al., 1998).

In a subsequent experiment (Joseph et al., 1999) we found that dietary supplementation (for 8 wk) with spinach, strawberry, or blueberry (BB) extracts in an AIN-93 diet was effective in reversing age-related deficits in neuronal and behavioral (cognitive, Morris water maze [MWM] performance) function in aged (19 mo) F344 rats. Only the BB-supplemented group exhibited improved performance on tests of motor function that assessed balance and coordination (e.g., rod walking and the accelerating rotarod), while none of the other supplemented groups differed from control on these tasks. Additional findings from a subsequent experiment (Joseph et al., 2004) suggest that cranberry or concord grape juice supplementations have beneficial effects on motor behavior similar to those seen with BBs. Recent data from our laboratory also suggest that cranberries may have similar beneficial effects on motor behavior.

Unlike the results seen with respect to motor behavior, the study by Joseph et al. (1999) showed that the animals in all supplemented groups (relative to controls) showed improved working memory (short-term memory) performance in the MWM, suggesting less selectivity among fruits and vegetables with respect to cognition than are seen with motor behavior. This may be the result of brain region selectivity of polyphenolic compounds from the various fruits and vegetables.

However, examinations of the striata from the supplemented groups showed minimal levels of antioxidant activity, which were insufficient to account for the observed significant beneficial effects of BB supplementation on motor and cognitive function. Findings from this (Joseph et al., 1999) and a subsequent study (Youdim et al., 2000) suggested that there are beneficial properties, in addition to those involving antioxidant or anti-inflammatory effects, of BBs on both motor and cognitive behavior; these may involve alterations in neuronal signaling and communication.

This was observed in a study (Joseph et al., 2003) carried out in APP/PS1 transgenic mice, which serve as a model for AD, since these mutations promote the production of amyloid β and subsequently Alzheimer-like plaques in several brain regions, accompanied in middle age by cognitive deficits. A group of these mice was given BB supplementation beginning at 4 mo of age (as in Joseph et al., 1999) and continued until they were 12 mo of age, when their performance was tested in a Y-maze. The results indicated that mice supplemented with BB exhibited Y-maze performance similar to that seen in nontransgenic mice and significantly better than that seen in the nonsupplemented transgenic animals. Interestingly, there was a dichotomy between the plaque burden and behavior in the BB-supplemented transgenic mice. No differences in the number of plaques between the supplemented and non-supplemented APP/PS1 mice were observed, even though behavioral declines were prevented in the BB-supplemented animals.

One possible reason that the behavior did not reflect the morphology may be that enhanced signaling in the BB-supplemented transgenic mice acted to prevent or circumvent any putative deleterious effects of the amyloid plaques on behavior. Evidence for this possibility is provided by data showing that the BB-supplemented APP/PS1 mice exhibited higher levels of hippocampal ERK as well as striatal and hippocampal PKCα than were seen in transgenic mice maintained on the control diet. As pointed out above, ERK and PKC have been shown to be important in mediating cognitive function, especially conversion of short-term to long-term memory (Micheau & Riedel, 1999). Enhancement was also seen in the BB-supplemented group in the sensitivity of muscarinic receptors (i.e., increasing striatal, carbachol-stimulated GTPase activity), which have been found to be associated with learning and memory in numerous studies.

7. CONCLUSION

These findings, combined with additional preliminary research showing that BB supplementation, in addition to altering ERK activity, may also increase hippocampal neurogenesis (Casadesus et al.), suggests that at least part of the effect of the BB supplementation may be a result of enhanced neuronal function in areas of the brain affected by aging or disease. This would allow more effective intra- and interarea communication and ultimately facilitate both cognitive and motor function.

REFERENCES

Afanas'ev, I. B., Dorozhko, A. I., Brodskii, A. V., Kostyuk, V. A., & Potapovitch, A. I. (1989). Chelating and free radical scavenging mechanisms of inhibitory action of rutin and quercetin in lipid peroxidation. *Biochemical Pharmacology, 38*, 1763–1769.

Baek, B. S., Kim, J. W., Lee, J. H., Kwon, H. J., Kim, N. D., Kang, H. S., Yoo, M. A., Yu, B. P., & Chung, H. Y. (2001). Age-related increase of brain cyclooxygenase activity and dietary modulation of oxidative status. *The Journals of Gerontology. Series A, Biological Sciences and Medical Sciences, 56*, B426–B431.

Bartus, R. T. (1990). Drugs to treat age-related neurodegenerative problems. The final frontier of medical science? *Journal of the American Geriatrics Society, 38*, 680–695.

Bartus, R. T., Dean, R. L., Beer, B., & Lippa, A. S. (1982). The cholinergic hypothesis of geriatric memory dysfunction. *Science, 217*, 408–417.

Battaini, F., Elkabes, S., Bergamaschi, S., Ladisa, V., Lucchi, L., De Graan, P. N., Schuurman, T., Wetsel, W. C., Travucchi, M., & Govoni, S. (1995). Protein kinase C activity, translocation, and conventional isoforms in aging rat brain. *Neurobiology of Aging, 16*, 137–148.

Berman, D. E., Hazvi, S., Rosenblum, K., Seger, R., & Dudai, Y. (1998). Specific and differential activation of mitogen-activated protein kinase cascades by unfamiliar taste in the insular cortex of the behaving rat. *Journal of Neuroscience, 18*, 10,037–10,044.

Bickford, P. (1993). Motor learning deficits in aged rats are correlated with loss of cerebellar noradrenergic function. *Brain Research, 620*, 133–138.

Bickford, P. C., Chadman, K., Williams, B., Shukitt-Hale, B., Holmes, D., Taglialatela, G., Joseph, J. A. (1999). Effect of normobaric hyperoxia on two indexes of synaptic function in Fischer 344 rats. *Free Radical Biology and Medicine, 26*, 817–824.

Bickford, P. C., Heron, C., Young, D. A., Gerhardt, G. A., & De La Garza, R. (1992). Impaired acquisition of novel locomotor tasks in aged and norepinephrine-depleted F344 rats. *Neurobiology of Aging, 13*, 475–481.

Bindoli, A., Cavallini, L., & Siliprandi, N. (1977). Inhibitory action of silymarin of lipid peroxide formation in rat liver mitochondria and microsomes. *Biochemical Pharmacology, 26*, 2405–2409.

Bourtchuladze, R., Frenguelli, B., Blendy, J., Cioffi, D., Schutz, G., & Silva, A. J. (1994). Deficient long-term memory in mice with a targeted mutation of the cAMP-responsive element-binding protein. *Cell, 79*, 59–68.

Boxall, A. R., & Lancaster, B. (1998). Tyrosine kinases and synaptic transmission. *The European Journal of Neuroscience, 10*, 2–7.

Cao, G., Sofic, E., & Prior, R. L. (1996). Antioxidant capacity of tea and common vegetables. *Journal of Agricultural and Food Chemistry, 44*, 3426–3431.

Carney, J. M., Smith, C. D., Carney, A. M., & Butterfield, D. A. (1994). Aging- and oxygen-induced modifications in brain biochemistry and behavior. *Annals of the New York Academy of Sciences, 738*, 44–53.

Casadesus, G., Shukitt-Hale, B., & Joseph, J. A. (2002). Qualitative versus quantitative caloric intake: Are they equivalent paths to successful aging? *Neurobiology of Aging, 23*, 747–769.

Casolini, P., Catalani, A., Zuena, A. R., & Angelucci, L. (2002). Inhibition of COX-2 reduces the age-dependent increase of hippocampal inflammatory markers, corticosterone secretion, and behavioral impairments in the rat. *Journal of Neuroscience Research, 68*, 337–343.

Cavallini, M. L., Bindoli, A., & Siliprandi, N. (1978). Comparative evaluation of antiperoxidative action of silymarin and other flavonoids. *Pharmacological Research Communications, 10*, 133–136.

Chang, H. N., Wang, S. R., Chiang, S. C., Teng, W. J., Chen, M. L., Tsai, J. J., Huang, D. F., Lin, H. Y., & Tsai, Y. Y. (1996). The relationship of aging to endotoxin shock and to production of TNFα. *Journals of Gerontology. Series A, Biological Sciences and Medical Sciences, 51*, M220–M222.

Chang, L., & Karin, M. (2001). Mammalian MAP kinase signalling cascades. *Nature, 410*, 37–40.

Chang, M. S., Yoo, H. Y., & Rho, H. M. (1999). Positive and negative regulatory elements in the upstream region of the rat Cu/Zn-superoxide dismutase gene. *The Biochemical Journal, 339*, 335–341.

Chang, R. C., Chen, W., Hudson, P., Wilson, B., Han, D. S., & Hong, J. S. (2001). Neurons reduce glial responses to lipopolysaccharide (LPS) and prevent injury of microglial cells from over-activation by LPS. *Journal of Neurochemistry, 76*, 1042–1049.

Chen, K., & Maines, M. D. (2000). Nitric oxide induces heme oxygenase-1 via mitogen-activated protein kinases ERK and p38. *Cellular and Molecular Biology, 46*, 609–617.

Colombo, P. J., Wetsel, W., & Gallagher, M. G. (1997). Spatial memory is related to hippocampal subcellular concentrations of calcium-dependent protein kinase C isoforms in young and aged rats. *Proceedings of the National Academy of Sciences of the United States of America, 94*, 1495–1499.

Das, K. C., Lewis-Molock, Y., & White, C. W. (1995). Activation of NF-kappa B and elevation of MnSOD gene expression by thiol reducing agents in lung adenocarcinoma (A549) cells. *The American Journal of Physiology, 269*, L588–L602.

Denisova, N. A., Erat, S. A., Kelly, J. F., & Roth, G. S. (1998). Differential effect of aging on cholesterol modulation of carbachol stimulated low-Km GTPase in striatal synaptosomes. *Experimental Gerontology, 33*, 249–265.

De Sarno, P., Shestopal, S. A., King, T. D., Zmijewska, A., Song, L., & Jope, R. S. (2003). Muscarinic receptor activation protects cells from apoptotic effects of DNA damage, oxidative stress, and mitrochondrial inhibition. *Journal of Biological Chemistry, 278*, 11,086–11,093.

Devan, B. D., Goad, E. H., & Petri, H. L. (1996). Dissociation of hippocampal and striatal contributions to spatial navigation in the water maze. *Neurobiology of Learning and Memory, 66*, 305–323.

English, J. D., & Sweatt, J. D. (1996). Activation of p42 mitogen-activated protein kinase in hippocampal long-term potentiation. *Journal of Biological Chemistry, 271*, 24,329–24,332.

English, J. D., & Sweatt, J. D. (1997). A requirement for the mitogen-activated protein kinase cascade in hippocampal long-term potentiation. *Journal of Biological Chemistry, 272*, 19,103–19,106.

Fisher, A., Pittel, Z., Haring, R., Bar-Ner, N., Kliger-Spatz, M., Natan, N., Egozi, I., Sonego, H., Marcovitch, I., & Brandeis, R. (2003). M1 muscarinic agonists can modulate some of the hallmarks in Alzheimer's disease: Implications in future therapy. *Journal of Molecular Neuroscience, 20*, 349–356.

Floyd, R. A. (1999). Antioxidants, oxidative stress, and degenerative neurological disorders. *Proceedings of the Society for Experimental Biology and Medicine, 222*, 236–245.

Floyd, R. A., & Hensley, K. (2002). Oxidative stress in brain aging. Implications for therapeutics of neurodegenerative diseases. *Neurobiology of Aging, 23*, 795–807.

Fordyce, D. E., & Wehner, J. M. (1993). Effects of aging on spatial learning and hippocampal protein kinase C in mice. *Neurobiology of Aging, 14*, 309–317.

Frigo, D. E., Duong, B. N., Melnik, L. I., Schief, L. S., Collins-Burow, B. M., Pace, D. K., McLaughlan, J. A., & Burow, M. E. (2002). Flavonoid phytochemicals regulate activator protein-1 signal transduction pathways in endometrial and kidney stable cell lines. *Journal of Nutrition, 132*, 1848–1853.

Gilissen, E. P., Jacobs, R. E., & Allman, J. M. (1999). Magnetic resonance microscopy of iron in the basal forebrain cholinergic structures of the aged mouse lemur. *Journal of Neurological Sciences, 168*, 21–27.

Graves, J. D., Campbell, J. S., & Krebs, E. G. (1995). Protein serine/threonine kinases of the MAPK cascade. *Annals of the New York Academy of Sciences, 766*, 320–343.

Hauss-Wegrzyniak, B., Dobrzanski, P., Stoehr, J. D., & Wenk, G.L. (1998). Chronic neuroinflammation in rats reproduces components of the neurobiology of Alzheimer's disease. *Brain Research, 780*, 294–303.

Hauss-Wegrzyniak, B., Vannucchi, M. G., & Wenk, G. L. (2000). Behavioral and ultrastructural changes induced by chronic neuroinflammation in young rats. *Brain Research, 859*, 157–166.

Hauss-Wegrzyniak, B., Vraniak, P., & Wenk, G. L. (1999). The effects of a novel NSAID on chronic neuroinflammation are age dependent. *Neurobiology of Aging, 20*, 305–313.

Hauss-Wegrzyniak, B., Willard, L. B., Del Soldato, P., Pepeu, G., & Wenk, G.L. (1999). Peripheral administration of novel anti-inflammatories can attenuate the effects of chronic inflammation within the CNS. *Brain Research, 815*, 36–43.

Herman, J. P., Chen, K. C., Booze, R., & Landfield, P. W. (1998). Up-regulation of alpha1D $Ca2^{+}$ channel subunit mRNA expression in the hippocampus of aged 344 rats. *Neurobiology of Aging, 19*, 581–587.

Ho, L., Pieroni, C., Winger, D., Purohit, D. P., Aisen, P. S., & Pasinetti, G. M. (1999). Regional distribution of cyclooxygenase-2 in the hippocampal formation in Alzheimer's disease. *Journal of Neuroscience Research, 57*, 295–303.

Hoozemans, J. J., Bruckner, M. K., Rozemuller, A. J., Veerhuis, R., Eikelenboom, P., & Arendt, T. (2002). Cyclin D1 and cyclin E are co-localized with cyclo-oxygenase 2 (COX-2) in pyramidal neurons in Alzheimer disease temporal cortex. *Journal of Neuropathology and Experimental Neurology, 61*, 678–678.

Hoult, J. R., Moroney, M. A., & Paya, M. (1994). Actions of flavonoids and coumarins on lipoxygenase and cyclooxygenase. *Methods in Enzymology, 234*, 443–454.

Huidobro, A., Blanco, P., Villalba, M., Gomez-Puertas, P., Villa, A., Pereira, R., Bogonez, E., Martinez-Serrano, A., Aparicio, J. J., & Satrustegui, J. (1993). Age-related changes in calcium homeostatic mechanisms in synaptosomes in relation with working memory deficiency. *Neurobiology of Aging, 14*, 479–486.

Ingram, D. K., Jucker, M., & Spangler, E. (1994). Behavioral manifestations of aging. In: Mohr U., Cungworth D. L., & Capen C. C. (Eds.), *Pathobiology of the aging rat* (Vol. 2, pp. 149–170). Washington DC: ILSI.

Joseph, J. A. (1992). The putative role of free radicals in the loss of neuronal functioning in senescence. *Integrative Physiological and Behavioral Science, 27*, 216–227.

Joseph, J. A., Arendash, G., Gordon, M., Diamond, D., Shukitt-Hale, B., & Morgan, D. (2003). Blueberry supplementation enhances signaling and prevents behavioral deficits in an Alzheimer disease model. *Nutritional Neuroscience, 6*, 153–163.

Joseph, J. A., Bartus, R. T., Clody, D. E., Morgan, D., Finch, C., Beer, B., & Sesack, S. (1983). Psychomotor performance in the senescent rodent: Reduction of deficits via striatal dopamine receptor up-regulation. *Neurobiology of Aging, 4*, 313–319.

Joseph, J. A., Denisova, N., Fisher, D., Bickford, P., Prior, R., & Cao, G. (1998). Age-related neurodegeneration and oxidative stress: Putative nutritional intervention. *Neurologic Clinics, 16*, 747–755.

Joseph, J. A., Denisova, N. A., Fisher, D., Shukitt-Hale, B., Bickford, P., Prior, R., & Cao, G. (1998). Membrane and receptor modifications of oxidative stress vulnerability in aging: Nutritional considerations. *Annals of the New York Academy of Sciences, 854*, 268–276.

Joseph, J. A., Erat, S., & Rabin, B. M. (1998). CNS effects of heavy particle irradiation in space: Behavioral implications. *Advances in Space Research, 22*, 209–216.

Joseph, J. A., Fisher, D. R., Carey, A., & Szprengiel, A. (2004). The M3 muscarinic receptor i3 domain confers oxidative stress protection on calcium regulation in transfected COS-7 cells. *Aging Cell, 3*, 263–271.

Joseph, J. A., Fisher, D. R., & Strain J. (2002). Muscarinic receptor subtype determines vulnerability to oxidative stress in COS-7 cells. *Free Radical Biology and Medicine, 32*, 153–161.

Joseph, J. A., Hunt, W. A., Rabing, B. M., & Dalton, T. K. (1992). Possible "accelerated striatal aging" induced by 56Fe heavy-particle irradiation: Implications for manned space flights. *Radiation Research, 130*, 88–93.

Joseph, J. A., Shukitt-Hale, B., Denisova, N. A., Bielinski, D., Martin, A., McEwen, J. J., & Bickford, P. C. (1999). Reversals of age-related declines in neuronal signal transduction, cognitive and motor behavioral deficits with blueberry, spinach or strawberry dietary supplementation. *Journal of Neuroscience, 19*, 8114–8121.

Joseph, J. A., Shukitt-Hale, B., Denisova, N. A., Martin, A., Perry, G., & Smith, M. A. (2001). Copernicus revisited: Amyloid beta in Alzheimer's disease. *Neurobiology of Aging, 22*, 131–146.

Joseph, J. A., Shukitt-Hale, B., Denisova, N. A., Prior, R. L., Cao, G., Martin, A., Taglialatela, G., & Bickford, P.C. (1998). Long-term dietary strawberry, spinach or vitamin E supplementation retards the onset of age-related neuronal signal-transduction and cognitive behavioral deficits. *Journal of Neuroscience, 18*, 8047–8055.

Joseph, J. A., Shukitt-Hale, B., McEwen, J. J., & Rabin, B. M. (2000). CNS-induced deficits of heavy particle irradiation in space: The aging connection. *Advances in Space Research, 25*, 2057–2064.

Joseph, J. A., Villalobos-Molina, R., Denisova, N., Erat, S., Cutler, R., & Strain, J. G. (1996). Age differences in sensitivity to H_2O_2- or NO-induced reductions in K^+-evoked dopamine release from superfused striatal slices: Reversals by PBN or Trolox. *Free Radical Biology and Medicine, 20*, 821–830.

Josselyn, S. A., Shi, C., Carlezon, W. A. Jr., Neve, R. L., Nestler, E. J., & Davis, M. (2001). Long-term memory is facilitated by cAMP response element-binding protein overexpression in the amygdala. *Journal of Neuroscience, 21*, 2404–2412.

Kaasinen, V., Vilkman, H., Hietala, J., Nagren, K., Helenius, H., Olsson, H., Farde, L., & Rinne, J. (2000). Age-related dopamine D2/D3 receptor loss in extrastriatal regions of the human brain. *Neurobiology of Aging, 21*, 683–688.

Kalt, W., Forney, C. F., Martin, A., & Prior, R. L. (1999). Antioxidant capacity, vitamin C, phenolics, and anthocyanins after fresh storage of small fruits. *Journal of Agricultural and Food Chemistry, 47*, 4638–4644.

Kaufmann, J. L., Bickford, P. C., & Taglialatela, G. (2001). Oxidative-stress dependent up-regulation of Bcl-2 expression in the central nervous system of aged Fisher 344 rats. *Journal of Neurochemistry, 76*, 1099–1108.

Kimura, Y., Okuda, H., Taira, Z., Shoji, M., Takemoto, T., & Arichi, S. (1984). Studies on *Scutellariae radix*. IX. New component inhibiting lipid peroxidation in rat liver. *Planta Medica, 50*, 290–295.

Kluger, A., Gianutsos, J. G., Golomb, J., Ferris, S. H., George, A. E., Frannssen, E., & Reisberg, B.(1997). Patterns of motor impairment in normal aging, mild cognitive decline, and early Alzheimer's disease. *Journal of Gerontology, 52*, 28–39.

Kushner, I. (2001). C-reactive protein elevation can be caused by conditions other than inflammation and may reflect biologic aging. *Cleveland Clinical Journal of Medicine, 68*, 535–537.

Lamprecht, R. (1999). CREB message to remember. *Cellular and Molecular Life Sciences, 55*, 554–563.

Leahy, J. C., Luo, Y., Kent, C. S., Meiri, K. F., & Vallano, M. L. (1993). Demonstration of presynaptic protein kinase C activation following long-term potentiation in rat hippocampal slices. *Neuroscience, 52*, 563–574.

Lynch, D. R., & Dawson, T. M. (1994). Secondary mechanisms in neuronal trauma. *Current Opinion in Neurology, 7*, 510–516.

Manev, H., & Uz, T. (1999). Primary cultures of rat cerebellar granule cells as a model to study neuronal 5-lipoxygenase and FLAP gene expression. *Annals of the New York Academy of Sciences, 890*, 183–190.

Manev, H., Uz, T., Sugaya, K., & Qu, T. (2000). Putative role of neuronal 5-lipoxygenase in an aging brain. *The FASEB Journal, 14*, 1464–1469.

Maridonneau-Parini, I., Braquet, P., & Garay, R. P. (1986). Heterogeneous effect of flavonoids on K^+ loss and lipid peroxidation induced by oxygen free radicals in human red cells. *Pharmacological Research Communications, 18*, 61–72.

Martin, S., Favot, L., Matz, R., Lugnier, C., & Andriantsitohaina, R. (2003). Delphinidin inhibits endothelial cell proliferation and cell cycle progression through a transient activation of ERK-1/-2. *Biochemical Pharmacology, 65*, 669–675.

Matsumoto, A. (2000). Age-dependent changes in phosphorylated cAMP response element-binding protein immunoreactivity in motorneurons of the spinal nucleus of the bulbocavernosus of male rats. *Neuroscience Letters, 279*, 117–120.

Mattson, M. P. (2000). Emerging apoptosis in neurodegenerative disorders. *Nature Reviews. Molecular Cell Biology, 1*, 120–129.

Mazzucchelli, C., & Brambilla, R. (2000). Ras-related and MAPK signalling in neuronal plasticity and memory formation. *Cellular and Molecular Life Sciences, 57*, 604–611.

McDonald, R. J., & White, N. M. (1994). Parallel information processing in the water maze: Evidence for independent memory systems involving dorsal striatum and hippocampus. *Behavioral and Neural Biology, 61*, 260–270.

McGeer, P. L., & McGeer, E. G. (1995). The inflammatory response system of the brain: implications for therapy of Alzheimer and other neurodegenerative diseases. *Brain Research. Brain Research Reviews, 21*, 195–218.

Micheau, J., & Riedel, G. (1999). Protein kinases: Which one is the memory molecule? *Cellular and Molecular Life Science, 55*, 534–548.

Muir, J. L. (1997). Acetylcholine, aging, and Alzheimer's disease. *Pharmacology, Biochemistry, and Behavior, 56*, 687–696.

Nyakas, C., Oosterink, B. J., Keijser, J., Felszeghy, K., de Jong, G. I., Korf, J., & Luiten, D. G. (1997). Selective decline of 5-HT1A receptor binding sites in rat cortex, hippocampus and cholinergic basal forebrain nuclei during aging. *Journal of Chemical Neuroanatomy, 13*, 53–61.

Olanow, C. W. (1992). An introduction to the free radical hypothesis in Parkinson's disease. *Annals of Neurology, 32*, S2–S9.

Oliveira, M. G., Bueno, O. F., Pomarico, A. C., & Gugliano, E. B. (1997). Strategies used by hippocampal- and caudate-putamen-lesioned rats in a learning task. *Neurobiology of Learning Memory, 68*, 32–41.

Prior, R. L., Cao, G., Martin, A., Sofic, E., McEwen, J., O'Brien, C., Lischer, N., Ehlenfeldt, M., Kalt, W., Krewer, G., & Mainland, M. C. (1998). Antioxidant capacity as influenced by total phenolic and anthocyanin content, maturity and variety of Vaccinium species. *Journal of Agricultural and Food Chemistry, 46*, 2586–2593.

Rabin, B. M., Joseph, J. A., & Erat, S. (1998). Effects of exposure to different types of radiation on behaviors mediated by peripheral or central systems. *Advances in Space Research, 22*, 217–225.

Rabin, B. M., Joseph, J. A., Shukitt-Hale, B., & McEwen, J. (2000). Effects of exposure to heavy particles on a behavior mediated by the dopaminergic system. *Advances in Space Research, 25*, 2065–2074.

Rosenman, S. J., Shrikant, P., Dubb, L., Benveniste, E. N., & Ransohoff, R. M. (1995). Cytokine induced expression of vascular cell adhesion molecule-1 (VCAM-1) by astrocytes and astrocytoma cell lines. *Journal of Immunology, 154*, 1888–1899.

Rosenzweig, M. R., Bennett, E. L., Colombo, P. J., Lee, D. W., & Serrano, P. A. (1993). Short-term, intermediate-term, and long-term memories. *Behavioural Brain Research, 57*, 193–198.

Rozovsky, I., Finch, C. E., & Morgan, T. E. (1998). Age-related activation of microglia and astrocytes: In vitro studies show. *Neurobiology of Aging, 19*, 97–103.

Sadoul, R. (1998). Bcl-2 family members in the development and degenerative pathologies of the nervous system. *Cell Death and Differentiation, 5*, 805–815.

Sato, M., Bagchi, D., Tosaki, A., & Das, D. K. (2001). Grape seed proanthocyanidin reduces cardiomyocyte apoptosis by inhibiting ischemia/reperfusion-induced activation of JNK-1 and C-JUN. *Free Radical Biology and Medicine, 31*, 729–737.

Savory, J., Rao, J. K., Huang, Y., Letada, P. R., & Herman, M. M. (1999). Age-related hippocampal changes in Bcl-2:Bax ratio, oxidative stress, redox-active iron and apoptosis associated with aluminum-induced neurodegeneration: Increased susceptibility with aging. *Neurotoxicology, 20*, 805–817.

Schafe, G. E., Nadel, N. V., Sullivan, G. M., Harris, A., & LeDoux, J. E. (1999). Memory consolidation for contextual and auditory fear conditioning is dependent on protein synthesis, PKA, and MAP kinase. *Learning and Memory, 6*, 97–110.

Schipper, H. M. (1996). Astrocytes, brain aging, and neurodegeneration. *Neurobiology of Aging, 17*, 467–480.

Schroeter, H., Clinton, B., Spencer, J. P., Williams, R. J., Cadenas, E., & Rice-Evans, C. (2002). MAPK signalling in neurodegeneration:Influences of flavonoids and of nitric oxide. *Neurobiology of Aging, 23*, 861–880.

Seeram, N. P., Bourquin, L. D., & Nair, M. G. (2001). Degradation products of cyanidin glycosides from tart cherries and their bioactivities. *Journal of Agricultural and Food Chemistry, 491*, 4924–4929.

Seeram, N. P., Cichewicz, R. H., Chandra, A., & Nair, M. G. (2003). Cyclooxygenase inhibitory and antioxidant compounds from crabapple fruits. *Journal of Agricultural and Food Chemistry, 51*, 1948–1951.

Seeram, N. P., Momin, R. A., Bourquin, L. D., & Nair, M. G. (2001). Cyclooxygenase inhibitory and antioxidant cyanidin glycosides in cherries and berries. *Phytomedicine, 8*, 362–369.

Seeram, N. P., Schutzki, R., Chandra, A., & Nair, M. G. (2002). Characterization, quantification, and bioactivities of anthocyanins in *Cornus* species. *Journal of Agricultural and Food Chemistry, 50*, 2519–2523.

Selcher, J. C., Atkins, C. M., Trzaskos, J. M., Paylor, R., & Sweatt, J. D. (1999). A necessity for MAP kinase activation in mammalian spatial learning. *Learning and Memory, 6*, 478–490.

Serrano, P. A., Beniston, D. S., Oxonian, M. G., Rodriguez, W. A., Rosenzweig, M. R., & Bennett, E. L. (1994). Differential effects of protein kinase inhibitors and activators on memory formation in the 2-day-old chick. *Behavioral and Neural Biology*, 61, 60–72.

Sgambato, V., Pages, C., Rogard, M., Besson, M. J., & Caboche, J. (1998). Extracellular signal-regulated kinase (ERK) controls immediate early gene induction on corticostriatal stimulation. *Journal of Neuroscience, 18*, 8814–8825.

Shukitt-Hale, B. (1999). The effects of aging and oxidative stress on psychomotor and cognitive behavior. *Age, 22*, 9–17.

Shukitt-Hale, B., Casadesus, G., McEwen, J. J., Rabin, B. M., & Joseph, J. A. (2000). Spatial learning and memory deficits induced by exposure to iron-56-particle radiation. *Radiation Research, 154*, 28–33.

Shukitt-Hale, B., Denisova, N. A., Strain, J. G., & Joseph J. A. (1997). Psychomotor effects of dopamine infusion under decreased glutathione conditions. *Free Radical Biology and Medicine, 23*, 412–418.

Shukitt-Hale, B., Erat, S. A., & Joseph, J. A. (1998). Spatial learning and memory deficits induced by dopamine administration with decreased glutathione. *Free Radical Biology and Medicine, 24*, 1149–1158.

Shukitt-Hale, B., Mouzakis, G., & Joseph J. A. (1998). Psychomotor and spatial memory performance in aging male Fischer 344 rats.*Experimental Gerontology, 33*, 615–624.

Sorata, Y., Takahama, U., & Kimura, M. (1984). Protective effect of quercetin and rutin on photosensitized lysis of human erythrocytes in the presence of hematoporphyrin. *Biochimica et Biophysica Acta, 29*, 313–317.

Spaulding, C. C., Walford, R. L., & Effros, R. B. (1997). Calorie restriction inhibits the age-related dysregulation of the cytokines TNF-α and IL-6 in C3B10RF1 mice. *Mechanisms of Ageing and Development, 93*, 87–94.

Steffen, B., Breier, G., Butcher, E., Schulz, M., & Engelhardt, B. (1996). VCAM-1, and MAdCAM-1 are expressed on choroid plexus epithelium but not endothelium and mediate binding of lymphocytes in vitro. *American Journal of Pathology,148*, 1819–1838.

Stella, N., Estelles, A., Siciliano, J., Tence, M., Desagher, S., Piomelli, D., Glowinksi, J., & Premont, J. (1997). Interleukin-1 enhances the ATP-evoked release of arachidonic acid from mouse astrocytes. *Journal of Neuroscience, 17*, 2939–2946.

Swank, M. W., & Sweatt, J. D. (2001). Increased histone acetyltransferase and lysine acetyltransferase activity and biphasic activation of the ERK/RSK cascade in insular cortex during novel taste learning. *Journal of Neuroscience, 21*, 3383–3391.

Sweatt, J. D. (2001). Memory mechanisms: The yin and yang of protein phosphorylation. *Current Biology, 11*, R391–R394.

Toescu, E. C., & Verkhratsky, A. (2000). Parameters of calcium homeostasis in normal neuronal ageing. *Journal of Anatomy, 197*, 563–569.

Van der Zee, E. A., Compaan, J. C., Bohus, B., & Luiten, P. G. (1995). Alterations in the immunoreactivity for muscarinic acetylcholine receptors and colocalized PKC gamma in mouse hippocampus induced by spatial discrimination learning. *Hippocampus, 5*, 349–362.

Vannucci, R. C., Brucklacher, R. M., & Vannucci, S. J. (2001). Intracellular calcium accumulation during the evolution of hypoxic-ischemic brain damage in the immature rat. *Brain Research. Developmental Brain Research, 126*, 117–120.

Volpato, S., Guralnik, J. M., Ferrucci, L., Balfour, J., Chaves, P., Fried, L. P., & Harris, T. B. (2001). Cardiovascular disease, interleukin-6, and risk of mortality in older women: The women's health and aging study. *Circulation, 103*, 947–953.

Wang, H., Cao, G., & Prior, R. (1996). Total antioxidant capacity of fruits. *Journal of Agricultural and Food Chemistry, 44*, 701–705.

Wang, H., Nair, M. G., Strasburg, G. M., Chang, Y., Booren, A. M., Gray, J. I., & DeWitt, D. L. (1999). Antioxidant and anti-inflammatory activities of anthocyanins and their aglycon, cyanidin, from tart cherries. *Journal of Natural Products, 62*, 294–296.

West, R. L. (1996). An application of pre-frontal cortex function theory to cognitive aging. *Psychological Bulletin, 120*, 272–292.

Woodroofe, M. (1995). Cytokine production in the central nervous system. *Neurology, 45*, S6–S10.

Yamada, K., Komori, Y., Tanaka, T., Senzaki, K., Nikai, T., Sugihara, H., Kameyama, T., & Nabeshima, T. (1999). Brain dysfunction associated with an induction of nitric oxide synthase following an intracerebral injection of lipopolysaccharide in rats. *Neuroscience, 88*, 281–294.

Youdim, K. A., Shukitt-Hale, B., Martin, A., Wang, H., Denisova, N., & Joseph, J. A. (2000). Short-term dietary supplementation of blueberry polyphenolics: Beneficial effects on aging brain performance and peripheral tissue function. *Nutritional Neuroscience, 3*, 383–397.

Yu, B. P. (1994). Cellular defenses against damage from reactive oxygen species. *Physiological Reviews, 76*, 139–162.

Zhang, L., & Jope, R. S. (1999). Oxidative stress differentially modulates phosphorylation of ERK, p38 and CREB induced by NGF or EGF in PC12 cells. *Neurobiology of Aging, 20*, 271–278.

Zhen, X., Uryu, K., Cai, G., Johnson, G., & Friedman, E. (1999). Age-associated impairment in brain MAPK signal pathways and the effect of restriction in Fischer 344 rats. *The Journals of Gerontology. Series A, Biological Sciences and Medical Sciences, 54*, B539–B548.

Zippe, L. M., & Mulcahy, R. T. (2000). Inhibition of ERK and p38 MAP kinases inhibits binding of Nrf2 and induction of GCS genes. *Biochemical and Biophysical Research Communications, 278*, 484–492.

Zyzak, D. R., Otto, T., Eichenbaum, H., & Gallagher, M. (1995). Cognitive decline associated with normal aging in rats: A neuropsychological approach. *Learning and Memory, 2*, 1–16.

5 Effects of Stress and Nutrition on Blood–Brain Barrier Functions

Akihiko Urayama and William A. Banks

KEY POINTS

- Several kinds of barriers exist between the body and brain.
- Outlines the anatomical features of the blood–brain barrier and how it works physiologically.
- There are adaptive neuroendocrine responses to stress that are mediated through the blood–brain barrier.
- Stress can induce the disruption of the blood–brain barrier.
- Diet can affect transport-related changes in amino acid patterns within the brain.

1. INTRODUCTION: WHAT IS THE BLOOD–BRAIN BARRIER?

Over the past two decades, dramatic progress has been made in understanding the physiology and functions of the blood–brain barrier (BBB). The BBB is made up of brain microvessel endothelial cells, astroglia, pericytes, perivascular macrophages, and basal lamina. Brain microvessel endothelial cells are characterized by tight intercellular junctions restricting the passage of most molecules from the circulation to the brain. The brains of vertebrates are perfused by a dense microvascular network formed by the capillary endothelial cells within the brain (Pardridge, 2002). The density of the microvasculature in the brain is so intricate that no neuron or glial cell is more than 20 μm from a neighboring capillary (Bar, 1980). Therefore, every neuron is virtually perfused by its own microvessel. Once a circulating solute crosses the brain microvascular wall, it can be immediately utilized by every neuron within the brain.

In humans, approx 400 miles of capillaries perfuse the brain, and the surface area of the brain microvascular endothelium is approx 20 m^2 (Pardridge, 2001). Despite the vast surface area of the human BBB, the barrier itself is very thin; the total intracellular volume of the brain capillary endothelium is only 5 mL in the human and 1 μL in the rat (Fig. 1). Brain capillary endothelial cells are approx 200–300 nm thick. This very thin cellular barrier has some of the most restrictive permeability properties of any biological membrane (Oldendorf, 1971).

The BBB regulates the passage of solutes between the central nervous system (CNS) and the blood. The BBB not only restricts the entry of serum proteins into the CNS, but also controls the passage of nutrients, electrolytes, vitamins, minerals, free fatty acids,

From: *Nutrients, Stress, and Medical Disorders*
Edited by: S. Yehuda and D. I. Mostofsky

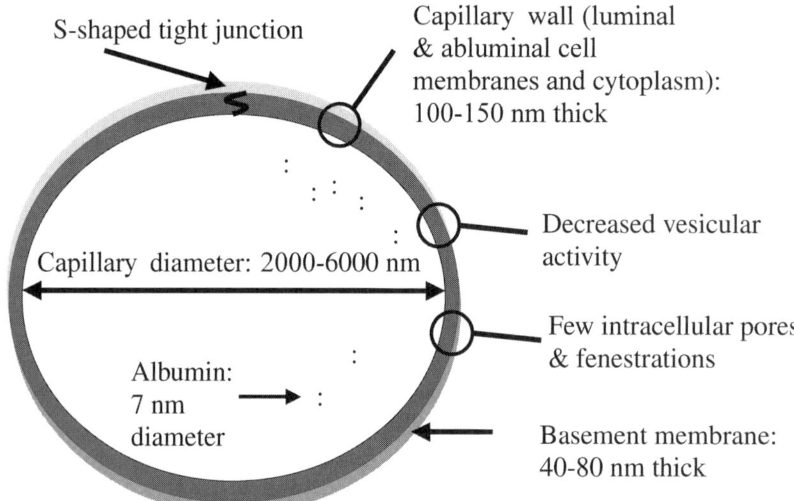

Fig. 1. Architectural sketch of the brain vascular wall.

peptides, and regulatory proteins in both the brain-to-blood and blood-to-brain directions (Davson & Segal, 1996). The BBB performs these functions through a number of nonsaturable and saturable transport mechanisms. For example, efflux (brain-to-blood direction) systems regulate the levels of nutrients and minerals in the cerebrospinal fluid (CSF) and secrete brain-originating substances into the blood. Influx systems control the homeostatic environment of the CNS, supply the brain with nutrients, and help to integrate CNS and peripheral functions (Banks, 1999).

The entry of substances into the brain from blood is restricted at the BBB through multiple mechanisms, including a physical endothelial barrier, an enzymatic barrier, and an efflux barrier. This multifunctional property of the BBB arises from the multicellularity of the brain microvasculature, which is formed by capillary endothelial cells, capillary pericytes, and a perivascular astrocyte foot process, from the multiple functions each cell type can perform, and from a complexity of intercellular interactions (Pardridge, 2001). The endothelium and pericyte share a common microvascular basement membrane, and 99% of the surface of capillary basement membrane is invested by the end feet of processes extending from astrocytic cell bodies originating within the brain parenchyma (Pardridge, 2002).

Capillaries perfusing peripheral organs have porous endothelial walls. Peripheral capillaries have open interendothelial junctional spaces, intracellular fenestrations, and are actively engaged in pinocytosis. These characteristics form paracellular and transcellular routes for the free diffusion of molecules from the blood to the interstitial space of the organ. By comparison, brain capillary endothelial cells express epithelial-like high-resistance tight junctions, which eliminate the paracellular pathway, and have minimal pinocytosis and no intracellular fenestrations, which eliminate the nonspecific transcellular route from the blood to the brain (Broadwell & Banks, 1993). The combination of the very-high-resistance endothelial tight junctions, minimal endothelial pinocytosis, and lack of fenestrations forms a physical barrier to the entry of many substances into the brain from the blood. There is another barrier to circulating substances, in addition to the physical barrier formed by the endothelial tight junctions: the capillary endothelial cells, capillary pericytes, and astrocyte foot processes all express a variety of ectoenzymes on the cellular plasma membranes, including aminopeptidases, carboxypeptidases, endopeptidases, cholinesterases, and others, which inactivate many endogenous and exogenous substances that may pass the endothelial barrier (el-Bacha & Minn, 1999).

The protective function of the BBB can be altered during various disease states of the CNS. Damage to the BBB leads to increased entry of the vascular components, such as serum proteins, into the brain, changes in the homeostasis and metabolic activities of the brain, and alterations in the vesicular activity and morphology of brain capillary endothelial cells (Wisniewski, Vorbrodt, & Wegiel, 1997).

2. ASPECTS OF STRESS THAT AFFECT THE BBB

Stress is a common experience of daily life, and all organisms have evolved mechanisms and strategies to deal with crucial alterations in their internal and external environment. A limited stress can actually exert beneficial effects on brain function, particularly promotion of plasticity and enhancement of learning and memory formation (Fuchs & Flugge, 1998). However, it is known that a persistent or overwhelming stress can cause deleterious effects on the brain, including effects on the BBB (Bryan, 1990; Sharma, Cervos-Navarro, & Dey, 1991). The potential mechanisms by which stress alters the BBB include stimulation of central catecholaminergic neurons and release of noradrenaline, an increased local activation and release of serotonin, changes in the circulating levels of corticosteroids, and increased cerebral blood flow and energy metabolism (Bryan, 1990). In addition, exposure to a significant acute or chronic stress causes neuroendocrine alterations, including activation of vasoactive mediators such as histamine released from perivascular brain mast cells (Esposito et al., 2001; Zhuang, Silverman, & Silver, 1990), activation of the hypothalamic–pituitary–adrenal (HPA) axis through the release of corticotropin-releasing hormone (CRH) resulting in the secretion of glucocorticoids and catecholamines leading to neuronal injury (Barryd, Yoramfinkelstein, Koffler, & Gilad 1985; Chrousos, 1995), and interaction of glucocorticoid and catecholamine effects with glutamatergic neurotransmission (Gilad, gilad, Wyatt, & Tizabi, 1990). All of these phenomena can affect the functions of the BBB and the CNS.

During exposure to stress stimuli, the body responds physiologically with increased activity of both the HPA axis and the sympathoadrenal system (Vanitallie, 2002). The main feature of stress reaction is activation of the HPA axis. In the brain, the hippocampus is involved in the integration of sensory information, the interpretation of environmental information, and the execution of appropriate behavioral and neuroendocrine responses (Vinogradova, 2001). The amygdala is an executor of stress-related behavioral, autonomic, and neuroendocrine responses (Carrasco & Van de Kar, 2003). CRH in the paraventricular nucleus (PVN) of the hypothalamus is responsible for initiating the response of the HPA axis to stress (Carrasco & Van de Kar, 2003). The negative-feedback regulation of stress hormones, local hypothalamic circuits, and cytokines are involved in the regulation of HPA activation (Fig. 2). At first, stress induces the release of CRH from the hypothalamus, which in turn results in the release of adrenocorticotropic hormone (ACTH) into the general circulation. ACTH then acts on the adrenal cortex,

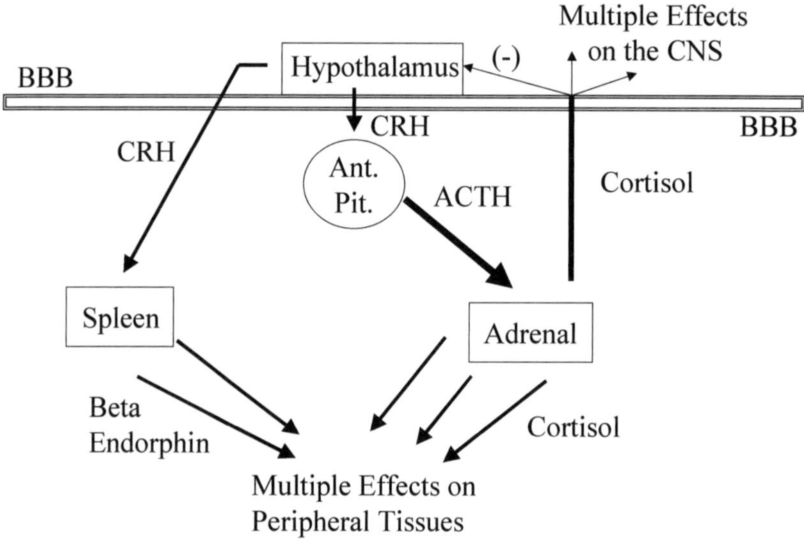

Fig. 2. The HPA axis: classic and revised.

stimulating the release of glucocorticoids into the blood. Glucocorticoids act in a negative-feedback fashion to terminate the release of CRH (Carrasco & Van de Kar, 2003; Makino, Hashimoto, & Gold, 2002). The body uses this elegant negative-feedback loop to maintain glucocorticoid levels within physiological boundaries. Interference at any level of the HPA axis will influence the other components via the feedback loop. Stress can alter or even disrupt the normal homeostasis of the HPA axis.

3. DISRUPTION OF THE BBB BY STRESS

With the multifaceted nature of both the stress response and BBB function, one might expect that interactions would occur at many levels. Although this seems to be true, most work has focused on only one aspect of BBB function: its disruption. It has been shown experimentally that alterations of physiological functions under emotional and physical stress depend on particular regulatory properties of the CNS. In acutely immobilized animals used as a model of stress, it has been observed that variation of catecholamine levels in the brain nuclei correlates with blood pressure changes (Majewski, Alade, & Rand, 1986). Several lines of evidence indicate that catecholamine content is not only a function of the metabolism of nuclei, but also may be related to their fluxes from the circulation (Hendley, Burrows, Robinson, Heidenreich, & Bulman, 1977; Nakagawa, Tanaka, Kohno, Noda, & Nagasaki, 1981). Although there is both a physical and an enzymatic barrier to catecholamines—the latter formed by decarboxylate inactivation of catecholamines within the brain endothelial cell—catecholamines can still disrupt the BBB to macromolecules, leading to the extravasation of serum proteins, such as albumin (Oztas, Erkin, Dural, & Isbir, 2000). Under physiological conditions, albumin is nearly totally excluded from the CNS by the BBB, with a CSF-to-blood ratio of about 1:200. However, a marked increase in BBB permeability to albumin in several brain regions was observed after the onset of immobilization stress (Skultetyova, Tokarev, & Jezova, 1998).

The exposure of animals to long-lasting stress conditions, such as immobilization for 4–8 h (Belova & Jonsson, 1982), heat stress for 4 h (Sharma, Nyberg, Cervos-Navarro, & Dey, 1992), prolonged hypoglycemia (Oztas, Kucuk, & Sandalci, 1985), or starvation (Angel, 1969), was shown to result in disruption of the BBB. Furthermore, it has been observed that short immobilization stress (30 min) was enough to induce increased extravasation of serum albumin into the brain tissue. The permeability of albumin across the BBB under stress was markedly increased in different brain regions such as the hippocampus, brainstem, and cerebellum (Skultetyova et al., 1998). These results confirmed previous findings showing that immobilization stress induced increased barrier permeability in the hypothalamus, as measured by histochemical analysis using horseradish peroxidase, another substance used to estimate the integrity of the BBB (Jezova et al., 1989). In comparison, there is little increase in the extravasation of endogenous albumin into either the cerebral cortex or the striatum. Different quantitative changes in individual brain regions might be caused by differences in vulnerability of microvasculatures in respective areas. Also, these data are consistent with previous findings of increased BBB permeability in the hypothalamus, hippocampus, and cerebellum following 30 min of forced swimming (Sharma, Westman, Navarro, Day, & Nyberg, 1995). Increased BBB permeability was shown in the cortex in some studies using different stress models and different methods for the evaluation for BBB integrity (Saija, Princi, De Pasquale, & Costa, 1988; Sharma et al., 1995). This inconsistent regional variation in BBB disruption suggests a stressor-specific effect, since different experimental conditions were employed.

One of the factors inducing BBB disruption is acute elevation of arterial blood pressure related to stress (Johansson, Li, Olsson, & Klatzo, 1970). Other factors, such as metabolic changes found in animals subjected to stress, might be important. Another possible mechanism of BBB disruption is change in the vascular tone mediated by vasoactive substances released during stress, such as epinephrine and norepinephrine (Borges, Shi, Azevedo, & Audus, 1994). Exposure to stress increases extracecllular glutamate levels in the brain (Lowy, Wittenberg, & Yamamoto, 1995; Moghaddam, 1993). Recent studies suggest that glutamate might be involved in the regulation of BBB permeability. Whcn glutamate receptors in the cerebral capillaries are overstimulated, a breakdown of the BBB may occur. High doses of glutamate can also induce convulsions, which in turn disrupt the BBB (Nemeroff & Crisley, 1975).

Stress activates the HPA axis through the release of CRH, leading to production of glucocorticoids that downregulate immune responses (Chrousos, 1995). CRH is synthesized predominantly in the PVN of hypothalamus and mediates its effects through at least three types of CRH receptors (CRHRs): CRHR-1; CRHR-2α; CRHR-2β (Hillhouse, Randeva, Ladds, & Grammatopoulos, 2002; Lawrence, Krstew, Dautzenberg, & Ruhmann, 2002). Stress worsens a number of neuro-inflammatory disorders (Rosch, 1979), and CRH release leads to inflammation (Karalis et al., 1991), mediated through the activation of mast cells (Theoharides et al., 1998). It has been shown that mast cells play a key role to inflammatory reactions by releasing histamine and cytokines (Galli, 1993; Metcalfe, Baram, & Mekori, 1997). In the brain, mast cells are predominantly in a perivascular location, especially in the thalamus and hypothalamus (Cirulli, Pistillo, de Acetis, Alleva, & Aloe, 1998). It has been suggested that BBB permeability induced by acute restraint stress involves CRH because the increase in the permeability by CRH is inhibited by pretreatment with the CRH receptor antagonist antalarmin and is induced by the intracranial injection of CRH into the PVN (Esposito et al., 2002). Furthermore, the stress-induced increase in BBB permeability requires mast cells since it is absent in mast-cell-deficient mice (Esposito et al., 2002). In addition to the expression of CRH in hypothalamus, it is also detected in extrahypothalamic regions, such as the central and medial nuclei of the amygdala, the olfactory bulb, the cortex, and the deep cerebellar nuclei of the cerebellum (Dieterich, Lehnert, & De Souza, 1997; Fellmann et al., 1984). Although CRH activates the HPA axis, it could have other effects because CRHRs exist in many brain regions. CRHR-1 expression is very high in the cerebral cortex, striatum, amygdala, and cerebellum, whereas CRHR-2 expression is generally confined to subcortical regions such as the lateral septal nucleus, several nuclei of the hypothalamus, and the choroid plexus (Chalmers, Lovenberg, Grigoriadis, Behan, & De Souza, 1996). It has been demonstrated that CRH mediates the degranulation of dura mast cells and skin mast cells and increases vascular permeability (Theoharides et al., 1995, 1998). Stress-induced behavioral and endocrine responses (Deak et al., 1999) were inhibited by the treatment of antalarmin, which has higher selectivity for CRHR-1 subtype (Webster et al., 1996).

Mast cells are localized around the cerebral microvasculature, and cerebral microvessels forming the BBB align closely with nerves throughout the brain. In addition, mast cells have also been identified close to CRH-positive neurons in the median eminence (Theoharides et al., 1995). The effects of mast cells on the BBB is also demonstrated by several studies that mast-cell-derived histamine increases BBB permeability determined by the extravasations of circulating substances (Boertje, Le Beau, & Williams, 1989) and by electrical resistance in brain microvessel endothelial cells (Butt & Jones, 1992). In fact, it is possible that both histamine and serotonin affect BBB permeability because pretreatment with cyproheptadine, a dual antagonist for histamine (H1) and serotonin (5-HT2) receptors suppressed the increase in BBB permeability induced by acute forced swimming (Sharma et al., 1991). These results indicate that brain mast cell activation and CRH release are involved in the increase in BBB permeability induced by acute stress. Also, whereas CRH deficiency virtually impaired the HPA axis responsiveness, certain behavioral and endocrine responses to stress were still observed in CRH knockout mice (Jacobson, Muglia, Weninger, Pacale, & Majzoub, 2000). Certain hypothalamic mast cell mediators may independently activate the HPA axis. In fact, histamine increases CRH expression in the PVN (Kjaer, Larsen, Knigge, Jorgensen, & Warberg, 1998), and interleukin-6 has the aspect of CRH-independent stimulator of the HPA axis during immune system activation (Bethin, Vogt, & Muglia, 2000). In addition, both BBB permeability and mast cell activation were inhibited by cromoglycate, a mast cell stabilizer (Esposito et al., 2001). These results demonstrate that CRH and mast cells are involved in stress-induced disruption of the BBB.

Activation of the HPA axis depends on the secretion of CRH, an intact pituitary, and the ventral adrenergic bundle innervating the hypothalamic PVN. Thus, the neuroendocrine mechanisms mentioned above that may contribute to the disruption of the BBB include the stress response of the HPA axis.

4. OTHER INTERACTIONS BETWEEN STRESS AND THE BBB

Effects of stress on other aspects of BBB function have not been extensively studied. However, enough work exists to illustrate that stress has effects on several BBB transporters. Unlike disruption, which likely represents an extreme pathological endpoint, changes in transporter functions may represent adaptive responses to stress. Restraint, fasting, and sickness behavior provide examples of interactions between aspects of stress and BBB function. Restraint, but not fasting (Banks, Kastin, & Nager, 1988), reduces the transport of Tyr-MIF-1 in the brain-to-blood direction. In contrast, starvation affects the blood-to-brain influx of leptin (Kastin & Akerstrom, 2000). This is likely a protective mechanism against starvation, as the decreased transport would attenuate the CNS-mediated anorectic effects of leptin. Sickness behavior occurs with infection and is recognized by a loss of energy and interests in one's surrounding (Bluthe, Parnet, Dantzer, & Kelley, 1991; Dantzer & Kelley, 1989). It is also associated with a loss of cognitive abilities, which are known to be mediated through interleukin-1 (Larson & Dunn, 2001). The ability of blood borne interleukin-1 to mediate these cognitive effects depends, at least in part, on its ability to cross the BBB and act at the posterior division of the septum (Banks, Farr, La Scola, & Morley, 2001).

HPA axis and BBB interaction may have results other than BBB disruption. One hypothesis suggests that decreased CRH production is an early event in the development of chronic fatigue syndrome, preceding and leading to alterations in serotonin and interleukin-1 levels (Kastin et al., 1997). An efflux system separate from that of the hypophyseal circulation transports CRH directly from brain tissue into the bloodstream (Martins, Kastin, & Banks, 1996, 1997a, 1997b). The levels secreted are high enough to affect peripheral responses, including enhanced secretion of β-endorphin by the spleen into the blood. This may represent an additional arm in the classic HPA axis (Fig. 2).

5. COMPETITION AMONG AMINO ACIDS FOR TRANSPORT INTO THE BRAIN: RELATIONSHIPS WITH DIET

Macronutrients in the diet and nutrient levels in the blood can affect amino acid and nutrient transport across the BBB. It has been reported that animals increase their alcohol intake when fed nutrient-deficient diets or after a stressful experience. Alcohol, stress-related hormones, such as arginine and vasopressin, feeding peptides, and neurotoxins can alter the rate of amino acid transport into the brain (Branchey, Shaw, & Leiber, 1981; Brust, 1986; Chance, Balasubramaniam, Thomas, & Fischer, 1992; Eriksson & Carlson, 1980; Grammas, Kwaiser, & Caspers, 1992). The levels of neurotransmitters in the brain, in turn, are a function of the levels of amino acid precursors in brain. The levels of tryptophan in the brain, for example, correlate with levels of brain serotonin (Branchey et al., 1981; Fernstrom & Wurtman, 1971). Thus, diet and stress-related hormones can directly affect the levels of brain neurotransmitters, which in turn can have profound effects on behavior and stress responses.

It has long been known that administration of certain amino acids alters the concentration of other amino acids in the brain (Oldendorf & Szabo, 1976). It is also known that there are several classes of amino acid transport systems across the BBB and that competition for transport occurs among the amino acids of a given transport system (Fernstrom & Wurtman, 1972; Peng, Gubin, Harper, Varich, & Kemmerer, 1973). The affinities for amino acid transport across the BBB are similar to physiological concentrations of amino acids in the plasma (Pardridge & Oldendorf, 1975; Pratt, 1976); hence, changes in plasma amino acid concentrations might be expected to alter their rate of passage from blood to brain.

The concentration of histidine in the brain is decreased by approx 80% within 12 h after feeding of a low-histidine, low-protein diet also supplemented with the remaining essential amino acids (Peng, Tews, & Harper, 1972). Lutz, Tews, and Harper (1975) used brain slices as a model to study competition for amino acid entry into these tissues. Histidine transport was also significantly inhibited by large neutral amino acids at concentrations present in plasma of rats fed a low-histidine diet. Small neutral and basic amino acids were less inhibitory (Peng et al., 1972). Threonine transport into brain slices was most strongly inhibited by other small neutral amino acids such as serine, alanine, and α-amino-*n*-butyric acid (AABA), whereas the large neutral amino acids were only moderately inhibitory, and the basic amino acid lysine was without effect (Tews, Good, & Harper, 1978). Adding serine or AABA to a low-protein diet low in threonine markedly reduced brain threonine content by about 40 or 55%, respectively (Tews, Kim, & Harper, 1980). In another trial, rats were fed a low-protein diet limited in lysine and containing extra arginine, a basic amino acid that competes with lysine for its transport into brain slices (Tews, Bradford, & Harper, 1981).

Entry into the brain of large neutral amino acids such as valine and histidine was most severely inhibited by amino acid analogs such as norleucine, norvaline, and α-aminooctanoate, whereas basic amino acids and isomer of α-aminooctanoate had little effect on the transport of large neutral amino acids (Oldendorf & Szabo, 1976; Tews & Harper, 1983). Lysine entry was markedly inhibited by other basic amino acids and by the analog homoarginine, whereas various large neutral amino acids were relatively ineffective. Feeding a single meal of a diet low in lysine and containing homoarginine reduced brain content of lysine by 65% (Tews, 1986).

Diet-induced changes in the levels of amino acids in brain occur because of alterations in the absolute and relative levels of amino acids in serum that share a common BBB transporter. The results of these studies show that diet can induce transport-related changes in brain amino acid patterns as well as deplete pools of amino acids. These effects may be important in the regulation of feeding behavior, inasmuch as many dietary treatments that alter brain amino acid patterns are associated with depressed food intake.

Amino acids can also affect other BBB transport systems. The branched-chain amino acids, for example, can influence peptide transport system (PTS)-1, which transports Tyr-MIF-1 and methionine enkephalin out of the brain (Banks & Kastin, 1986). Brain levels of methionine enkephalin, in turn, are inversely correlated with voluntary alcohol intake and alcohol withdrawal seizures (Blum, Briggs, Wallace, Hall, & Trachtenberg, 1987; Blum, Elston, DeLallo, Briggs, & Wallace, 1983; Koide, Onishi, Katayama, Kai, & Yamagami, 1995). Not surprisingly, branched-chain amino acids affect alcohol intake (Avogaro et al., 1986).

6. CONCLUSION

The BBB regulates the passage of solutes between the CNS and the blood. The BBB not only restricts the entry of serum proteins into the CNS, but also controls the passage of nutrients, electrolytes, vitamins, minerals, free fatty acids, peptides, and regulatory proteins in both the brain-to-blood and blood-to-brain directions. The BBB performs these functions through a number of nonsaturable and saturable transport mechanisms. Exposure to a stress causes neuroendocrine alterations and activation of the HPA axis through release of CRH. The negative feedback regulation of stress hormones, local hypothalamic circuits, and cytokines are involved in the regulation of HPA activation. These neuroendocrine alterations may result in the disruption of the BBB, leading to an increased entry of vascular components into the brain and changes in the homeostasis and metabolic activities of the brain.

Changes in transporter functions across the BBB may represent adaptive responses to stress. The levels of neurotransmitters in the brain are a function of the amount of amino acid precursors in the brain. Macronutrient and nutrient levels can affect amino acid and nutrient transport across the BBB. It has been reported that animals increase their alcohol intake when fed nutrient-deficient diets or after a stressful experience. Thus, diet and stress-related hormones can directly affect the levels of brain neurotransmitters, which in turn can have profound effects on behavior and stress responses.

REFERENCES

Angel C. (1969). Starvation, stress and the blood-brain barrier. *Diseases of the Nervous System, 30*, 94–97.

Avogaro, A., Cibin, M., Croatto, T., Rizzo, A., Gallimberti, L., & Tiengo, A. (1986). Alcohol intake and withdrawal: Effects on branched chain amino acids and alanine. *Alcoholism: Clinical and Experimental Research, 10*, 300–304.

Banks, W. A. (1999). Physiology and pathology of the blood-brain barrier: Implications for microbial pathogenesis, drug delivery and neurodegenerative disorders. *Journal of NeuroVirology, 5*, 538–555.

Banks, W. A., Farr, S. A., La Scola, M. E., & Morley, J. E. (2001). Intravenous human interleukin-1α impairs memory processing in mice: Dependence on blood-brain barrier transport into posterior division of the septum. *Journal of Pharmacology and Experimental Therapeutics, 299*, 536–541.

Banks, W. A., and Kastin, A. J. (1986). Modulation of the carrier-mediated transport of the Tyr-MIF-1 across the blood-brain barrier by essential amino acids. *Journal of Pharmacology and Experimental Therapeutics, 239*, 668–672.

Banks, W. A., Kastin, A. J., and Nager, B. J. (1988). Analgesia and the blood-brain barrier transport system for Tyr-MIF-1/enkephalins: Evidence for a dissociation. *Neuropharmacology, 27*, 175–179.

Bar, T. (1980). The vascular system of the cerebral cortex. *Advances in Anatomy, Embryology, and Cell Biology, 59*, 1–62.

Barryd, G. G., Yoramfinkelstein, M., Koffler, B., & Gilad, V. (1985). Stress-induced activation of the hippocampal cholinergic system and the pituitary-adrenocortical axis. *Brain Research, 347*, 404–408.

Belova, T. I., & Jonsson, G. (1982). Blood-brain barrier permeability and immobilization stress. *Acta Physiologica Scandinavica, 116*, 21–29.

Bethin, K. E., Vogt, S. K., & Muglia, L. J. (2000). Interleukin-6 is an essential, corticotropin-releasing hormone-independent stimulator of the adrenal axis during immune system activation. *Proceedings of the National Academy of Sciences, 97*, 9317–9322.

Blum, K., Briggs, A. H., Wallace, J. E., Hall, C. W., & Trachtenberg, M. A. (1987). Regional brain [Met]-enkephalin in alcohol-preferring and non-alcohol-preferring inbred strains of mice. *Experientia, 43*, 408–410.

Blum, K., Elston, S. F. A., DeLallo, L., Briggs, A. H., & Wallace, J. E. (1983). Ethanol acceptance as a function of genotype amounts of brain [met]-enkephalin. *Proceedings of the National Academy of Sciences, 80*, 6510–6512.

Bluthe, R. M., Parnet, P., Dantzer, R., & Kelley, K. W. (1991). Interleukin-1 receptor antagonist blocks effects of IL-1α and IL-1β on social behavior and body weight in mice. *Neuroscience Research Communications, 15*, 151–158.

Boertje, S. B., Le Beau, D., & Williams, C. (1989). Blockade of histamine-stimulated alterations in cerebrovascular permeability by the H2-receptor antagonist cimetidine. *Neuropharmacology, 28*, 749–752.

Borges, N., Shi, F., Azevedo, I., & Audus, K. L. (1994). Changes in brain microvessel endothelial cell monolayer permeability induced by adrenergic drugs. *European Journal of Pharmacology, 269*, 243–248.

Branchey, L., Shaw, S., & Lieber, C. S. (1981). Ethanol impairs tryptophan transport into the brain and depresses serotonin. *Life Sciences, 29*, 2751–2755.

Broadwell, R. D., & Banks, W.A. (1993). Cell biological perspective for the transcytosis of peptides and proteins through the mammalian blood-brain fluid barriers. In W.M. Pardridge (Ed.), *The blood-brain barrier.* (pp. 165–199). New York: Raven.

Brust, P. (1986). Changes in regional blood-brain transfer of L-leucine elicited by arginine-vasopressin. *Journal of Neurochemistry, 46*, 534–541.

Bryan, R. M. (1990). Cerebral blood flow and energy metabolism during stress. *American Journal of Physiology, 259*, H269–H280.

Butt, A. M., & Jones, H. C. (1992). Effect of histamine and antagonists on electrical resistance across the blood-brain barrier in rat brain-surface microvessels. *Brain Research, 569*, 100–105.

Carrasco, G. A., & Van de Kar, L. D. (2003). Neuroendocrine pharmacology of stress. *European Journal of Pharmacology, 463*, 235–272.

Chalmers, D. T., Lovenberg, T. W., Grigoriadis, D. E., Behan, D. P., & De Souza, E. B. (1996). Corticotrophin-releasing factor receptors: From molecular biology to drug design. *Trends in Pharmacological Science, 17*, 166–172.

Chance, W. T., Balasubramaniam, A., Thomas, I., & Fischer, J. E. (1992). Amylin increases transport of tyrosine and tryptophan into the brain. *Brain Research, 593*, 20–24.

Chrousos, G. P. (1995). The hypothalamic-pituitary-adrenal axis and immune-mediated inflammation. *New England Journal of Medicine, 322*, 1351–1362.

Cirulli, F., Pistillo, L., de Acetis, L., Alleva, E., & Aloe, L. (1998). Increased number of mast cells in the central nervous system of adult male mice following chronic subordination stress. *Brain, Behavior, and Immunity, 12*, 123–133.

Dantzer, R., & Kelley, K. W. (1989). Stress and immunity: An integrated view of relationships between the brain and the immune system. *Life Sciences, 44*, 1995–2008.

Davson, H., & Segal, M. B. (1996). Special aspects of the blood-brain barrier. In *Anonymous physiology of the CSF and blood-brain barriers.* (pp. 303–485). Boca Raton, FL: CRC.

Deak, T., Nguyen, K. T., Ehrlich, A. L., Watkins, L. R., Spencer, R. L., Maier, S. F., Licinio, J., Wong, M. L., Chrousos, G. P., Webster, E., & Gold, P. W. (1999). The impact of the nonpeptide corticotropin-releasing hormone antagonist antalarmin on behavioral and endocrine responses to stress. *Endocrinology, 140*, 79–86.

Dieterich, K. D., Lehnert, H., & De Souza, E. B. (1997). Corticotropin-releasing factor receptors: an overview. *Experimental and Clinical Endocrinology & Diabetes, 105*, 65–82.

el-Bacha, R. S., & Minn, A. (1999). Drug metabolizing enzymes in cerebrovascular endothelial cells afford a metabolic protection to the brain. *Cellular and Molecular Biology, 45*, 15–23.

Eriksson, T., & Carlsson, A. (1980). Ethanol-induced increase in brain concentrations of administered neutral amino acids. *Naunyn-Schmiedeberg's Archives of Pharmacology, 314*, 47–50.

Esposito, P., Chandler, N., Kandere, K., Basu, S., Jacobson, S., Connolly, R., Tutor, D., & Theoharides, T. C. (2002). Corticotropin-releasing hormone and brain mast cells regulate blood-brain-barrier permeability induced by acute stress. *Journal of Pharmacology and Experimental Therapeutics, 303*, 1061–1066.

Esposito, P., Gheorghe, D., Kandere, K., Pang, X., Connolly, R., Jacobson, S., & Theoharides, T. C. (2001). Acute stress increases permeability of the blood-brain barrier through activation of brain mast cells. *Brain Research, 888*, 117–127.

Fellmann, D., Bugnon, C., Bresson, J. L., Gouget, A., Cardot, J., Clavequin, M. C., & Hadjiyiassemis, M. (1984). The CRF neuron: Immunocytochemical study. *Peptides, 5*, 19–33.

Fernstrom, J. D., & Wurtman, R. J. (1971). Brain serotonin content: Physiological dependence on plasma tryptophan levels. *Science, 173*, 149–152.

Fernstrom, J. D., & Wurtman, R. J. (1972). Brain serotonin content: physiological regulation by plasma neutral amino acids. *Science, 178*, 414–416.

Fuchs, E., & Flugge, G. (1998). Stress, glucocorticoids and structural plasticity of the hippocampus. *Neuroscience and Biobehavioral Revues, 23*, 295–300.

Galli, S. J. (1993). New concepts about the mast cell. *New England Journal of Medicine, 328*, 257–265.

Gilad, G. M., Gilad, V. H., Wyatt, R. J., & Tizabi, Y. (1990). Region-selective stress-induced increase of glutamate uptake and release in rat brain. *Brain Research, 525*, 335–338.

Grammas, P., Kwaiser, T. M., & Caspers, M. L. (1992). Regulation of amino acid uptake into cerebral microvessels. *Neuropharmacology, 31*, 409–412.

Hendley, E. D., Burrows, G. H., Robinson, E. S., Heidenreich, K. A., & Bulman, C. A. (1977). Acute stress and the brain norepinephrine uptake mechanism in the rat. *Pharmacology, Biochemistry, and Behavior, 6*, 197–202.

Hillhouse, E. W., Randeva, H., Ladds, G., & Grammatopoulos, D. (2002). Corticotropin-releasing hormone receptors. *Biochemical Society Transactions, 30*, 428–432.

Jacobson, L., Muglia, L. J., Weninger, S. C., Pacak, K., & Majzoub, J. A. (2000). CRH deficiency impairs but does not block pituitary-adrenal responses to diverse stressors. *Neuroendocrinology, 71*, 79–87.

Jezova, D., Johansson, B. B., Olsson, Y., Oprsalova, Z., Kiss, A., Jurcovicova, J., Grassler, J., Westergren, I., & Vigas, M. (1989). Can catecholamines and other neurotransmitters cross the blood-brain barrier and modify neuroendocrine function during stress? In G. R. Van Loon, R. Kvetnansky, R. McCarty, & J. Axelrod (Eds.), *Stress: Neurochemical and humoral mechanisms*, (pp. 325–337). New York: Gordon and Breach Sciences.

Johansson, B., Li, C. L., Olsson, Y., & Klatzo, I. (1970). The effect of acute arterial hypertension on the blood-brain barrier to protein tracers. *Acta Neuropathologica (Berlin), 16*, 117–124.

Karalis, K., Sano, H., Redwine, J., Listwak, S., Wilder, R. L., & Chrousos, G. P. (1991). Autocrine or paracrine inflammatory actions of corticotropin-releasing hormone in vivo. *Science, 254*, 421–423.

Kastin, A. J., & Akerstrom, V. (2000). Fasting, but not adrenalectomy, reduces transport of leptin into the brain. *Peptides, 21*, 679–682.

Kastin, A. J., Olson, R. D., Martins, J. M., Olson, G. A., Zadina, J. E., & Banks, W. A. (1997). Chronic fatigue syndrome: Possible integration of hormonal and immunological observations. In S. Yehuda, & D. I. Mostofsky (Eds.), *Chronic fatigue syndrome* (pp. 161–192). New York: Plenum.

Kjaer, A., Larsen, P. J., Knigge, U., Jorgensen, H., & Warberg, J. (1998). Neuronal histamine and expression of corticotropin-releasing hormone, vasopressin and oxytocin in the hypothalamus: Relative importance of H1 and H2 receptors. *European Journal of Endocrinology, 139*, 238–243.

Koide, S., Onishi, H., Katayama, M., Kai, T., & Yamagami, S. (1995). HPLC/RIA analysis of bioactive methionine enkephalin content in the seizure-suseptible E1 mouse brain. *Neurochemistry Research, 20*, 1115–1118.

Larson, S. J., & Dunn, A. J. (2001). Behavioral effects of cytokines. *Brain, Behavior, and Immunity, 15*, 371–387.

Lawrence, A. J., Krstew, E. V., Dautzenberg, F. M., & Ruhmann, A. (2002). The highly selective CRF(2) receptor antagonist K41498 binds to presynaptic CRF(2) receptors in rat brain. *British Journal of Pharmacology, 136*, 896–904.

Lowy, M. T., Wittenberg, L., & Yamamoto, B. K. (1995). Effect of acute stress on hippocampal glutamate levels and spectrin proteolysis in young and aged rats. *Journal of Neurochemistry, 65*, 268–274.

Lutz, J., Tews, J. K., & Harper, A. E. (1975). Stimulated amino acid imbalance and histidine transport in rat brain slices. *American Journal of Physiology, 229*, 229–234.

Majewski, H., Alade, P. I., & Rand, M. J. (1986). Adrenaline and stress-induced increases in blood pressure in rats. *Clinical and Experimental Pharmacology and Physiology, 13*, 283–288.

Makino, S., Hashimoto, K., & Gold, P. W. (2002). Multiple feedback mechanisms activating corticotropin-releasing hormone system in the brain during stress. *Pharmacology, Biochemistry, and Behavior, 73*, 147–158.

Martins, J. M., Banks, W. A., & Kastin, A. J. (1997a). Acute modulation of the active carrier-mediated brain to blood transport of corticotropin-releasing hormone. *American Journal of Physiology, 272*, E312–E319.

Martins, J. M., Banks, W. A., & Kastin, A. J. (1997b). Transport of CRH from mouse brain directly affects peripheral production of β-endorphin by the spleen. *American Journal of Physiology, 273*, E1083–E1089.

Martins, J. M., Kastin, A. J., & Banks, W. A. (1996). Unidirectional specific and modulated brain to blood transport of corticotropin-releasing hormone. *Neuroendocrinology, 63*, 338–348.

Metcalfe, D. D., Baram, D., & Mekori, Y. A. (1997). Mast cells. *Physiology Revues, 77*, 1033–1079.

Moghaddam, B. (1993). Stress preferentially increases extraneuronal levels of excitatory amino acids in the prefrontal cortex: Comparison to hippocampus and basal ganglia. *Journal of Neurochemistry, 60*, 1650–1657.

Nakagawa, R., Tanaka, M., Kohno, Y., Noda, Y., & Nagasaki, N. (1981). Regional responses of rat brain noradrenergic neurones to acute intense stress. *Pharmacology, Biochemistry, and Behavior, 14*, 729–732.

Nemeroff, C. B., & Crisley, F. D. (1975). Monosodium L-glutamate-induced convulsions: Temporary alteration in blood-brain barrier permeability to plasma proteins. *Environmental Physiology and Biochemistry, 5*, 389–395.

Oldendorf, W. H. (1971). Brain uptake of radio-labelled amino acids, amines and hexoses after arterial injection. *American Journal of Physiology, 221*, 1629–1639.

Oldendorf, W. H., & Szabo, J. (1976). Amino acid assignment to one of three blood-brain barrier amino acid carriers. *American Journal of Physiology, 230*, 94–98.

Oztas, B., Erkin, E., Dural, E., & Isbir, T. (2000). Influence of antioxidants on blood-brain barrier permeability during adrenaline-induced hypertension. *International Journal of Neuroscience, 105*, 27–35.

Oztas, B., Kucuk, M., & Sandalci, U. (1985). Effect of insulin-induced hypoglycemia on blood-brain barrier permeability. *Experimental Neurology, 87*, 129–136.

Pardridge, W. M. (2001). *Brain drug targeting: The future of brain drug development.* Cambridge, UK: Cambridge University Press.

Pardridge, W. M. (2002). Drug and gene delivery to the brain: The vascular route. *Neuron, 36*, 555–558.

Pardridge, W. M., & Oldendorf, W. H. (1975). Kinetic analysis of blood-brain barrier transport of amino acids. *Biochimica et Biophysica Acta, 401*, 128–136.

Peng, Y., Gubin, J., Harper, A. E., Vavich, M. G., & Kemmerer, A. R. (1973). Food intake regulation: Amino acid toxicity and changes in rat brain and plasma amino acids. *Journal of Nutrition, 103*, 608–617.

Peng, Y., Tews, J. K., & Harper, A. E. (1972). Amino acid imbalance, protein intake, and changes in rat brain and plasma amino acids. *American Journal of Physiology, 222*, 314–321.

Pratt, O. E. (1976). The transport of metabolizable substances into the living brain. *Advances in Experimental Medicine and Biology, 69*, 55–75.

Rosch, P. J. (1979). Stress and illness. *Journal of the American Medical Association, 242*, 417–418.

Saija, A., Princi, P., De Pasquale, R., & Costa, G. (1988). High intensity light exposure increases blood-brain barrier transport in rats. *Pharmacological Research Communications, 20*, 553–559.

Sharma, H. S., Cervos-Navarro, J., & Dey, P. K. (1991). Increased blood brain barrier permeability following acute short-term swimming exercise in conscious normotensive young rats. *Neuroscience Research, 10*, 211–221.

Sharma, H. S., Nyberg, F., Cervos-Navarro, J., & Dey, P. K. (1992). Histamine modulates heat stress-induced changes in blood-brain barrier permeability, cerebral blood flow, brain oedema and serotonin levels: An experimental study in conscious young rats. *Neuroscience, 50*, 445–454.

Sharma, H. S., Westman, J., Navarro, J. C., Dey, P. K., & Nyberg, F. (1995). Probable involvement of serotonin in the increased permeability of the blood-brain barrier by forced swimming. An experimental study using Evans blue and ^{131}I-sodium tracers in the rat. *Behavior and Brain Research, 72*, 189–196.

Skultetyova, I., Tokarev, D., & Jezova, D. (1998). Stress-induced increase in blood-brain barrier permeability in control and monosodium glutamate-treated rats. *Brain Research Bulletin, 45*, 175–178.

Tews, J. K. (1986) Competition among amino acids for transport into brain: Relationships with diet. *Federal Proceedings, 45*, 2445–2447.

Tews, J. K., Bradford, A. M., & Harper, A. E. (1981). Induction of lysine imbalance in rats: Relationships between tissue amino acids and diet. *Journal of Nutrition, 111*, 968–978.

Tews, J. K., Good, S. S., & Harper, A. E. (1978). Transport of threonine and tryptophan by rat brain slices: Relation to other amino acids at concentrations found in plasma. *Journal of Neurochemistry, 31*, 581–589.

Tews, J. K., & Harper, A. E. (1983). Atypical amino acids inhibit histidine, valine, or lysine transport into rat brain. *American Journal of Physiology, 245*, R556–R563.

Tews, J. K., Kim, Y. W., & Harper, A. E. (1980). Induction of threonine imbalance by dispensable amino acids: Relationships between tissue amino acids and diet in rats. *Journal of Nutrition, 110*, 394–408.

Theoharides, T. C., Singh, L. K., Boucher, W., Pang, X., Letourneau, R., Webster, E., & Chrousos, G. (1998). Corticotropin-releasing hormone induces skin mast cell degranulation and increased vascular permeability, a possible explanation for its proinflammatory effects. *Endocrinology, 139*, 403–413.

Theoharides, T. C., Spanos, C., Pang, X., Alferes, L., Ligris, K., Letourneau, R., Rozniecki, J. J., Webster, E., & Chrousos, G. P. (1995). Stress-induced intracranial mast cell degranulation: A corticotropin-releasing hormone-mediated effect. *Endocrinology, 136*, 5745–5750.

Vanitallie, T. B. (2002). Stress: A risk factor for serious illness. *Metabolism, 51*, 40–45.

Vinogradova, O. S. (2001). Hippocampus as comparator: Role of the two input and two output systems of the hippocampus in selection and registration of information. *Hippocampus, 11*, 578–598.

Webster, E. L., Lewis, D. B., Torpy, D. J., Zachman, E. K., Rice, K. C., & Chrousos, G. P. (1996). In vivo and in vitro characterization of antalarmin, a nonpeptide corticotropin-releasing hormone (CRH) receptor antagonist: Suppression of pituitary ACTH release and peripheral inflammation. *Endocrinology, 137*, 5747–5750.

Wisniewski, H. M., Vorbrodt, A. W., & Wegiel, J. (1997). Amyloid angiopathy and blood-brain barrier changes in Alzheimer's disease. *Annals of the New York Academy of Sciences, 826*, 161–172.

Zhuang, X., Silverman, A. J., & Silver, R. (1990). Brain mast cell degranulation regulates blood-brain barrier. *Journal of Neurobiology, 31*, 393–403.

II Nutrients and Stress

6 Essential Fatty Acids and Stress

Shlomo Yehuda, Sharon Rabinovitz, and David I. Mostofsky

KEY POINTS

- Polyunsaturated fatty acid effects are mediated by changes in the neuronal membrane.
- Cortisol levels are reduced and hippocampal receptors are protected by polyunsaturated fatty acids.
- Polyunsaturated fatty acids exert direct effects on brain neurotransmitters.
- Polyunsaturated fatty acids may act as signal transducers in the membrane and synapse.
- Effective clinical changes by polyunsaturated fatty acid supplementation in a number of serious neurological disorders have been demonstrated, and the potential for human application appears promising.

1. INTRODUCTION

This chapter reviews the role of fatty acids (FA) in the neurobiology of stress, the psychological and medical consequences of FA deficiency, and the treatment potential for FA supplementation.

2. ESSENTIAL FATTY ACIDS

The popular press routinely reports medical advisories urging the public to dramatically reduce the amount of fat they consume in order to combat risks associated with cardiovascular disease, diabetes, and other chronic disorders. Paradoxically, deficiencies in fat intake are likely to contribute to health hazards, including increased risk of infection, dysregulation of chronobiological activity, and impaired cognitive and sensory functions, especially in infants (Yehuda, Rabinovitz, & Mostofsky, 1997). The conflicting roles of cholesterol (e.g., "good" cholesterol and "bad" cholesterol) have been reviewed elsewhere (Joseph, Villalobos-Molinas, Denisova, Erat, & Strain, 1997). A consensus from recent research suggests that it is not so much the amount of fat we eat as the balance of the different types of fats that is significant. The type of dietary fat affects how well the cell can perform its vital functions and its ability to resist disease.

Linoleic and α-linolenic acids (ALAs), both polyunsaturated fatty acids (PUFAs), are necessary for good health. They are called essential fatty acids (EFAs) because the body

From: *Nutrients, Stress, and Medical Disorders*
Edited by: S. Yehuda and D. I. Mostofsky © Humana Press Inc., Totowa, NJ

cannot manufacture or synthesize them—they must be provided by nutritional intake. EFAs are involved in energy production, transfer of oxygen from the air to the bloodstream, and the manufacture of hemoglobin. Above all they are essential for normal nerve impulse transmission and brain function. They are also involved in growth, cell division, and nerve function and are found in high concentrations in the brain.

EFAs have beneficial effects when available in moderation. Excesses of the otherwise beneficial FAs may, however, exert harmful effects, with high intakes of saturated and hydrogenated fats being linked to an increase in a number of health risks, including degenerative diseases, cardiovascular disease, cancer, and diabetes.

3. POLYUNSATURATED FATTY ACIDS

Linoleic acid is a member of the family of ω-6 (*n*-6) FAs, whereas ALA is an ω-3 (*n*-3) FA. These terms refer to characteristics in the chemical structure of the FAs. Other ω-6 FAs, such as γ-linolenic acid (GLA), dihomo-GLA (DHGLA), and arachidonic acid (AA), can be manufactured in the body using linoleic acid as a starting point. Similarly, other ω-3 FAs that are manufactured in the body, using ALA as a starting point, include eicosapentaenoic acid (EPA) and docosahexaenoic acid (DHA).

Among the significant components of cell membranes are the phospholipids, which contain FAs. The types of FAs in the diet determine the types of FAs that are available for the composition of cell membranes. A phospholipid made from a saturated fat has a different structure and is less fluid than one that incorporates an EFA. In addition, linoleic acids and ALAs *per se* have an effect on the neuronal membrane fluidity index. They are able to decrease the cholesterol level in the neuronal membrane, which would otherwise decrease membrane fluidity, which in turn would make it difficult for the cell to carry out its normal functions and increase its susceptibility to injury and death. These effects on cell function are not restricted to absolute levels of FAs alone, rather it appears that the relative amounts of ω-3 FAs and ω-6 FAs in the cell membranes are responsible for affecting cellular function. At a more molar level, the behavioral and physiological effects of a specific ratio of *n*-3/*n*-6 compound (1:4) correlate with changes in the FA profile and with changes in the cholesterol level (Yehuda, Rabinovitz, & Mostofsky, 1999).

At least six categories of PUFA effects on brain functions have been noted and discussed elsewhere namely (a) modifications of membrane fluidity, (b) modifications of the activity of membrane-bound enzymes, (c) modifications of the number and affinity of receptors, (d) modifications of the function of ion channels, (e) modifications of the production and activity of neurotransmitters, and (f) signal transduction, which controls the activity of neurotransmitters and neuronal growth factors (Yehuda et al., 1999).

The symptoms of EFA deficiency include fatigue, dermatological problems, immune problems, weakness, gastrointestinal disorders, heart and circulatory problems, growth retardation, and sterility. In addition, a lack of dietary EFAs has been implicated in the development or aggravation of breast cancer, prostate cancer, rheumatoid arthritis, asthma, preeclampsia, depression, schizophrenia, and attention deficit and hyperactivity disorders (ADHD) (Yehuda et al., 1997). This list is neither exhaustive nor conclusive.

4. PROSTAGLANDINS

EFAs are a special class of unsaturated FAs that act as precursors of yet other types of FAs. Most prostaglandins are derivatives of AA, itself derived from *n*-6, and all of them have a high physiological hormone-like activity level. They are involved in numerous brain functions, such as regional blood flow and permeability of various biological membranes. It has been suggested that prostaglandins are also involved in the activity of cyclic AMP (cAMP), a second messenger in the cells (Joo, 1993). It is a promising conjecture that a compound of *n*-3/*n*-6 at a 1:4 ratio may affect the prostaglandin system as well and may mediate the behavioral and biochemical changes observed in the rat. There is also evidence that prostaglandin (PG) D2 has a profound effect on sleep (Fadda, Martellotta, De Montis, Gessa, & Fratta, 1992; Fradda, Martellotta, Gessa, & Fratta, 1993; Gabbita, Butterfield, Hensley, Shaw, & Carney, 1995; Ongini, Bonizzoni, Ferri, Milani, & Trampus, 1995). Prostaglandins enhance corticotropin-releasing factor (CRF) activity (Behan et al., 1996, Lacroix & Rivest, 1996; Thompson, Keelan, & Clandinin, 1991; Watanabe, Clark, Ceriani, & Lipton, 1994), and CRF induces release of prostaglandins (Petraglia et al., 1995). Prostaglandins enhance thyrotropin-releasing hormone (TRH) release and stimulate dopaminergic and noradrenergic receptor activity (Murray & Lynch, 1998, Yamaguchi & Hama, 1993), whereas β-endorphin inhibits prostaglandin synthesis (Gelfand, Wepsic, Parker, & Jadus, 1995).

5. CHOLESTEROL AND FATTY ACIDS

Cholesterol, a complex lipid, is involved with many functions of the membrane. Cholesterol decreases the membrane fluidity index, with consequences on the activity of ion channels and receptor functions, and is involved in dopamine release. Moreover, cholesterol is a key molecule in the end product of the CRF–adrenocorticotropic hormone (ACTH) axis. Because steroids are derivatives of cholesterol, it is notable that various FAs have different effects on cholesterol metabolism. Huang, Koba, Horrobin, and Sugano (1993) cited studies confirming that the administration of *n*-6 FAs reduces cholesterol levels in the blood serum. However, *n*-6 FAs and *n*-3 FAs differ in their mode of action in cholesterol reduction, such that *n*-6 FAs redistribute cholesterol, whereas *n*-3 FAs, actually reduce the levels of cholesterol in the neuronal membrane (Horrocks & Harder, 1983). This may explain why a decrease in cholesterol level in the blood is found in humans who consume *n*-3 FA supplements. It has been demonstrated that *n*-3 EFAs are more effective in reducing cholesterol levels in macrophages than *n*-6 EFAs, probably because of the effects on acyl-coenzyme A (acyl-CoA) activity. However, Horrocks and Harder (1983) indicated that cholesterol-esterifying enzymes that incorporate free FAs into cholesterol esters without the participation of CoA are also present in the rat brain.

The mechanism by which *n*-3 FAs are able to reduce cholesterol levels is unclear, although several hypotheses have been proposed. For example, Bourre et al. (1991) claim that ALA controls the composition of nerve membranes, which implies an inverse relationship between ALA and cholesterol level. Salem and Niebylski (1995) propose that DHA (22:6 *n*-3) controls the level of cholesterol as well as the composition and function of the neuronal membrane. We recently reviewed a number of studies that provide support for a reduction in neuronal membrane cholesterol by dietary supplementation of an *n*-3/*n*-6 compound of 1:4 (Yehuda & Carasso, 1993). It is possible that such a ratio optimizes the uptake of PUFAs into the brain and promotes FA incorporation into the neuronal membranes.

6. SPECIFIC FATTY ACIDS AND THE RATIO BETWEEN VARIOUS FATTY ACIDS

Various FAs operate differently in the nervous system and in the body, and it has been suggested that the nervous system has an absolute molecular species requirement for its proper function (Salem & Niebylski, 1995). Studies in our laboratory seem to confirm this suggestion and provide an added qualifying requirement, namely, the need for a proper ratio between the EFAs. We tested our hypothesis that the ratio of *n*-3 and *n*-6 may be a key factor in modulating behavioral and neuropharmacological effects of PUFAs, and attempted to identify the optimal ratio (Yehuda & Carasso, 1993). To avoid the variations in the composition of FAs that occur in commercially prepared oils and to exclude the possible confounding effects of other FA or lipid admixtures, we used highly purified α-linolenic and linoleic acids. We tested a wide range of α-linolenic/linoleic acid (1:3, 1:3.5, 1:4, 1:4.5, 1:5, 1:5.5, 1:6 [vol/vol]) ratios, which were administered as dietary supplements. We found that a mixture of α-linolenic and linoleic acids at a 1:4 ratio was most effective in improving learning performance (as assessed by the Morris water maze), elevating pain threshold, improving sleep, and improving thermoregulation (Yehuda & Carasso, 1993; Yehuda, Rabinovitz, & Mostofsky, 1997). This compound was also able to correct learning deficits induced by the neurotoxins AF64A and 5,7-dihydroxytryptamine (Yehuda, Carasso, & Mostofsky, 1995) and to provide protection from seizures induced by pentylenetetrazol (Yehuda, Carasso, & Mostofsky, 1994). The special supplement also provided protection from blepharospasm, which could otherwise be induced by Ro4-1284 (Yehuda et al., 1999). In addition, our study showed that the administration of this compound exerted beneficial effects in rats given a diluted dose of the experimental allergic encephalomyelitis (EAE) toxin. The untreated EAE rats showed learning and motor deficits as well as major changes in the FA profile and cholesterol level in frontal cortex synaptosomes. FA treatment was able to rehabilitate the changes induced by EAE toxin to a significant degree, but was unable to completely reverse the deficits to the level of normal controls (Yehuda et al., 1999). In addition, although old (22–24 mo) rats performed very poorly in the Morris water maze, following pretreatment with SR-3 their level of performance was substantially improved.

The importance of differentiation among the various types of FAs may be appreciated from noting their effects on immunological factors: *n*-3 FAs suppress the synthesis of interleukin (IL)-1and IL-6 and enhance the synthesis of IL-2, whereas *n*-6 FAs have the opposite effect. It should be recalled that both IL- 6 and IL-1(and to a lesser degree IL-2) promote CRF release via AA (Cambronero, Rivas, Borrell, and Guaza, 1992; Karanath, Lyson, Aguila, & McCann, 1995; Rivier, 1995). However, CRF inhibits the stimulating effect of IL-1 on prostaglandin synthesis (Fleisher-Berkovich & Danon, 1995; Oka, Aou, & Hori, 1993).

7. PEPTIDE INTERACTIONS WITH $P450_{SCC}$, PROSTAGLANDINS, CHOLESTEROL, AND FATTY ACIDS

In light of the studies reviewed above, it seems that the various FAs and lipids play a major role in the synthesis, release, and function of several peptides, especially those connected with releasing factors. For example, in the analysis of the CRF–ACTH–steroid axis, metabolism of enzyme P450 and cholesterol has been shown to exert profound effects on dopamine at the beginning of the axis and on steroids at the end of the axis (Makita, Falck, & Capdevila, 1996). Prostaglandins are derivatives of FAs, but their metabolism is modulated by P450. Prostaglandins are involved in the metabolism and functions of all neurotransmitters (including dopamine), CRF, and steroids. The interaction between prostaglandins and ACTH is not yet clear. Cholesterol is a major molecule in the membrane, and an elevated level of cholesterol results in a decrease in membrane fluidity and a disturbance of membrane function. In addition, steroids are derivatives of cholesterol. Many studies have demonstrated the role of specific FAs (mainly essential FAs of *n*-3 and *n*-6 groups) in all aspects of synthesis, release, and receptor functions of dopamine, CRF, ACTH, and steroids.

8. EFA RATIO AND STRESS

We examined the effects of a mixture of FAs on cortisol and cholesterol levels under laboratory conditions of stress (Yehuda et al., 1999). A compound of free nonesterified unsaturated FAs α-linolenic and linolenic acids at a 1:4 ratio was administered for 3 wk prior to the injection of cortisone (10 mg/kg) or prior to immersion of rats in a 10°C saline bath. The results confirmed the expected elevation of cortisol and cholesterol levels in stress, but more importantly the treatment prevented the elevation of blood levels of cortisol and cholesterol found in untreated control animals. Similarly, Morris water maze learning performance among the pretreated animals did not reflect deficits that usually accompany such stressful conditions and that can be observed in the absence of the SR-3 pretreatment.

9. PUFAS AND THE IMMUNE SYSTEM

Repeated demonstrations that PUFAs can modify the production and activity of various components of the immune system have left unexplained the mode of action by which they exert their effects. PUFA mediation of immunological functions and cytokine level is evident in several disorders such as Alzheimer's disease and schizophrenia (Yao & Van Kammen, 2004). Several mechanisms had been proposed, including membrane fluidity (changes that might effect the capability of cytokines to bind to their respective receptors on the cell membrane), lipid peroxidation (decrease in free-radical-induced tissue damage); prostaglandin production (an indirect mechanism whereby prostaglandins, which are derivatives of PUFAs, modify cytokine activity); and regulation of gene expression (PUFA influences on the signal transudation pathways and modified mRNA activity). The role of PUFAs in immune function is complicated by the fact that *n*-3 and *n*-6 have differential effects on various immune components. In a recent review, Singer and Richterheinrich (1991) indicated that *n*-3 FAs induce a decrease in lymphocyte proliferation in humans and rats, a decrease in IL-1 production, and a decrease in IL-2 production in both humans and animals. In addition, *n*-3 FAs decrease tumor necrosis factor (TNF)-α production in humans but increases it in mice macrophages and also decreases natural killer (NK) cell activity. On the other hand, *n*-6 increases the production of IL-2 in mice and decreases TNF-α production and NK cell activity. Still other studies have shown that linoleic acid (*n*-6) decreases the activity of IL-2 and increases IL-1 production and tissue response to cytokines (Yehuda et al., 1997), whereas *n*-3 generally decreases IL-1 production and activity (Grimble, 1998). Despite some disagreement among studies, it seems that *n*-3 FAs (ALA, DHA, EPA) decrease the production and activity of the pro-inflammatory cytokines (IL-1, IL-6, TNF-α) (Blok et al., 1997; Chavali, Zhong, & Forse, 1998; Hughes & Pinder, 1997; Yano, Kishida, Iwasaki, Shosuke, & Masuzawa, 2000) and that the *n*-6 family has the opposite effect (Caughey, Mantzioris, Gibson, Cleland, & James, 1996; James, Gibson & Cleland, 2000; Grimble, 1998). The ability of *n*-3 PUFAs to reduce pro inflammatory cytokines and prostaglandin (Chavali & Forse, 1999) led to the proposal for the use of fish oil to relieve pain. Indeed, fish oil rich in *n*-3 PUFAs has been shown to decrease IL-6, IL-10, IL-12, TNF-α, and PG E_2 (Denisova, Cantuti-Castelvetri, Hassan, Paulson, & Joseph, 2001).

Increasingly, the salutary effects of PUFAs are being examined not only with respect to their absolute level in diet, supplementation, or serum and tissue content, but also with respect to their proportional relationship to other FAs. One example of the critical nature and importance of a proper ratio can be seen in the level of anti-inflammatory IL-2 production, which increases following treatment with a mixture of FAs (*n*-3:*n*-6 ratio 1:3) (Yehuda et al., 1999) together with an increase in *n*-3 in the tissue (James et al., 2000).

10. STRESS

In psychology and biology the term "stress" is applied to describe a strain or interference that disturbs and jeopardizes the functioning of an organism. Organisms, including humans, respond to physical and psychological stress with behavioral and physiological defenses. If the stress is too powerful, too prolonged, or is perceived as too threatening, or if the defenses are inadequate, then a somatic or comparable dysfunction may be expressed.

Outside the laboratory stress is accepted as an unavoidable effect of living and is an especially complex phenomenon in the modern technological society. Although many may profess to thrive in a stressful environment, there is little doubt that an individual's success or failure in controlling stressful situations (real or perceived) can have a profound effect on his or her ability to function. The ability to cope successfully with stress has figured prominently in anxiety and psychosomatic research. Stress has figured prominently in discussions of areas of health psychology or behavioral medicine. A statistical link between coronary heart disease and individuals with a particular personality profile characterized by a behavioral pattern that manifests a lifestyle of impatience, a sense of time urgency, hard-driving competitiveness, and a preoccupation with vocational and related deadlines (type A personality) (Rosenman, 1997) has been widely reported. Similar correlations with other behavior profiles have suggested potential links to cancer, diabetes, and other chronic medical conditions. Although different types of stress can be identified, the following discussion is limited to psychological stress.

11. EFAS AND STRESS

As early as 1964, Back and Bogdanoff (1964) reported elevations of free FAs and cholesterol among stressed persons. Rosenman (1997) summarized many years of research on cholesterol levels among type A behavior subjects. Subsequent studies confirmed the correlation between stressful situations and an increased level of cholesterol and free FAs (Arbogast, Neumann, Arbogast, Leeper, & Kostrzema, 1994; Brennan, Cobb, Silbert, Watkins, & Maier, 1996; Clark, Moore, & Adams, 1998; Mills, Prkachin, Harvey, & Ward, 1989). It is not surprising, therefore, to observe that dietary intake of soybean oil and fish oil has stress-reduction properties (Ulmann, Mimouni, Roux, Porsolt, & Poisson, 2001). A striking exception is the report that stressed medical students exhibited lower levels of linoleic and AAs (*n*-6), with no change in *n*-3 FAs (Ohno, Ohinata, Ogawa, & Kuroshima, 1996; Williams, Kiecolt Glaser, Horrocks, Hillhouse, & Glaser, 1992). Stress was also shown to modify several key steps in FA and lipid metabolism (Matsmoto et al., 1999; Mills, Huang, Narce, & Poisson, 1994). It is of interest to note that the hormones released during stress (both catecholamines and glucocorticoids) serve as strong inhibitors of the first desaturase reaction, which converts linoleic and ALAs to longer-chained FAs. Mills et al. (1994) reported this finding in rats subjected to psychosocial stress. One way to overcome the blocked biochemical step is to administer GLA to stressed patients, which bypasses the blocked step in the *n*-6 essential FA pathway and thereby reduces the elevated blood pressure and elevated catecholamine levels (Mills et al., 1989). On the other hand, administration of linoleic and ALAs reduced the elevated cortisol level (Youdim, Martin, & Joseph, 2000).

In addition, during stress the cardiac uptake of free FAs was shown to be reduced (Bagger, Botker, Thomassen, & Nielsen, 1997). Administration of DHA (an *n*-3 derivative) improved cardiac response to stress (Rossetti, Seiler, DeLuca, Laposata, & Zurier, 1997), decreased the level of aggression (Hamazaki et al.,1996; Sawazaki, Hamazaki, Yazawa, & Kobayashi, 1999), decreased stress responses (Hamazaki et al., 1999; Sawasaki et al., 1999; Singer & Richterheinrich, 1991), and decreased the level of prostaglandin E2 (Deutch, 1995; Rossetti et al., 1997).

12. MEMBRANE FLUIDITY

Membrane fluidity is dependent on lipid composition. The protein component is very stable, but the lipid component has a high turnover rate. More specifically, fluidity depends on (a) the transition temperature (i.e., the temperature at which the membrane is converted from the fluid to the gel state) and (b) tight packing (where unsaturated FAs lower the transition temperature and cholesterol changes the sharp transition temperature and disturbs packing by membrane insertion). It seems that the critical transition temperature may change during aging along with an increase in cholesterol. The membrane fluidity index can also be regulated by neurons in a number of ways, such as (a) desaturation of FAs or (b) transferring of FAs between molecules (e.g., Colles et al., 1995; Regev, Assaraf, & Eytan, 1999; Strosznajder, Chalimoniuk, Strosznajder, Albanese, & Alberghina, 1996). It is interesting to note that pretreatment with an *n*-6 PUFA diet prevents the fluidizing effect of alcohol on the neuronal membrane (Meehan, Beauge, Choquart, & Leonard, 1995). Local anesthetics (Kopeikina, Kamper, Siafaka, & Stavridis, 1997) and several peptides (Giorgi, Biraghi & Kantar, 1998) can also fluidize the membrane. Finally, factors such as rapid eye movement (REM) sleep deprivation and stress may also induce rigidity in the neural membrane (Mallick, Thakkar, & Gangabhagirathi, 1995).

13. HIPPOCAMPAL VULNERABILITY AND AGING

The hippocampus is centrally involved in spatial learning and memory. Decreased volume and function of the hippocampus have been reported in aged organisms and among Alzheimer's patients. There are sufficient data to conclude that chronic elevation of corticosteroid levels might lead to hippocampal regeneration (de Kloet, Vreugdenhil,

Oitzl, & Joels, 1998), in that high levels of corticosterone and cortisol are toxic to the hippocampus, whereas estradiol protects it. The intact hippocampus plays a major role in the overall inhibitory activity of hypothalamus–pituitary–adrenal (HPA) axis activities. Accordingly, it has a protective role in stress situations. The response to stress mediated via CRF, ACTH, or corticosterone (or cortisol) is enhanced and prolonged in aging, compared to young animals. In addition, the level of the involved molecules in aging animals returned very slowly to normal. Even without a stressor, the level of corticosterone in aged rats is elevated. De Kloet et al. (1998) found a reduced number of mineralocorticoid receptors (MRs) and glycocorticoid receptors (GRs) in the aged hippocampus. He proposed that the normal feedback mechanism is disintegrated in the hippocampus of aged rats. Only MR-type receptors are involved in stress responses. A preliminary study from our laboratory showed that treatment with a FA compound could prevent structural changes in the hippocampus, decrease corticosterone level, and prevent a decrease in MR-type receptors in stressed young and old rats.

14. CONCLUSION

Although it seems that many studies confirm the involvement of PUFAs in all stages of onset, maintenance, prevention of, and recovery from stress, the mode of action is still unknown. Our own work points to PUFA effects as being mediated via modifications in the neuronal membrane, although it is quite possible that other mechanisms might also be involved. PUFAs are able to reduce cortisol levels and protect hippocampal receptors and have a direct effect on brain neurotransmitters. Our studies have indicated the effects of PUFAs on the brain dopaminergic system. Recently, the role of γ-aminobutyric acid in the control of DHA, cortisol, and CRH levels in stressful situations has been confirmed (Takeuchi, Iwanaga & Harada, 2003). The possible mechanism whereby PUFAs can act as signal transducers in the membrane and in synapses requires further study. Together with the elucidation of this role of PUFAs and platelet-activating factor (Bazan, 2003), new directions for future research have been opened.

ACKNOWLEDGMENTS

We would like to thank the William Farber Center for Alzheimer Research and the Rose K. Ginsburg Chair for Research into Alzheimer's disease for their support.

REFERENCES

Arbogast, B. W., Neumann, J. K., Arbogast, L. Y., Leeper, S. C., & Kostrzema, R. M. (1994). Transient loss of serum protective activity following short-term stress: A possible biochemical link between stress and atherosclerosis. *Journal of Psychosomatic Research, 38*, 871–884.

Back, K. W., & Bogdanoff, M. D. (1964). Plasma lipid response to leadership, conformity and deviation. In: P. H. Leiderman, & D. Shapiro (Eds.), *Psychological approach to social behavior* (pp. 24–42). London: Tavistock Publishers.

Bagger, J. P., Botker, H. E., Thomassen, A., & Nielsen, T. T. (1997). Effects of ranolizine on ischemic threshold, coronary sinus blood flow, and myocardial metabolism in coronary artery disease. *Cardiovascular Drugs and Therapy, 11*, 479–484.

Bazan, N. (2003). Synaptic lipid signaling: Significance of polyunsaturated fatty acids and platelet-activating factor. *Journal of Lipid Research, 44*, 2221–2233.

Behan, D. P., Grigoriadis, D. E, Lovenberg, T., Chalmers, D., Heinrichs, S., Liaw, C., & De Souza, E. B. (1996). Neurobiology of corticotropin releasing factor (CRF) receptors and CRF-binding protein: Implications for the treatment of CNS disorders. *Molecular Psychiatry, 1*, 265–277.

Blok, W. L., Deslypere, J. P., Demacker, P. N., van der Ven-Jongekrijg, J., Hectors, M. P., van der Meer, J. W., & Katan, M.B. (1997). Pro- and anti-inflammatory cytokines in healthy volunteers fed various doses of fish oil for 1 year. *European Journal of Clinical Investigation, 27*, 1003–1008.

Bourre, J. M., Dumont, O., Piciotti, M., Clement, M., Chaudiere, J., Bonneil, M., Nalbone, G., Lafont, H., Pascal, G., & Durand, G. (1991). Essentiality of w3 fatty acids for brain structure and function. *World Review of Nutrition, 66*, 103–117.

Brennan, F. X., Cobb, C. L., Silbert, L. E., Watkins, L. R., & Maier, S. F. (1996). Peripheral beta-adrenoreceptors and stress-induced hypercholesterolemia in rats. *Physiology and Behavior, 60*, 1307–1310.

Cambronero, J. C., Rivas, F. J., Borrell, J., & Guaza, C. (1992). Role of arachidonic acid metabolism on corticotropin-releasing factor (CRF)-release induced by interleukin-1 from superfused rat hypothalami. *Journal of Neuroimmunology, 39*, 57–66.

Caughey, G. E., Mantzioris, E., Gibson, R. A., Cleland, L. G., & James, M. J. (1996). The effect on human tumor necrosis factor alpha and interleukin-1 beta production of diets enriched in n-3 fatty acids from vegetable oil or fish oil. *The American Journal of Clinical Nutrition, 63*, 116–122.

Chavali, S. R., & Forse, R. A. (1999). Decreased production of interleukin-6 and prostoglandin E2 associated with inhibition of delta-5 desaturation of omega-6 fatty acids in mice fed safflower oil diets supplemented with sesamol. *Prostaglandins, Leukotrienes, and Essential Fatty Acids, 61*, 347–352.

Chavali, S. R., Zhong, W. W., & Forse, R. A. (1998). Dietary alpha-linolenic acid increases TNF_{alpha}, and decreases IL-6, IL-10 in response to LPS: effects of sesamin on the delta-5 desaturation of omega-6 and omega-3 fatty acids in mice. *Prostaglandins, Leukotrienes, and Essential Fatty Acids, 58*, 185–191.

Clark, V. R., Moore, C. L., & Adams, J. H. (1998). Cholesterol concentrations and cardiovascular reactivity to stress in African American college volunteers. *Journal of Behavioral Medicine, 21*, 505–515.

Colles, S., Wood, W. G., Myers-Payne, S. C., Igbavboa, U., Avdulov, N. A., Joseph, J., & Schroeder, F. (1995). Structure and polarity of mouse brain synaptic plasma membrane: effects of ethanol in vitro and in vivo. *Neuroscience Research, 22*, 117–122.

de Kloet, E. R., Vreugdenhil, E., Oitzl, M. S., & Joels, M. (1998). Brain corticosteroid receptor balance in health and disease. *Endocrine Reviews, 19*, 269–301.

Denisova, N. A., Cantuti-Castelvetri, I., Hassan, W. N., Paulson, K. E. & Joseph, J. A. (2001). Role of membrane lipids in regulation of vulnerability to oxidative stress in PC12 cells: Implication for aging. *Free Radical Biology & Medicine, 30*, 671–678.

Deutch, B. (1995). Menstrual pain in Danish women correlated with low n-3 polyunsaturated fatty acid intake. *European Journal of Clinical Nutrition, 49*, 508–516.

Fadda, P., Martellotta, M. C., De Montis, M. G., Gessa, G. L., & Fratta, W. (1992). Dopamine D1 and opioid receptor binding changes in the limbic system of sleep deprived rats. *Neurochemistry International, 20*, 153S–156S.

Fadda, P., Martellotta, M. C., Gessa, G. L., & Fratta, W. (1993). Dopamine and opioids interactions in sleep deprivation. *Progress in Neuro Psychopharmacology Biological Psychiatry, 17*, 269–278.

Fleisher-Berkovich, S., & Danon, A. (1995). Effect of corticotropin-releasing factor on prostaglandin synthesis in endothelial cells and fibroblasts. *Endocrinology, 136*, 4068–4072.

Gabbita, S. P., Butterfield, D. A., Hensley, K., Shaw, W., & Carney, J. M. (1997). Aging and caloric restriction affect mitochondrial respiration and lipid membrane status: An electron paramagnetic resonance investigation. *Free Radical Biology & Medicinem, 23*, 191–201.

Gelfand, R. A., Wepsic, H. T., Parker, L. N., & Jadus, M. R. (1995). Prostaglandin E2 induces up-regulation of murine macrophage beta-endorphin receptors. *Immunology Letters, 45*, 143–148.

Grimble, R. F. (1998). Dietary lipids and the inflammatory response. *The Proceedings of the Nutrition Society, 57*, 535–542.

Giorgi, P. L., Biraghi, M., & Kantar, A. (1998). Effect of desmopressin on rat brain synaptosomal membranes: A pilot study. *Current Therapeutic Research, Clinical and Experimental, 59*, 172–178.

Hamazaki, T., Sawazaki, S., Itomura, M., Asaoka, E., Nagao, Y., Nishimura, N., Yazawa, K., Kuwamori, T., & Kobayashi, M. (1996). The effect of docosahexaenoic acid on aggression in young adults. A placebo- controlled double- blind study. *The Journal of Clinical Investigation, 97*, 1129–1133.

Hamazaki, T., Sawazaki, S., Nagasawa, T., Nagao, Y., Kanagawa, Y., & Yazawa, K. (1999). Administration of docosahexaenoic acid influence behavior and plasma catecholamine levels at times of psychological stress. *Lipids, 34*, S33–S37.

Horrocks, L. A., & Harder, H. W. (1983). Fatty acids and cholesterol. In A. Lajtha, (Ed.), *Handbook of neurochemistry* (pp. 1–16). New York: Plenum.

Huang, Y. S., Koba, K., Horrobin, D. F., & Sugano, M. (1993). Interrelationship between dietary protein, cholesterol and n-6 polyunsaturated fatty acid metabolism. *Progress in Lipid Research, 32*, 123–137.

Hughes, D. A., & Pinder, A. C. (1997). N-3 polyunsaturated fatty acids modulate the expression of functionally associated molecules on human monocytes and inhibit antigen- presentation in vitro. *Journal of Clinical and Experimental Psychopathology, 110*, 516–523.

James, M. J., Gibson, R. A., & Cleland, L. G. (2000). Dietary polyunsaturated fatty acids and inflammatory mediator production. *American Journal of Clinical Nutrition, 71*, 343s–348s.

Joo, F. Brain microvascular cyclic nucleotides and protein phosphorylation. In W. M. Pardridge (Ed.) *Blood brain barrier, cellular and molecular biology* (pp. 267–287). New York: Raven.

Joseph, J. A., Villalobos-Molinas, R., Denisova, N. A., Erat, S., & Strain, J. (1997). Cholesterol: A two-edged sword in brain aging. *Free Radical Biology & Medicine, 22*, 455–462.

Karanath, S., Lyson, K., Aguila, M. C., & McCann, S. M. (1995). Effects of lutenizing-hormone-releasing hormone, alpha-melanocyte-stimulating hormone, naloxone, dexamethasone and indomethacin on interleukin-2-induced corticotropin-releasing factor release. *Neuroimmunomodulation, 2*, 166–173.

Kopeikina, L. T., Kamper, E. F., Siafaka, I., & Stavridis, J. (1997). Modulation of synaptosomal plasma membrane-bound enzyme activity through the perturbation of plasma membrane lipid structure by bupivacaine. *Anesthesia and Analgesia, 85*, 1337–1343.

Lacroix, S., & Rivest, S. (1996). Role of cyclo-oxygenase pathways in the stimulatory influence of immune challenge on the transcription of a specific CRF receptor subtype in the rat brain. *Journal of Chemical Neuroanatomy, 10*, 53–71.

Makita, K., Falck, J. R., & Capdevila, J. H. (1996). Cytochrome P450, the arachidonic acid cascade, and hypertension: New vistas for an old enzyme system. *The FASEB Journal, 10*, 1456–1463.

Mallick, B. N., Thakkar, M., & Gangabhagirathi, R. (1995). Rapid eye movement sleep deprivation decreases membrane fluidity in the rat brain. *Neuroscience Research, 22*, 117–122.

Matsmoto, K., Yobimoto, K., Huong, N. T., Abdel- Fattah, M., Van Hien, T., & Watanabe, H. (1999). Psychological stress-induced enhancement of brain lipid peroxidation via nitric oxide systems and its modulation by anxiolytic and anxiogenic drugs in mice. *Brain Research, 839*, 74–84.

Meehan, E., Beauge, F., Choquart, D., & Leonard, B. E. (1995). Influence of an n-6 polyunsaturated fatty acid-enriched diet on the development of tolerance during chronic ethanol administration in rats. *Alcoholism, Clinical and Experimental Research, 1*, 1441–1446.

Mills, D. E., Huang, Y. S., Narce, M., & Poisson, J. P. (1994). Psychosocial stress catecholamines, and essential fatty acid metabolism in rats. *Proceedings of the Society for Experimental Biology and Medicine, 205*, 56–61.

Mills, D. E., Prkachin, K. M., Harvey, K. A., & Ward, R. P. (1989). Dietary fatty acid supplementation alters stress reactivity and performance in man. *Journal of Human Hypertension, 3*, 111–116.

Murray, C. A., & Lynch, M. A. (1998). Evidence that increased hippocampal expression of the cytokine interleukin-1 beta is a common trigger for age- and stress-induced impairments in long-term potentiation. *Journal of Neuroscience, 18*, 2974–2981.

Ohno, T., Ohinata, H., Ogawa, K., & Kuroshima, A. (1996) Fatty acid profiles of phospholipids in brown adipose tissue from rats during cold acclimation and repetitive intermittent immobilization. With special reference to docosahexaenoic acid. *Japanese Journal of Physiology, 46*, 265–270.

Oka, T., Aou, S., & Hori, T. (1993). Intracerebroventriculaer injection of interleukin-1 beta induces hyperalgesia in rats. *Brain Research, 624*, 61–68.

Ongini, E., Bonizzoni, E., Ferri, N., Milani, S., & Trampus, M. (1993). Differential effects of dopamine D-1 and D-2 receptor antagonist antipsychotics on sleep-wake patterns in the rat. *The Journal of Pharmacology and Experimental Therapeutics, 266*, 726–731.

Petraglia, F., Benedetto, C., Florio, P., D'Ambrogio, G., Genazzani, A. D., Marozio, L., & Vale, W. (1995). Effect of corticotropin-releasing factor-binding protein on prostaglandin release from cultured maternal decide and on contractile activity of human myometrium in vitro. *The Journal of Clinical Endocrinology and Metabolism, 80*, 3073–3076.

Regev, R., Assaraf, Y. G., & Eytan, G. D. (1999). Membrane fluidization by ether, other anesthetics, and certain agents abolishes P-glycoprotein ATPase activity andmodulates efflux from multidrug-resistant cells. *European Journal of Biochemistry, 258*, 18–24.

Rivier, C. (1995). Influence of immune signals on the hypothalamic-pituitary axis of the rodent. *Frontiers in Neuroendocrinology, 16*, 151–182.

Rosenman, R. H. (1997). Do environmental effects on human emotions cause cardiovascular disorders? *Acta Physiologica Scandinavica. Supplementum, 640*, 133–136.

Rossetti, R. G., Seiler, C. M., DeLuca, P., Laposata, M., & Zurier, R. B. (1997). Oral administration of unsaturated fatty acids: Effects on human peripheral blood T lymphocyte proliferation. *Journal of Leukocyte Biology, 62*, 438–443.

Salem, N., Jr., & Niebylski, C. D. (1995). The nervous system has an absolute molecular species requirement for proper function. *Molecular Membrane Biology, 12*, 131–134.

Sawazaki, S., Hamazaki, T., Yazawa, K., & Kobayashi, M. (1999). The effect of docosahexoaenoic acid on plasma catecholamine concentrations and glucose tolerance during long-lasting psychological stress: A double blind placebo-controlled study. *Journal of Nutritional Science and Vitaminology, 45*, 655–665.

Singer, P., & Richterheinrich, E. (1991). Stress and fatty liver—possible indications for dietary long-chain n-3 fatty acids. *Medical Hypotheses, 36*, 90–94.

Strosznajder, J., Chalimoniuk, M., Strosznajder, R. P., Albanese, V., & Alberghina, M. (1996). Arachidonate transport through the blood-retina and blood-brain barrier of the rat during aging. *Neuroscience Letters, 209*, 145–148.

Takeuchi, T., Iwanaga, M., & Harada, E. (2003). Possible regulatory mechanism of DHA-induced anti-stress reaction in rats. *Brain Research, 964*, 136–143.

Thompson, A. B. R., Keelan, M., & Clandinin, M.T. (1991). Feeding rats a diet enriched with saturated fatty acids presents the inhibitory effects of acute and chromic ethanol exposure on the in vitro uptake of hexoses and lipids. *Biochimica et Biophysica Acta, 1084*, 122–128.

Ulmann, L., Mimouni, V., Roux, S., Porsolt, R., & Poisson, J.P. (2001). Brain and hippocampus fatty acid composition in phospholipid classes of aged-relative cognitive deficit rats. *Prostaglandins, Leukotrienes, and Essential Fatty Acids, 64*, 189–195.

Watanabe, T., Clarck, W. G., Ceriani, G., & Lipton, J.M. (1994). Elevation of plasma ACTH concentration in rabbits made febrile by systemic injection of bacterial endotoxin. *Brain Research, 652*, 201–206.

Williams, L. L., Kiecolt Glaser, J. K., Horrocks, L. A., Hillhouse, J. T., & Glaser, R. (1992). Quantitative association between altered plasma esterfied omega-6 fatty-acid proportions and psychological stress. *Prostaglandins, Leukotrienes, and Essential Fatty Acids, 47*, 165–170.

Yamaguchi, K., & Hama, H. (1993). Evaluation for roles of brain prostaglandins in the catecholamine-induced vasopressin secretion in conscious rats. *Brain Research, 607*, 149–153.

Yano, M., Kishida, E., Iwasaki, M., Shosuke, K., & Masuzawa, Y. (2000). Docosahexaenoic acid and vitamin E can reduce human monocytic U937 cell apoptosis induced by tumor necrosis factor. *Journal of Nutrition, 130*, 1095–1101.

Yao, J. K., & Van Kammen, D. P. (2004). Membrane phospholipids and cytokine interaction in schizophrenia. *International Review of Neurobiology, 59*, 297–326.

Yehuda, S., & Carasso, R. L. (1993). Modulation of learning, pain threshold, and thermoregulation in the rat by preparations of free purified alpha-linoleic and linoleic acids: Determination of optimal n-3 to n-6 ratio. *Proceedings of the National Academy of Sciences of the United States of America, 90*, 10,345–10,349.

Yehuda, S., Carasso, R. L., & Mostofsky, D. I. (1994). Essential fatty acid preparation (SR-3) raises the seizure threshold in rats. *European Journal of Pharmacology, 254*, 193–198.

Yehuda, S., Carasso, R. L., & Mostofsky, D.I. (1995). Essential fatty acid preparation (SR-3) rehabilitates learning deficits induced by AF64A and 5,7-DHT. *NeuroReport, 6*, 511–515.

Yehuda, S., Rabinovitz, S., & Mostofsky, D. I. (1997). Effects of essential fatty acids preparation (SR-3) on brain biochemistry and on behavioral and cognitive functions. In S. Yehuda, & D. I. Mostofsky (Eds.), *Handbook of essential fatty acids biology: biochemistry physiology and behavioral neurobiology* (pp. 427–452). Totowa, NJ: Humana.

Yehuda, S., Rabinovitz S., & Mostofsky, D. I. (1999). Essential fatty acids are mediators of brain biochemistry and cognitive functions. *Journal of Neuroscience Research, 56*, 565–570.

Youdim, K. A., Martin, A., & Joseph, J. A. (2000). Essential fatty acids and the brain: Possible health implications. *International Journal of Developmental Neuroscience, 18*, 383–399.

7 Stress, Glucocorticoids, and the Brain

R. H. DeRijk and E. R. de Kloet

KEY POINTS

- Corticosteroids function to optimize the stress response and are thus essential for the organism to cope with the stressor.
- Corticosteroid signaling is mediated by two receptors: the high-affinity mineralocorticoid receptor and the low-affinity glucocorticoid receptor.
- Imbalance between central glucocorticoid and mineralocorticoid receptor affects the secretion of corticosteroids and has profound consequences for adaptation to stress.
- Single nucleotide polymorphisms in the glucocorticoid receptor gene affect not only corticosteroid production and secretion but also the effects of corticosteroids in different physiological and behavorial systems.
- Other influences such as trauma can permanently alter the glucocorticoid/mineralocorticoid receptor balance.

1. INTRODUCTION

1.1. Stress and Homeostasis

When deviations in physiological or behavioral parameters exceed a certain threshold, central release of corticotropin-releasing hormone (CRH) from the parvocellular neurons of the hypothalamic paraventricular nucleus (PVN) is triggered. CRH activates, in the specific context of the stressor, the sympathetic nervous system and the hypothalamic–pituitary–adrenal (HPA) axis, which promote a series of physiological and behavioral adaptations in order to reestablish homeostasis (McEwen, 1998). Multiple afferents can activate CRH neurons, each conveying specific stressful information. These afferents can be ascending direct innervations from the brainstem that relay stressors of systemic origin (metabolic demands, fluid loss, pain, inflammation). Sensory cognitive and emotional information also reaches via a complex transsynaptic pathway—the PVN (Herman et al., 2003). The summation of all inputs to the PVN provides an output that can be measured as the threshold for activation of these neurons as well as the rate of onset, magnitude and duration of the response. The type of afferent input additionally determines the composition of the cocktail of adrenocorticotropic hormone (ACTH) secretagogs released with CRH in interaction with other stress hormones (e.g., norepinephrine [NE] and epinephrine [E]) (Goldstein, 2003; Herman et al., 2003; Romero &

From: *Nutrients, Stress, and Medical Disorders*
Edited by: S. Yehuda and D. I. Mostofsky © Humana Press Inc., Totowa, NJ

Sapolsky, 1996). This initial CRH-mediated stress reaction is counterbalanced by the stress-induced elevation in circulating levels of glucocorticoids and by parasympathetic nervous system activity. Recently it has been suggested that the CRH-2 receptor system is prominent in the coordination of these later slow responses, facilitating the recovery of homeostasis (Hsu & Hsueh, 2001; Reul & Holsboer, 2002).

1.2. HPA Axis Regulation

Corticosteroids are secreted from the adrenal gland under the control of ACTH of pituitary origin. In turn, ACTH is mainly under the regulatory influence of hypothalamic CRH. In addition, the hippocampus, a limbic brain structure involved in behavioral adaptation, exerts a tonic inhibitory control over these secretagogs. Furthermore, a strong negative feedback effect influences the secretion of ACTH and CRH exerted by cortisol at the level of the pituitary and PVN respectively. Three features with respect to the regulation of the HPA axis need further attention.

First, depending on the nature of the stressor, it seems that different cocktails of ACTH secretagogs, with respect to absolute and relative concentrations, are released from the PVN. ACTH then enters the circulation and induces the production and secretion of corticosteroids from the adrenal glands—predominantly cortisol in humans and corticosterone in rodents. Both physical and psychosocial stimuli—real, anticipated, or imagined—that modulate emotional and cognitive processes can be stressors. This processing of psychosocial information occurs in the so-called limbic structures, including the amygdala, hippocampus, and frontal cortex, which modulate CRH release transsynaptically via a γ-aminobutyric acid (GABA)-ergic network surrounding the PVN (Herman, Cullinan, Ziegler, & Tasker, 2002). Collectively, the PVN integrates the inhibitory and excitatory signals producing its cocktail of ACTH secretagogs (Windle, Wood, Shanks, Lightman, & Ingram, 1998; Goldstein, 2003).

A second important feature of the HPA axis is the existence of an ultradian rhythm of about one pulse per hour resulting in phasic release of hormones (Lightman et al., 2000). It is unlikely that levels of CBG are changing rapidly enough to counteract the dynamic fluctuation in total plasma corticosteroids, suggesting the same large fluctuations for free plasma corticosteroids (Windle et al., 1998). The pulse generator seems localized in the hypothalamus, but its identity is largely unknown. However, at the level of the adrenals important modulations occur through a transsynaptic descending pathway from the suprachiasmatic pacemaker (Kalsbeek & Buijs, 2002). This nervous input changes adrenal sensitivity to ACTH in a circadian fashion. Altered ultradian rhythms are observed, and recent studies suggest that previous early experiences as well as the nature of the stressor are important determinants for HPA axis pulsatility. It is thought that the pattern (e.g., fast short-lasting vs slow long-lasting increase) rather than the absolute amount of circulating stress hormone is the important determinant in adaptive or maladaptive effects of HPA axis activation.

Third, corticosteroids target those stress centers in the brain involved in adaptive responses and regulation of the HPA axis. These actions exerted by corticosteroids proceed in different time domains. The rapid nongenomic corticosteroid action modulating the HPA axis pulse and associated behaviors is still poorly understood. It may involve at the membrane rapid assembly of molecular aggregates or second messenger signaling cascades. The genomic actions of corticosteroids are much better documented. These actions are mediated by high-affinity mineralocorticoid receptors (MRs) and lower-affinity glucocorticoid receptors (GRs), which are co-localized in abundance, particularly in limbic neurons, such as the hippocampus. Because of the stress-induced signaling cascades that occur in the various afferents to the PVN, the actions of corticosteroids mediated by these two different types of receptors present with enormous diversity. We postulated that the balance in MR- and GR-mediated actions is essential for homeostasis, adaptation, and resilience (de Kloet, 1991; de Kloet, Vreugdenhil, Oitzl, & Joëls, 1998). Via MR-mediated actions, corticosteroids set signaling pathways at a certain threshold, which determines how and how fast the response to stress occurs. This helps in the appraisal of the nature and the severity of the stressor and facilitates the retrieval of an appropriate physiological response and/or behavioral coping style. GRs promote recovery and adaptation while facilitating the behavioral response in order to be prepared at the next encounter.

A large part of our knowledge leading to the MR/GR balance concept has been obtained by selective blockade of one or the other receptor type following intracerebral application of antagonists, which have been tested using different behavioral paradigms (Oitzl & de Kloet, 1992; Oitzl, Fluttert, & de Kloet, 1994). In addition, mouse mutants in which the GR or MR have been knocked out (Oitzl, Reichard, Joëls, & de Kloet, 2001; Reichard et al., 1998) or downregulated have been used (Montkowski et al., 1995). In testing stress system regulation, investigators are faced with the problem that the significance of MR- and GR-mediated actions in the various brain circuits and afferent inputs to the PVN is still largely unknown. Therefore, it is important to identify the search for factors that may change the MR/GR balance (*see* Fig. 1). Defining these signaling pathways will help to determine the predisposition and pathogenesis of stress-related disorders.

2. MR/GR BALANCE

2.1. Intracellular Level

Since the MR in the brain has a very high affinity for corticosterone (and aldosterone), the 1-h pulses of corticosterone in the ultradian adrenal rhythm are predicted to maintain a stable, near-saturation, occupancy of the MR in brain (de Kloet, 1975). In contrast, the GR has too low an affinity to become activated by low nonstress concentrations of corticosterone in vivo. Only following stress levels of corticosteroids does activation occur, and receptor translocation to the nucleus varies in parallel with the circulating corticosterone levels (Kitchener, Di Blasi, Borelli, & Piazza, 2004). These receptor studies are performed mainly with hippocampal tissue in which MR and GR are co-localized (van Steensel et al., 1996). The MR seems to be predominantly located in the nuclear compartment, even under basal resting pulsatile conditions, whereas GR only translocates during the peaks of corticosterone pulses (van Steensel et al., 1996). As a result of the differential corticosteroid receptor locations, different patterns of corticosteroid genes are affected. Using a paradigm of (a) absence of, (b) low, and (c) high corticosterone, we discriminated MR-responsive, MR + GR-responsive, and GR-responsive genes in the rat hippocampus (Fig. 2) (Datson, van der Perk, de Kloet, & Vreugdenhil, 2001). This indicates that, depending on relative MR and GR activity, distinct patterns of gene activity are induced.

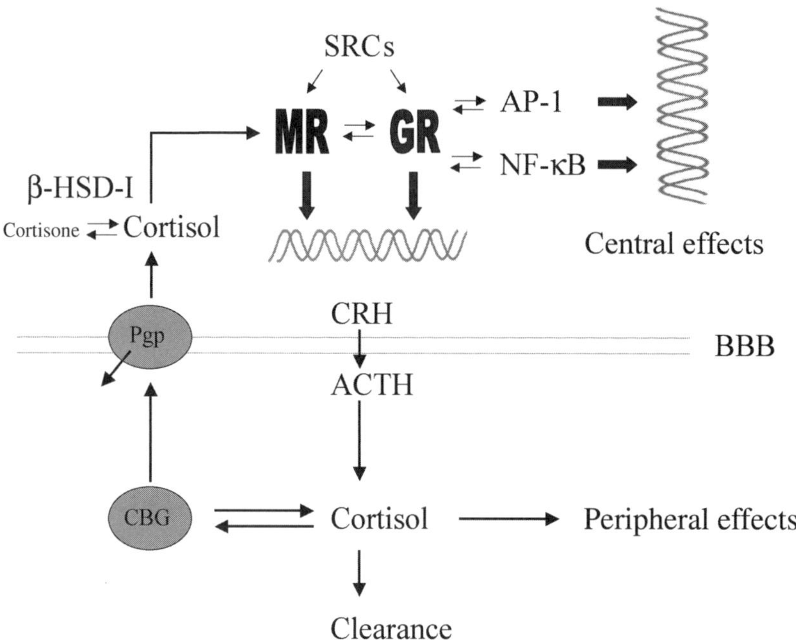

Fig. 1. Factors involved in central corticosteroid-signaling—the MR/GR balance. CRH is the main driving hypothalamic secretagog inducing ACTH secretion from the pituitary gland. In turn, ACTH induces increased production and secretion of cortisol from the adrenals. In the circulation, cortisol is bound to cortisol-binding globulin (CBG), limiting the concentration of free cortisol (the active fraction) and clearence by the liver. In case of central effects, cortisol access is further limited by the Pgp located at the BBB, which excludes cortisol to a certain extent from the brain. Additional regulation is accomplished by two 11β-HSD isoenzymes: 11β-HSD-1 regenerates cortisol from (inactive) cortisone, while 11β-HSD-II does the opposite. Cortisol binds with high affinity to the MR and with approx 10 × lower affinity to the GR. Genomic activity is modified by direct DNA binding or by interaction with other transcription factors such as AP-1 or NF-κB. Direct DNA binding is influenced by SRCs and the composition of the target promotor region. These factors influence the MR/GR balance and their effects on, for example, target gene expression (*see* Fig. 2). In addition, genetic variability can influence protein expression and amino acid sequence. Changes in amino acid sequence could hypothetically induce changes in phosphorylation capacity, higher affinity, or diminished dimerization. As a result, corticosteroid effects will shift towards a certain effect/direction (e.g., NF-κB interaction) and away from another (e.g., direct DNA binding), leading to a condition with a less favourable metabolic profile, more HPA axis reactivity, high blood pressure, or being inflammatory-prone. Abbreviations: ACTH, adrenocorticotropic hormone; AP-1, activation protein-1; BBB, blood–brain barrier; CRH, corticotropin-releasing hormone; 11βHSD-I, 11β-hydroxysteroid dehydrogenase, active as a reductase; CBG, cortisol-binding globulin; HPA, hypothalamic–pituitary–adrenal; GR, glucocorticoid receptor; MR, mineralocorticoid receptor; NF-κB, nuclear factor κB; Pgp, P glycoprotein; SRCs, steroid receptor coactivators.

2.2. Cellular Level

Using the CA1 pyramidal neurons in the hippocampal slice as a model, two general principles were revealed (Joëls & de Kloet, 1989, 1992, 1994). First, the control exerted by MR and/or GR appeared to proceed in a U-shaped manner. Maximal ion conductance

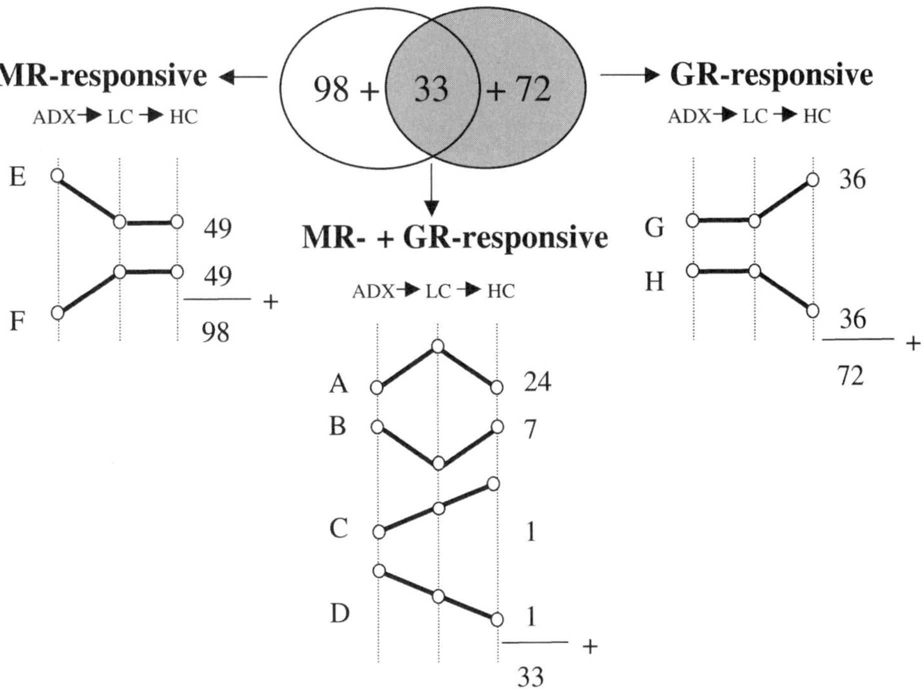

Fig 2. MR- and GR-responsive genes in the rat hippocampus. Following adrenalectomy (ADX), rats were supplied with low (LC) or high levels (HC) of corticosterone. The transition from depleted to low corticosterone levels will involve MR activity because no GRs will be occupied. Ninety-eight genes were identified to be exclusively MR-responsive, being induced (F; 49) or downregulated (E; 49). Seventy-two genes were found to be exclusively GR-responsive—36 upregulated (G; 36) and 36 downregulated (H; 36). Interestingly, 33 genes were both MR- and GR-responsive, showing down- and upregulation (A–D). Changes in MR or GR expression, intrinsic activity (owing to gene polymorphism), corticosteroid availability, cofactors, and other transcription factors will direct the pool of corticosteroid-responsive genes in a certain direction: e.g., predominant MR activity in combination with low GR activity will skew gene regulation to the 98 and 33 pools, away from the 72 pool. One result will be that the exclusively GR-responsive genes will lack control by high stress levels of corticosteroids, possibly leading to an overreactive stress response, with all the accompanying dangers. (Reprinted with permission from Datson et al., 2001.)

and transmitter responses were seen in the absence of corticosterone when no receptor was active. The same pattern was observed in the presence of very high supraphysiological concentrations of the steroid when both receptors were active. Intermediate corticosterone concentrations occupying predominantly MR and little GR minimize the cell responses. These concentrations are thought to represent the average steroid concentration during the day. Second, these responses form the mechanistic basis for phenomena on the network level such as long-term potentiation (LTP), which also have been demonstrated to show a U-shaped dose-responsiveness to corticosterone (Diamond, Bennett, Fleshner, & Rose, 1992). Thus, at least in hippocampal neurons, cellular work demonstrates that MR stabilizes excitability on the cell and circuit level in the hippocampus, and GR modulates excitability transiently raised by stimulatory stimuli.

The aforementioned MR- and GR-mediated changes in excitability in the hippocampus have consequences for the excitatory output of the system. Changes in MR-regulated thresholds can increase or decrease responsiveness of neurons critical for the regulation of the PVN. It is thought that MR maintains a high excitatory tone mediated by glutamate, which can be attenuated by transient GR activation. The excitatory outflow is thought to activate the GABA-ergic network around the PVN. A few studies have shown that the GABA-ergic input to the PVN changes as a function of corticosteroid exposure both in characteristics and the number of synaptic contacts (Joëls, Verkuyl, & van Riel, 2003).

2.3. Behavioral Level

On the behavioral level, the brain site and circuit activated, the context of the stressor, and the activity of the central corticosteroid receptors determine the final outcome. Thus, if MR is blocked in the medial amygdala or the circumventricular organs, one typically interferes with mineralocorticoid control of salt appetite (Sakai, Ma, Zhang, McEwen, & Fluharty, 1996), because these sites contain aldosterone-selective MR. However, if MR is blocked elsewhere, a plethora of effects has been observed that can be summarized as follows.

MR blockade attenuates autonomic outflow (Rahmouni, Barthelmebs, Grima, Imbs, & de Jong, 2003; van den Berg, de Kloet, & de Jong, 1994; van den Buuse, van Acker, Fluttert, & de Kloet, 2002) in regulation of cardiovascular and renal function. MR antagonists block the conservation/withdrawal response if animals are exposed to a severe stressor (Korte, 2002) and disrupts conditioning processes as observed in the forced extinction of an inhibitory avoidance response (Bohus & de Kloet, 1981). These responses suggest rapid anxiolytic effects of centrally administered MR antagonists, which proceed independently from direct interaction with the GABA-A receptor. Also, with a time delay of only a few minutes MR activation enhances aggressive behavior of a resident mouse towards an intruder (Haller, Millar, & Kruk, 1998). In spatial learning tests MR rapidly affects interpretation of environmental information and selection of the appropriate behavioral response to deal with the challenge. Experimental evidence for this thesis comes from the findings that administration of a few nanograms of mineralocorticoid antagonist icv immediately before testing altered the behavioral pattern of an animal in a maze to find food that it had learned to locate the previous day or to search for an escape route (Oitzl et al., 1994). How these mostly rapid MR-mediated effects occur is not known.

Blockade of brain GR impairs the storage of new information (Loscertales, Rose, & Sandi, 1997; Oitzl & de Kloet, 1992). A glucocorticoid antagonist administered around the time of learning in the hippocampus or in the amygdala impaired the consolidation of newly acquired information (Roozendaal, Griffith, Buranday, Quervain, & McGaugh, 2003). As a consequence 24 h later the rat is unable to retrieve the information learned the previous day and has to learn the maze problem all over again. Likewise, mutant mice with a point mutation in GR that obliterates binding to DNA are unable to store learned information (Oitzl et al., 2001). This suggests that corticosteroid-induced cognitive performance requires transactivation, as was previously found in the cellular responses to corticosterone in hippocampus (Karst et al., 2000), because such mutants lack the direct activation of GRs, but still have a GR that can interact with other transcription factors (Reichardt, Tuckermann, Bauer, & Schütz, 2000). Transgenic mice with downregulated

GRs (knockdown) show cognitive defects and elevated plasma ACTH and corticosterone concentrations in response to stress (Müller, Holsboer, & Kellendonk, 2002).

The above studies are based mostly on observations in rodents, but observations in humans largely agree (Buchanan & Lovallo, 2001; Lupien et al., 2002; Schmidt, Fox, Goldberg, Smith, & Schulkin, 1999; Wolkowitz et al., 1990). In general, the data show that MR plays a role in the interpretation of environmental stimuli and affects the animal's reactivity and behavioral response pattern. These effects are mostly rapid, but the underlying (nongenomic) mechanism is not known. Much confusion has been created in the literature about the role of GR. Blockade of the GR clearly demonstrates its facilitatory role in the storage of new information. However, if the receptor is stimulated beyond the context of the learning experience (e.g., at retrieval) the learned response is considered no longer relevant, and the animal switches to a more opportune response. Mice exposed to chronic stress and high corticosterone concentrations deteriorate in spatial learning, whereas the reverse occurs after chronic treatment with GR antagonists. Chronic GR blockade in brain appears to result in enhancement of cognitive performance (Oitzl, Fluttert, Sutanto, & de Kloet, 1998).

2.4. Neuroendocrine Control

Intracerebral blockade of MRs and GRs using selective antagonists exerts a profound and differential effect on HPA axis activity. We also distinguished the blockade of GRs in the HPA core (i.e., pituitary corticotrophs and PVN microenvironment) from the blockade of MRs and/or GRs in stressor-specific afferents from prefrontal cortex, hippocampus, brainstem, amygdala-locus coeruleus, and other forebrain structures. The latter blockade interferes with processing of information and behavioral responses and leads to subsequent changes in HPA regulation. Thus, exposure to a novel environment was used as a stressor, since the limbic-cortical brain circuits involved in responding to a novel situation (e.g., fear, attention, appraisal, and reward) abundantly express MRs and GRs.

In adrenal intact animals, the results showed that application of the MR antagonist RU 28318 icv causes a rise in basal trough and peak levels of HPA activity during basal nonstress conditions as well as an enhanced response to the novelty stressor (Ratka, Sutanto, Bloemers, & de Kloet, 1989). In humans MR blockade enhances HPA activity (Deuschle et al., 1998; Dodt, Kern, Fehm, & Born, 1993; Heuser, Deuschle, Weber, Stalla, & Holsboer, 2000; Young, Lopez, Murphy-Weinberg, Watson, & Akil, 1998). As expected, the GR antagonist mifepristone had no effect on basal trough activity because no GR is occupied under these conditions. Rather a prolonged response to the novelty stressor was observed after GR blockade (Ratka et al., 1989). The attenuation of the novelty-induced response was mimicked with antagonist application in the dorsal hippocampus, whereas the prolonged response required GR blockade in the PVN (de Kloet, de Kock, Schild, & Veldhuis, 1988; Oitzl, van Haarst, Sutanto, & de Kloet, 1995; van Haarst, Oitzl, & de Kloet, 1997). After continuous infusion of a few nanograms of mifepristone icv the amplitude of the circadian rhythm became greatly enhanced after 4 d because the peak rather than the trough levels in HPA axis activity increased (van Haarst, Oitzl, Workel, & de Kloet, 1996). As is the case in the rat, chronic mifepristone enhanced the amplitude of the flattened circadian rhythm in cortisol characteristic of the disease (Belanoff et al., 2002).

3. ACCESS TO CORTICOSTEROID RECEPTORS

3.1. Corticosteroid-Binding Globulin

Only a small proportion of circulating corticosteroids is free, which is the active fraction. Several proteins in the circulation are capable of binding corticosteroids, but, corticosteroid-binding globulin (CBG) is the most important. CBG circulates during young and adult life, but is virtually absent from the circulation during the first 2 wk of life. This may account for the very strong postnatal glucocorticoid feedback signal observed. CBG-bound steroid is thought to be bio-inactive, and according to this view CBG serves as a pool from which glucocorticoids are made available. CBG is expressed in liver but also at low levels in a range of glucocorticoid target tissues. Besides its "buffer" function, CBG is a member of the serine protease inhibitors and is a substrate for neutrophil elastase (SERPINS). There is evidence suggesting a specific interaction between CBG and elastase on the surface of neutrophils, which may promote the delivery of glucocorticoids at sites of inflammation or perhaps other tissues affected by stress (Hammond, Smith, Paterson, & Sibbald, 1990). The role of CBG in the delivery of glucocorticoids to the brain is not known, although high levels have been found in the pituitary gland.

3.2. 11β-Hydroxy-Oxido-Reductase

Two isoenzymes exist for 11β-steroid dehydrogenase (Seckl & Walker, 2001). 11β-Steroid dehydrogenase type 2 is an NAD(H)-dependent enzyme that functions as an oxidase and is found co-localized with MR in tissues that selectively respond to the mineralocorticoid aldosterone. Aldosterone circulates at approx 1000 times lower concentrations as compared to corticosteroids, which makes it necessary to "protect" these tissues from high levels of corticosterone/cortisol. Type 2 is localized in kidney and in brain circumventricular organs, where it conveys aldosterone selectivity because of local intracellular metabolic conversion of the naturally occurring glucocorticoids cortisol and corticosterone (Edwards et al., 1988; Seckl & Walker, 2001). 11β-steroid dehydrogenase type 1 is an NADP(H)-dependent enzyme that functions mainly as a reductase in the cell to generate active cortisol and corticosterone from inactive 11-dehydrocorticosterone. The type-1 enzyme is widely distributed. The enzyme is also located in brain, where it may regenerate bioactive corticosteroids.

3.3. Multidrug-Resistance P-Glycoprotein

Dexamethasone in low concentrations penetrates the brain poorly, but is accumulated in pituitary corticotrophs (de Kloet, 1975; Meijer et al., 1998). We have shown that the synthetic steroid is extruded by multidrug-resistance P-glycoprotein (mdr Pgp) and related proteins in the blood–brain barrier. These Pgps play a role in mdr, such as with cancer. Using Pgp knockout mice a 10-fold higher accumulation of ^{3}H-dexamethasone was observed in the brain of the mutants. ^{3}H-cortisol, not naturally occurring in rat and mouse, is also poorly retained in wild type rodent brains and appears as a Pgp substrate. In the Pgp mutants profound labeling of hippocampal neurons occurs with cortisol, as is the case with corticosterone. To our surprise, human mdr also recognizes cortisol rather than corticosterone as substrate, and liquid chromatography–mass spectrometry analysis of postmortem human brain samples revealed that corticosterone is preferred by the human brain more often than cortisol (Karssen et al., 2001). In plasma the ratio of cortisol to corticosterone is approx 20, whereas in brain it was oftcn 3.3. Thus, it is possible that human mdr differs in specificity for cortisol and corticosterone.

3.4. Transcription Factors and Coregulators

On binding ligand, MRs and GRs can both bind to glucocorticoid response elements (GREs, consensus sites located on the DNA), but only GRs can interact with transcription factors (protients) such as activating protein (AP-1) and nuclear factor-κB (NF-κB) (Auphan, DiDonato, Rosette, Helmberg, & Karin, 1995; De Bosscher, Vanden Berghe, & Haegeman, 2003). It is now known that they achieve this blockade through interaction of the GR monomers with transcription factors activated by signaling cascades driven by several stress factors. This finding provides a firm mechanistic underpinning to the concept advanced by Tausk (1951) and Munck, Guyre, and Holbrook (1984) that a major action of glucocorticoids is to block primary stress reactions.

Recently, coregulator molecules were identified that appeared to be powerful modulators of nuclear receptor function (Meijer, Steenbergen, & de Kloet, 2002). Members of the steroid receptor coactivator (SRC) family of proteins promote agonist-induced receptor activation by permitting recruitment of, for example, CBP/p300 transcription activators. The corepressor molecules do the opposite and promote repression of gene transcription. The GR antagonist mifepristone (RU 486) with the receptors provides an interesting example of the possible modes of interaction with steroid receptor signaling. This antagonist only acts as an antagonist (at GREs) if sufficient corepressor is available. In vitro transfection experiments suggest that variable stoechiometry of corepressors and co-activators may underlie differential MR/GR functioning.

4. VARIANTS OF THE GLUCOCORTICOID RECEPTOR

In 1985 two different human (h)GR cDNAs were cloned: hGRα and hGRβ cDNA, which were later shown to encode the α and β isoforms of the receptor (Hollenberg et al., 1985) (Fig. 3). hGRα and hGRβ mRNA both contain exons 1–8 but have different versions of exon 9 as a result of alternative splicing; hGRα mRNA contains exon 9α, whereas hGRβ mRNA contains exon 9β (Oakley, Sar, & Cidlowski, 1996). In addition, hGR mRNA may contain five different versions of exon 1. Through the usage of the three different promoters, three different exons 1 can be transcribed (1A, 1B, and 1C), and alternative splicing of exon 1A can result in yet three different versions (1A1, 1A2, 1A3) (Breslin, Geng, & Vedeckis, 2001). Like other members of the steroid receptor family, the hGR contains three major domains (Giguere, Hollenberg, Rosenfeld, & Evans, 2001; Weinberger, Hollenberg, Rosenfeld, & Evans, 1985). The most N-terminal domain is called the immunogenic domain, which in hGR consists of amino acids (AAs) 1–420. AAs 421–488 form the DNA-binding domain (DBD) of hGRα, and its C-terminal ligand-binding domain (LBD) consists of AAs 527–777, of which the last 50 AAs are encoded by exon 9α. The LBD of hGRβ is similar to that of hGRα until AA 727, at which point the last 15 AA are encoded by exon 9β. After that hGRα and hGRβ diverge, and 15 unique AAs form the most C-terminal part of hGRβs LBD.

Recently it has been shown that alternative translation initiation results in the presence of two different isoforms (A and B) of hGRα (Yudt & Cidlowski, 2001). An alternative start site for translation is formed at codon 27, encoding methionine. This results in a

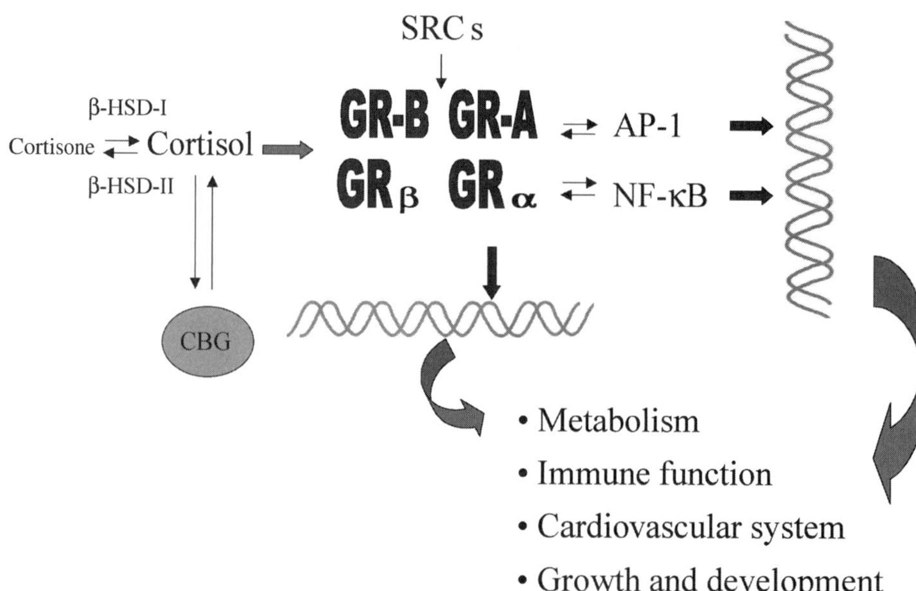

Fig. 3. Factors involved in corticosteroid signaling. Cortisol is released from the adrenal glands binds to cortisol-binding globulin (CBG) in the circulation, thereby protecting the hormone against degradation by liver P450 enzymes. In the target tissue, cortisol can be converted to the inert cortisone by 11β-HSD-II or reactivated by 11β-HSD-I. At the GR level, the amount, degree of phosphorylation, and affinity (the latter being influenced by binding of the unliganded GR to several heat shock proteins) directly determine corticosteroid responsiveness. Several variants of the GR exist, of which GRβ is thought to function as a natural inhibitor of the classical GR, GRα (Bamberger, Bamberger, de Castro, & Chrousos, 1995; DeRijk, Sternberg, & de Kloet, 1997). In addition, two translationary variants exist, GR-A and GR-B, using two different translation start sites, both at the beginning of exon 2 (Yudt & Cidlowski, 2001). GR-B seems to be even more active as compared to the classic GR(α)-A. At the DNA level, a "simple" glucocorticoid-responsive element (GRE) can exert a positive or negative action on gene transcription after direct binding of GR homodimers. This mode of action seems to be most important in metabolic actions, such as activation of the enzyme phosphoenol pyruvate carboxykinase (PEP-CK). In contrast to direct binding to DNA, GR can interact with other transcription factors such as AP-1, NF-κB, or cAMP-responsive element-binding protein (CREB), often resulting in mutual inhibition (De Bosscher et al., 2003). These activities are important in immune function, cardiovascular control, growth and development, and behavior. Finally, chromatin structure or modulation of chromatin structure, e.g., by histones, determines access of the receptors to nuclear-binding sites.

protein that is 751 AAs in length (the B isoform), in addition to the originally identified 777-AA-long isoform of hGRα (the A isoform). A similar mechanism of alternative translation initiation has been proposed for hGRβ, but this has not yet been demonstrated.

Mutations within the GR gene are not compatible with life or result in severe corticosteroid-resistance syndrome. This is owing to their pleiotropic actions (*see* Figs. 1 and 3), and their effects on almost every physiological and behavioral system. The corticosteroid-resistance syndrome is characterized by hypertension, excess androgens, and increased plasma cortisol concentration in the absence of the stigmata of Cushing's syndrome (Brönnegård & Carlstedt-Duke, 1995; Charmandari et al., 2004; Chrousos, Detera-Wadleigh, & Karl, 1993; Lamberts, Huizenga, de Lange, de Jong, & Koper,

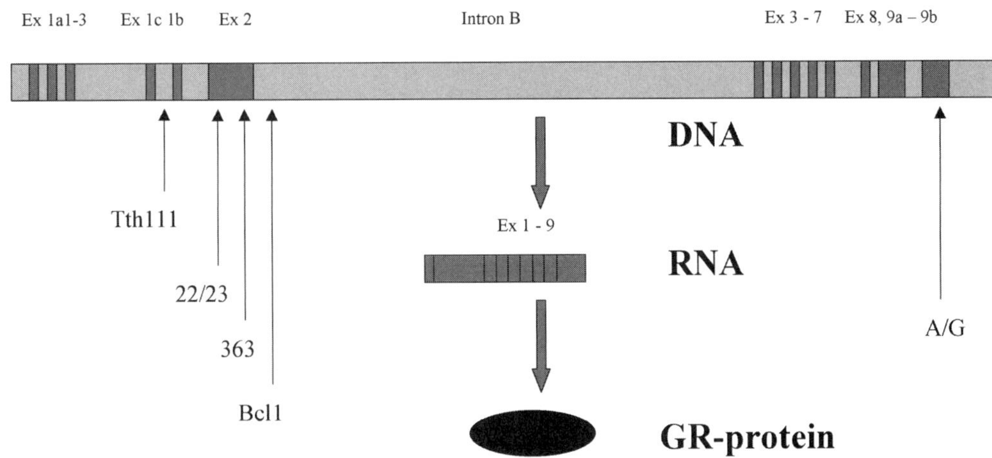

Fig. 4. Single-nucleotide polymorphisms (SNPs) in the GR gene. Schematic overview of the GR gene. Translation starts at the beginning of exon 2 and ends in exon 9. Several splice variants exist: different exon 1s have been described (Breslin et al., 2001), whereas exon 8 can join exon 9α or 9β, giving rise to GRα or GRβ, respectively. Recently, Yudt and Cidlowski (2001) described a GR-translation variant, designated GR-B, with a potential high effect on gene expression. Depicted are Tth111 located between exon 1c and 1b, ER22/23EK at the beginning of exon 2, N363S at the end of exon 2, Bcl 1 site downstream of exon 2, being an allele spanning almost the entire intron B (±80 kB) and the A to G in exon 9β in the ATTTA site. For the effects of these SNPs, *see* text.

1996). Moreover, several GR-gene mutations have been found in human malignancies, including Cushing's disease (for review, *see* DeRijk, Schaaf, & de Kloet, 2002). In addition, naturally occurring GR-gene polymorphisms have been found that are not directly associated with overt disease (Lamberts et al., 1996) (Fig. 4; Table 1). However, some GR-gene single-nucleotide polymorphisms (SNPs) have been associated with diseases such as obesity, cardiovascular diseases, and autoimmunity (Table 1). Three GR-gene polymorphisms have received much attention: ER22/23EK, located at the beginning of exon 2; N363S, located at the end of exon 2; and the Bcl1-restriction site, located ±650 bp downstream of exon 2 in intron B (Table 1). Highly important, associations of these polymorphisms with the (central) regulation of the HPA axis have recently been described that will affect the whole body (Stevens et al., 2004; Wüst et al., 2004).

4.1. Cardiovascular Control

Glucocorticoids have long been associated with increased vascular tone and cardiac output. Furthermore, in human hypertension a strong genetic component has been inferred, which has nourished the search for GR-gene mutations in human hypertension.

The Bcl1 polymorphism was originally identified using Southern blot techniques (Murray, Smith, Ardinger, & Weinberger, 1987) and was recently characterized as a G/C transversion 647 base pairs downstream of exon 2, in intron B (Fleury, Beaulieu, Primeau, Sinnett, & Krajinovic, 2003; van Rossum & Lamberts, 2004). Originally, this polymorphism was detected using Southern blotting in combination with the Bcl1 restriction enzyme. Lack of the Bcl1 site due to the polymorphism resulted in a larger band in the Southern blot. This polymorphism was found to be associated with increased corticosteroid sensitivity using a budesonide skin-bleaching test (Panarelli et al., 1998).

Table 1
Functional Human GR-Gene Polymorphisms Associated With HPA Axis Regulation or Metabolic Aspects

Region	*Position*	*Nucleotide change*	*AA change*	*Characteristics of the hGR-SNP*	*Ref.*
Promoter	Ex1B–Ex1C	Tth111L-site C → T		Presently not associated with any pathology, may be involved in regulation of basal levels of cortisol, especially detectable at night trough levels. No changes in DST or following other stimulation. Frequency: wt, 40%; heterozygote, 45%; homozygote, 16%.	Detera-Wadleigh, Encio, & Rollins, 1991; Rosmond et al., 2000a; van Rossum & Lamberts, 2004
Exon 2	198	GAG → GAA	Glu22Glu	ER22/23EK = GAGAGG(GluArg)-GAAAAG(GluLys)	Koper et al., 1997
Exon 2	200	AGG → AAG	Arg23Lys	Relative steroid resistance and Dex escape. Lower insulin and lower cholesterol, a more favorable metabolic profile. Male carriers are taller, have more muscle mass, and are stronger. Increased frequency in older population. Decreased risk of dementia. Frequency: heterozygote ± 5–10%.	Koper et al., 1997; van Rossum & Lamberts, 2004; van Rossum et al., 2003a
Exon 2	1220	ATT → AGT	Asn363Ser	Increased cortisol sensitivity to 1 mg Dex, still suppression after 0.25 mg Dex. Associated with strong cortisol response following psychological stress (TSST). Increased BMI and other metabolic disturbances, increased insulin response following Dex. Frequency: heterozygote ± 8%.	Dobson et al., 2001; Di Blasio et al., 2001; de Lange et al., 1997; Huizinga et al., 1998; Koper et al., 1997; Lin et al., 1999a, Wüst et al., 2004
Intron B	IVS2 + 646	TGATCA → TGATGA Bcl-1-site Allele spanning intron B		Corticosteroid sensitivity increase in skin bleaching test. Low cortisol levels following the 0.25 mg Dex test. Low HPA axis reactivity psychological stress (TSST), and higher cortisol following lunch. Increased BMI, increased BMI and LDL following overeating (young Swedish population), decreased BMI (elderly Dutch population). Associated with increased blood pressure. Heterozygote frequency ± 30–52%; homozygote frequency ± 0–7%, depending on ethnicity.	Buemann et al., 1997; Detera-Wadleigh et al., 1991; Fleury et al, 2003; Murray et al., 1987; Panarelli et al., 1998; Rosmond et al., 2000b; Stevens et al., 2004; Tremblay et al., 2003; Ukkola, Rosmond, et al., 2001; van Rossum et al., 2003b; Wüst et al., 2004

Dst, dexamethasone suppression test; Dex, dexamethasone; TSST, Trier social stress test; BMI, body mass index; HPA, hypothalamic–pituitary–adrenal; LDL, low-density lipoprotein.

Recently it was shown that this Bcl1 polymorphisms is a marker of a large allele, or haplotype, spanning almost the entire intron B (±80 kbp), located between exon 2 and exon 3 of the GR gene (Stevens et al., 2004). The gene frequency of this haplotype is between 15 and 33%, depending on ethnicity, making it in potention highly important (Fleury et al., 2003). Watt et al. (1992) described the BclI restriction fragment to be associated with high blood pressure; homozygotes for the larger allele had higher blood pressure scores than homozygotes for the alternative allele (wild types), whereas heterozygotes were intermediates. As described below, in another study of this locus Weaver, Hitman, & Kopelman (1992) reported that the larger allele was associated with severe hyperinsulinemic obesity, a phenotype feature that, in a milder form, is common in patients with essential hypertension.

The N363S polymorphism (Asn363Ser, an AAT-to-AGT transition in codon 363 in exon 2) in the GR gene was originally detected by Koper et al. (1997) and was recently found to be associated with coronary artery disease (CAD), independent of the presence of overweight (Lin, Wang, & Morris, 2003). In addition, unstable angina further increased the association. However, in a previous study by the same group, no such association was detected (Lin, Wang, & Morris, 1999a, 1999b). This has led to fierce debate with respect to the validity of these associations and SNP association studies in general. It has been proposed that functionality of the SNP under study should be revealed through in vitro testing (Daly & Day, 2001; Emahazion et al., 2001; Rosmond, 2003a; Zondervan & Cardon, 2004). Unfortunately, in vitro tests of SNP functionality in cells are also of somewhat limited value, because (a) they exclude the influence of variables from physiology, and (b) the effect of the SNP is heavily dependent on the cellular context (e.g., promoter region, presence of other transcription factors, etc.) (De Bosscher et al., 2003).

4.2. Immune Function

Large-scale application of synthetic corticosteroids to suppress rheumatoid arthritis was initially the therapy of choice in the field of autoimmunity. With respect to the molecular mechanism of corticosteroid sensitivity in immune tissue, much research has focused on the GR. GRβ, the putative natural antagonist of GRα, has received the most attention in this field as compared to other GR-gene variants (DeRijk et al., 2002). We described a variant in GRβ to be associated with rheumatoid arthritis and possibly with systemic lupus erythematosus (SLE) (DeRijk et al., 2001). Importantly, this variant was found in vitro to stabilize GRβ mRNA and to increase GRβ expression (Schaaf & Cidlowski, 2002a). It was proposed that this SNP could contribute to the process of autoimmunity by decreasing corticosteroid sensitivity. The expression of the GRβ variant was found to be very low, although several days of exposure of immune cells to cytokines increased the GRα/GRβ ratio to levels at which the dominant activity of the GRβ could become important (Schaaf & Cidlowski, 2002b). In line with this notion is the finding of associations of GRβ expression and corticosteroid resistance in active immune tissue (for overview, see DeRijk et al., 2002). However, in human postmortem hippocampal tissue we detected only very low levels of GRβ expression, as determined by both mRNA expression and immuncytochemistry (DeRijk et al., 2003). Moreover, in this brain region GRβ immune-reactive-positive cells were found to be of bloodborne origin. Thus, at present it is unclear if GRβ plays any role in centrally mediated processes such as behavior or HPA axis regulation.

4.3. Behavior

Although both experimental animal research and studies with human subjects clearly show a profound role of corticosteroids in behavior, few studies have addressed the relationship between GR expression or GR-gene variants and human behavior. An important role of corticosteroid signaling in behavior has been inferred, as described extensively in this chapter; for example, changes in HPA axis reactivity in healthy family members of patients with affective disorders are documented, suggesting a genetic contribution through cortisol regulation (Ellenbogen, Hodgins, & Walker, 2004; Holsboer, Lauer, Schreiber, & Krieg, 1995). Van Rossum and Lamberts (2004) reported in an abstract that carriers of the linked polymorphisms ER22/23EK (GAG AGG [GluArg or ER] g GAA AAG [GlyLys or EK] [Koper et al., 1997]) had a lower risk of dementia as well as fewer white matter lesions in the brain and better performance on psychomotor speed tests. No associations between GR-polymorphisms and psychiatric diseases have been described, although it has to be mentioned that Binder et al. (2004) recently found an association between better treatment efficacy and increased recurrence with a FKBP5, a GR-regulating cochaperone of hsp-90. Psychiatric diseases are considered multigenetic diseases with great environmental influence. Also, little consensus exists with respect to subtle phenotypic determination of psychiatric patients, which is almost a prerequisite to study genetic determinants. Taken together, much attention has to be paid to phenotypic determination and the regulation of the HPA axis in order to minimize variation when studying genetic polymorphisms in psychiatric disorders.

4.4. HPA Axis Regulation

Several GR-gene SNPs have been associated with changes in HPA axis regulation. Human carriers of the Bcl1 polymorphism showed an allele dosage effect; with respect to increased dexamathasone suppression of plasma cortisol (Panarelli et al., 1998; van Rossum & Lamberts, 2004), indicating increased corticosteroid sensitivity in these subjects. The same pattern was found for human carriers of the N363S polymorphism (Huizinga et al., 1998). In contrast, ER22/23EK showed the opposite effect: a decreased sensitivity to dexamethasone and thus a higher postdexamethasone cortisol level (van Rossum & Lamberts, 2004).

Recently, Wüst (2004) showed a strong genetic effect of the N363S and the Bcl1 variant on psychological stress- and ACTH-induced cortisol responses. More precise, carriers of N363S had higher ACTH and cortisol responses following the Trier Social Stress Test (TSST, a psychological stressor) and also higher cortisol following ACTH administration as compared to wild type subjects. Subjects genotyped as Bcl1 heterozygotes had fewer high responses for both cortisol and ACTH following psychological challenge than the N363 carriers, but they were still higher as compared to wild type individuals. Unexpectedly, the Bcl1 homozygotes had lower cortisol responses as compared to wild types, following both TSST and ACTH administration. It is conceivable that the presence of two Bcl1 alleles exceeds a threshold, followed by a downward resetting of the HPA axis, through an unknown mechanism. It is also possible that Bcl1 carriers additionally have ER22/23EK, but too few subjects with this genotype were available.

Interestingly, Stevens et al. (2004), found the Bcl1 site to be in linkage disequilibrium with two other polymorphism both located downstream, showing an allele spanning almost the entire intron B (between exon 2 and exon 3) (*see* Fig. 4). Still, the molecular mechanism of this SNP is unknown; it could be that this SNP has an effect on mRNA splicing or stability. An association was established between the presence of this allele and relatively low postdexamethasone (0.25 mg) plasma cortisol levels, compared to noncarriers. These findings indicate that the BclI SNP is associated with a relative increased corticosteroid sensitivity.

The Tth111I variant was found to be located in the promoter region between exons 1b and 1c, 3807 bp upstream of the GR mRNA start site (van Rossum & Lamberts, 2004). Rosmond et al. (2000a) did find an association between this variant and higher total and evening cortisol concentrations, although not with metabolic parameters. In contrast, the group of Lamberts et al. (1996) could not find any association of this polymorphism with dexamethasone-induced cortisol suppression or with antropomorphic markers, cholesterol, glucose, or insulin levels (van Rossum & Lamberts, 2004). As suggested by van Rossum and Lamberts (2004), this discrepancy could be explained by the finding that carriers of ER22/23EK also seem to have the T-variant of the Tth111I site.

Recently we found an allele in the MR gene to be associated with increased saliva and plasma cortisol responsiveness in healthy human subjects during the TSST (DeRijk et al., 2005). However, the full impact of this MR-gene SNP on HPA axis regulation has still to be explored.

Taken together, these data and especially the recent studies by Wüst and Stevens suggest that GR-gene polymorphisms can, by changing the setting and reactivity of the HPA axis, affect peripheral cortisol availability. This will almost certainly have an effect on peripheral tissue reactivity during stress.

4.5. Metabolism

Glucocorticoid effects on metabolism are numerous and complex. In the acute phase, glucocorticoids increase blood glucose by facilitating the flow of substrates through intermediary metabolism and activating the process of gluconeogenesis. AAs are released from skeletal muscle while fatty acids and glycerol are released from adipose tissue. In the liver the enzyme phosphoenol pyruvate carboxykinase (PEP-CK) is induced, resulting in enhanced gluconeogenesis. In addition, peripheral glucose uptake and utilization is inhibited, partly as a result of decreased translocation to the cell surface of GLUT 4 glucose transporters (Barthel & Schmoll, 2003; Reynolds & Walker, 2003). Furthermore, corticosteroids inhibit glucose-stimulated insulin release from pancreatic β-cells, and it has been proposed that cortisol has a regulatory, predominantly inhibitory, effect on plasma leptin concentrations.

Prolonged high levels of glucocorticoids, as opposed to short-term acute elevations, are associated with insulin resistance and peripheral fat depositions. This is most clearly depicted in patients with Cushing's syndrome, who have high levels of circulating cortisol, often owing to an ACTH-producing tumor. In contrast, patients with Addison's disease, a deficiency of adrenal cortisol production, are extremely thin and display increased insulin sensitivity.

Human obesity is characterized by excess body fat, whereas the metabolic syndrome describes a constellation of cardiovascular risk factors such as insulin resistance or type 2 diabetes, dislipidemia. and hypertension. It has been proposed that abdominally obese individuals display subtle abnormalities in the regulation of the HPA axis (Rosmond, Dallman, & Björntorp, 1998) and that this dysregulation plays a causative role in the pathogenesis of human obesity and insulin resistance (Björntorp, 1993). However, additional research has suggested that only minor, if any, changes in the regulation of the HPA axis exist (Seckl, Morton, Chapman, & Walker, 2004). In patients with obesity, levels of cortisol are in fact slightly decreased, probably owing to increased metabolism of cortisol (Stewart et al., 1999). Alternatively, local effects of corticosteroids may result in obesity and the metabolic syndrome.

First, the activity of 11β-HSD type-1, predominantly a 11-ketoreductase, reactivating inert cortisone into cortisol, could be upregulated, resulting in increased corticosteroid efficacy in adipose tissue. In a mouse model exhibiting a two- to threefold overexpression of 11β-HSD type-1 in adipose tissue, modest obesity, glucose intolerance, insulin resistance, dyslipidemia, increased leptin serum levels, and hypertension were observed (Masuzaki et al., 2001). These data suggest that 11β-HSD type-1 activity is involved in the metabolic syndrome, and it is suggested that 11β-HSD type-1 is a pharmacological target in the human metabolic syndrome (Seckl et al., 2004).

Second, GR-gene polymorphism may affect corticosteroid sensitivity of the target tissues. Several studies have found associations of the Bcl1 haplotype with changes in metabolism, including hyperinsulimia, higher abdominal fat, higher body mass index (BMI), higher leptin levels, and greater increases in body weight following experimentally induced overfeeding, in carriers of the C genotype (Buemann et al., 1997; Di Blasio et al., 2003; Rosmond et al., 2000b; Ukkola, Pérusse, Chagnon, Després, & Bouchard, 2001; Ukkola, Rosmond, Tremblay, & Bouchard, 2001; van Rossum et al., 2003b; Weaver et al., 1992). In a long prospective study, the increase in subcutaneous fat over 12 yr was more than doubled in females genotyped as heterozygotes as compared to the wild types and homozygotes (Tremblay et al., 2003). The same trend was observed in males but did not reach statistical significance. Some controversy about associations can possible be explained by an age-dependent effect: van Rossum and Lamberts (2004) described a lower BMI in carriers of this genotype with higher age, probably due to increased muscle atrophy (decreased lean mass) in these subjects.

N363S is possibly related to increased corticosteroid sensitivity. Associations have been found with metabolic changes such as higher BMI, waist-to-hip ratio, and insulin response following administration of 0.25 mg dexamethasone (Dobson, Redfern, Unwin, & Weaver, 2001; Huizinga et al., 1998; Lin et al., 1999a). In a severely obese Italian population, the N363S variant was associated with increased BMI (Di Blasio et al., 2003). However, in a Swedish population no such association with either BMI or weight-to-height ratio was found (Rosmond, Bouchard, & Björntorp, 2001), which has led to discussion about the validity of the findings (Rosmond, 2003b). Importantly, in the Swedish study no association was found between the N363S variant and an increased sensitivity towards dexamethasone, in contrast with the previous study by Huizenga et al. (1998). This suggests that the central effects of N363S, e.g., on HPA axis regulation (Wüst et al., 2004), in addition to local tissue-specific effects also play a role in the observed phenotypic changes.

Codons 22 and 23 of exon 2 are possibly related to corticosteroid resistance (Koper et al., 1997). This ER22/23EK polymorphism was associated with a favorable metabolic profile: lower fasting insulin and low-density lipoprotein cholesterol concentrations (van Rossum et al., 2003a). Interestingly, in line with these favorable metabolic parameters, the frequency of this polymorphism was higher in the older population.

Peripheral metabolic status seems to be a factor in the regulation of the HPA axis. Adrenalectomy (ADX) increases the expression of central CRH and other neurotransmitters, probably due to the lack of negative inhibition. Dallman et al. showed that ADX rats drinking saline and glucose appear normal with respect to metabolism and CRH expression (Laugero, Gomez, Manalo, & Dallman, 2002). This suggests that the basal negative feedback signal by corticosteroids on the HPA axis is mediated through peripheral glucose (Dallman et al., 2002). Also, as discussed above, chronic high levels of corticosteroids affect central stress circuits leading to changes in behavior, including increased feeding. It is proposed that chronic stress, as present in western society, leads to increased craving for so-called comfort food, which functions to downregulate central stress systems (Dallman et al., 2003). Indeed, symptoms of depression and anxiety are positively related to anthropometric and metabolic parameters in humans. For example, men with abdominal obesity have symptoms of depression and anxiety (Ahlberg et al., 2002). Moreover, depression (classified according to DSM-IV, not subgrouped in atypical vs melancholic), is associated with increased intra-abdominal fat, resistance to insulin, and impaired glucose tolerance (Roberts, Deleger, Strawbridge, & Kaplan, 2003; Weber, Schweiger, Deuschle, & Heuser, 2000; Weber-Hamann et al., 2002). If depression is further subdivided into melancholic and atypical depression (characterized by lethargy, fatigue, hypersomnia, and hyperphagia), the latter has been found to be associated with low levels of cortisol and probably low levels of CRH and noradrenaline from the Locus Ceruleus (Gold & Chrousos, 2002), suggesting that the hyperphagia functions to downregulate the central stress system. Finally, it was found that plasma glucose levels influence TSST-induced cortisol responses. High levels of glucose, induced by drinking water with 100 g glucose after a night fasting, were associated with much higher saliva cortisol responses as compared to non-glucose-loaded subjects when exposed to the TSST (Kirschbaum et al., 1997).

Although far from clear, there seems to be a bidirectional interaction between the HPA axis and peripheral metabolism. This interaction could have important implications for pathological states such as obesity, the metabolic syndrome, and depression (Eaton, 2002).

5. CONCLUSIONS

Resilience and adaptation seem dependent on the balance of central MR- and GR-mediated actions (de Kloet, 2003; de Kloet et al., 1998). It is thought that the MR activates signaling pathways that stabilize homeostasis by facilitating the selection of a stressor-appropriate coping strategy. On the other hand, the GR represents a mechanism to recover from stress. The receptor activates signaling pathways that facilitate adaptation, in processes such as metabolic demand, immune function, cardiovascular control, and behavior. In the case of behavior, an adequate coping strategy is stored for use at the next encounter. Accordingly, aberrant GR-mediated processes are thought to cause stress-related brain disorders and therefore present targets for therapy. In addition, MR-mediated processes may present an opportunity to design therapeutic approaches for prevention of certain mental diseases.

An aberrant MR/GR balance may lead to a condition of neuroendocrine dysregulation and metabolic, cardiovascular, and behavioral pathology. An additional aspect of aberrant MR/GR balance is a central dysregulation of the HPA axis, which will affect the whole body (Chrousos, Charmandari, & Kino, 2004; de Kloet, 1991; de Kloet et al.,

1998). Many determinants are involved in the MR/GR balance. Bioavailability of corticosteroids and access to their receptors, receptor properties, and numbers as well as the stochiometry with transcription factors and coregulators are important. Moreover, splice variants of the GR gene, GR variants, and SNPs in the GR gene may alter central and local corticosteroid sensitivity. It implies that in case of imbalance the individual loses the ability to maintain homeostasis, if challenged by an adverse event. It is in this arena that the conversion of good vs bad corticosteroid effects may occur. If coping with stress fails corticosteroids fail to optimize stress reactions and targets are exposed to improper corticosteroid concentrations for a prolonged period of time. This condition is thought to sustain reverberating positive feedback loops that further aggravate the condition of imbalance (Gold & Chrousos, 2002).

In addition to genetic influences on the regulation of the HPA axis, traumatic life events can permanently alter the setpoint of the HPA axis (Bremner et al., 2003; Heim et al., 2001; Rinne et al., 2002; Yehuda, 2002; Yehuda, Halligan, Grossman, Golier, & Wong, 2002). It is conceivable that certain GR-gene SNPs modulate the vulnerability to these severe life events and HPA axis regulation with global consequences for metabolism, immune function, cardiovascular regulation, and behavior.

ACKNOWLEDGMENTS

The editorial assistance of Ellen M. Heidema is gratefully acknowledged. The research in this review was supported by de Hersenstichting Nederland (project no: 10F02[2].37: Single nucleotide polymorphism in the HPA axis and in corticosteroid-responsive genes: implications for depression) and the Netherlands Foundation for Advanced Research NWO, Rivierduinen (psychiatric hospital), and the Royal Academy of Arts and Sciences.

REFERENCES

Ahlberg, A.-C., Ljung, T., Rosmond, R., McEwen, B. S., Holm, G., Akesson, H. S., & Björntorp, P. (2002). Depression and anxiety symptoms in relation to anthropometry and metabolism in men. *Psychiatry Research, 112*, 101–110.

Auphan, N., DiDonato, J. A., Rosette, C., Helmberg, A., & Karin, M. (1995). Immunosuppression by glucocorticoids: Inhibition of NF-kappa B activity through induction of I kappa B synthesis. *Science, 270*, 286–290.

Bali, B., & Kovacs, K. J. (2003). GABAergic control of neuropeptide gene expression in parvocellular neurons of the hypothalamic paraventricular nucleus. *European Journal of Neuroscience, 18*, 1518–1526.

Bamberger, C. M., Bamberger, A. M. , de Castro, M., & Chrousos, G. P. (1995). Glucocorticoid receptor beta, a potential endogenous inhibitor of glucocorticoid action in humans. *Journal of Clinical Investigation, 95*, 2435–2441.

Barthel, A., & Schmoll, D. (2003). Novel concepts in insulin regulation of hepatic gluconeogenesis. *American Journal of Physiology, Endocrinology and Metabolism, 285*, E685–E692.

Belanoff, J. K., Rothschild, A. J., Cassidy, F., DeBattista, C., Baulieu, E. E., Schold, C., & Schatzberg, A. F. (2002). An open trial of C-1073 (mifepristone) for psychotic major depression. *Biological Psychiatry, 52*, 386–392.

Binder, E. B., Salyakina, D., Lichtner, P., Wochnik, G. M., Ising, M., Putz, B., Papiol, S., Seaman, S., Lucae, S., Kohli, M. A., Nickel, T., Kunzel, H. E., Fuchs, B., Majer, M., Pfennig, A., Kern, N., Brunner, J., Modell, S., Baghai, T., Deiml, T., et al. (2004). Polymorphisms in FKBP5 are associated with increased recurrence of depressive episodes and rapid response to antidepressant treatment. *Nature Genetics, 36*, 1319–1325.

Bjorntorp, P. (1993). Visceral obesity: A "civilization syndrome." *Obesity Research, 1*, 206–222.

Bohus, B., & de Kloet, E. R. (1981). Adrenal steroids and extinction behavior: Antagonism by progesterone, deoxycorticosterone and dexamethasone of a specific effect of corticosterone. *Life Science, 28*, 433–440.

Bremner, J. D., Vythilingam, M., Anderson, G., Vermetten, E., McGlashan, T., Heninger, G., Rasmusson, A., Southwick, S. M., & Charney, D. S. (2003). Assessment of the hypothalamic–pituitary–adrenal axis over a 24-hour diurnal period and in response to neuroendocrine challenges in women with and without childhood sexual abuse and posttraumatic stress disorder. *Biological Psychiatry, 54*, 710–718.

Breslin, M. B., Geng, C. D., & Vedeckis, W. V. (2001). Multiple promoters exist in the human GR gene, one of which is activated by glucocorticoids. *Molecular Endocrinology, 15*, 1395.

Brönnegård, M., & Carlstedt-Duke, J. (1995). The genetic basis of glucocorticoid resistance. *Trends in Endocrinology and Metabolism, 6*, 160–164.

Buchanan, T. W. & Lovallo, W. R. (2001). Enhanced memory for emotional material following stress-level cortisol treatment in humans. *Psychoneuroendocrinology, 26*, 307–317.

Buemann, B., Vohl, M. C., Chagnon, M., Gagnon, J., Perusse, L., Dionne, F., Despres, J. P., Tremblay, A., Nadeau, A., & Bouchard, C. (1997). Abdominal visceral fat is associated with a BclI restriction fragment length polymorphism at the glucocorticoid receptor gene locus. *Obesity Research, 5*, 186–192.

Charmandari, E., Kino, T., Souvatzoglou, E., Vottero, A., Bhattacharyya, N., & Chrousos, G. P. (2004). Natural glucocorticoid receptor mutants causing generalized glucocorticoid resistance: Molecular genotype, genetic transmission, and clinical phenotype. *Journal of Clinical Endocrinology and Metabolism, 89*, 1939–1949.

Chrousos, G. P., Charmandari, E., & Kino, T. (2004). Glucocorticoid action networks—an introduction to systems biology. *Journal of Clinical Endocrinology and Metabolism, 89*, 563–564.

Chrousos, G. P., Detera-Wadleigh, S., & Karl, M. (1993). Syndromes of glucocorticoid resistance. *Annals of Internal Medicine, 119*, 1113–1124.

Dallman, M. F., Pecoraro, N., Akana, S. F., la Fleur, S. E., Gomez, F., Houshyar, H., Bell, M. E., Bhatnagar, S., Laugero, K., & Manalo, S. (2003). Chronic stress and obesity: A new view of "comfort food." *Proceedings of the National Academy of Sciences, 100*, 11,696–11,701.

Dallman, M. F., Viau, V. G., Bhatnagar, S., Gomez, F., Laugero, K., & Bell, M. E. (2002). Corticotropin-releasing factor, corticosteroids, stress and sugar: Energy balance, the brain and behavior. In D. Pfaff (Ed.), *Hormones, brain and behavior* (Vol. 1, pp. 571–631). New York: Elsevier.

Daly, A. K., & Day, C. P. (2001). Candidate gene case-control association studies: advantages and potential pitfalls. *British Journal of Clinical Pharmacology, 52*, 489–499.

Datson, N. A., van der Perk, J., de Kloet, E. R., & Vreugdenhil, E. (2001). Identification of corticosteroid-responsive genes in rat hippocampus using serial analysis of gene expression. *European Journal of Neuroscience, 14*, 675–689.

De Bosscher, K., Vanden Berghe, W., & Haegeman, G. (2003). The interplay between the glucocorticoid receptor and nuclear factor-kappaB or activator protein-1: Molecular mechanisms for gene repression. *Endocrine Reviews, 24*, 488–522.

de Kloet, E. R. (1975). Differences in corticosterone and dexamethasone binding to rat brain and pituitary. *Endocrinology, 96*, 598–609.

de Kloet, E. R. (1991). Brain corticosteroid receptor balance and homeostatic control. *Frontiers in Neuroendocrinology, 12*, 95–164.

de Kloet, E. R. (2003). Hormones, brain and stress. *Endocrine Regulations, 37*, 51–68.

de Kloet, E. R., de Kock, S., Schild, V., & Veldhuis, H. D. (1988). Antiglucocorticoid RU 38486 attenuates retention of a behaviour and disinhibits the hypothalamic-pituitary adrenal axis at different brain sites. *Neuroendocrinology, 47*, 109–115.

de Kloet, E. R., Vreugdenhil, E., Oitzl, M. S., & Joels, M. (1998). Brain corticosteroid receptor balance in health and disease. *Endocrine Reviews, 19*, 269–301.

de Lange, P., Koper, J. W., Huizinga, N. A. T. M., Brinkman, A. O., de Jong, F. H., Karl, M., Chrousos, G. P., & Lamberts, S. W. (1997). Differential hormone-dependent transcriptional activation and repression by naturally occurring human glucocorticoid receptor variants. *Molecular Endocrinology, 11*, 1156–1164.

DeRijk, R. H., Schaaf, M., & de Kloet, E. R. (2002). Glucocorticoid receptor variants: Clinical implications. *Journal of Steroid Biochemistry and Molecular Biology, 81*, 103–122.

DeRijk, R. H., Schaaf, M., Stam, F. J., Jong, I. E. M., Swaab, D. F., Ravid, R., Vreugdenhil, E., de Kloet, E. R., & Lucassen, P. J. (2003). Very low levels of the glucocorticoid receptor b isoform in the human hippocampus as shown by Tagman RT-PCR and immunocytochemistry. *Molecular Brain Research, 116*, 17–26.

DeRijk, R. H., Schaaf, M., Turner, G., Datson, N. A., Vreugdenhil, E., Cidlowski, J. A., de Kloet, E. R., Emery, P., Sternberg, E. M., & Detera-Wadleigh, S. (2001). A glucocorticoid receptor variant that increases the stability of the glucocorticoid receptor b-isoform is associated with rheumatoid arthritis. *Journal of Rheumatology, 28*, 2383–2388.

DeRijk, R. H., Sternberg, E. M., & de Kloet, E. R. (1997). Glucocorticoid receptor function in health and disease. *Current Opinion in Endocrinology and Diabetes, 4*, 185–193.

DeRijk, R. H., Wüst, S., Meijer, O. C., Zennaro, C., Vreugdenhil, E., Federenko, I., Gao, Y., Hellhammer, D., & de Kloet, E. R. A common polymorphism mineralocorticoid receptor determines stress-responsivity to a psychosocial challenge in humans. Abstract presented at the 4th Dutch Endo-Neuro-Psycho meeting. Doorwerth, Netherlands: May 31–June 3, 2005.

Detera-Wadleigh, S., Encio, I. J., & Rollins, D. Y. (1991). A TthIII1 polymorphism on the 5' flanking region of the glucocorticoid receptor gene (GRL) [Abstract]. *Nucleic Acid Research, 19*, 1960.

Deuschle, M., Weber, B., Colla, M., Müller, M., Kniest, A., & Heuser, I. J. (1998). Mineralocorticoid receptor also modulates basal activity of hypothalamus–pituitary–adrenocortical system in humans. *Neuroendocrinology, 68*, 355–360.

Diamond, D. M., Bennett, M. C., Fleshner, M., & Rose, G. M. (1992). Inverted-U relationship between the level of peripheral corticosterone and the magnitude of hippocampal primed burst potentiation. *Hippocampus, 2*, 421–430.

Di Blasio, A. M., van Rossum, E. F. C., Maestrini, S., Berselli, M. E., Tagliaferri, M., Podesta, F., Koper, J. W., Liuzzi, A., & Lamberts, S. W. (2003). The relation between two polymorphisms in the glucocorticoid receptor gene and body mass index, blood pressure and cholesterol in obese patients. *Clinical Endocrinology, 59*, 68–74.

Dobson, M. G., Redfern, C. P. F., Unwin, N., & Weaver, J. U. (2001). The N363S polymorphism of the glucocorticoid receptor: Potential contribution to central obesity in men and lack of association with other risk factors for coronary heart disease and diabetes mellitus. *Journal of Clinical Endocrinology and Metabolism, 86*, 2270–2274.

Dodt, C., Kern, W., Fehm, H. L., & Born, J. (1993). Antimineralocorticoid Canrenoate enhances secretory activity of the hypothalamus-pituitary-adrenocortical (HPA) axis in humans. *Neuroendocrinology, 58*, 570–574.

Eaton, W. W. (2002). Epidemiological evidence on the comorbidity of depression and diabetes. *Journal of Psychosomatic Research, 53*, 903–906.

Edwards, C. R., Steward, P. M., Burt, D., Brett, L., McIntyre, M. A., Sutanto, W., de Kloet, E. R., & Monder, C. (1988). Localisation of 11 beta-hydroxysteroid dehydrogenase—tissue specific protector of the mineralocorticoid receptor. *The Lancet, 2*, 986–989.

Ellenbogen, M. A., Hodgins, S., & Walker, C. D. (2004). High levels of cortisol among adolescent offspring of parents with bipolar disorder: A pilot study. *Psychoneuroendocrinology, 29*, 99–106.

Emahazion, T., Feuk, L., Jobs, M., Sawyer, S. L., Fredman, D., St Clair, D., Prince, J. A., & Brookes, A. J. (2001). SNP association studies in Alzheimer's disease highlight problems for complex disease analysis. *Trends in Genetics, 17*, 407–413.

Fleury, I., Beaulieu, P., Primeau, M., Sinnett, D., & Krajinovic, M. (2003). Characterization of the BclI polymorphism in the glucocorticoid receptor gene. *Clinical Chemistry, 49*, 1528–1531.

Giguere, V., Hollenberg, S. M., Rosenfeld, M. G., & Evans, R. M. (2001). Functional domains of the human glucocorticoid receptor. *Cell, 46*, 645–652.

Gold, P. W., & Chrousos, G. P. (2002). Organization of the stress system and its dysregulation in melancholic and atypical depression: High vs low CRH/NE states. *Molecular Psychiatry, 7*, 254–275.

Goldstein, D. S. (2003). Catecholamines and stress. *Endocrine Regulations, 37*, 69–80.

Haller, J., Millar, S., & Kruk, M. R. (1998). Mineralocorticoid receptor blockade inhibits aggressive behavior in male rats. *Stress, 2*, 201–207.

Hammond, G. L., Smith, C. L., Paterson, N. A. M., & Sibbald, W. J. (1990). A role for corticosteroid binding globulin in delivery of cortisol to activated neutrophils. *Journal of Clinical Endocrinology and Metabolism, 71*, 34–39.

Heim, C., Newport, D. J., Heit, S., Graham, Y. P., Wilcox, M., Bonsall, R., Milller, A. H., & Nemeroff, C. B. (2001). Pituitary-adrenal and autonomic responses to stress in woman after sexual and physical abuse in childhood. *Journal of the American Medical Association, 284*, 592–597.

Herman, J. P., Cullinan, W. E., Ziegler, D. R., & Tasker, J. G. (2002). Role of the paraventricular nucleus microenvironment in stress integration. *European Journal of Neuroscience, 16*, 381–385.

Herman, J. P., Figueiredo, H., Mueller, N. K., Ulrich-Lai, Y., Ostrander, M. M., Choi, D. C., & Cullinan, W. E. (2003). Central mechanisms of stress integration: Hierarchical circuitry controlling hypothalamo-pituitary-adrenocortical responsiveness. *Frontiers in Neuroendocrinology, 24*, 151–180.

Heuser, I., Deuschle, M., Weber, B., Stalla, G. K., & Holsboer, F. (2000). Increased activity of the hypothalamus-pituitary-adrenal system after treatment with the mineralocorticoid receptor antagonist spironolactone. *Psychoneuroendocrinology, 25*, 513–518.

Hollenberg, S. M., Weinberger, C., Ong, E. S., Cerelli, G., Oro, A., Lebo, R., Thompson, E. B., Rosenfeld, M. G., & Evans, R. M. (1985). Primary structure and expression of a functional glucocorticoid receptor cDNA. *Nature, 318*, 635–641.

Holsboer, F., Lauer, C. J., Schreiber, W., & Krieg, J.-C. (1995). Altered hypothalamic-pituitary-adrenocortical regulation in healthy subjects at high familial risk for affective disorders. *Neuroendocrinology, 62*, 340–347.

Hsu, S. Y., & Hsueh, A. J. (2001). Human stresscopin and stresscopin-related peptide are selective ligands for the type 2 corticotropin-releasing hormone receptor. *Nature Medicine, 7*, 605–611.

Huizinga, N. A. T. M., Koper, J. W., de Lange, P., Pols, H. A. , Stolk, R. P., Burger, H., Grobbee, D. E., Brinkman, A. O., de Jong, F. H., & Lamberts, S. W. (1998). A polymorphism in the glucocorticoid receptor gene may be associated with an increased sensitivity to glucocorticoids. *Journal of Clinical Endocrinology and Metabolism, 83*, 144–151.

Joëls, M., & de Kloet, E. R. (1989). Effects of glucocorticoids and norepinephrine on the excitability in the hippocampus. *Science, 245*, 1502–1505.

Joëls, M., & de Kloet, E. R. (1992). Control of neuronal excitability by corticosteroid hormones. *Trend in Neurosciences, 15*, 25–30.

Joëls, M., & de Kloet, E. R. (1994). Mineralocorticoid and glucocorticoid receptors in the brain. Implications for ion permeability and transmitter systems. *Progress in Neurobiology, 43*, 1–36.

Joëls, M., Verkuyl, J. M., & van Riel, E. (2003). Hippocampal and hypothalamic function after chronic stress. *Annals of the New York Academy of Sciences, 1007*, 367–378.

Kalsbeek, A., & Buijs, R. M. (2002). Output pathways of the mammalian suprachiasmatic nucleus: Coding circadian time by transmitter selection and specific targeting. *Cell Tissue Research, 309*, 109–118.

Karssen, A. M., Meijer, O. C., van der Sandt, I., Lucassen, P. J., de Lange, E. C., de Boer, A. G., & de Kloet, E. R. (2001). Multidrug resistance P-glycoprotein hampers the access of cortisol but not of corticosterone to mouse and human brain. *Endocrinology, 142*, 2686–2694.

Karst, H., Karten, Y. J., Reichard, H. M., de Kloet, E. R., Schütz, G., & Joels, M. (2000). Corticosteroid actions in hippocampus require DNA binding of glucocorticoid receptor homodimers. *Nature Neuroscience, 3*, 977–978.

Kirschbaum, C., Bono, E. G., Rohleder, N., Gessner, C., Pirke, M., Salvador, A., & Hellhammer, D. (1997). Effects of fasting an glucose load on free cortisol responses to stress and nicotine. *Journal of Clinical Endocrinology and Metabolism, 82*, 1101–1105.

Kitchener, P., Di Blasi, F., Borelli, E., & Piazza, P. V. (2004). Differences between brain structures in nuclear translocation and DNA binding of the glucocorticoid receptor during stress and the circadian cycle. *European Journal of Neuroscience, 19*, 1837–1846.

Koper, J. W., Stolk, R. P., de Lange, P., Huizenga, N. A. T., Molijn, G. J., Pols, H. A., Grobbee, D. E., Karl, M., de Jong, F. H., Brinkmann, A. O., & Lamberts, S. W. (1997). Lack of association between five polymorphisms in the human glucocorticoid receptor gene and glucocorticoid resistance. *Human Genetics, 99*, 663–668.

Korte, S. M. (2002). Corticosteroids in relation to fear, anxiety and psychopathology. *Neuroscience & Biobehavioral Reviews, 25*, 117–142.

Lamberts, S. W., Huizenga, N. A. T. M., de Lange, P., de Jong, F. H., & Koper, J. W. (1996). Clinical aspects of glucocorticoid sensitivity. *Steroids, 61*, 157–160.

Laugero, K., Gomez, F., Manalo, S., & Dallman, M. F. (2002). Corticosterone infused intracerebroventricularly inhibits energy storage and stimulates the hypothalamo-pituitary axis in adrenalectomized rats drinking sucrose. *Endocrinology, 143*, 4552–4562.

Lightman, S., Windle, R. J., Julian, M. D., Harbuz, M. S., Shanks, N., Wood, S. A., Kershaw, Y. M., & Ingram, C. D. (2000). Significance of pulsatility in the HPA axis. *In Mechanisms and biological significance of pulsatile hormone secretion* (pp. 244–260). Chichester: Wiley.

Lin, R. C. Y., Wang, W. Y. S., & Morris, B. J. (1999a). High penetrance, overweight and glucocorticoid receptor variant: Case-control study. *British Medical Journal, 319*, 1337–1338.

Lin, R. C. Y., Wang, W. Y. S., & Morris, B. J. (1999b). Association and linkage analysis of glucocorticoid receptor gene markers in essential hypertension. *Hypertension, 34*, 1192.

Lin, R. C. Y., Wang, X. L., & Morris, B. J. (2003). Association of coronary artery disease with the glucocorticoid receptor N363S variant. *Hypertension, 41*, 404–407.

Loscertales, M., Rose, S. P., & Sandi, C. (1997). The corticosteroid synthesis inhibitors metyrapone and aminoglutethimide impair long-term memory for a passive avoidance task in day-old chicks. *Brain Research, 769*, 357–361.

Lupien, S. J., Wilkinson, D. W., Brière, S., Ménard, C., Ng Ying Kin, N. M. K., Nair, N. P. V. (2002). The modulatory effects of corticosteroids on cognition: Studies in young human populations. *Psychoneuroendocrinology, 27*, 401–416.

Masuzaki, H., Paterson, J., Shinyama, H., Morton, N. M., Mullins, J. J., Seckl, J. R., & Flier, J. S. (2001). A transgenic model of visceral obesity and the metabolic syndrome. *Science, 294*, 2166–2170.

McEwen, B. S. (1998). Protective and damaging effects of stress mediators. *New England Journal of Medicine, 338*, 171–179.

Meijer, O. C., de Lange, E. C. M., Breimer D.D., de Boer, A. G., Workel, J. O., & de Kloet, E. R. (1998). Penetration of dexamethasone into brain glucocorticoid targets is enhanced in mdr1a-Pglycoprotein knockout mice. *Endocrinology, 139*, 1789–1793.

Meijer, O. C., Steenbergen, P. J., & de Kloet, E. R. (2002). Differential expression and regional distribution of steroid receptor coactivators SRC-1 and SRC-2 in brain and pituitary. *Endocrinology, 141*, 2192–2199.

Montkowski, A., Barden, N., Wotjak, C., Stec, I. E., Ganster, J., Meaney, M. J., Engelmann, M., Reul, J. M., Landgraf, R., & Holsboer, F. (1995). Long-term antidepressant treatment reduces behavioural deficits in transgenic mice with impaired glucocorticoid receptor function. *Journal of Neuroendocrinology, 7*, 841–845.

Müller, M. B., Holsboer, F., & Kellendonk, C. (2002). Genetic modification of corticosteroid receptor signaling: Novel insights into pathophysiology and treatment strategies of human affective disorders. *Neuropeptides, 36*, 117–131.

Munck, A., Guyre, P. M., & Holbrook, N. J. (1984). Physiological functions of glucocorticoids in stress and their relation to pharmacological actions. *Endocrine Reviews, 5*, 25–44.

Murray, J. C., Smith, R. F., Ardinger, H. A., & Weinberger, C. (1987). RFLP for the glucocorticoid receptor (GRL) located at 5q11-5q13. *Nucleic Acid Research, 15*, 6765.

Oakley, R. H., Sar, M., & Cidlowski, J. A. (1996). The human glucocorticoid receptor beta isoform. Expression, biochemical properties, and putative function. *Journal of Biological Chemistry, 271*, 9550–9559.

Oitzl, M. S., & de Kloet, E. R. (1992). Selective corticosteroid antagonists modulate specific aspects of spatial orientation learning. *Behavioral Neuroscience, 106*, 62–71.

Oitzl, M. S., Fluttert, M., & de Kloet, E. R. (1994). The effect of corticosterone on reactivity to spatial novelty is mediated by central mineralocorticoid receptors. *European Journal of Neuroscience, 6*, 1072–1079.

Oitzl, M. S., Fluttert, M., Sutanto, W., & de Kloet, E. R. (1998). Continuous blockade of brain glucocorticoid receptors facilitates spatial learning and memory in rats. *European Journal of Neuroscience, 10*, 3759–3766.

Oitzl, M. S., Reichard, H. M., Joëls, M., & de Kloet, E. R. (2001). Point mutation in the mouse glucocorticoid receptor preventing DNA binding impairs spatial memory. *Proceedings of the National Academy of Sciences, 98*, 12,790–12,795.

Oitzl, M. S., van Haarst, A. D., Sutanto, W., & de Kloet, E. R. (1995). Corticosterone, brain mineralocorticoid receptors (MRs) and the acitivity of the hypothalamic-pituitary-adrenal (HPA) axis: The Lewis rat as an

example of increased central MR capacity and a hyporesponsive HPA axis. *Psychoneuroendocrinology, 20*, 655–675.
Panarelli, M., Holloway, C. D., Fraser, R., Connell, J. M. C., Ingram, M., Anderson, N. N., & Kenyon, C. J. (1998). Glucocorticoid receptor polymorphism, skin vasoconstriction and other metabolic intermediate phenotypes in normal subjects. *Journal of Clinical Endocrinology and Metabolism, 83*, 1846–1852.
Rahmouni, K., Barthelmebs, M., Grima, M., Imbs, J. L., & de Jong, W. (2003). Influence of sodium intake on the cardiovascular and renal effects of brain mineralocorticoid receptor blockade in normotensive rats. *Journal of Hypertension, 20*, 1829–1834.
Ratka, A., Sutanto, W., Bloemers, M., & de Kloet, E. R. (1989). On the role of the brain type I and type II corticosteroid receptors in neuroendocrine regulation. *Neuroendocrinology, 50*, 117–123.
Reichard, H. M., Kaestner, K. H., Tuckermann, J., Kretz, O., Wessely, O., Bock, R., Gass, O., Schmid, W., Herrlich, P., Angel, P., & Schütz, G. (1998). DNA binding of the glucocorticoid receptor is not essential for survival. *Cell, 93*, 531–541.
Reichardt, H. M., Tuckermann, J., Bauer, A., & Schütz, G. (2000). Molecular genetic dissection of glucocorticoid receptor function in vivo. *Zeitschrift für Rheumatologie, 59*, 1–5.
Reul, J. M., & Holsboer, F. (2002). Corticotropin-releasing factor receptors 1 and 2 in anxiety and depression. *Current Opinion in Pharmacology, 2*, 23–33.
Reynolds, R. M., & Walker, B. R. (2003). Human insulin resistance: The role of glucocorticoids. *Diabetes, Obesity and Metabolism, 5*, 5–12.
Rinne, T., de Kloet, E. R., Wouters, L., Goekoop, J. G., DeRijk, R. H., & Brink, W. (2002). Hyperresponsiveness of hypothalamic–pituitary–adrenal axis to combined dexamethasone/corticotropin-releasing hormone challenge in female borderline personality disorder subjects with a history of sustained childhood abuse. *Biological Psychiatry, 52*, 1102–1112.
Roberts, R. E., Deleger, S., Strawbridge, W. J., & Kaplan, G. A. (2003). Prospective association between obesity and depression: Evidence from the Alameda County Study. *International Journal of Obesity, 27*, 514–521.
Romero, L. M., & Sapolsky, R. M. (1996). Patterns of ACTH secretagog secretion in response to psychological stimuli. *Journal of Neuroendocrinology, 8*, 243–258.
Roozendaal, B., Griffith, Q. K., Buranday, J., Quervain, D. J.-F., & McGaugh, J. L. (2003). The hippocampus mediates glucocorticoid-induced impairment of spatial memory retrieval: Dependence on the basolateral amygdala. *Proceedings of the National Academy of Sciences, 100*, 1328–1333.
Rosmond, R. (2003a). Glucocorticoid receptor gene and coronary artery disease: Right idea, wrong gene variant? *Hypertension, 42*, e3–e4.
Rosmond, R. (2003b). Glucocorticoid receptor N363S variant in obesity: comes into vanity and goes into darkness [Letter]. *Obesity Research, 11*, 1606–1607.
Rosmond, R., Bouchard, C., & Björntorp, P. (2001). Tsp509I polymorphism in exon 2 of the glucocorticoid receptor gene in relation to obesity and cortisol secretion: Cohort study. *British Medical Journal, 322*, 652–653.
Rosmond, R., Chagnon, Y. C., Chagnon, M., Pérusse, L., Bouchard, C., & Björntorp, P. (2000a). A polymorphism of the 5'-flanking region of the glucocorticoid receptor gene locus is associated with basal cortisol secretion in men. *Metabolism, 49*, 1197–1199.
Rosmond, R., Chagnon, Y. C., Holm, G., Chagnon, M., Pérusse, L., Lindell, K., Carlsson, B., Bouchard, C., & Björntorp, P. (2000b). A glucocorticoid receptor gene marker is associated with abdominal obesity, leptin, and dysregulation of the hypothalamic-pituitary-adrenal axis. *Obesity Research, 8*, 211–218.
Rosmond, R., Dallman, M. F., & Björntorp, P. (1998). Stress-related cortisol secretion in men: Relationships with abdominal obesity and endocrine, metabolic and hemodynamic abnormalities. *Journal of Clinical Endocrinology and Metabolism, 83*, 1853–1859.
Sakai, R. R., Ma, L. Y., Zhang, D. M., McEwen, B. S., & Fluharty, S. J. (1996). Intracerebral administration of mineralocorticoid receptor antisense oligonucleotides attenuate adrenal steroid-induced salt appetite in rats. *Neuroendocrinology, 64*, 425–429.
Schaaf, M., & Cidlowski, J. A. (2002a). AUUUA motifs in the 3'UTR of human glucocorticoid receptor alpha and beta mRNA destabilize mRNA and decrease receptor protein expression. *Steroids, 67*, 627–636.
Schaaf, M., & Cidlowski, J. A. (2002b). Molecular mechanisms of glucocorticoid action and resistance. *Journal of Steroid Biochemistry and Molecular Biology, 83*, 37–48.

Schmidt, L. A., Fox, N. A., Goldberg, M. C., Smith, C. C., & Schulkin, J. (1999). Effects of acute prednisone administration on memory, attention and emotion in healthy human adults. *Psychoneuroendocrinology, 24*, 461–483.

Seckl, J. R., Morton, N. M., Chapman, K. E., & Walker, B. R. (2004). Glucocorticoid and 11beta-hydroxysteroid dehydrogenase in adipose tissue. *Recent Progress in Hormone Research, 59*, 359–393.

Seckl, J. R., & Walker, B. R. (2001). Minireview: 11Beta-hydroxysteroid dehydrogenase type 1—a tissue-specific amplifier of glucocorticoid action. *Endocrinology, 142*, 1371–1376.

Stevens, A., Ray, D. W., Zeggini, E., John, S., Richards, H. L., Griffiths, C. E. M., & Donn, R. (2004). Glucocorticoid sensitivity is determined by a specific glucocorticoid receptor haplotype. *Journal of Clinical Endocrinology and Metabolism, 89*, 892–897.

Stewart, P. M., Boulton, A., Kumar, S., Clark, P. M. S., Shahidi, H., & Shackleton, C. H. L. (1999). Cortisol metabolism in human obesity: Impaired cortisone → cortisol conversion in subjects with central adiposity. *Journal of Clinical Endocrinology and Metabolism, 84*, 1027.

Tremblay, A., Bouchard, L., Bouchard, C., Despres, J. P., Drapeau, V., & Perusse, L. (2003). Long-term adiposity changes are related to a glucocorticoid receptor polymorphism in young females. *Journal of Clinical Endocrinology and Metabolism, 88*, 3141–3145.

Ukkola, O., Pérusse, L., Chagnon, M., Després, J. P., & Bouchard, C. (2001). Interactions among the glucocorticoid receptor, lipoprotein lipase and adrenergic receptor genes and abdominal fat in the Quebec Family Study. *International Journal of Obesity and Related Metabolic Disorders, 25*, 1332–1339.

Ukkola, O., Rosmond, R., Tremblay, A., & Bouchard, C. (2001). Glucocorticoid receptor Bcl I variant is associated with an increased atherogenic profile in response to long-term overfeeding. *Atherosclerosis, 157*, 221–224.

van den Berg, D. T., de Kloet, E. R., & de Jong, W. (1994). Central effects of mineralocorticoid antagonist RU-28318 on blood pressure of DOCA-salt hypertensive rats. *American Journal of Physiology, 267*, E927–E933.

van den Buuse, M., van Acker, S. A., Fluttert, M., & de Kloet, E. R. (2002). Involvement of corticosterone in cardiovascular responses to an open-field novelty stressor in freely moving rats. *Physiology & Behavior, 75*, 207–215.

van Haarst, A. D., Oitzl, M. S., & de Kloet, E. R. (1997). Facilitation of feedback inhibition through blockade of glucocorticoid receptors in the hippocampus. *Neurochemical Research, 22*, 1323–1328.

van Haarst, A. D., Oitzl, M. S., Workel, J. O., & de Kloet, E. R. (1996). Chronic brain glucocorticoid receptor blockade enhances the rise in circadian and stress-induced pituitary-adrenal activity. *Endocrinology, 137*, 4935–4943.

van Rossum, E. F. C., Koper, J. W. , Huizenga, A. T., Uitterlinden, A. G., Janssen, J. A. M. J. L., Brinkmann, A. O., Grobbee, D. E., de Jong, F. H., van Duyn, C. M., Pols, H. A. P., & Lamberts, S. W. (2003a). A polymorphism in the glucocorticoid receptor gene, which decreases sensitivity to glucocorticoids in vivo, is associated with low insulin and cholesterol levels. *Diabetes, 51*, 3128–3134.

van Rossum, E. F. C., Koper, J. W. , van den Beld, A. W., Uitterlinden, A. G., Arp, P., Ester, W., Janssen, J. A. M. J. L., Brinkman, A. O., de Jong, F. H., Grobbee, D. E., Pols, H. A., & Lamberts, S. W. (2003b). Identification of the BclI polymorphism in the glucocorticoid receptor gene: Association with sensitivity to glucocorticoids in vivo and body mass index. *Clinical Endocrinology, 59*, 585–592.

van Rossum, E. F. C., & Lamberts, S. W. (2004). Polymorphisms in the glucocorticoid receptor gene and their associations with metabolic parameters and body composition. *Recent Progress in Hormone Research, 59*, 333–357.

van Steensel, B., van Binnendijk, E. P., Hornsby, C. D., van der Voort, H. T., Krozowski, Z. S., de Kloet, E. R., & van Driel, R. (1996). Partial colocalization of glucocorticoid and mineralocorticoid receptors in discrete compartments in nuclei of rat hippocampus neurons. *Journal of Cell Science, 109*, 787–792.

Watt, G. C. M., Harrap, S. B., Foy, C. J. W., Holton, D. W., Edwards, H. V., Davidson, H. R., Conner, J. M., Lever, A. F., & Fraser, R. (1992). Abnormalities of glucocorticoid metabolism and the renin-angiotensin system: A four corner approach to the identification of genetic determinants of blood pressure. *Journal of Hypertension, 10*, 473–482.

Weaver, J. U., Hitman, G. A., & Kopelman, P. G. (1992). An association between a BclI restriction fragment length polymorphism of the glucocorticoid receptor locus and hyperinsulinaemia in obese woman. *Journal of Molecular Biology, 9*, 295–300.

Weber, B., Schweiger, U., Deuschle, M., & Heuser, I. (2000). Major depression and impaired glucose tolerance. *Experimental and Clinical Endocrinology and Diabetes, 108*, 187–190.

Weber-Hamann, B., Hentschel, F., Kniest, A., Deuschle, M., Colla, M., Lederbogen, F., & Heuser, I. (2002). Hypercortisolemic depression is associated with increased intra-abdominal fat. *Psychosomatic Medicine, 64*, 274–277.

Weinberger, C., Hollenberg, S. M., Rosenfeld, M. G., & Evans, R. M. (1985). Domain structure of human glucocorticoid receptor and its relationship to the v-erb-A oncogene product. *Nature, 318*, 670–672.

Windle, R. J., Wood, S. A., Shanks, N., Lightman, S., & Ingram, C. D. (1998). Ultradian rhythm of basal corticosterone release in the female rat: Dynamic interaction with the response to acute stress. *Endocrinology, 139*, 443–450.

Wolkowitz, O. M., Reus, V. I., Weingartner, H., Thompson, K., Breier, A., Doran, A., Rubinow, D., & Pickar, D. (1990). Cognitive effects of corticosteroids. *American Journal of Psychiatry, 147*, 1297–1303.

Wüst, S., van Rossum, E. F. C., Federenko, I., Koper, J. W., Kumsta, R., & Hellhammer, D. (2004). Common polymorphisms in the glucocorticoid receptor gene are associated with adrenocortical responses to psychosocial stress. *Journal of Clinical Endocrinology and Metabolism, 89*, 563–564.

Yehuda, R. (2002). Post-traumatic stress disorder. *New England Journal of Medicine, 346*, 108–114.

Yehuda, R., Halligan, S. L., Grossman, R., Golier, J. A., & Wong, C. (2002). The cortisol and glucocorticoid receptor response to low dose dexamethasone administration in aging combat veterans and Holocaust survivors with and without posttraumatic stress disorder. *Biological Psychiatry, 52*, 393–403.

Young, E. A., Lopez, J. F., Murphy-Weinberg, V., Watson, S. J., & Akil, H. (1998). The role of mineralocorticoid receptors in hypothalamic-pituitary-adrenal axis regulation in humans. *Journal of Clinical Endocrinology and Metabolism, 83*, 3339–3345.

Yudt, M. R., & Cidlowski, J. A. (2001). Molecular identification and characterization of A and B forms of the glucocorticoid receptor. *Molecular Endocrinology, 15*, 1093–1103.

Zondervan, K. T., & Cardon, L. R. (2004). The complex interplay among factors that influence allelic association. *Nature Reviews Genetics, 5*, 89–101.

8 Herbal Products, Stress, and the Mind

David Wheatley

KEY POINTS

- Seminal components of the stress vicious circle are depression, anxiety, heart, sleep, sex, and memory.
- St. John's wort—the Baptist's herb and depression.
- Kavakava may be in disgrace, but it does work for anxiety and insomnia.
- Valerian—to sleep, perchance to dream.
- Putative sleep-inducers include lavender, chamomile, ylang-ylang, melissa, passion-flower, and hops.
- Ginkgo biloba—memories are made of this.
- Enigma variations: Why do herbal plants exist?

1. INTRODUCTION

One individual's lucid thoughts spell confusion to another unless logically explained from conception. I will therefore commence my preamble to this chapter, with some definitions, as I interpret them, of key aspects of my subject.

Herbs perform two important functions in humans: nutritional and medicinal. The two may be inexorably entwined, or they may be separate and distinct. I concern myself primarily with the medicinal uses of herbal products, and by this token, I mean any substance that has been seminally derived from any form of plant life, be that borne by, or born from, root, tuber, bulb, seed, stem, trunk, bark, leaf, bud, flower, or fruit.

One person's stress is another's inspiration. By stress I mean any life stimulus, mental or physical, that the individual perceives as unpleasant or harmful. Because it is so perceived, be that real or illusionary, it may exert adverse effects on the individual's health. For example, retirement comes as a blessed relief from a life of tedious toil to many, but denies the fulfillment of achievement to others. In the first case there is relief of stress; in the second, a totally new stress is created—depending on the individual's reaction to the new life situation. Therefore, stress is very much in the eye of the beholder.

The mind is both a happy and a sad place, and both basic emotions play appropriate parts in the regulation of the individual's day-to-day life. As in the case of stress, what is sadness to one may be happiness to another, depending upon both the individual and the circumstances. I am concerned with ailments of the mind as they affect the individual

From: *Nutrients, Stress, and Medical Disorders*
Edited by: S. Yehuda and D. I. Mostofsky © Humana Press Inc., Totowa, NJ

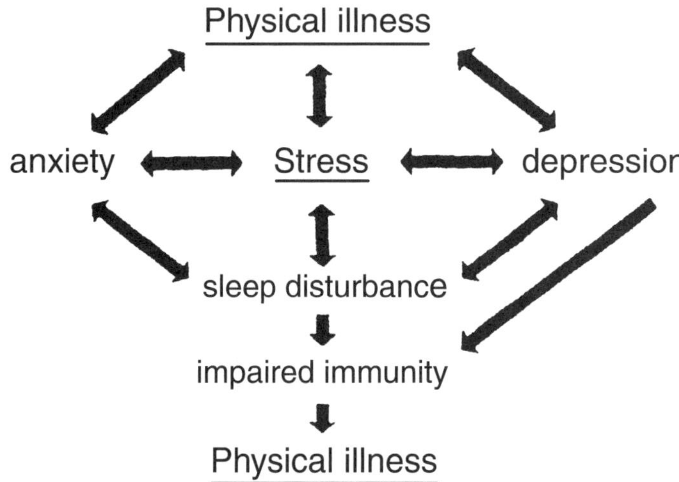

Fig. 1. The stress–illness vicious circle. This is multidimensional and can be interpreted clockwise, anticlockwise, horizontally, or vertically, with equal validities.

and the role that herbal products can play in easing these and thereby curing "dis-ease." But such compounds have another very important function: improving age- or circumstance-related changes in bodily functions. For example, ginkgo biloba can help to restore the failing memory of old age and improve it in the young to help them meet certain life challenges. A paradigm is the use of coffee to ensure alertness and cognitive perfection when taking examinations: gilding the lily perhaps, but it might equally well be termed a means of "logging-on" to a normal mental reserve function. The end result is the same: the individual is better enabled to cope with whatever stress may confront him or her.

2. STRESS AND PSYCHIATRIC DISORDERS

The impact of stress is, *de novo*, on the mind, and that which starts as a physiological response to the environment may become established as a pathological process. In order to fully appreciate this concept, it is important to consider the physiological changes initiated in a stress situation and their consequences on human functioning, or, as I have termed it, the stress vicious circle (Fig. 1) (Wheatley, 1990).

2.1. The Stress Vicious Circle

All higher living organisms are programmed with the "fight-or-flight" reaction to stress (Selye, 1936). In the wild, constant fear of attacks by predators creates an existence fraught by ever-present anxiety. It can be aptly said that the animal's "stress jungle" is simply transformed into the human "anxiogenic jungle" (Wheatley, 1997). Thus, anxiety both causes and is caused by stress, thus creating more stress and even physical illness. Singly or combined, such noxious effects may initiate depression in a susceptible individual, an integral component of which is sleep disturbance, with resultant impairment of immunity (Mendelson et al., 1984; Palmblad et al., 1986), which may cause or aggravate physical illness (Jacobs et al., 1969). So, we have come round full circle, and we perceive that the model is, in reality, a two-dimensional one, which can be read from left to right or from top to bottom or, conversely, with equal validity.

In peacetime, life-threatening stress is not often encountered by human beings, but it has been replaced by other, more subtle stresses that may exert far-reaching effects. Furthermore, unlike the situation in the wild, where the stress responses return to normal once the threat has passed, in humans these are often perpetuated when there is a failure to cope with them. One example would be an individual whose employment depends on working under a beligerant supervisor, a continuing and inescapable source of stress. In consequence, physiological stress responses may become established, resulting in illnesses such as anxiety states, panic disorder, phobias, and depression. Of all these consequences of stress, the last-named is undoubtedly the most deadly.

2.2. Depression: Emotion or Illness?

Under the cloak of continuing anxiety symptoms, the aptly designated "masked depression" may insidiously develop and remain undetected by patient and physician alike (Hordern, 1976). As Hordern commented: "suicide is the mortality of depression." So we are indeed dealing with a potentionally deadly outcome if the condition is not diagnosed and treated promptly. But the mood of depression is a normal expression of grief. When then does it become an illness? This can be best determined by the use of appropriate psychiatric and diagnostic rating scales, which are beyond the scope of this chapter (*see* Frances et al., 1994; Hamilton, 1960). However, a pragmatic guide is provided by the appropriateness of the circumstances of the depressed mood.

It is appropriate for someone who has suffered a bereavement to feel depressed about it (mood), but it is not appropriate for someone who is emotionally and financially buoyant and carefree to do so (illness). It would be inappropriate to treat depressed *mood* with chemical antidepressant drugs, but it is imperative to do so in the case of depressive *illness*. The distinction need not apply to herbal antidepressant compounds such as St. John's wort (SJW), which can be used for both mood and illness, as will be discussed in the next section. When treating depression with either chemical antidepressants, such as selective serotonin reuptake inhibitors (SSRIs) or SJW, it is of utmost importance to achieve patient cooperation in drug taking during the first critical 3–4 wk of treatment. It is an inexplicable fact that all antidepressants, chemical and herbal alike, require this amount of time before any benefit ensues that is apparent to the patient. In the face of side effects that frequently occur with chemical drugs, patients may stop a treatment that is perceived as making them worse. Or they may reduce doses to inadequate levels. Since SJW is virtually devoid of side effects, the physician's task is rendered that much easier in this respect. Other aspects of depression may also be directly benefited by herbal products, notably anxiety and sleep.

2.3. The Anxious Heart

The main impact of the fight-or-flight reaction to stress is manifested through the cardiovascular system (Wheatley, 1981). Catecholamine release results in an increase in pulse rate, a rise in blood pressure, and a redistribution of blood flow to muscles and brain at the expense of the gut. Once the stress is over, these rapidly return to normal. But in the case of long-continuing stress, albeit of lesser degree, this may not happen, and so this becomes a factor in the establishment of cardiac disease and hypertension. Under these circumstances, drugs such as β-adrenergic blockers become particularly useful—both improving cardiac function and relieving anxiety (Wheatley, 1969). Tranquilization can also be achieved with herbal products, such as valerian, and these may provide a more acceptable alternative to anxiolytic drugs such as the benzodiazepines, with all their problems of addiction and dependence.

2.4. To Sleep, Perchance to Dream

An adequate amount of quality sleep is essential to the maintenance of good health (Horne,1988). Benzodiazepine hypnotics suffer from the same problems as their counterparts, the anxiolytics, and do not even produce "normal" sleep, as evidenced by sleep polysomnography, being deficient in the deep stages (Wheatley, 1992). Although this deficiency has been remedied by the introduction of the nonbenzodiazepine drugs zopiclone (UK), zolpidem, and zaleplon (UK and US), these drugs are by no means free of dependence problems. On the other hand, valerian not only improves deep sleep but would appear to be free of this disadvantage.

The reason for this emphasis on the deep stages of sleep (stages 3 and 4, short-wave or δ sleep) is because these embody the restorative value of sleep (Adam & Oswald, 1983), deprivation of which leads to impaired physical and mental performance (Pilcher & Huffcutt, 1996). Thus, insomnia is a key factor in the stress vicious circle and restoration of deep sleep a major contribution to breaking it. But what of dreaming? Described as the "cinema of the mind" (Horne, 1988), its natural purpose remains a mystery, but it is an essential contributor to health.

Although kavakava has been withdrawn in most countries because of hepatoxicity (Escher & Desmeules, 2001), I am including some comment concerning this compound since it has been so well established over many decades and in the remote possibility that this verdict may be reversed at some time in the future.

2.5. Sex: The Trigger of Life

Without sex, we would not be. Therefore, it behooves us to nurture this seminal function well. Sexual problems are a potent cause of stress and, of course, are often a consequence of it. The paradigm in the round again! And sexual impairment is a common core symptom of depression, anxiety, and allied states and, with some notable exceptions, including SJW, is worsened by antidepressant drugs (Segraves, 1998; Wheatley, 1998)—another advantage for the herbal product. Partner support can be a vital element in motivating the depressed patient to continue with treatment, even when the latter threatens the harmony of the relationship itself. Freedom from this impediment provides a boost indeed to curing the illness.

2.6. Forgotten Memories

Life experiences are the essence of that life, without which we could not function in temporal time, neither could we profit from their experience or enjoy, in retrospect, those that were pleasurable. When memory is impaired, as in cerebral arteriosclerosis or Alzheimer's disease, or even when a stimulus is required for "normal" memory function, drugs can prove effective. The slow progressive decline in memory that is the inevitable accompaniment of senescence can be retarded by anti-Alzheimer drugs such as donepezil and memantine in circumstances other than dementia. The stimulant effects (including memory) of caffeine and amphetamine drugs are well known as those taking examinations, attending conferences, or going into battle know full well. A vivid specific example has been provided by Yesavage et al. (2002), who assessed 18 pilots in a flight simulator of a single-engined aircraft and faced with various complex tasks and emergency procedures, depending on memory for their correct execution. The trial was double-blinded between donepezil and placebo, administered over a period of 30 d; the active drug was significantly better, particularly when landing and facing emergencies. The herbal preparation ginkgo biloba has been shown to be effective in improving memory both in normal subjects and various dementia states, including Alzheimer's disease. These will be considered in the next section. Therefore, by improving memory, we are not just gilding the lily, but enabling the human organism to bring into play hidden reserves to combat extreme stress situations that otherwise would be, perversely, denied by nature.

3. ST. JOHNS WORT: THE BAPTIST'S HERB

A number of herbal remedies have important medicinal properties and offer advantages over conventional chemical drugs, especially as far as patient acceptability and side effects are concerned. Of these, one of the most important is SJW, the popular name for the plant *Hypericum perforatum*, which has been known since biblical times when it was used by St. John the Baptist (Grigson, 1958). It was collected on St. John's day (June 26) and used to ward off "goblins, devils and witches." Among other properties, including being a "healer of wounds," it was known for its effects on the mind as a "cure for demoniacs" (Porcher, 1970).

3.1. Role in Psychopharmacology

The extract is also known as *hypericum*, and it is standardized as to *hypericin* content, although the active principle is thought to be *hyperforin* (Laakmann et al., 1998). The usual dose for mild-moderate depression is 900 mg daily, but doses up to 1800 mg have been used with benefit in more severe cases (Vorbach et al., 1997). With the exception of rare skin hypersensitivity (but only in those with sun allergy, who should not take it anyway), it is virtually free of side effects in comparison to placebo. In a meta-analysis of 1757 patients treated with SJW, there were only two dropouts (0.8%) for adverse events compared to seven (5%) with the comparator drugs used in these trials (Linde et al., 1996). Furthermore, the overall incidence with SJW was only 19.8%, as compared to a massive 52.8% with the latter. In another study on 3250 patients treated with SJW for 6 wk, the incidence of side effects was a mere 2.4%, and only 1.5% had to discontinue treatment because of them (Woelk et al., 1994). There has been no report of death from overdose: contrast this with a suicide risk in depressed patients that is 13–30 times greater than in the normal population (Hagnell et al., 1981) and the fact that most of these result from antidepressant drug overdose (Starkey & Lawson, 1980). Hypomania is a well-known possibility with antidepressant drugs, and three such instances have been reported with SJW (O'Breasail & Arguarch, 1998).

3.2. Modus Operandi

Rat experiments have shown that reuptake of serotonin, dopamine, and noradrenaline (norepinephrine) are all inhibited by SJW with equal potency; that is comparable to chemical antidepressants (Muller et al., 1997). Furthermore, SJW exerts effects similar to other antidepressants in a number of experimental animal models of depression (Ozturk, 1997). The pituitary–adrenal axis has been thought for many years to be implicated in the etiology of depression, although the exact mechanism by which this is achieved has always eluded research workers. In rat brain SJW has been shown to reduce cortisol and corticosterone (Franklin et al., 2004), which led the authors to speculate on a putative association with its antidepressant effect.

3.3. Evidence Base: SJW

Well over 50 double-blind controlled trials have been published comparing SJW to both placebo and standard antidepressant drugs, including the SSRIs fluoxetine (Prozac) (Schrader et al., 2000) and sertraline (Lustral [UK], Zoloft [US]) (Brenner & Azbel, 2000). A number of earlier trials have been reviewed by Linde et al. (1996), who concluded that "there is evidence that extracts of hypericum are more effective than placebo for the treatment of mild-moderately severe depressive disorders." These advantages of SJW were mirrored in my own double-blind comparison to amitriptyline (AMI) (Wheatley, 1997). In that study, adverse events were recorded after direct questioning. Table 1 shows the incidence in the two treatment groups.

The incidence of patients with side effects was considerably less with SJW—32 (37%)—than AMI—50 (64%) ($p < 0.05$). The differences were even more significant in the cases of the two most important ones: dry mouth—5% with SJW but 41% with AMI ($p < 0.001$)—and drowsiness—2% with SJW but 24% with AMI ($p < 0.001$). But what of clinical effectiveness?

3.4. Antidepressant Efficacy

My study was a randomized, double-blind comparison between SJW and AMI given to 165 mild-moderately depressed patients for 6 wk (Wheatley, 1997). The results on the mean Hamilton depression scale (HAM-D) (Hamilton, 1960) are shown in Fig. 2.

The HAM-D can be used in three fundamental ways to interpret the results of clinical trials: statistical comparison of baseline mean scores to the latter at endpoint, comparison of between-group mean scores at different time points during the trial, and using defined criteria to designate endpoint clinical outcomes. Both SJW and the control drug AMI showed a highly significant reduction in mean HAM-D score ($p < 0.0001$) from 2 wk onward and no between-group differences, except at wk 6 in favor of AMI ($p < 0.05$). Responders were defined as having a final HAM-D score of <10 or a reduction of >50% by the end of the trial. There were 60% of such cases with SJW as compared to 78% on AMI (NS) at endpoint. Treatment was continued for at least 6 mo. At that follow-up time, there was no longer a significant between-group difference. Therefore, despite the slight disparity in 6-wk scores, SJW was shown to be equivalent to amitriptyline in antidepressive effectiveness. The mirror simply reflects the true image: need more be said?

4. KAVAKAVA: THE DRUG THAT WAS

Kavakava (or simply Kava) is derived from the root of the Polynesian plant *Piper methysticum* and is used in the South Pacific for its sedative, aphrodisiac, and stimulatory effects, both recreationally and in religious ceremonies (Singh, 1992). Currently its use is compromised owing to the danger of toxicity (reviewed by Wheatley, 2005), but the basic data are as follows.

Table 1
Side Effects Occurring More Than Once in a Double-Blind Trial Comparing St. John's Wort to Amitriptyline[a]

Side effect	*St. John's wort (n = 87)*	*Amitriptyline (n = 78)*	*Significance (p)*
None	55 (63%)	28 (36%)	> 0.05
Dry mouth	4 (5%)	32 (41%)	> 0.001
Drowsiness	3 (2%)	19 (24%)	> 0.001
Nausea/vomiting	6 (7%)	6 (8%)	NS
Headache	6 (7%)	2 (3%)	NS
Constipation	4 (5%)	1 (1%)	NS
Pruritus	2 (2%)	1 (1%)	NS
Dizziness	1 (1%)	6 (8%)	NS
Tiredness	1 (1%)	3 (4%)	NS

NS, not significant.
[a]St. John's wort, 900 mg; amitriptyline, 75 mg. Both were given daily for 6 wk.
Source: Wheatley, 1997.

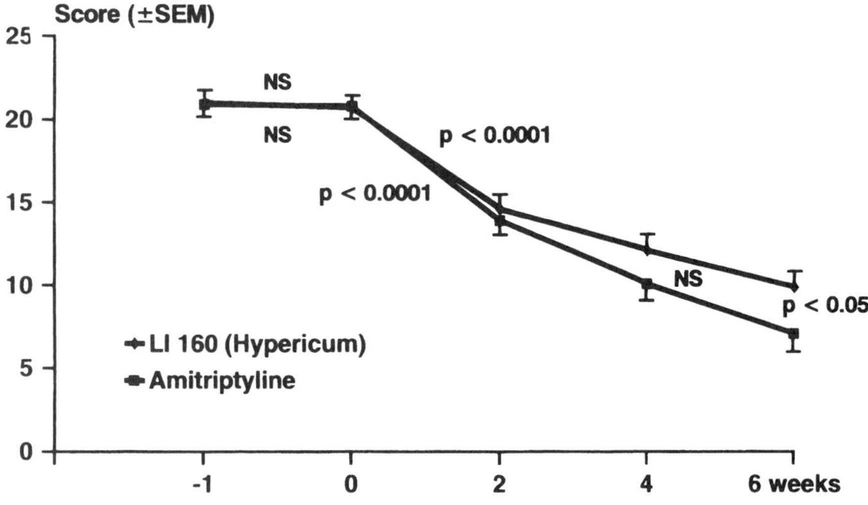

Fig. 2. Reduction in severity of mean Hamilton Depression rating scores (HAM-D) in two groups of patients treated for 6 wk with St. John's Wort (SJW, LI 160, Hypericum) 900 mg and amitriptyline 75 mg daily, respectively (±SEM).

4.1. Basic Facts

Kava contains a number of active compounds, among which are the kava pyrones, kawain, dihydrokawain, methysticin, dihydromethysticin, yangonin, and desmethoxyyangonin, although it is not known which of these is responsible for any anxiolytic actions it may have (Hansel & Haas, 1984; Walden et al.,1997). There is also evidence for serotonergic and calcium antagonistic potencies of the kava pyrone kawain, and in discussing effects on GABA-ergic transmission, it was later concluded that "the cellular actions of the kawain appear heterogeneous, but all of them counter excitation" (Grunze & Walden, 1999). This led the authors to suggest that it might prove useful in the treat-

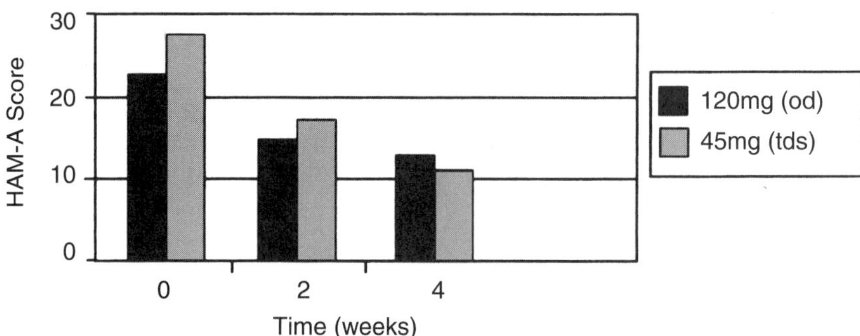

Fig. 3. Reduction in severity of mean Hamilton Anxiety rating scores (HAM-A) in an open crossover trial of kava 2 wk each on doses of 120 mg once daily (od) and 45 mg thrice daily (tid).

ment of epilepsies, bipolar disorder, depression, and anxiety, all conditions characterized by increased cellular excitability. Evidence for a protective action against the human response to stress has been provided by Cropley et al. (2002), who investigated psychological stress induced under laboratory conditions. They found that both kava and valerian protected healthy volunteers against the adverse effects of doing a mental task.

4.2. *Hepatoxicity*

Were it not for the specter of this potentionally fatal side effect (Escher & Desmeules, 2001), including five patients requiring liver transplantation (Gruenwalde & Feder, 2002), the reported incidence of adverse events has been low overall (see Schulz et al., 2000). Thus, the incidence has varied between 1.5% in 4049 patients in one study to 2.3% in 3029 patients in another. The adverse events that occurred were described as "mild and reversible" but did include 31 cases of gastrointestinal disturbances and 31 cases of allergic reactions.

4.3. *Anxiolytic and Hypnotic*

A number of clinical trials have been undertaken in anxiety and insomnia, both pilot and controlled studies against both placebo and standard anxiolytics (Schulz et al., 2000). These have demonstrated effectiveness for kava in both therapeutic roles, comparable to its chemical counterparts; it does not appear to have dependence potential. I completed a pilot study in generalized anxiety disorder (GAD) using the Hamilton anxiety rating scale (HAM-A) (Wheatley 2001a). The results are shown in Fig. 3.

This was a trial in 24 patients treated for 4 wk (Wheatley, 2001a), and two dose schedules were compared: 120 mg once daily (od) and 45 mg thrice daily (tid), in a randomized-order crossover design. There were highly significant reductions in mean HAM-A scores (Hamilton, 1959) ($p < 0.001$), irrespective of dose schedule, treatment order, or sex of the patients. The impact of side effects was relatively low, and only one patient had to omit treatment on tid dosage because of nausea. No side effects were experienced by nine patients (37%) on tid or by five (22%) on od dosages, but daytime drowsiness occurred in eight (33%) on tid and two (9%) on od. There were 13 patient preferences for od and 8 for tds doses, with no preferences in the remaining 2 cases.

However, a double-blind comparative trial was required to verify these results, which was conducted by Connor et al. (2000), who treated 35 patients with kava 280 mg daily for 4 wk, in a double-blind placebo-controlled trial. Results were significantly better with the active drug, which was "well-tolerated and not associated with withdrawal at the doses administered." But no more of kava.

5. VALERIAN: THE DRUG THAT IS

Derived from the flowering plant *Valeriana officinalis*, over 100 constituents of valerian have been identified, and their concentrations are subject to seasonal variation (Bos et al., 1998). It is uncertain which of these may be responsible for any anxiolytic and hypnotic actions it may have (Hansel & Haas, 1984; Walden et al., 1997). Significantly, valerian binds to benzodiazepine receptors in the brain (Holz & Godot, 1989).

A number of clinical and polysomnographic trials have been undertaken, including double-blind trials against both placebo and standard chemical hypnotics . Schulz et al. (2000) reviewed a number of these and concluded that "valerian is not a suitable agent for the *acute* treatment of insomnia." The essential value of valerian may lie in its ability to promote natural sleep after several weeks of use, with no risk of dependence or adverse health effects. Most importantly, valerian improves deep sleep (Donath et al., 2000), and studies have been undertaken in comparison with the benzodiazepine hypnotic oxazepam. One of these was a randomized parallel-group study (Lindhal & Lindwall, 1989), which treated 202 insomniac patients for 6 wk with either valerian 600 mg or oxazepam 10 mg, taken nightly. The authors found that "both treatments markedly increased sleep quality compared with baseline ($p < 0.01$)." Reference has already been made to relief of psychological stress in the laboratory by valerian (as well as kava) (Cropley et al., 2002). But what of personal experience?

5.1. Stress-Induced Insomnia

I have undertaken an unblinded pilot study on 24 patients with stress-induced insomnia to compare valerian to kava and the combination of both, with patients acting as their own controls (Wheatley, 2001b). Insomniac patients, of whom there were 24, were first treated for 6 wk with kava 120 mg/d, followed by 2 wk off treatment, and then treated for another 6 wk with valerian 600 mg. After a further 2 wk off treatment, there was a final 6 wk treatment with both drugs combined. Stress was measured in three areas: social, personal, and life events. Insomnia was also measured in three areas: time to fall asleep, hours slept, and waking mood.

Total severity of stress, as well as insomnia, was significantly relieved by both compounds ($p < 0.01$), with no significant differences between them (Figs. 4, 5). There was also further improvement with the combination, significant in the case of insomnia ($p < 0.05$). These results were considered to be promising and to demonstrate the rapid onset of effect with kava (redundant though this now is) and the slower, but appreciable effect of valerian in the promotion and maintenance of sleep. However, this tentative conclusion must be viewed with reserve in view of the fact that the trial was not double-blind, although patients were randomized to treatment. There is now a need for longer-term studies on a double-blind basis to determine whether the effect is maintainable and safe.

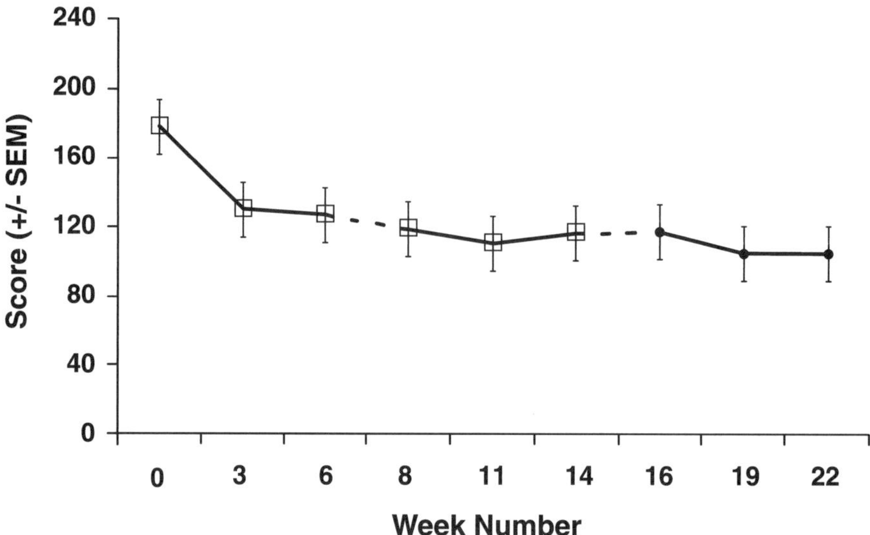

Fig. 4. Reduction in severity of mean stress ratings on the scale devised for the crossover trial comparing kava 120 mg to valerian 600 mg nightly to the combination of the two with intervening no-treatment periods.

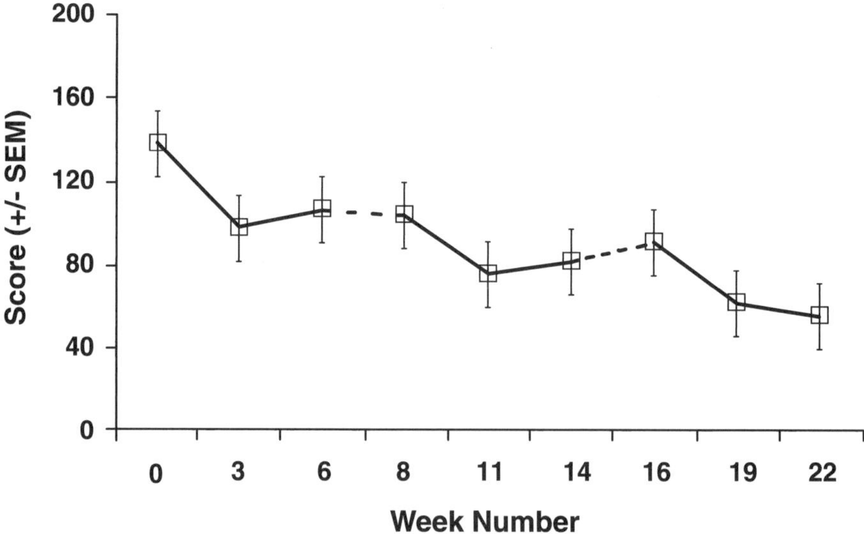

Fig. 5. Reduction in severity of mean sleep ratings on the scale devised for the crossover trial comparing kava 120 mg to valerian 600 mg nightly to the combination of the two with intervening no-treatment periods.

5.2. And What of Dreaming?

Only a few minor side effects have been reported with valerian (Schulz, Hansel, & Tyler, 2000), and many of the published clinical trials do not record any at all. In my study on stress-induced insomnia, the most common side effect was vivid dreams with kava + valerian (4 cases, 21%) and with valerian alone (3 cases, 16%). Vivid dreams is an unusual side effect and did not occur on kava alone, so may well be specific to valerian and possibly related to the drug's known polysomnographic effects, as outlined previously. The dreams were in no way unpleasant, simply impressing the patients as being particularly lifelike and well remembered on awakening. Valerian is recorded as increasing rapid eye movement (REM) sleep (Donath et al., 2000), and so this may account for these comments. But are there any other herbal remedies that may assist the natural function of sleep?

6. AROMATHERAPY: THE SCENT IS SWEET

A popular way to induce a state of tranquilty, the necessary substrate for the induction of sleep, is by the inhalation of certain volatile oils. The most notable of these are lavender, chamomile and ylang-ylang.

6.1. Lavender

Lavender oil is produced from the fresh flowering tops of the plants by steam inhalation, the main components being linalyl acetate and linalool (Schulz et al., 2000). In mice, anticonvulsant effects have been demonstrated by Lis-Balchin and Hart (1999), together with diminution in spontaneous activity and additive effects when combined with several narcotics (Atanossova-Shopova & Roussinov, 1970). These authors also noted that exposure of mice to a lavender atmosphere in a dark cage resulted in depression of motor activity. Furthermore, lavender oil has been shown to inhibit the stimulant effects of caffeine (Buchbauer et al., 1991). In a clinical study on four benzodiazepine-dependent geriatric patients (Hardy et al., 1995), on stopping this treatment there was a significant decrease in sleep duration, which was restored to previous levels by substitution of aromatherapy with lavender oil. Other clinical studies have confirmed these effects (Schulz et al., 2000). Therefore, there would appear to be some evidence for the belief that lavender inhalation may act as an aid to sleep.

6.2. Chamomile

Usually taken in the form of a tea, inhalation of the resultant vapor is an important element of any sedative effect that chamomile flowers may have. The sedative effects may be due to the flavonoid apigenin, which binds to benzodiazepine receptors in the brain. Studies in mice and rats have shown anticonvulsant and central nervous system depressant effects, respectively (Avallone et al., 1996). Clinical trials are notable for their absence, although 10 cardiac patients are reported to have "immediately fallen into a deep sleep lasting for 90 minutes" after drinking it (Gould et al., 1973).

6.3. Ylang-Ylang

Derived from the tropical tree *Cananga Odorata var. gemima*, ylang-ylang is reputed to have calming effects in humans. In a recent study on 144 healthy adults (Moss et al., 2003), participants were divided into three groups in cubicles infused, respectively, with ylang-ylang, peppermint (a reputed stimulant), or no odor. On various psychological tests, those in the ylang-ylang atmosphere reported increased levels of calmness, but at the expense of impaired memory and attention. The evidence suggests that aromatherapy may have some merits in inducing a state of mind conducive to sleep, but whether the technique has any direct hypnotic effect is uncertain.

6.4. Other Putative Sedative Herbs

A number of compounds are traditionally credited with sedative or mood-calming properties, but there is little scientific evidence to support such claims. The most notable are *Melissa* (balm leaves, lemon balm), passionflower, and hops.

6.4.1. Melissa

Derived from the dried leaves of the plant *Melissa officinalis*, the preparation contains volatile oils—citronellal, geranial, and neral—and was shown to possess "nonspecific" sedative effects (Wagner et al., 1984). More recently a randomised, double-blind, placebo-controlled trial (Kennedy et al., 2003) demonstrated *Melissa* to be "beneficial in moderating subjective mood in response to mild psychological stress." Although no sleep measurements were made, this does suggest that the compound is capable of inducing a mood state compatible with the induction of sleep.

6.4.2. Passionflower

Passionflower extracts reduce spontaneous locomotor activity and prolong sleep in mice (Speroni & Minghetti,1988). Apart from one study showing a hypnotic-sedative effect (Maluf et al.,1991), there do not appear to have been any clinical studies in humans. However, this one study also showed "signs of hepatotoxicity and pancreatotoxicity," so that clearly a considerable amount of research is required before even considering this compound for clinical use.

6.4.3. Hops

"Hop-picker fatigue" is thought to result from transfer of hop resin from hand to mouth or even inhalation of the volatile oil of the hop plant (Tyler, 1987). An experimental study in mice found "no demonstrable sedative effects" (Hansel & Wagener, 1967). Furthermore, a study in 15 human subjects for 5 d, recorded "no sleep-inducing effects in any of the subjects tested" (Stocker, 1967). Perhaps sedation from hops is better confined to that product derived from them—alcohol.

7. GINKGO BILOBA: A DRUG TO REMEMBER

"The richness of life lies in memories we have forgotten," according to Cesare Pavese (1961), and how relevant are these words to the problem of declining memory with increasing old age. Ginkgo biloba (or ginko) is an herbal tree extract that has been extensively researched for its memory-enhancing properties in normal subjects, the elderly, and patients with dementia owing to both cerebral arteriosclerosis and Alzheimer's disease (Diamond et al., 2000). As these authors commented: "Ginkgo has shown activity centrally and peripherally, affecting electrochemical, physiologic, and vascular systems in animals and humans with few adverse side-effects or drug interactions. Ginkgo shows promise in patients with dementia, normal aging, and cerebrovascular-related disorders. Clinical indications include memory, informatiom processing, and ADL." What better qualifications could there be for countering the chronic effects of the stress vicious circle?

7.1. Evidence Base: Ginkgo

The foundations for efficacy are firm, but I will confine my comments to some notable studies in normal subjects (Table 2).

Table 2
Ginko Biloba in Normal Subjects: Double-Blind vs Placebo Trials, 2000–2003

No. of patients	*Age group (yr)*	*Trial period*	*Dose (mg)*	*Result vs placebo*	*Ref.*
214	82–83 yr	24 wk	120–240	=	van Dongen et al., 2000
262	67–68 yr	6 wk	180	>	Mix & Crews, 2002
61	18–40 yr	30 d	120	>	Stough et al.. 2001
20	21 yr	1 d	120–360	>	Kennedy et al., 2003

These were all double-blind, placebo-controlled trials, and in only one of these was there no difference from placebo (Van Dongen et al., 2000). This study was on the oldest group reported (82–83 yr), and so perhaps it is not surprising, as cerebral atrophy might already be established in such an age group (Fox & Schott 2004). In the other three studies, with patients ranging progressively downwards from 67–68 yr (Mix & Crews 2002) through 18–40 yr (Stough, Clarke, Lloyd, & Nathan, 2001) to 21 yr (Kennedy et al., 2002), ginkgo was significantly better than placebo in improving memory. So, memory really can be stimulated beyond the peak adult norm! And how essential this is in the defense against stress.

But in disease processes such as arteriosclerotic dementia and Alzheimer's disease, this may not be possible: or is it?

7.2. The Demented Patient

A number of published reports affirm that with ginkgo biloba it is possible to reverse the inexorable decline in memory that is the hallmark of the demented individual. One of the most notable of these was that undertaken by Le Bars et al. (1997), who treated 309 patients with Alzheimer's disease or multi-infarct dementia for 1 yr in a double-blind, placebo-controlled trial. The dose used was 120 mg daily, and significant differences in favor of ginkgo were recorded on a number of standard measures. These results are particularly impressive in view of the long duration of the trial and the sustained effect from a relatively small dose (240 mg is now considered the optimum dose for conditions such as these). There were no significant differences between ginkgo and placebo in respect to incidence or severity of side effects. The authors concluded that their study demonstrated that ginkgo had improved cognitive performance and, in consequence, the social functioning of a substantial number of their patients. A tribute indeed to herbal therapy! It would be of great interest to undertake a comparison between ginkgo and the two most effective chemical drugs for these indications, namely donepezil (Burns et al., 1999) and memantine (Reisberg et al., 2003).

7.3. Sex Imperfect

In depressive illness, impairment of libido, other sexual functions, and, in the male, erection and ejaculation are integral components of the illness. Even when depression responds to treatment with antidepressant drugs, sexual function does not improve, often being impaired by those very drugs themselves. This may occur in as many as 67% of patients (Segraves, 1998). A report of successful treatment of this problem with ginkgo biloba (Cohen & Bartlik, 1998) led me to conduct a small pilot study on 12 such patients (Wheatley, 1999). There was significant relief of symptoms, but clearly such a study would not suffice, and so I then undertook a triple-blind, placebo-controlled trial with 24 patients treated for 6 wk with a 12-wk follow-up (Wheatley, 2004). Triple-blind means that in addition to investigator and patient, the statistician was also blind until the final analysis had been completed, simply being presented with two sets of data, distinguished only by symbols. The dose of ginkgo was 240 mg daily. Alas, the results were completely negative: ginkgo was no better than placebo! And so the choice of treatment for depression remains one of forming a balance between two sources of stress: depression and sex.

8. ENIGMA VARIATIONS

Stress is not really an enigma at all: the enigma is to understand why we have conscious control over many of the destinies in our lives and how we cope with them, but over others we exert little influence at all, being dependent instead on genetically determined reflexes. The fight-or-flight reaction is perfectly designed to cope with acute stress in the wild, but fails woefully when translated to the milieu of modern-day civilization, in which case it may cause more harm than good, particularly where the mind is concerned. Perhaps nature (or whatever higher being you may choose to believe in), from which we have inherited this situation, has provided the means in the natural world to find many solutions to our medical problems. But we must look for them. Surely it is a measure of human beings' intellectual purpose on this planet that we should set about this diligently on two parallel tracks: innovative research in the laboratory and by the bedside, but equally by endeavouring to identify and metamorphose that which is there before our eyes but awaiting our recognition.

9. CONCLUSIONS

Stress is a self-perpetuating vicious circle involving depression, anxiety, sleep and dreams, sex, and memory among its most important components. The individual is better enabled to cope with stress if this circle can be broken; one way of doing this is by means of herbal medicine. The prime example is the "Baptist's herb," St. John's wort, comparable in its effect to relieve depressive illness to the most effective chemical drugs available—and much safer! Kavakava, that exotic migrant from Polynesia, is no longer available to us due to reported hepatotoxicity, although its efficacy as an anxiolytic and hypnotic is not in doubt. No such problems would seem to exist in the case of valerian, with that compound's unique effects in improving deep sleep (short-wave, δ) and consequent carry-over effects on depression and immunity. Associated with sleep is sex, the impairment of which is another potent stress factor. The importance of good-quality sleep cannot be overemphasized, and aromatherapy may provide another means of achieving this. Perhaps the greatest stress of all is failing memory, with which the consolation of life's achievements is denied to the aging individual. But again an herb, ginkgo biloba, may hold promise for the past and future alike.

REFERENCES

Adam, K., & Oswald, I. (1983). Protein synthesis, bodily renewal and the sleep-wake cycle. *Clinical Science, 65*, 561–567.

Atanossova-Shopova, S., & Roussinov, K. S. (1970). On certain central neurotropic effects of lavender essential oil. *Bulletin of the Institute of Physiology, 8*, 69–76. (Quoted in V. Schulz et al., 2000, qv.)

Avallone, R., Zanoli, P., Corsi, L., et al. (1995). Benzodiazepine compounds and GABA in flower heads of matricaria chamomilla. *Lancet, 346*, 701.

Bos R., Woerdenbag, H. J., Van Putten, P. M. S., et al. (1998). Seasonal variations of the essential oil, valerenic acid and derivatives, and valepotriates in valeriana officinalis roots and rhizomes, and the selection of plants suitable for phytomedicines. *Planta Medica, 64*, 143–147.

Brenner, R., & Azbel, V. (2000). Comparison of an extract of hypericum (LI 160) and sertraline in the treatment of depression: A double-blind, randomised pilot study. *Clinical Therapeutics, 22*(4), 411–419.

Buchbauer, G., Jirovet, L., Jager, W., et al. (1991). Aromatherapy: Evidence for sedative effects of the essential oil of lavender after inhalation. *Zeitung Naturforsche, 46c*, 1067–1072.

Burns, A., Rossor, M., Hecker, J., et al. (1991). The effects of donepezil in Alzheimer's disease—results from a multinational trial. *Dementia and Geriatric Cognitive Disorders, 10*, 237–244.

Cohen, A. J., & Bartlik, B. (1998). Ginkgo biloba for antidepressant-induced sexual dysfunction. *Journal of Sex and Marital Therapy, 24*, 139–143.

Connor, K. M., Watkins, L. L., & Davidson, J. R. T. (2000). A study of an herbal anxiolytic. In *39th Annual Meeting of the American College of Neuropsychopharmacology 2000.*

Cropley, M., Cave, Z., Ellis, J., et al. (2002). Effect of kava and valerian on human physiological and psychological responses to mental stress assessed under laboratory conditions. *Phytotherapy Research, 16*, 23–27.

Diamond, B. J., Shiflett, S. C., Feweil, N., et al. (2000). Ginkgo biloba extract: Mechanisms and clinical indications. *Archives of Physical Medicine and Rehabilitation, 81*, 668–678.

Donath, F., Quispe, S., Diefenbach K., et al. (2000). Clinical evaluation of the effect of valerian extract on sleep structure and sleep quality. *Pharmacopsychiatry, 33*, 47–53.

Escher, M., & Desmeules, J. (2001). Hepatitis associated with kava, an herbal remedy for anxiety. *British Medical Journal, 322*, 139.

Fox N. C., & Schott J. M. (2004). Imaging cerebral atrophy: Normal aging to Alzheimer's disease. *Lancet 363*, 392–394.

Frances, A., Pincus, H. A., & First, M.B. (1994). *Diagnostic and statistical manual of psychiatric disorders (3rd ed.).* Washington, DC: American Psychiatric Association.

Franklin, M., Reed, A., & Murck, H. (2004). Sub-chronic treatment with an extract of *Hypericum perforatum* (St. John's wort) significantly reduces cortisol and corticosterone in rat brain. *European Psychopharmacology, 14*, 7–10.

Gould, L., Reddy, C. V. R., & Comprecht, R. F. (1973). Cardiac effect of chamomile tea. *Journal of Clinical Pharmacology, 13*, 475–479.

Grigson, G. (1958). *The Englishman's Flora.* London: Hart-Davis, MacGibbon.

Gruenwald, J., & Feder, J. (2002). Kava, the present European situation. *Nutriceuticals World, Jan/Feb*, 22–24.

Grunze, H., & Walden, J. (1999). Kawain limits excitation in CA 1 pyramidal neurons of rats by modulating ionic currents and attenuating excitatory synaptic transmission. *Human Psychopharmacology: Clinica-l and Experimental, 14*, 63.

Guillmain, J., Rousseau, A., & Delaveau, P. (1989). Effets neurodepresseurs de l'huile essentielle de lavandula augustifolia. *Mill. Ann. Pharmaceutiques, 47*, 337–343.

Hagnell, O., Lanke, J., & Rorsman, B. (1981). Suicide rates in the Lundby study; mental illness as a risk factor for suicide. *Neuropsychology, 7*, 248–253.

Hamilton, M. (1959). The assessment of anxiety states by rating. *British Journal of Medical Psychology, 32*, 50–55.

Hamilton, M. (1960). Development of a rating scale for primary depressive illness. *British Journal of Social and Clinical Psychology, 6*, 278–296.

Hansel, R., & Haas, H. (1984). *Therapie mit Phytopharmaka.* Heidelberg: Springer-Verlag.

Hansel, R., & Wagener, H. H. (1967). Versuche: Sedativ-hypnotische Wirkstoffe im Hopfen Nachzuweisen. *Arzheim-Forsche/Drug Research, 17*, 79–81.

Hardy, M., Kirk-Smith, M. D., & Stretch, D. D. (1995). Replacement of drug treatment for insomnia by ambient odour. *Lancet, 346*, 701.

Holz, J., & Godot P. (1989). Receptor binding studies with valeriana officinalis on the benzodiazepine receptor. *Planta Medica, 65*, 642.

Hordern, A. (1976). *Tranquility denied.* Adelaide: Rigby.

Horne, J. (1988). *Why we sleep.* Oxford: Oxford University Press.

Jacobs, M. A., Spilken, A., & Norman, N. (1969). Relationship of life-change, maladaptive aggression and upper respiratory infections in male college students. *Psychosomatic Medicine, 31*, 31–34.

Kennedy, D. O., Little, W., & Scholey, A. B. (2002). Effects of Melissa officinalis (lemon balm) on mood changes during acute psychological stress. *Pharmacology, Biochemistry and Behavior, 72*, 953–964.

Laakmann, G., Schule, C., Baghai T., et al. (1998). St John's wort in mild-moderate depression: The relevance of hyperforin for clinical efficacy. *Pharmacopsychiatry, 31 (Suppl.)*, 54–59.

Le Bars, P. L., Katz, M. M., Berman N., et al. (1997). A placebo-controlled, double-blind, randomised trial of an extract of ginkgo biloba for dementia. *Journal of the American Medical Association, 278*(16), 1327–1332.

Lindahl, O. & Lindwall, L. (1989). Double-blind study of a valerian preparation. *Pharmacology, Biochemistry and Behavior, 32*, 1065–1066.

Linde, K., Ramirez, G., Mulrow, C. D., et al. (1996). St. John's wort for depression: An overview and meta-analysis of randomised clinical trials. *British Medical Journal, 315*, 255–258.

Lis-Balchin, M., & Hart, S. (1999). Studies on the mode of action of essential oil lavender (lavandula angustifolia P. Miller). *Phytotherapy Research, 13*, 540–542.

Maluf, E., Barros, H. M. T., Prochtengarten, M. L., et al. (1991). Assessment of the hypnotic/sedative effects and toxicity of passiflora edulis aqueous extract in rodents and humans. *Phytotherapy Research, 5*, 262–265.

Mendelson, W. V., Garnet, G., Gilling, J. C., et al. (1984). The experience of insomnia and daytime and night-time functioning, *Psychosomatic Research, 12*, 235–250.

Mix, J. A., & Crews, W. D. (2002). A double-blind, placebo-controlled, randomized trial of ginkgo extract EGb 761 in a sample of cognitively intact older adults: Neuropsychological findings. *Human Psychopharmacology: Clinical and Experimental, 17*, 267–277.

Moss, M. C., Hewitt, S., Wesnes, K., & Goford, J. (2003). Modulation of cognition and mood by the aromas of ylang-ylang and peppermint essential oils. Poster presented by the University of Manchester at the summer meeting of the *British Association for Psychopharmacology, 2003.*

Muller, W. E., Rolli, M., Schafer, C., et al. (1997). Effects of hypericum extract (LI 160) in biochemical models of antidepressant activity. *Pharmacopsychiatry 30 (Suppl. 2)*, 202–207.

O'Breasail, A. M., & Arguarch, S. (1998). Hypomania and St.John's wort. *Canadian Journal of Psychiatry, 43*(7), 746–747.

Ozturk, Y. (1997). Testing of antidepressant effects of hypericum species on animal models. *Pharmacopsychiatry, 30 (Suppl. 2)*, 125–128.

Palmblad, J., Petrini, B., Wasserman, J., et al. (1986). Lymphocyte and granulocyte reactions during sleep deprivation. *Psychosomatic Medicine, 41*, 273–278.

Pavese, C. (1961). *This business of living: Diaries 1935–1950.* London: Peter Owen.

Pilcher, J. J., & Huffcutt, A. I. (1996). Effects of sleep deprivation on performance: A meta-analysis. *Sleep, 19,* 316–326.

Porcher, F. P. (1970). *Resources of the southern fields and forests: Medical, economical and agricultural: Prepared and published by order of the Surgeon-General 1863.* New York: Amo.

Reisberg, B., Doody, R., Stoffler, A., et al. (2003). Memantine in moderate-to-severe Alzheimers disease. *New England Journal of Medicine, 348*, 1333–1334.

Schrader, E. (2000). Equivalence of St. John's wort extract (Ze 117) and fluoxetine: A randomised, controlled study in mild-moderate depression. *Clinical Psychopharmacology, 15*, 61–68.

Schulz, V., Hansel, R., & Tyler, V. E. (2000). *Rational phytotherapy.* Berlin: Springer-Verlag.

Segraves, R. T. (1998). Antidepressant-induced sexual dysfunction. *Journal of Clinical Psychiatry 59, (Suppl. 4)*, 48–54.

Selye, H. (1936). A syndrome produced by diverse noxious agents. *Nature, 146*, 37–45.

Singh, Y. N. Kava: An overview. (1992). *Journal of Ethnopharmacology, 37*, 13–45.

Speroni, E., & Minghetti, A. (1988). Neuropharmacological activity of extracts from passiflora incarnata. *Planta Medica, 54*, 488–491.

Starkey, I. R., & Lawson, A. A. (1980). Psychiatric aspect of acute poisoning with tricyclic and related antidepressants. A ten year revue. *Scottish Medical Journal, 25*, 303–308.

Stocker, H. R. (1967). Sedative und hypnogenie Wirkung des Hopfens. *Schweizer Brauerei Rundschau, 78*, 80–89.

Stough, C., Clarke, J., Lloyd, J., & Nathan, P. J. (2001). Neuropsychological changes after 30-day Ginkgo biloba administration in healthy participants. *International Journal of Neuropsychopharmacology, 4*, 131–134.

Tyler, V. E. (1987). *The new honest herbal: A sensible guide to herbs and related substances* (2nd ed., pp. 125–126). Philadelphia: Suckly Co.

van Dongen, M. C., van Rossum, M., & Knipschild, P. (2000). In T .A. van Beek, (Ed.). *Ginkgo biloba.* Amsterdam: Harwood Academic.

Vorbach, E. U., Arnoldt, K. H., & Hubner, W. D. (1997). Efficacy and tolerability of St. John's wort extract LI 160 versus imipramine in patients with severe depressive episodes according to ICD-10. *Pharmacopsychiatry, 30 (Suppl.)*, 19–23.

Wagner, H., Sprinkmeyer, L., Koch-Heitzmann, I., & Schultze, W. (1984). Melissa officinalis. Eine alte Arzneipilance mit neuen therapeutischen Wirkungen. *Deutsche Apotheker-Zeitung, 124*, 2137–2145.

Walden, J., von Wegerer, J., Winter, U., et al. (1997) Effects of kawain and dihydromethisticin on field potential changes in the hippocampus. *Progress in Neuropsychopharmacology and Biological Psychiatry, 21*, 697–706.

Wheatley, D. (1969). Comparative effects of propranolol and chlordiazepoxide in anxiety states. *British Journal of Psychiatry, 115*, 1411–1412.

Wheatley, D. (1981). *Stress and the heart (2nd ed.).* New York: Raven.

Wheatley, D. (1990). *The anxiolytic jungle: Where next?* Chichester: John Wiley & Sons.

Wheatley, D. (1992). Prescribing short-acting hypno-sedatives, current recommendations from a safety perspective. *Drug Safety, 7*(2), 106–115.

Wheatley, D. (1997). LI 160, an extract of St John's wort, versus amitriptylline in mildly-moderately depressed outpatients—a controlled clinical trial in outpatients. *Pharmacopsychiatry, 30*(2), 77–80.

Wheatley, D. (1998). Sex, stress and sleep. *Stress Medicine, 14*, 245–248.

Wheatley, D. (1999). Ginkgo biloba in the treatment of sexual dysfunction due to antidepressant drugs. *Human Psychopharmacology: Clinical and Experimental, 14*, 511–513.

Wheatley, D. (2001a). Kava-kava in the treatment of generalized anxiety disorder. *Primary Care Psychiatry, 7*, 97–100.

Wheatley, D. (2001b). Stress-induced insomnia treated with kava and valerian singly and in combination. *Human Psychopharmacology, 16*, 353–356.

Wheatley, D. (in press). Medicinal plants for insomnia: A review of their pharmacology, efficacy and tolerability. *CNS Drugs.*

Wheatley, D. (2004). Triple-blind placebo-controlled trial of Ginkgo biloba in sexual dysfunction due to antidepressant drugs. *Human Psychopharmacology, 19*, 545–548.

Woelk, H., Burkard, G., & Grunwald, J. G. (1994). Benefits and risks of the hypericum extract LI 160: Drug monitoring study with 3250 patients. *Journal of Geriatric and Psychiatric Neurology, 7 (Suppl. 1)*, 34–38.

Yesavage, J. A., Mumenthaler, M. S., Taylor J. L., et al. (2002). Donepezil and flight simulator performance: Effects on retention of complex skills. *Neurology, 59*, 123–125.

9 Stress and Food Craving

Sharon Rabinovitz

KEY POINTS

- Cravings for drugs and cravings for food share several important features, including overlapping neural pathways and conditioned cue reactivity.
- Dysphoric mood and stress precede food craving and binge eating in bulimia nervosa.
- Carbohydrate food cravings in the perimenstruum as self-medication for stress and depression due to decreased brain serotonin is critically discussed.
- Future research into how activation of the hypothalamic–pituitary–adrenal axis impacts food cravings using drug-craving research paradigms will result in the identification of more effective treatment for eating disorders.

1. INTRODUCTION

Cravings are generally defined as intense desires or urges to consume particular substances, most notably drugs (e.g., Miller & Goldsmith, 2001). While the exact nature of craving remains a controversial subject, craving is commonly believed to be a subjective state capable of motivating behavior (Rogers & Smit, 2000; Tiffany, 1990). Similarly to the hypothesized causal relationship between drug cravings and compulsive drug use (Tiffany, 1990), the construct of food cravings has been important for theories and treatments of eating disorders and of ingestive behaviors (Cepeda-Benito, Fernandez, & Moreno, 2003). This chapter will briefly describe the scientific evidence on food craving and stress, focusing primarily on overlapping between food and drug cravings.

The most commonly used definition of food craving is that it is an intense desire to eat a specific food (Kozlowski & Wilkinson, 1987; Rozin, 1976; Weingarten & Elston, 1990). To distinguish food cravings from ordinary food choices, the desire should be intense, something that we might go out of our way for (although *see* Cepeda-Benito, Gleaves, Williams, & Ertath, 2000; Gendall, Joyce, & Sullivan, 1997; Rogers & Smit, 2000 for alternative views). Food craving is not to be mistaken with hunger: presumably any of a variety of foods can satisfy hunger, but there is a specific (probably sensory) template that must be matched in order to satisfy a food craving (Pelchat, 2002). Furthermore, craving (or pathological wanting) and liking for drug effects are separate: as drugs come to be wanted more and more, they often come to be liked less and less (Robinson & Berridge, 1993, 2003). However, Robinson and Berridge assert that for natural rewards (such as food), craving and liking are more closely linked. Features of intensity of craving

From: *Nutrients, Stress, and Medical Disorders*
Edited by: S. Yehuda and D. I. Mostofsky © Humana Press Inc., Totowa, NJ

include difficulty resisting eating, feeling anxious when the craved food is unavailable, and a change in the speed of consumption (Gendall, Joyce, et al., 1997).

Drug craving and relapse to drug use present the greatest obstacles to successful treatments for addictions. Indeed, despite high levels of motivation and weeks or months of abstinence, recovering addicts often experience intense, overpowering urges that may rekindle drug-seeking behavior, excessive or inappropriate drug use, and relapse to using drugs after quitting (Jellinek, 1955; Robinson and Berridge, 1993; Shiffman, 2000).

Analogously, food cravings may promote greater dietary variety under conditions of dietary monotony such as a repetitive diet in a military setting (Kamen & Peryam, 1961). Food cravings are also widely believed to influence snacking behavior, compliance with dietary restrictions, early dropout from weight-loss treatments, and overeating and binge eating in obese individuals (e.g., Basdevant, Craplet, & Guy-Grand, 1993; Drewnowski, 1991; Gendall, Sullivan, Joyce, Fear, & Bulik, 1997), all generally viewed as undesirable effects of cravings. Food cravings have also been blamed for binge eating in bulimia nervosa (*see* review by Cepeda-Benito et al., 2000). The effectiveness of pharmacotherapy in reducing compulsive or binge eating has been attributed to the possibility that serotonin-enhancing drugs either block or reduce food cravings (Fluoxetine Bulimia Nervosa Collaborative Study Group, 1992; Wurtman & Wurtman, 1995). Moreover, some cognitive-behavioral interventions for binge eating also target cravings through cue-exposure methods (Carter, Bulik, McIntosh, & Joyce, 2002; Toro et al., 2003). However, few researchers have indicated that food cravings are not necessarily pathological, as suggested by the high incidence of sweet food (in females, mostly) and savories (mostly in males) cravings in normal individuals (Rozin, Levine, & Stoes, 1991; Zellner, Garriga-Trillo, Rohm, Centeno, & Parker, 1999) and the fact that many individuals experience cravings as a simple desire for specific type of food (Gendall, Sullivan, et al., 1997; Weingarten & Elston, 1991).

Despite the important role of craving in both drug addictions and eating disorders, little research has been done to directly examine the relationship between cravings for drugs and cravings for foods.

2. OVERLAPPING CHARACTERISTICS BETWEEN FOOD AND DRUG CRAVINGS

2.1. Craving Following Abstinence?

Cravings for drugs and cravings for food have been shown to share several important features, including their tendency to intensify following abstinence. In the case of food, craving can be triggered by restricted intake (Mitchell, Hatsukami, Eckert, & Pyle, 1985). People who limit their food consumption report increased urges for food (Warren & Cooper, 1988). Food deprivation was also found to elicit both physiological responses to food stimuli (Drobes et al., 2001) and reported craving (Nederkoorn, Smulders, & Jansen, 2000). In the case of drugs, craving can be triggered by abrupt discontinuation of drug use (Jellinek, 1955; Marlatt, 1978; Shiffman, 1979). Alsene, Li, Chaverneff, and De Wit (2003) found that overnight smoking abstinence increased craving for cigarets and overnight food abstinence increased craving for food. However, it has also been observed that craving often returns after an extended period of abstinence, long after alleviation of withdrawal symptoms (Robinson & Berridge, 1993; Wise & Bozarth, 1987), indicating that abstinence may not be the only requirement for the induction of craving.

2.2. Cue Reactivity and Craving

Cravings for food and drugs also share the capacity to be elicited by conditioned stimuli. The importance of conditioned stimuli in addictive behavior and relapse to drug use was first proposed by Wikler (1948), who noted that abstinent opiate addicts were able to function without symptoms of withdrawal or craving while in a drug-free environment, but they experienced marked feelings of withdrawal and craving upon returning to the environment they associated with drug taking. Models based on classical conditioning mechanisms propose that stimuli (e.g., drug paraphernalia, sight of drug-use locality) that have been paired repeatedly with the drug administration become conditioned stimuli, which are then capable of producing physiological and psychological responses or states associated with drug use (Anton, 1999; Childress et al., 1999; Singleton & Gorelick, 1998). Like drug cravings, food cravings are readily triggered by exposure to the sight, smell, or imagery of the craved food (Fedoroff, Polivy, & Herman, 1997). This phenomenon reflects conditioned craving, and conditioned responses to drug cues have been studied extensively with several drugs, including cocaine, nicotine, and alcohol (Carter & Tiffany, 1999). Alsene et al. (2003) found that presentation of food-related stimuli increased craving for food regardless of the motivational state of the individual, in a similar way in which cigaret cues further increased craving for smoking. Conditioned food cues and conditioned hunger appear to elicit eating and hunger in the absence of a biological state of food deprivation (Mattes, 1997; Nederkoorn et al., 2000) and even under satiated condition (Cornell et al., 1989).

2.3. Overlapping Neural Pathways Between Food and Drug Cravings

In view of the extensive evidence for conditioning effects of drugs in animals (Pavlov, 1927; Stewart, De Wit, & Eikelboom, 1984), it is likely that neural adaptations underlying pavlovian learning mechanisms may be critical to the processes of craving and relapse (O'Brien, Childress, Ehrman, & Robbins, 1998). Schroeder et al. reported that opiate-associated cues (Shroeder, Holahan, Landry, & Kelley, 2000) and nicotine cues (Shroeder, Binzak, & Kelley, 2001) elicit conditioned neuronal activation (via the expression of the immediate-early gene, Fos) of corticolimbic regions, particularly prefrontal and cingulate cortices. These findings, as well as several other reports with cocaine in both animals and humans (Childress et al., 1999; Franklin & Druhan, 2000), suggest that mere exposure to drug-paired contextual cues is sufficient to engender an activation of particular neural pathways that may reflect a specific motivational state. This pattern of gene expression displays interesting similarities—especially in the prefrontal cortex—to that elicited by conditioning to a natural reward, the highly palatable food chocolate (Schroeder et al., 2001). Moreover, conditioned increases in dopamine efflux are observed in both prefrontal cortex and nucleus accumbens when cues associated with food are presented to food-deprived animals (Ahn & Phillips, 1999; Phillips, Atkinson, Blackburn, & Blaha, 1993). However, in non-food-deprived animals, food-associated cues increased only in the prefrontal cortex (Bassareo & Di Chiara, 1997). Using positron emission tomography (PET), Wang, Volkow, Thanos, & Fowler (2004) found in pathologically obese subjects reductions in striatal dopamine D2 receptors similar to reductions found in drug-addicted subjects. They postulated that decreased levels of dopamine-D2-receptors predisposed subjects to search for reinforcers as a means to temporarily compensate for a decreased sensitivity of dopamine D2-regulated reward circuits.

Interestingly, work in brain-damaged humans indicates that regions of the orbital prefrontal cortex are important for decision making based on future outcome (Bechara et al., 1999). Similarly, in relapse to drug use, individuals fail to make a rational choice or exert voluntary control when confronted by drug cues despite their apparent knowledge of a poor future outcome. Several studies have demonstrated that dysfunction in frontal regions is associated with the maladaptive behavior characteristic of substance abusers (London, Ernst, Grant, Bonson, & Weinstein, 2000; O'Brien et al., 1998).

Obsessive thoughts and feelings of loss of control or compulsion to consume are salient characteristics of both food and drug cravings (O'Brien et al., 1998; Volkow & Fowler, 2000). Activity in the orbitofrontal cortex, which is implicated in the pathology of obsessive–compulsive disorder (Insel, 1992) and which receives projections from reward circuits (e.g., nucleus accumbens and ventral tegmental area), is also associated with cocaine and alcohol craving (e.g., Volkow & Fowler, 2000). Similarly, Uher et al. (2004) have found that in response to food stimuli, women with eating disorders had greater activation in the left medial orbitofrontal and anterior cingulate cortices and less activation in the lateral prefrontal cortex, inferior parietal lobule, and cerebellum relative to the comparison group. Moreover, the orbitofrontal cortex is activated by the two major sensory components of flavor: gustatory (e.g., Baylis, Rolls, & Baylis, 1995) and olfactory stimuli (Wiesman et al., 2001). There is also a higher than expected co-occurrence of obsessive–compulsive disorder and anorexia and bulimia (Bellodi et al., 2001). Individuals with an obsessive–compulsive disorder diagnosis also report higher than normal levels of carbohydrate craving (O'Rourke et al., 1994).

Many of the same neurotransmitter systems are implicated in both food cravings and in cravings for drugs of abuse. A number of excellent reviews have recently been published on endogenous neurotransmitter involvement in increased responding for both food and drugs (Pelchat, 2002), including specific papers on food and opiates (Grigson, 2002; Kelley et al., 2002), neuropeptide Y and leptin (Kalra & Kalra, 2004), cannabinoids (Harrold & Williams, 2003), and dopamine (Cannon & Bseikri, 2004; Carr, 2002), and the reader is encouraged to consult these articles for a more thorough understanding of the subject, which is beyond the space limitations of this chapter.

3. STRESS AND CRAVING

Little research has been done to examine the direct relationship between stress and food cravings. Most of the studies have focused on two specific subjects: the effects of negative emotional states on food craving and binge eating in bulimia nervosa and the relationship between premenstrual emotional tension and sweet food cravings.

3.1. Emotional State Effects on Food Craving and Binge Eating in Bulimia Nervosa

Dysphoric mood was found to precede food craving (Cooper & Bowskill, 1986) and binge eating in bulimics (Davis, Freeman, & Solyom, 1985; Lingswiler, Crowther, & Stephens, 1989). Laberg, Wilson, Eldredge, and Nordly (1991) reported both enhanced attention to pictures of food and an increase in craving in bulimic patients when they experienced negative affect. Bulimic patients also rated themselves as having an increased desire to binge when confronted with interpersonal stressors (Cattanach, Malley, & Rodin,

1988; Tuschen-Caffier & Vögele, 1999) and binged less when treated with a guided-imagery relaxation technique (Esplen, Garfinkel, Olmsted, Gallop, & Kennedy, 1998). Similarly, Waters, Hill, and Waller (2001) found that food cravings leading to binge eating in bulimic patients were associated with higher tension, lower mood, and lower hunger than those cravings not leading to binge. When craving was followed by a binge, a further deterioration of mood followed, while the tension was not reduced. Mood affected binge eating when in a state of food craving, rather than hunger. According to Marlatt's classical conditioning model (1978), hunger can be seen as a motivational state arising from a general awareness of caloric deprivation. In contrast, food craving is a motivational state associated with a strong desire for an expected positive outcome, in which the target substance offering relief from the aversive state is known to the individual. Thus, the function of food craving will be to initiate binging as a means of obtaining relief from the aversive state of intolerable negative effect.

3.2. Sweet Craving Secondary to Premenstrual Tension

Approximately half of the 40–50% of North American women who crave chocolate or sweets do so principally in the perimenstruum, the part of the menstrual cycle surrounding the onset of menstruation, and food cravings are considered to be a symptom of the premenstrual syndrome (PMS) (American Psychiatric Association, 1994; York, Freeman, Lowery, & Strauss, 1989). Some researchers have suggested that women seek out and consume carbohydrates or sweets (Smith & Sauder, 1969) to alleviate premenstrual dysphoria. Thus, craving is seen as a psychological reaction to negative mood or stress, a form of "comfort eating" that has no direct biological bases (e.g., Hill, Weaver, & Blundell, 1991). Others have suggested that women self-medicate for any depression with sweets or chocolate (Schuman, Gitlin, & Fairbanks, 1987). This explanation understands food craving and the increased intake of sweet (carbohydrate-rich) food that follows as a device to restore well-being by increasing the availability of brain serotonin (5HT) (Spring, Chiodo, & Bowen, 1987; Wurtman, Brzezinski, Wurtman, & Laferrere, 1989).

On the other hand, premenstrual chocolate cravings (Tomelleri & Grunewald, 1987) and general food cravings (Bancroft, Cook, & Williamson, 1988) can occur in women who do not suffer any change in mood in the perimenstruum and were also reported in the absence of depression (Dye, Warner, & Bancroft, 1995). Clearly, not all premenstrual food cravings are secondary to mood change. With respect to stress, Dye et al. (1995) failed to find any effect of stress or happiness on food craving once the effect of depression was accounted for. Michener, Rozin, Freeman, and Gale (1999) also failed to prove that dysphoria or tension in the perimenstruum triggers sweet cravings, as alprazolam (a tranquillizer) did not decrease chocolate or sweet craving. Earlier factor analyses suggested that food craving does not load onto the negative mood factor in PMS (e.g., Freeman, DeRubeis, & Rickels, 1996). These findings do not support the hypothesis that chocolate is craved for a possible antidepressant effect of exogenous phenylethylamine (Liebowitz & Klein, 1979) or for a possible anxiolytic effect of exogenous anandamide or its analogs in chocolate (di Tomaso, Beltramo, & Piomelli, 1996). However, more research is needed before any final conclusion can be made as to the relationship between premenstrual emotional tension and sweet food cravings.

3.3. Effect of Stress on Drug Craving: What Can We Learn About Food Craving?

During abstinence, exposure to stressors or drug-associated cues can stimulate the hypothalamic–pituitary–adrenal (HPA) axis to remind the individual about the effects of the abused substance, thus producing craving and promoting relapse. Although exposure to the stressor itself may be aversive, the net result is reflected as an increased sensitivity to the drug (for review, *see* Goeders, 2003). Therefore, if certain individuals are more sensitive to stress (Piazza & Le Moal, 1998; Piazza, Deminiere, Le Moal, & Simon, 1990) and/or if they find themselves in an environment where they do not feel that they have adequate control over this stress (Levine, 2000), these individuals may be more likely to engage in substance abuse or to experience craving.

High-stress reactivity has been identified as a reliable psychological vulnerability associated with the risk status for eating disorders (Leon, Fulkerson, Perry, & Cudeck, 1993), and the premorbid characteristics of patients with eating disorders include clear evidence of mood-related disorders (e.g., Deep, Nagy, Weltzin, Rao, & Kaye, 1995). A related finding is that anxious and depressive mood states have consistently been identified as psychological precursors of drug addiction (*see* Jaffe & Clouet, 1982, for a review).

Reinstatement is a preclinical approach that is widely regarded as an animal model of the propensity to relapse to drug taking, involving mechanisms related to the development and expression of craving (Gerber & Stretch, 1975; Stewart and De Wit, 1987). In a typical reinstatement experiment, previously drug-trained rats undergo extinction during which responding is no longer followed by drug delivery. After significant extinction is observed, rats are then exposed to an event expected to reinstate drug-seeking behavior (Shaham, Shalev, Lu, De Wit, & Stewart, 2003). This reinstatement of drug-seeking behavior can be elicited in several ways, including exposure to brief periods of intermittent electric foot shock stress in rats (e.g., Shaham, Erb, & Stewart, 2000). The presentation of stress-related imagery (Sinha, Fuse, Aubin, & O'Malley, 2000) has also been identified as a potent event for provoking relapse to drug seeking in humans. Norepinephrine and corticotropin-releasing hormone, mediators of the activation of the sympathetic nervous system and HPA axis, respectively, are involved in stress-induced reinstatement (Weiss et al., 2001). These findings suggest a causal role for stressful events in relapse to drug self-administration and corroborate clinical observations that have associated stressful events or negative mood states with relapse or an enhanced craving for the abused drug (Sinha, 2001). However, the effects of stress-induced reinstatement on food-seeking behavior is yet to be determined, because only one study to date has examined this subject (Ahmed & Koob, 1997).

4. CONCLUSION

In light of the overlapping characteristics between food cravings and drug cravings, continued investigations into how stress and the subsequent activation of the HPA axis impact food cravings will result in the identification of more effective and efficient treatment for eating disorders in humans. Stress reduction and coping strategies, either alone or in combination with pharmacotherapies targeting the HPA axis, may prove beneficial in reducing cravings in individuals seeking treatment for eating disorders.

REFERENCES

Ahmed, S. H., & Koob, G. F. (1997). Cocaine- but not food-seeking behavior is reinstated by stress after extinction. *Psychopharmacology, 132*, 289–295.

Ahn, S., & Phillips, A.G., (1999). Dopaminergic correlates of sensory-specific satiety in the medial prefrontal cortex and nucleus accumbens of the rat. *Journal of Neuroscience, 19*, RC29.

Alsene, K. M., Li, Y., Chaverneff, F., & De Wit, H. (2003). Role of abstinence and visual cues on food and smoking craving. *Behavioral Pharmacology, 14*, 145–151.

American Psychiatric Association. (1994). *Diagnostic and statistical manual of mental disorders,* 4th ed., revised. Washington, DC.

Anton, R. F. (1999). What is craving? Models and implications for treatment. *Alcohol Research and Health, 23*, 165–173.

Bancroft, J., Cook, A., & Williamson, L. (1988). Food craving, mood and the menstrual cycle. *Psychological Medicine, 18*, 855–860.

Basdevant, A., Craplet, C., & Guy-Grand, B. (1993). Snacking patterns in obese French women. *Appetite, 21*, 17–23.

Bassareo, V., & Di Chiara, G. (1997). Differential influence of associative and nonassociative learning mechanisms on the responsiveness of prefrontal and accumbal dopamine transmission to food stimuli in rats fed ad libitum. *Journal of Neuroscience, 17*, 851–861.

Baylis, L. L., Rolls, E. T., & Baylis, G. C. (1995). Afferent connections of the caudolateral orbitofrontal cortex taste area. *Neuroscience, 64*, 801–812.

Bechara, A., Damasio, H., Damasio, A. R. & Lee, G. P. (1999). Different contributions of the human amygdala and ventromedial prefrontal cortex to decision-making. *Journal of Neuroscience, 19*, 5473–5481.

Bellodi, L., Cavallini, M. C., Bertelli, S., Chiapparino, D., Riboldi, C., & Smeraldi, E. (2001). Morbidity risk for obsessive–compulsive spectrum disorders in first-degree relatives of patients with eating disorders. *American Journal of Psychiatry, 158*, 563–569.

Cannon, C. M., & Bseikri, M. R. (2004). Is dopamine required for natural reward? *Physiology and Behavior, 81*, 741–748.

Carr, K. D. (2002). Augmentation of drug reward by chronic food restriction: behavioral evidence and underlying mechanisms. *Physiology and Behavior, 76*, 353–64.

Carter, B. L., & Tiffany, S. T. (1999). Meta-analysis of cue-reactivity in addiction research. *Addiction, 94*, 327–340.

Carter, F. A., Bulik, C. M., McIntosh, V. V., & Joyce, P.R. (2002). Cue reactivity as a predictor of outcome with bulimia nervosa. *International Journal of Eating Disorders, 31*, 240–250.

Cattanach, L., Malley, R., & Rodin, J. (1988). Psychologic and physiologic reactivity to stressors in eating disordered individuals. *Psychosomatic Medicine, 50*, 591–599.

Cepeda-Benito, A., Fernandez, M. C., & Moreno, S. (2003). Relationship of gender and eating disorder symptoms to reported cravings for food: Construct validation of state and trait craving questionnaires in Spanish. *Appetite, 40*, 47–54.

Cepeda-Benito, A., Gleaves, D. H., Williams, T. L., & Ertath, S. T. (2000). The development and validation of the state and trait food cravings questionnaire. *Behavior Therapy, 31*, 151–173.

Childress, A.R., Mozley, P.D., McElgin, W., Fitzgerald, J., Reivich, M., & O'Brien, C.P. (1999). Limbic activation during cue-induced cocaine craving. *American Journal of Psychiatry, 156*, 11–18.

Cooper, P. J., & Bowskill, R. (1986). Eating disorders. In E. Miller & P. J. Cooper (Eds.), *Adult abnormal psychology* (pp. 268–298). London: Churchill Livingstone.

Cornell, C. E., Rodin, J., & Weingarten, H. (1989). Stimulus-induced eating when satiated. *Physiology and Behavior, 45*, 695–704.

Davis, R., Freeman, R., & Solyom, L. (1985). Mood and food: An analysis of bulimic episodes. *Journal of Psychiatric Research, 19*, 331–335.

Deep, A. L., Nagy, L. M., Weltzin, T. E., Rao, R., & Kaye, W. H. (1995). Premorbid onset of psychopathology in long-term recovered anorexia nervosa. *International Journal of Eating Disorders, 17*, 291–297.

di Tomaso, E., Beltramo, M., & Piomelli, D. (1996). Brain cannabinoids in chocolate. *Nature, 382*, 677–678.

Drewnowski, A. (1991). Obesity and eating disorders: Cognitive aspects of food preference and food aversion. *Bulletin of the Psychon Society, 29*, 261–264.

Drobes, D. J., Miller, E. J., Hillman, C. H., Bradley, M. M., Cuthbert, B. N., & Lang, P. J. (2001). Food deprivation and emotional reactions to food cues: Implications for eating disorders. *Biological Psychology, 57*, 153–177.

Dye, L., Warner, P., & Bancroft, J. (1995). Food craving during the menstrual cycle and its relationship to stress, happiness of relationship and depression; a preliminary enquiry. *Journal of Affective Disorders, 34*, 157–164.

Esplen, M. J., Garfinkel, P. E., Olmsted, M., Gallop, R. M., & Kennedy, S. A. (1998). Randomized controlled trial of guided imagery in bulimia nervosa. *Psychological Medicine, 28*, 1347–1357.

Fedoroff, I. C., Polivy, J., & Herman, P. C. (1997). The effect of pre-exposure to food cues on the eating bahavior of restrained and unrestrained eaters. *Appetite, 28*, 33–47.

Fluoxetine Bulimia Nervosa Collaborative Study Group. (1992). Fluoxetine in the treatment of bulimia nervosa: A multicenter, placebo-controlled, double-blind trial. *Archives of General Psychiatry, 49*, 139–147.

Franklin, T. R., & Druhan, J. P. (2000). Expression of Fos-related antigens in the nucleus accumbens and associated regions following exposure to a cocaine-paired environment. *European Journal of Neuroscience, 12*, 2097–2106.

Freeman, E. W., DeRubeis, R. J., & Rickels, K. (1996). Reliability and validity of a daily diary for premenstrual syndrome. *Psychiatry Research, 65*, 97–106.

Gendall, K. A., Joyce, P. R., & Sullivan, P. F. (1997). Impact of definition on prevalence of food cravings in random sample of young women. *Appetite, 28*, 33–47.

Gendall, K. A., Sullivan, P. F. Joyce, P. R., Fear, J. L., & Bulik, C. M. (1997). Psychopathology and personality of young women who experience food cravings. *Addictive Behaviors, 22*, 545–555.

Gerber, G. J., & Stretch, J. R. (1975). Drug-induced reinstatement of extinguished self-administration behavior in monkeys. *Pharmacology, Biochemistry and Behavior, 3*, 1055–1061.

Goeders, N. E. (2003). The impact of stress on addiction. *European Neuropsychopharmacology, 13*, 435–441.

Grigson, P. S. (2002). Like drugs for chocolate: Separate rewards modulated by common mechanisms? *Physiology and Behavior, 76*, 389–395.

Harrold, J. A., & Williams, G. (2003). The cannabinoid system: A role in both the homeostatic and hedonic control of eating? *British Journal of Nutrition, 90*, 729–734.

Hill, A. J., Weaver, C. F. L., & Blundell, J. E. (1991). Food craving, dietary restraint and mood. *Appetite, 17*, 187–197.

Insel, T. R. (1992). Towards a neuroanatomy of obsessive–compulsive disorder. *Archives of General Psychiatry, 49*, 739–744.

Jaffe, J. H., & Clouet, D. H., (1982). Opioid dependence: Links between biochemistry and behavior. In H. M. Van Praag (Ed.) *Handbook of biological psychiatry: Part IV* (pp. 277–308). New York: Marcel Dekker.

Jellinek, E. M. (1955). The "craving" for alcohol. *Quarterly Journal of Studies on Alcohol, 16*, 35–38.

Kalra, S. P., & Kalra, P. S. (2004). Overlapping and interactive pathways regulating appetite and craving. *Journal of Addictive Diseases, 23*, 5–21.

Kamen, J. M., & Peryam, D. R. (1961). Acceptability of repetitive diets. *Food Technology, 15*, 173–177.

Kelley, A. E., Bakshi, V. P., Haber, S. N., Steininger, T. L., Will, M. J., & Zhang, M. (2002). Opioid modulation of taste hedonics within the ventral striatum. *Physiology and Behavior, 76*, 365–377.

Kozlowski, L., & Wilkinson, D. A. (1987). Use and misuse of the concept of craving by alcohol, tobacco, and drug researchers. *British Journal of Addiction, 82*, 31–36.

Laberg, J. C., Wilson, G. T., Eldredge, K., & Nordly, H. (1991). Effects of mood on heart rate reactivity in bulimia nervosa. *International Journal of Eating Disorders, 10*, 169–178.

Leon, G. R., Fulkerson, J. A., Perry, C. L., & Cudeck, R. (1993). Personality and behavioral vulnerabilities associated with risk status for eating disorders in adolescent girls. *Journal of Abnormal Psychology, 102*, 438–444.

Levine, S. (2000). Influence of psychological variables on the activity of the hypothalamic–pituitary adrenal axis. *European Journal of Pharmacology, 405*, 149–160.

Liebowitz, M. R., & Klein, D. F. (1979). Hysteroid dysphoria. *The Psychiatric Clinics of North America, 2*, 555–575.

Lingswiler, V. M., Crowther, J. H., & Stephens, M. A. P. (1989). Affective and cognitive antecendents to eating episodes in bulimia and binge eating. *International Journal of Eating Disorders, 8*, 533–539.
London, E. D., Ernst, M., Grant, S., Bonson, K., & Weinstein, A. (2000). Orbitofrontal cortex and human drug abuse: Functional imaging. *Cerebral Cortex, 10*, 334–342.
Marlatt, G. A. (1978). Craving for alcohol, loss of control, and relapse: Cognitive-behavioral analysis. In: Nathan, P. E., Marlatt, G. A., & Loberg, T. (Eds.), *Alcoholism: New directions in behavioral research and treatment* (pp. 271–314). New York: Guilford.
Mattes, R. D. (1997). Physiological responses to sensory stimulation by food: Nutritional implications. *Journal of the American Dietetic Association, 97*, 406–410.
Michener, W., Rozin, P., Freeman, E., & Gale, L. (1999). The role of low progesterone and tension as triggers of perimenstrual chocolate and sweets craving: Some negative experimental evidence. *Physiology and Behavior, 67*, 417–420.
Miller, N. S., & Goldsmith, R. J. (2001). Craving for alcohol and drugs in animals and humans: Biology and behavior. *Journal of Addictive Disorders, 20*, 87–104.
Mitchell, J. E., Hatsukami, D., Eckert, E. D., & Pyle, R. L. (1985). Characteristics of 275 patients with bulimia. *American Journal of Psychiatry, 142*, 482–485.
Nederkoorn, C., Smulders, F. T. Y., & Jansen, A. (2000). Cephalic phase responses, craving and food intake in normal subjects. *Appetite, 35*, 45–55.
O'Brien, C. P., Childress, A. R., Ehrman, R., & Robbins, S. J. (1998). Conditioning factors in drug abuse: Can they explain compulsion? *Journal of Psychopharmacology, 12*, 15–22.
O'Rourke, D. A., Wurtman, J. J., Wurtman, R. J., Tsay, R., Gleason, R., Baer, L., & Jenike, M. A. (1994). Aberrant snacking patterns and eating disorders in patients with obsessive compulsive disorder. *Journal of Clinical Psychiatry, 55*, 445–447.
Pavlov, I. P. (1927). *Conditioned reflexes*. London: Oxford University.
Pelchat, M. L. (2002). Food craving, obsession, compulsion, and addiction. *Physiology and Behavior, 76*, 347–352.
Phillips, A. G., Atkinson, L. J., Blackburn, J. R., & Blaha, C.D. (1993). Increased extracellular dopamine in the nucleus accumbens of the rat elicited by a conditional stimulus for food: An electrochemical study. *Canadian Journal of Physiology and Pharmacology, 71*, 387–393.
Piazza, P. V., Deminiere, J. M., Le Moal, M., & Simon, H. (1990). Stress- and pharmacologically-induced behavioral sensitization increases vulnerability to acquisition of amphetamine self-administration. *Brain Research, 514*, 22–26.
Piazza, P. V., & Le Moal, M. (1998). The role of stress in drug self-administration. *Trends in Pharmacological Science, 19*, 67–74.
Robinson, T. E., & Berridge, K. C. (1993). The neural basis of drug craving: An incentive-sensitization theory of addiction. *Brain Research: Brain Research Review, 18*, 247–291.
Robinson, T. E., & Berridge, K. C. (2003). Addiction. *Annual Reviews in Psychology, 54*, 25–53.
Rogers, P. J., & Smit, H. J. (2000). Food craving and food "addiction": A critical review of the evidence from a biopsychosocial perspective. *Pharmacology, Biochemistry, and Behavior, 66*, 3–14.
Rozin, P. (1976). The selection of food by rats, humans and other animals. In J. Rosenblatt, R. A. Hinde, C. Beer, & E. Shaw (Eds.), *Advances in the study of behavior* (pp. 21–76). New York: Academic .
Rozin, P., Levine, E., & Stoes, C. (1991). Chocolate craving and liking. *Appetite, 17*, 199–212.
Schroeder, B. E., Binzak, J. M., & Kelley, A. E. (2001). A common profile of prefrontal cortical activation following exposure to nicotine- or chocolate-associated contextual cues. *Neuroscience, 105*, 535–545.
Schroeder, B. E., Holahan, M. R., Landry, C. F., & Kelley, A. E. (2000). Morphine-associated environmental cues elicit conditioned gene expression. *Synapse, 37*, 146–158.
Schuman, M., Gitlin, M. J., & Fairbanks, L. (1987). Sweets, chocolate, and atypical depressive traits. *Journal of Nervous and Mental Disease, 175*, 491–495.
Shaham, Y., Erb, E., & Stewart, J. (2000). Stress-induced relapse to heroin and cocaine seeking in rats: A review. *Brain Research Review, 33*, 13–33.
Shaham, Y., Shalev, U., Lu, L., De Wit, H., & Stewart, J. (2003). The reinstatement model of drug relapse: History, methodology and major findings. *Psychopharmacology, 168*, 3–20.
Shiffman, S. M. (1979). The tobacco withdrawl syndrome. *NIDA Research Monographs, 23*, 158–184.

Shiffman, S. M. (2000). Comments on craving. *Addiction, 95*, S171–S175.

Singleton, E. G., & Gorelick, D. A. (1998). Mechanisms of alcohol craving and their clinical implications. *Recent Developments in Alcoholism, 14*, 177–195.

Sinha, R. (2001). How does stress increase risk of drug abuse and relapse? *Psychopharmacology, 158*, 343–359.

Sinha, R., Fuse, T., Aubin, L. R., & O'Malley, S. S. (2000). Psychological stress, drug-related cues and cocaine craving. *Psychopharmacology, 152*, 140–148.

Smith, S. L., & Sauder, C. (1969). Food cravings, depression, and premenstrual problems. *Psychosomatic Medicine, 31,* 281–287.

Spring, B., Chiodo, J., & Bowen, D. J. (1987). Carbohydrates, tryptophan, and behavior: A methodological review. *Psychological Bulletin, 102*, 234–256.

Stewart, J., & De Wit, H. (1987). Reinstatement of drug-taking behavior as a method of assessing incentive motivational properties of drugs. In M.A. Bozarth (Ed.), *Methods of assessing the reinforcing properties of abused drugs*, (pp. 21–227). New York: Springer.

Stewart, J., De Wit, H., & Eikelboom, R. (1984). Role of unconditioned and conditioned drug effects in the self-administration of opiates and stimulants. *Psychological Reviews, 91*, 251–268.

Tiffany, S. (1990). A cognitive model of drug urges and drug-use behavior: Role of automatic and nonautomatic processes. *Psychological Reviews, 97*, 147–168.

Tomelleri, M. S., & Grunewald, K. K. (1987). Menstrual cycle and food cravings in young college women. *Journal of the American Dietetic Association, 87*, 311–315.

Tuschen-Caffier, B., & Vögele, C. (1999). Psychological and Physiological Reactivity to stress: An experimental study on bulimic patients, restrained eaters and controls. *Psychotherapy and Psychosomatics, 68*, 333–340.

Toro, J., Cervera, M., Feliu, M. H., Garriga, N., Jou, M., Martinez, E., & Toro, E. (2003). Cue exposure in the treatment of resistant bulimia nervosa. *International Journal of Eating Disorders, 34*, 227–234.

Uher, R., Murphy, T., Brammer, M. J., Dalgleish, T., Phillips, M. L., Ng, V. W., Andrew, C. M., Williams, S. C., Campbell, I. C., & Treasure, J. (2004). Medial prefrontal cortex activity associated with symptom provocation in eating disorders. *American Journal of Psychiatry, 161*, 1238–1246.

Volkow, N. D., & Fowler, J. S. (2000). Addiction, a disease of compulsion and drive: Involvement of the orbitofrontal cortex. *Cerebral Cortex, 10*, 318–325.

Wang, G. J., Volkow, N. D., Thanos, P. K., & Fowler, J. S. (2004). Similarity between obesity and drug addiction as assessed by neurofunctional imaging: A concept review. *Journal of Addictive Diseases, 23*, 39–53.

Warren, C., & Cooper, P. J. (1988). Psychological effects of dieting. *British Journal of Clinical Psychology, 27*, 269–270.

Waters, A., Hill, A., & Waller, G. (2001). Bulimics' responses to food cravings: Is binge-eating a product of hunger or emotional state? *Behavior Research and Therapy, 39*, 877–886.

Weingarten, H. P., & Elston, D. (1990). The phenomenology of food cravings. *Appetite, 15*, 231–246.

Weingarten, H. P., & Elston, D. (1991). Food cravings in a college population. *Appetite, 17*, 167–175.

Weiss, F., Ciccocioppo, R., Parsons, L. H., Katner, S., Liu, X., Zorrilla, E. P., Valdez, G. R., Ben-Shahar, O., Angeletti, S., & Richter, R. R. (2001). Compulsive drug-seeking behavior and relapse: Neuroadaptation, stress, and conditioning factors. *Annals of the New York Academy of Sciences, 937*, 1–26.

Wiesman, M., Yousry, I., Heuberger, E., Nolte, A., Ilmberger, H., Kobal, G., Yousry, T. A., Kettenmann, B., & Naidich, T. P. (2001). Functional magnetic resonance imaging of human olfaction. *Neuroimaging Clinics of North America, 11*, 237–250.

Wikler, A. (1948). Recent progress in research on neurophysiological basis of morphine addiction. *American Journal of Psychiatry, 105*, 329–338.

Wise, R. A., & Bozarth, M. A. (1987). A psychomotor stimulant theory of addiction. *Psychological Review, 94*, 469–492.

Wurtman, J. J., Brzezinski, A., Wurtman, R. J., & Laferrere, B. (1989). Effect of nutrient intake on premenstrual depression. *American Journal of Obstetrics and Gynecology, 161*, 1228–1234.

Wurtman, R. J., & Wurtman, J. J. (1995). Brain serotonin, carbohydrate-craving, obesity and depression. *Obesity Research, 3*, 477S–480S.

York, R., Freeman, E., Lowery B., & Strauss, J. F. (1989). Characteristics of premenstrual syndrome. *Obstetrics and Gynecology, 73*, 601–605.

Zellner, D. A., Garriga-Trillo, A., Rohm, E., Centeno, S., & Parker, S. (1999). Food liking and craving: A cross-cultural approach. *Appetite, 33*, 61–70.

10 Stress, Alcohol Consumption, and the Hypothalamic–Pituitary–Adrenal Axis

Maria M. Glavas and Joanne Weinberg

KEY POINTS

- Alcohol comsumption has often been associated with stress; models put forward to explain this relationship include the tension-reduction theory and the stress-response-dampening hypothesis.
- Effectiveness of alcohol in reducing stress depends on a number of factors including family history of alcoholism, individual personality characteristics, environmental situation, temporal relationship between stressor and alcohol comsumption, and dose of alcohol consumed.
- Acute alcohol exposure typically activates the hypothalamic–pituitary–adrenal axis but may blunt subsequent hypothalamic–pituitary–adrenal responsivity to stressors and alcohol.
- Chronic alcohol exposure results in hypothalamic–pituitary–adrenal dysregulation, which persists long after cessation of alcohol abuse.
- Prenatal alcohol exposure results in hypothalamic–pituitary–adrenal hyperresponsiveness, lasting throughout the life span.
- Altered hypothalamic–pituitary–adrenal responsivity may play a role in promoting and maintaining alcohol abuse.

1. INTRODUCTION

It is a widely held belief that alcohol consumption can reduce stress, and individuals commonly use, or say they use, alcohol for this purpose. Stress is therefore thought to be a strong factor in the initiation and maintenance of alcohol consumption, and is considered to be a major contributor to alcohol dependence (Brady & Sonne, 1999; Pohorecky, 1981; Powers & Kutash, 1985). Consequently, the interaction between alcohol and stress has received much attention and interest from the scientific community and the literature on stress and alcohol interactions is extensive (Brady & Sonne, 1999; Pohorecky, 1981, 1990, 1991; Powers & Kutash, 1985). However, the interaction of alcohol and stress is complex. The effectiveness of alcohol in actually reducing stress appears to depend on

From: *Nutrients, Stress, and Medical Disorders*
Edited by: S. Yehuda and D. I. Mostofsky © Humana Press Inc., Totowa, NJ

both genetic and environmental factors. In addition, alcohol alters the activity of the hormonal stress response system, the hypothalamic–pituitary–adrenal (HPA) axis.

The present discussion will be a selective review that will touch on the use of alcohol consumption as a coping strategy to deal with stress, followed by a more in-depth discussion of the interactions of alcohol and the HPA axis and the possible role of the HPA axis in mediating the onset and maintenance of alcohol dependence.

2. STRESS AND ALCOHOL USE

Not only is the interaction between stress and alcohol use complex, but the definition and understanding of stress itself is also complex. The use of the term "stress" in the biological sense was popularized by Hans Selye (Selye, 1936, 1974), who defined it as the nonspecific response of the body to a challenge, whereas the internal or external challenges that elicit this stress response are referred to as"stressors." Stressors can range from real threats to survival, including immune challenges or physical stressors, such as cold or pain, to perceived threats such as psychological or social stressors. Within the alcohol-stress literature, the terms tension, anxiety and stress are often used interchangeably and the criteria used to define the terms have varied considerably. In the present text, the term "stress" will be used to refer to an individual's response to and appraisal of a stressor which is perceived to be harmful or threatening, whereas "tension" and "anxiety" will be used only in reference to studies that specifically used these terms.

Since alcohol consumption is commonly used as a coping strategy to deal with stress, one would expect that alcohol should reduce the stress response under various conditions. Much of the early work on stress–alcohol interactions revolved around the tension-reduction theory (TRT), based on the drive-reduction hypothesis put forward by Conger (1956). The TRT states that alcohol consumption reduces tension in an organism that is in a high state of drive/tension and that organisms drink alcohol for its tension-reducing properties (Cappell, 1975; Cappell & Herman, 1972). However, attempts to demonstrate the TRT empirically proved to be problematic (as reviewed by Cappell & Greeley, 1987; Greeley & Oei, 1999; and Sher, 1987). This was owing in part to a lack of consensus over the definition as well as the appropriate indices of tension as well as variability in, or a lack of control over, the initial degree of tension.

In an attempt to address some of the issues encountered with the TRT, Levenson, Sher, Grossman, Newman, and Newlin (1980) formulated the stress-response-dampening (SRD) hypothesis, which suggests that if alcohol consumption reduces the stress response, this effect will reinforce the consumption of alcohol in response to future stressors. The SRD model requires more specific indicators of a stress response than the TRT and suggests that SRD effects may vary greatly among individuals (Sher & Levenson, 1982). The SRD effect of alcohol refers to the degree to which alcohol consumption reduces an organism's stress response and may be measured by psychophysiological measures of stress, such as cardiovascular responses, glucocorticoid levels, skin conductance, and/or continuous self-reports of anxiety, prior to and following alcohol consumption (Levenson et al., 1980; Pohorecky, Rassi, Weiss, & Michalak, 1980).

The degree to which an individual may demonstrate an SRD effect varies widely from person to person, and in some instances no SRD effect or even an increased stress response may be observed with alcohol consumption (reviewed by Greeley & Oei, 1999). Whether or not an SRD effect occurs appears to depend on a number of factors, including genetic factors such as family history of alcoholism, whether or not the individual is an alcoholic, individual personality characteristics, the environmental situation, the temporal relationship between the stressor and alcohol consumption, and the dose of alcohol consumed. Each of these factors will be discussed briefly.

Alcoholism is a complex, multifactorial disorder involving multiple genes and gene–environment interactions. Twin and adoption studies have found that genetic influences account for 40–60% of the risk for alcoholism (Kendler, Prescott, Neale, & Pedersen, 1997; Prescott & Kendler, 1999; Schuckit, 1998, 2000). The genetics of alcoholism have also been investigated in animal models, primarily in rats and mice, using selected lines and inbred strains that differ in their free-choice alcohol intake (Crabbe, Belknap, & Buck, 1994; Grahame, 2000; Spanagel, 2000). These models include alcohol-preferring (P) and alcohol-non-preferring (NP) rat lines and high (HAD)- and low (LAD)-alcohol-drinking rats lines (Li et al., 1988; Lumeng, Hawkins, & Li, 1977), which have been selectively bred for preference differences, as well as the inbred mouse strains C57BL/6 and DBA/2, which demonstrate high and low preference for alcohol, respectively (McClearn & Rodgers, 1959). Although these animal models have been useful tools in the investigation of genetic and environmental contributions to the risk for alcohol dependence, they do not always parallel findings in humans since the genetic–environmental interactions are complex.

A positive family history of alcoholism (FHP), particularly if it spans more than one generation, is one of the strongest predictors of alcohol abuse and dependence (Goodwin, 1984), indicative of the genetic factor in the risk for alcoholism. Interestingly, a number of studies have shown that FHP, even in nonalcoholic individuals, is significantly correlated to a greater SRD effect of alcohol (Finn & Pihl, 1988; Levenson, Oyama, & Meek, 1987; Peterson, Pihl, Seguin, Finn, & Stewart, 1993). This finding has not been demonstrated unequivocally, however, and may be more prevalent with multigenerational alcohol abuse (Finn & Pihl, 1988; Sayette, Breslin, Wilson, & Rosenblum, 1994). A larger SRD effect in response to alcohol consumption, such as seen in FHP compared to family-history-negative (FHN) individuals, would likely be a stronger reinforcer for future alcohol consumption in the face of stress and may make such individuals more prone to alcoholism (Sher, 1987).

A number of individual or personality characteristics may also predict a greater SRD effect of alcohol. These include outgoing, aggressive, impulsive, or antisocial personalities (Sher & Levenson, 1982). Also, alcohol use in response to stressors may be more likely to occur in individuals who lack effective alternative coping strategies (Abrams & Niaura, 1987). Previous beliefs about the stress-reducing effects of alcohol, or positive alcohol expectancies, can also promote the consumption of alcohol in response to stress in some but not all individuals (as discussed by Pohorecky, 1991 and Powers & Kutash, 1985). However, the perception that alcohol consumption will reduce stress is clearly not the only factor influencing intake, since animals have also been shown to consume more alcohol in response to stressors. For example, rats consume more alcohol following exposure to an unpredictable schedule of isolation (Nash & Maickel, 1985), inescapable random shock (Mills, Bean, & Hutcheson, 1977), and restraint (Lynch, Kushner, Rawleigh, Fiszdon, & Carroll, 1999). Nonhuman primates also consume more alcohol in response to chronic stress or social separation, although consumption varies widely among individual monkeys (Elton, Greaves, Bunger, & Pyle, 1976; Kraemer &

McKinney, 1985). Thus, animal studies suggest that there are fundamental biological or physiological processes underlying the use of alcohol in response to stressors.

The temporal relationship between the stressor and alcohol consumption and the amount of alcohol consumed are important factors when considering the SRD effects of alcohol. For instance, alcohol consumption typically increases following but not during stressors (Conway, Vickers, Ward, & Rahe, 1981; Volpicelli, 1987). Some individuals may also consume alcohol in anticipation of a stressor, such as a social situation or an oral presentation, whereas others may not drink in the same situations for fear that alcohol may impair their cognition, speech, and/or judgment (Greeley & Oei, 1999). Such decisions likely depend on individual personality characteristics and alcohol expectancy beliefs. Finally, alcohol dose may determine whether or not SRD effects occur and their magnitude. For instance, dose-response studies have shown marked SRD effects (measured by cardiovascular reactivity) with higher doses of alcohol (in the range of 1 g/kg body weight) but no SRD effects with low alcohol doses (Sher & Walitzer, 1986; Stewart, Finn, & Pihl, 1992; Wilson, Abrams, & Lipscomb, 1980).

Experiments examining SRD effects of alcohol have used a wide array of paradigms and temporal relationships between the stressor and alcohol consumption, as well as numerous different types of stressors. All of these issues likely contribute to the lack of consistency in findings on alcohol's SRD effects in the literature. However, it appears likely that individuals exhibiting greater SRD effects in response to alcohol are more prone to alcoholism, particularly if they experience numerous or ongoing stressful life events (Sher, 1987).

Finally, the possible SRD effects of alcohol may differ in alcoholics vs nonalcoholics. Alcoholism may be defined as a loss of control over the amount of alcohol consumed as well as a preoccupation with obtaining alcohol. As discussed earlier, the risk for alcoholism appears to depend on a complex interaction of multiple genes and environmental factors, including stressors (Heath & Nelson, 2002; Pohorecky, 1991; Schuckit, 2000). Both casual drinkers and alcoholics may consume alcohol to reduce social anxiety or in response to a stressful life event. Timmer, Veroff, and Colten (1985) found that a number of stressors, including economic, marital, and job stressors, were significantly correlated with alcohol use. Because the relationship between stress and alcohol use in the human literature has been inconsistent, and not all individuals drink in response to stress, stress likely mediates alcohol-seeking behavior and consumption in only some individuals. Alcoholics not only consume more alcohol in response to stressful life events than nonalcoholics (Miller, Hersen, Eisler, & Hilsman, 1974), but they also generally experience more intense and more frequent stressors (O'Doherty, 1991; Williams, Calhoun, & Ackoff, 1982). In addition, alcoholism itself can increase the level of stress experienced by an individual, resulting from financial trouble or family, social, or work conflicts, related to their alcohol abuse. This can result in a vicious circle in which the individual consumes even greater amounts of alcohol in response to increased stress (O'Doherty, 1991; Powers & Kutash, 1985). Therefore, although alcohol may effectively reduce stress under some situations in casual drinkers who are at a low risk of developing alcoholism, in alcoholics alcohol may ultimately have the opposite effect.

Since the formulation of the SRD hypothesis, a number of models have been put forward that attempt to explain SRD effects through alcohol's effects on cognitive impairments. Hull's (1981) self-awareness model suggests that alcohol may reduce self-evaluation through impairment of cognitive processing and that this effect may reinforce alcohol consumption in self-conscious individuals. The attention-allocation model, formulated by Steele and Josephs (1988), suggests that alcohol-induced impairments in cognition result in the focusing of attention away from stressful cognitions and toward immediate, more pleasant distractions. The appraisal-disruption model (Sayette, 1993) suggests that alcohol interferes with an individual's ability to appraise a stressor by comparison with previous experiences and that this is most effective in producing SRD effects when alcohol is consumed prior to the stressor. These various models may help explain why SRD effects may be seen in some situations. However, it is likely that the underlying mechanisms of SRD effects vary greatly with the situation and the individual, and one global model may not be appropriate.

3. ALCOHOL CONSUMPTION AND STRESS-RESPONSE SYSTEMS

Alcohol-seeking behavior is a consequence of the interaction of genetic and environmental factors. As discussed above, an important environmental factor that may increase alcohol-seeking and consumption is exposure to stressors, and alcohol may effectively dampen the stress response under certain conditions. One biological system that has been widely investigated with respect to the stress–alcohol interaction is the HPA axis.

4. THE HPA AXIS AND THE β-ENDORPHIN SYSTEM

The hormonal response to a stressor is mainly mediated by two systems, namely, the locus coeruleus–sympathoadrenal medullary system and the HPA axis. The sympathoadrenal medullary system responds rapidly to a stressor with the secretion of norepinephrine from sympathetic nerves and epinephrine from the adrenal medulla. This system is involved in the "fight-or-flight" response and enables the organism to react rapidly and deal with the threat through various hemodynamic and metabolic effects including increased heart rate, vasoconstriction, and vasodilation. The HPA axis acts over a longer time frame than the sympathetic response and helps orchestrate the body's response and adaptation to the stressor through various physiological and metabolic effects in order to maintain homeostasis.

The HPA axis includes a number of brain areas, such as the paraventricular nucleus (PVN) of the hypothalamus, the anterior pituitary gland, and the adrenal cortex, which act together to produce a hormonal cascade in response to stressors. Corticotropin-releasing hormone (CRH) and arginine vasopressin (AVP) are synthesized in the parvocellular PVN (pPVN) and released into the median eminence, reaching the anterior pituitary via the hypophysial portal system. AVP is also present in large quantities in the magnocellular portion of the PVN (mPVN). CRH and AVP, originating in the pPVN, act synergistically at the anterior pituitary to stimulate the release of adrenocorticotropic hormone (ACTH) (Gillies, Linton, & Lowry, 1982). Although the main role of AVP neurons in the mPVN is the regulation of plasma osmolality, this population also exhibits some capacity to stimulate ACTH release (Holmes, Antoni, Aguilera, & Catt, 1986). In addition to ACTH, CRH also stimulates the release of the endogenous opioid β-endorphin from the anterior pituitary. Indeed, ACTH and β-endorphin share a common precursor protein, pro-opiomelanocortin (POMC), and are co-released in response to stressors (Guillemin et al., 1977). ACTH travels through the systemic circulation and acts at the adrenal cortex to stimulate the synthesis and release of glucocorticoids, namely, cortisol in humans and corticosterone (CORT) in rats. In addition to a variety of important physiological and metabolic actions throughout the body, CORT has a negative feedback function, which further inhibits HPA activity by acting at the anterior pituitary, the PVN, and other brain regions, particularly the hippocampus and prefrontal cortex. In response to stressors and circadian input, the HPA axis is activated at the level of the PVN, resulting in increased CRH and AVP secretion with subsequently increased release of ACTH and ultimately an increase in plasma glucocorticoid levels.

With respect to β-endorphin specifically, much research has focused on its role in the initiation and maintenance of alcohol consumption (for review, *see* Gianoulakis, 2001). In addition to the anterior pituitary, β-endorphin is present in the arcuate nucleus of the hypothalamus, and these neurons project to various brain regions, including those involved in the brain reward system (Khachaturian, Lewis, Schafer, & Watson, 1985). Alcoholics have been shown to exhibit lower β-endorphin levels during alcohol use even after as much as 10 yr of abstinence (Gianoulakis, Dai, & Brown, 2003; del Arbol et al., 1995). Interestingly, FHP nonalcoholic individuals also exhibit lower plasma levels of β-endorphin under normal conditions when no alcohol has been consumed, but following alcohol consumption they may exhibit greater β-endorphin levels compared to nonalcoholic FHN individuals (Dai, Tharundayil, & Gianoulakis, 2002a; Gianoulakis, Krishnan, & Tharundayil, 1996). In parallel to FHP individuals, ethanol-preferring C57BL/6 mice exhibit higher β-endorphin responses to ethanol compared to the ethanol-avoiding DBA/2 mice; however, unlike FHP individuals they exhibit higher, not lower, basal β-endorphin levels when no alcohol is consumed (Gianoulakis, 1996). Of possible clinical value, various β-endorphin antagonists, including naltrexone, have been shown to reduce alcohol consumption in both animals and humans (Froehlich, Harts, Lumeng, & Li, 1990; Myers et al., 1986; O'Malley, 1996). Furthermore, data suggest that β-endorphin may mediate some of ethanol's motivational and reinforcing effects through its effects on the dopaminergic brain reward system (Gianoulakis, 2001; Koob, 1992).

5. ACUTE ALCOHOL EXPOSURE AND HPA ACTIVITY

It has long been known that acute alcohol exposure alters the activity of the HPA axis. In rodents, acute alcohol exposure, producing blood alcohol levels above 100 mg%, has been shown to activate the HPA axis, resulting in elevated plasma levels of ACTH and CORT (Laszlo et al., 2001; Ogilvie, Lee, & Rivier, 1997a,b; Rivier & Lee, 1996; Zhou et al., 2000). This effect appears to be mediated primarily by CRH, because CRH antiserum (Rivier, Bruhn, & Vale, 1988), pituitary CRH receptor blockade (using the CRH antagonist astressin) (Rivier, Rivier, & Lee, 1996), and bilateral lesioning of the PVN (Rivest & Rivier, 1994) significantly reduce the ACTH response to alcohol. Also, CRH heteronuclear RNA (hnRNA) in the pPVN is rapidly increased in response to acute alcohol administration, although CRH mRNA appears to be unchanged (Rivier & Lee, 1996; Zhou et al., 2000). AVP also appears to play a role in alcohol-induced HPA activation. Acute alcohol exposure increases AVP mRNA in the PVN, although primarily within the magnocellular region (Rivier & Lee, 1996). Both AVP antiserum (Ogilvie et al., 1997a) and blockade of AVP receptors (Rivier & Lee, 1996) attenuate alcohol-induced ACTH secretion. The role of HPA activation in mediating the reinforcing effects of alcohol is unclear at present. However, evidence suggests that glucocorticoids may promote alcohol-seeking behavior. In rodents, alcohol self-administration is decreased by adrenalectomy, whereas CORT replacement restores alcohol consumption (Fahlke, Engel, Eriksson, Hard, & Soderpalm, 1994; Fahlke, Hard, & Hansen, 1996). These findings suggest that enhanced HPA activity may play some role in promoting alcohol consumption and support the suggestion that stressors can induce drinking.

In human nonalcoholics, HPA activation with acute alcohol exposure has not been shown consistently (Ida et al., 1992; Inder et al., 1995; Stott et al, 1987; Waltman, Blevins, Boyd, & Wand, 1993). The discrepancies in the literature may relate to alcohol dose, since HPA activation is seen more consistently in the studies that used higher alcohol doses (producing blood alcohol levels in the range of 100 mg%) (Wand, 1993). It has also been suggested that oral alcohol ingestion may result in HPA activation in some individuals as a result of gastrointestinal side effects, which would be more prevalent at higher alcohol doses (Inder et al., 1995). In addition, family history of alcoholism has been shown to affect HPA reactivity. For instance, FHP individuals who are drinkers but not alcohol dependent show a lesser cortisol increase in response to alcohol compared to FHN individuals (Schuckit, Tsuang, Anthenelli, Tipp, & Nurnberger, 1996). In addition, in the absence of alcohol, FHP nonalcoholic individuals exhibit lower basal plasma levels of β-endorphin, normal or lower cortisol levels, as well as lower responses to ovine CRH compared to FHN individuals (Gianoulakis, 1996; Gianoulakis et al., 1989; Waltman, McCaul, & Wand, 1994; Wand, Mangold, Ali, & Giggey, 1999). Similarly, studies in genetically selected P and NP rats have shown significantly lower CRH in the hypothalamus of the P compared to the NP rats (Ehlers et al., 1992). Whether or not blunted HPA responsivity to alcohol in genetically susceptible individuals may play a role in the development of alcoholism is not known.

Although acute alcohol exposure may activate the HPA axis in some cases, ACTH responses to alcohol, CRH, and various stressors presented immediately following acute alcohol exposure are consistently blunted in both animals and humans (Dai, Tharundayil, & Gianoulakis, 2002b; Rivier & Vale, 1988; Waltman et al., 1993). For instance, in one study in which rats were exposed to a mild, inescapable foot shock immediately after a 3-h intraperitoneal infusion of either alcohol or saline, alcohol-infused rats demonstrated a lower ACTH response to the foot shock compared to saline-infused rats (Rivier & Vale, 1988). Consistent with these data are results from a study conducted in individuals with no family history of alcoholism who performed a stress-inducing task involving a number of mathematical problems under the pressure of time and competition 30 min after consumption of either ethanol or placebo. Compared to placebo, prior ethanol consumption significantly reduced or abolished the stress-induced elevations in plasma ACTH and cortisol (Dai et al., 2002b). Even low doses of alcohol that do not stimulate ACTH or cortisol release in humans have been shown to blunt the HPA response to subsequent CRH administration (Waltman et al., 1993). Prior alcohol exposure thus may produce a cross-tolerance by altering the HPA responsivity to subsequent stimuli. One can speculate that this decreased HPA response to stressors may mediate alcohol-seeking behavior prior to a stressor in some individuals and in some situations.

6. CHRONIC ALCOHOL EXPOSURE AND HPA DYSREGULATION

Although acute alcohol exposure may activate the HPA axis, chronic alcohol consumption results in dysregulation of the HPA axis and may lead to the development of HPA tolerance to the stimulatory effects of alcohol. In addition, there may be differential effects of short-term vs long-term chronic exposure. Animal models of chronic alcohol exposure have used a wide range of exposure lengths, paradigms, and modes of alcohol delivery, making comparison more difficult. However, in virtually all instances chronic alcohol exposure clearly and consistently dysregulates HPA function.

Although rodents typically show elevated glucocorticoid levels after prolonged alcohol exposure, the magnitude of the elevation may decrease with time (Knych & Prohaska, 1981; Rivier, Imaki, & Vale, 1990; Spencer & McEwen, 1990; Tabakoff, Jafee, & Ritzmann, 1978; Zhou et al., 2000). Also, glucocorticoid receptors (GRs) have been shown to be decreased in rats in the PVN, hippocampus, and other brain regions after 15 d of ethanol exposure, possibly owing to receptor downregulation in the presence of elevated circulating glucocorticoid levels (Roy, Mittal, Zhang, & Pandey, 2002). In response to short-term chronic ethanol exposure (3–14 d), CRH mRNA in the PVN of rats is either increased (Rivier et al., 1990) or unchanged (Zhou et al., 2000). However, long-term (6 mo) ethanol exposure results in decreased CRH mRNA in the pPVN, suggesting that hormonal tolerance to ethanol may develop at the hypothalamic level (Silva, Paula-Barbosa, & Madeira, 2002). HPA responsivity to alcohol, CRH, and stressors is also affected by chronic ethanol exposure, demonstrated by blunted ACTH release and blunted CRH hnRNA responses, with no differences in AVP hnRNA (Lee et al., 2000a; Lee, Schmidt, Tilders, & Rivier, 2001; Wand, 1993).

In humans, elevated basal cortisol levels are seen only in some alcoholics (del Arbol et al., 1995; Gianoulakis et al., 2003; Wand & Dobs, 1991) and in the extreme may produce what is often referred to as pseudo-Cushing's syndrome (Rees, Besser, Jeffcoate, Goldie, & Marks, 1977; Veldman & Meinders, 1996). Normal cortisol levels in other alcoholics may be due in part to the development of hormonal tolerance in response to prolonged alcohol exposure. Inconsistencies are also seen in plasma ACTH levels of alcoholics, as various studies have reported either normal or low levels (del Arbol et al., 1995; Gianoulakis et al., 2003; Vescovi, DiGennaro, & Coiro, 1997). Similar to findings in animals, chronic alcoholics typically exhibit a blunted plasma ACTH response to CRH (Wand & Dobs, 1991). Thus, HPA dysregulation and therefore abnormal responsivity to other stimuli may occur following chronic alcohol exposure, possibly as a compensatory response mounted in an attempt to reestablish normal glucocorticoid levels.

7. HPA RESPONSIVITY AND SUSCEPTIBILITY TO ALCOHOL DEPENDENCE

Individuals with a family history of alcoholism, who are therefore at a high risk for alcoholism themselves, show differential HPA activity, including lower basal ACTH and β-endorphin levels as well as lower HPA responses to stress or alcohol consumption compared to those at a low risk of developing alcoholism (Dai et al., 2002a, 2002b; Gianoulakis et al., 1996; Schuckit, Gold, & Risch, 1987). Similarly, in a general population, a blunted cortisol response to alcohol has been shown to be predictive of alcohol dependence nearly a decade later (Schuckit et al., 1996). In addition to altered HPA responsivity to alcohol, differential HPA responses to stressors may play a role in predisposing an organism to alcohol abuse. For instance, monkeys that show a high plasma cortisol response to a social separation challenge in infancy show greater voluntary intake of alcohol in adulthood (Fahlke et al., 2000). Although individual differences in HPA responsivity to alcohol and to stressors may be in opposite directions, both may predispose an individual to, and possibly be predictive for, the development of alcoholism. In addition, adverse experiences in early life may also promote alcohol abuse later in life. For instance, early life stressors, including deleterious rearing experiences, have been shown to increase alcohol consumption in rats (Huot, Thrivikraman, Meany, & Plotsky, 2001; Weinberg, 1987) and nonhuman primates (Fahlke et al., 2000; Higley, Hasert, Suomi, & Linnoila, 1991). In addition, prenatal alcohol exposure, which will be discussed in more detail later, has been shown to increase alcohol preference in rats (Bond & Di Giusto, 1976) and increase the likelihood of alcohol problems in humans (Baer, Sampson, Barr, Connor, & Straissguth, 2003). Also, rats prenatally exposed to alcohol exhibit enhanced HPA responsivity to alcohol in adulthood (Taylor et al., 1981). Although both altered HPA activity and responsivity to alcohol appear to relate to alcohol use, the HPA–alcohol interaction is likely only one of many, including both genetic and environmental, factors that may increase the likelihood of developing alcohol dependence.

8. ALCOHOL WITHDRAWAL AND HPA FUNCTION

HPA dysregulation in alcoholics may persist up to several months after cessation of alcohol consumption. In the early stages, alcohol withdrawal appears to activate the HPA axis, as demonstrated by elevated plasma cortisol levels (Adinoff et al., 1991; Iranmanesh, Veldhuis, Johnson, & Lizarralde, 1989), although this may be owing in part to the stress of withdrawal itself in addition to the physiological readjustments that occur following withdrawal. However, cortisol levels are typically normalized or decreased within days to weeks of alcohol withdrawal (Costa et al., 1996; Vescovi et al., 1997). Although plasma ACTH levels may be normal in abstinent alcoholics (Vescovi et al., 1997), HPA responsivity to CRH and various stressors, as indicated by ACTH and cortisol responses, is blunted long after cessation of alcohol consumption (Costa et al., 1996; Ehrenreich et al., 1997; Vescovi et al., 1997). Interestingly, one study found that alcoholics who were abstinent for 12 wk showed blunted ACTH responses to systemic CRH, whereas the ACTH response to stressors had normalized at that time, suggesting possible compensatory mechanisms to enable normal responsivity to stressors in the face of HPA dysregulation (Ehrenreich et al., 1997). Blunted HPA responsivity is likely not mediated by increased glucocorticoid feedback since cortisol levels are typically not elevated with prolonged alcohol withdrawal. In addition, similar findings are reported following ethanol withdrawal in rats with no genetic predisposition for alcohol consumption, suggesting that these findings are at least partly owing to long-term effects of alcohol on HPA function (Rasmussen et al., 2000). The altered HPA responsivity seen following alcohol withdrawal resembles that seen in FHP nonalcoholics and may similarly play a role in the risk for relapse to alcohol abuse (Rasmussen et al., 2000).

9. GENDER DIFFERENCES IN ALCOHOL–HPA INTERACTIONS

Alcohol abuse occurs with less frequency in women than in men (Robins et al., 1984). However, adverse effects appear after a shorter duration of alcohol abuse in women and progress more rapidly, an effect that has been termed "telescoping" (Piazza, Vrbka, & Yeager, 1989; Randall et al., 1999). One study in which alcoholics were found to exhibit lower basal plasma ACTH levels compared to nonalcoholics additionally noted that this decrease was greater in females (Gianoulakis et al., 2003) and suggested that this may reflect a greater sensitivity to alcohol–HPA interactions in females. Studies in rats have shown that females exhibit greater ACTH and CORT responses to alcohol injection than males (Ogilvie & Rivier, 1996; Ogilvie & Rivier, 1997). Although this may partly reflect the normal sexual dimorphism of the HPA axis in response to stimuli, higher HPA responses to alcohol may exacerbate any detrimental effects associated with alcohol-induced HPA activation in females. These findings suggest that females may have a more labile HPA responsivity to alcohol and that this may strengthen any role that HPA activity plays in the development and/or maintenance of alcohol abuse. However, the fact that there are fewer female than male alcoholics (Corrigan, 1985; Hilton, 1987) suggests that this may not be a primary factor in the development of alcoholism.

10. PRENATAL ETHANOL EXPOSURE AND THE HPA AXIS

Because alcohol readily crosses the placenta, alcohol consumed during pregnancy can stimulate the fetal HPA axis, which is functional before birth (Eguchi, 1969). In addition, alcohol also stimulates the maternal HPA axis, resulting in elevated maternal plasma cortisol levels. Cortisol itself can, to some extent, cross the placenta in both directions and thus disrupt the development of the fetal HPA axis (Eguchi, 1969). Consequently, as a result of both direct and indirect influences, offspring of alcohol-consuming mothers exhibit altered development and responsiveness of the HPA axis throughout adult life.

Rats prenatally exposed to ethanol (E rats) exhibit significantly greater brain, plasma, and adrenal CORT levels and decreased corticosteroid-binding globulin (CBG) capacity at birth compared to controls (Kakihana, Butte, & Moore, 1980; Taylor, Branch, Kokka, & Poland, 1983; Weinberg, 1989). By 3–5 d of age, basal CORT levels are normalized. However, the HPA response to stress is blunted compared to that in controls, an effect that appears to persist throughout the preweaning period (Taylor, Branch, Nelson, Lane, & Poland, 1986; Weinberg, 1989). In contrast, following weaning and into adulthood, both male and female E rats exhibit hormonal hyperresponsiveness to stressors and to drugs such as ethanol or morphine (Kim, Osborn, & Weinberg, 1996; Lee, Schmidt, Tilders, & Rivier, 2000b; Taylor, Branch, Liu, & Kokka, 1982; Weinberg, 1988, 1993). In adult E rats, basal nonstress levels of plasma CORT, CBG, and ACTH are typically normal (Kim, Giberson, Yu, Zoeller, & Weinberg, 1999; Taylor et al., 1983; Weinberg & Gallo, 1982). However, in response to stressors including foot shock (Lee et al., 2000b; Nelson et al., 1986), novel environments (Weinberg, 1988), restraint (Weinberg, 1988, 1992), ether (Angelogianni & Gianoulakis, 1989; Weinberg & Gallo, 1982), cold (Angelogianni & Gianoulakis, 1989; Kim et al., 1999), and immune challenges (Lee & Rivier, 1996; Lee et al., 2000b), CORT and/or ACTH levels may show increased and/or prolonged elevations compared to controls. Sex differences in response to stressors are often observed and vary depending on the nature of the stressor and the time course and hormonal endpoint measured (Weinberg, 1985, 1992; Weinberg, Taylor, & Gianoulakis, 1996). For example, both male and female E rats exhibit increased CORT, ACTH, and/or β-endorphin (Weinberg, 1988, 1992; Weinberg et al., 1996) as well as immediate-early gene and CRH mRNA levels (Lee, Imaki, Vale, & Rivier, 1990; Lee et al., 2000b; Leo, Glavas, Yu, Ellis, & Weinberg, 2002) in response to stressors such as repeated restraint and foot shock and also show deficits in habituation to repeated stressors such as restraint (Weinberg et al., 1996). In contrast, in response to prolonged restraint or cold stress, HPA hyperactivity is seen primarily in male E rats (Kim et al., 1996; Weinberg, 1992), whereas in response to acute restraint or acute ethanol or morphine challenge, increased CORT and ACTH are found primarily in female E rats (Taylor et al., 1982, 1983; Taylor, Branch, van Zuylen, & Redei 1988; Weinberg, 1985, 1992; Weinberg & Gallo, 1982). This marked sexual dimorphism in fetal alcohol effects suggests a possible role for the gonadal steroids in mediating HPA hyperresponsiveness.

The mechanisms underlying hyperresponsiveness of the HPA axis in E rats are unknown at present. However, it appears that multiple mechanisms probably play a role and that these may differ to some extent in male and female E rats. In response to stressors, including foot shock and endotoxemia, immediate-early gene (c-fos and NGFI-B) and CRH hnRNA responses are greater in the pPVN of E compared to control animals (Lee et al., 2000b), suggesting that HPA hyperresponsiveness may be mediated by enhanced stimulatory inputs to the PVN. In addition, male E rats exhibit elevated CRH mRNA following adrenalectomy (Glavas, Ellis, Yu, & Weinberg, 2000), suggesting that this effect may be independent of CORT. Thus, similar to the effects of acute and chronic alcohol exposure, prenatal alcohol exposure effects on the HPA axis appear to be mediated primarily at the level of the PVN or higher.

11. CONSEQUENCES OF HPA DYSREGULATION

The ability to respond appropriately to stressors is an important adaptive mechanism, and HPA activation is known to be a central component of this response. In the short term, stress-induced increases in CORT enable the organism to respond to or cope with the stressor. Following termination of the stressor, high CORT levels help to initiate a recovery process by which the endocrine, metabolic, immune, and neural defensive reactions mobilized in response to stress are terminated. Prolonged or chronic CORT elevations can result in adverse physiological and behavioral consequences (e.g., obesity, metabolic disorders, cardiovascular disorders, depression, memory deficits, cognitive impairments) that could compromise health and even survival. Thus, elevated basal cortisol levels, as may occur in chronic alcoholics or during alcohol withdrawal, or enhanced reactivity to stress resulting from prenatal alcohol exposure may increase the vulnerability to illnesses later in life (De Kloet, Vreugdenhil, Oitzl, & Joels, 1998; O'Regan, Welberg, Holmes, & Seckl, 2001; Raber, 1998).

Early environmental events appear to play a major role in programming the HPA axis, resulting in permanent functional alterations in HPA responsivity that last throughout adulthood (Matthews, 2002). Since altered HPA responsivity has been shown to correlate with future alcohol abuse, it is possible that altered HPA reactivity resulting from early environmental factors, such as deleterious rearing conditions or prenatal alcohol exposure, may mediate the increased likelihood of future alcohol abuse.

An emerging model in the understanding of HPA dysregulation is the concept of allostatic load. Allostasis is a process of adaptation that allows an organism to maintain stability, or homeostasis, through change (Sterling & Eyer, 1988). In contrast to homeostasis, which is a steady-state condition with defined setpoints, allostasis is a dynamic condition without setpoints, which allows the organism to adapt to challenge, and the HPA axis is one system that mediates such adaptation (Sterling & Eyer, 1988). As suggested by Koob (2003), allostasis may lead to a new setpoint in brain reward systems and stress systems in alcoholics, and this may promote alcohol consumption and increase vulnerability to relapse. Allostatic load is a measure of the cumulative burden of challenges on an organism or the price of adaptation (McEwen, 1998; McEwen & Stellar,

1993; Seeman, McEwen, Rowe, & Singer, 2001). Over time, prolonged, repeated, or inadequate allostatic responses can result in allostatic load, leading to maladaptation and impaired responses to further challenges (Pacak & Palkovits, 2001). Allostatic load may therefore result in HPA dysregulation, or, alternatively, HPA dysregulation owing to genetic, environmental, or disease conditions may increase susceptibility to excessive allostatic load and lead to further dysfunction. Thus, not only may HPA dysregulation predispose an individual to alcohol dependence, but HPA dysregulation that results from chronic alcoholism or prenatal alcohol exposure can result in further impairments in the ability to respond and adapt to stressors, thus increasing allostatic load and vulnerability to illness.

12. CONCLUSIONS

The literature supports an interaction of stress and alcohol consumption; however, the mechanisms are complex and remain poorly understood. Although alcohol is often consumed in response to or in anticipation of a stressor, its effectiveness as a stress-reducing agent is inconsistent and appears to depend on numerous factors, including family history of alcoholism, whether or not the individual is an alcoholic, individual personality characteristics, the environmental situation, the temporal relationship between the stressor and alcohol consumption, and alcohol dose. Alcohol also alters the activity of the HPA axis, which may promote the maintenance of alcohol consumption and impair responsivity to subsequent stressors. In addition, chronic alcohol abuse results in HPA dysregulation, which may persist up to several months after the cessation of alcohol use. This dysregulation may also promote relapse to alcohol abuse in abstinent alcoholics. Alcohol consumption during pregnancy can permanently reprogram the developing fetal HPA axis, resulting in long-term HPA hyperresponsiveness in the offspring. Ultimately, although alcohol is often used to cope with stressors, alcohol abuse leads to an impaired ability to mount an appropriate HPA response to stressors. This can lead to serious detrimental health consequences and could compromise health and even survival.

REFERENCES

Abrams, D. B., & Niaura, R. S. (1987). Social learning theory. In H. T. Blane & K. E. Leonard (Eds.), *Psychological theories of drinking and alcoholism* (pp. 131–178). New York: Guilford.

Adinoff, B., Risher-Flowers, D., De Jong, J., Ravitz, B., Bone, G. H., Nutt, D. J., Roehrich, L., Martin, P. R., & Linnoila, M. (1991). Disturbances of hypothalamic–pituitary–adrenal axis functioning during ethanol withdrawal in six men. *American Journal of Psychiatry, 148*, 1023–1025.

Angelogianni, P., & Gianoulakis, C. (1989). Prenatal exposure to ethanol alters the ontogeny of the beta-endorphin response to stress. *Alcoholism: Clinical and Experimental Research, 13*, 564–571.

Baer, J. S., Sampson, P. D., Barr, H. M., Connor, P. D., & Streissguth, A. P. (2003). A 21-year longitudinal analysis of the effects of prenatal alcohol exposure on young adult drinking. *Archives of General Psychiatry, 60*, 377–385.

Bond, N. W., & Di Giusto, E. L. (1976). Effects of prenatal alcohol consumption on open-field behaviour and alcohol preference in rats. *Psychopharmacologia, 46*, 163–165.

Brady, K. T., & Sonne, S. C. (1999). The role of stress in alcohol use, alcoholism treatment, and relapse. *Alcohol Research and Health: the Journal of the National Institute on Alcohol Abuse and Alcoholism, 23*, 263–271.

Cappell, H. (1975). An evaluation of tension models of alcohol consumption. In R. J. Gibbins, Y. Israel, H. Kalant, R. E. Popham, W. Schmidt, & R. G. Smart (Eds.), *Research advances in alcohol and drug problems* (Vol. 2, pp. 177–210). New York: John Wiley & Sons.

Cappell, H., & Greeley, J. (1987). Alcohol and tension reduction: An update on research and theory. In H. T. Blake & K. E. Leonard (Eds.), *Psychological theories of drinking and alcoholism* (pp. 15–54). New York: Guilford.

Cappell, H., & Herman, C. P. (1972). Alcohol and tension reduction: A review. *Journal of Studies on Alcohol, 33*, 33–64.

Conger, J. J. (1956). Alcoholism: Theory, problem and challenge. II. Reinforcement theory and the dynamics of alcoholism. *Quarterly Journal of Studies on Alcohol, 13*, 296–305.

Conway, T. L., Vickers Jr., R. R., Ward, H. W., & Rahe, R. H. (1981). Occupational stress and variation in cigarette, coffee, and alcohol consumption. *Journal of Health and Social Behavior, 22*, 155–165.

Corrigan, E. M. (1985). Gender differences in alcohol and other drug use. *Addictive Behaviors, 10*, 313–317.

Costa, A., Bono, G., Martignoni, E., Merlo, P., Sances, G., & Nappi, G. (1996). An assessment of hypothalamic–pituitary–adrenal axis functioning in non-depressed, early abstinent alcoholics. *Psychoneuroendocrinology, 21*, 263–275.

Crabbe, J. C., Belknap, J. K., & Buck, K. J. (1994). Genetic animal models of alcohol and drug abuse. *Science, 264*, 1715–1723.

Dai, X., Thavundayil, J., & Gianoulakis, C. (2002a). Differences in the responses of the pituitary beta-endorphin and cardiovascular system to ethanol and stress as a function of family history. *Alcoholism: Clinical and Experimental Research, 26*, 1171–1180.

Dai, X., Thavundayil, J., & Gianoulakis, C. (2002b). Response of the hypothalamic–pituitary–adrenal axis to stress in the absence and presence of ethanol in subjects at high and low risk of alcoholism. *Neuropsychopharmacology, 27*, 442–452.

De Kloet, E. R., Vreugdenhil, E., Oitzl, M. S., & Joels, M. (1998). Brain corticosteroid receptor balance in health and disease. *Endocrine Reviews, 19*, 269–301.

del Arbol, J. L., Aguirre, J. C., Raya, J., Rico, J., Ruiz-Requena, M. E., & Miranda, M. T. (1995). Plasma concentrations of beta-endorphin, adrenocorticotropic hormone, and cortisol in drinking and abstinent chronic alcoholics. *Alcohol, 12*, 525–529.

Eguchi, Y. (1969). Interrelationships between the foetal and maternal hypophysial adrenal axes in rats and mice. In E. Bajusz (Ed.), *Physiology and pathology of adaptation mechanisms* (pp. 3–27). New York: Pergamon.

Ehlers, C. L., Chaplin, R. I., Wall, T. L., Lumeng, L., Li, T. K., Owens, M. J., & Nemeroff, C. B. (1992). Corticotropin releasing factor (CRF): Studies in alcohol preferring and non-preferring rats. *Psychopharmacology, 106*, 359–364.

Ehrenreich, H., Schuck, J., Stender, N., Pilz, J., Gefeller, O., Schilling, L., Poser, W., & Kaw, S. (1997). Endocrine and hemodynamic effects of stress versus systemic CRF in alcoholics during early and medium term abstinence. *Alcoholism: Clinical and Experimental Research, 21*, 1285–1293.

Elton, R. H., Greaves, D. A., Bunger, D. R., & Pyle, T. W. (1976). Drinking patterns of pigtailed macaques. *Journal of Studies on Alcohol, 37*, 1548–1555.

Fahlke, C., Engel, J. A., Eriksson, C. J., Hard, E., & Soderpalm, B. (1994). Involvement of corticosterone in the modulation of ethanol consumption in the rat. *Alcohol, 11*, 195–202.

Fahlke, C., Hard, E., & Hansen, S. (1996). Facilitation of ethanol consumption by intracerebroventricular infusions of corticosterone. *Psychopharmacology, 127*, 133–139.

Fahlke, C., Lorenz, J. G., Long, J., Champoux, M., Suomi, S. J., & Higley, J. D. (2000). Rearing experiences and stress-induced plasma cortisol as early risk factors for excessive alcohol consumption in nonhuman primates. *Alcoholism: Clinical and Experimental Research, 24*, 644–650.

Finn, P. R., & Pihl, R. O. (1988). Risk for alcoholism: A comparison between two different groups of sons of alcoholics on cardiovascular reactivity and sensitivity to alcohol. *Alcoholism: Clinical and Experimental Research, 12*, 742–747.

Froehlich, J. C., Harts, J., Lumeng, L., & Li, T. K. (1990). Naloxone attenuates voluntary ethanol intake in rats selectively bred for high ethanol preference. *Pharmacology, Biochemistry and Behavior, 35*, 385–390.

Gianoulakis, C. (1996). Implications of endogenous opioids and dopamine in alcoholism: Human and basic science studies. *Alcohol and Alcoholism, 31*, 33–42.

Gianoulakis, C. (2001). Influence of the endogenous opioid system on high alcohol consumption and genetic predisposition to alcoholism. *Journal of Psychiatry and Neuroscience, 26*, 304–318.

Gianoulakis, C., Beliveau, D., Angelogianni, P., Meaney, M., Thavundayil, J., Tawar, V., & Dumas, M. (1989). Different pituitary beta-endorphin and adrenal cortisol response to ethanol in individuals with high and low risk for future development of alcoholism. *Life Sciences, 45*, 1097–1109.

Gianoulakis, C., Krishnan, B., & Thavundayil, J. (1996). Enhanced sensitivity of pituitary beta-endorphin to ethanol in subjects at high risk of alcoholism. *Archives of General Psychiatry, 53*, 250–257.

Gianoulakis, C., Dai, X., & Brown, T. (2003). Effect of chronic alcohol consumption on the activity of the hypothalamic–pituitary–adrenal axis and pituitary beta-endorphin as a function of alcohol intake, age, and gender. *Alcoholism Clinical and Experimental Research, 27*, 410–423.

Gillies, G. E., Linton, E. A., & Lowry, P. J. (1982). Corticotropin releasing activity of the new CRF is potentiated several times by vasopressin. *Nature, 299*, 355–357.

Glavas, M. M., Ellis, L., Yu, W. K., & Weinberg, J. (2000). Corticotropin releasing hormone and vasopressin expression are altered in rats prenatally exposed to ethanol. *Alcoholism: Clinical and Experimental Research, 24*, 100A.

Goodwin, D. W. (1984). Studies of familial alcoholism: a review. *Journal of Clinical Psychiatry, 45*, 14–17.

Grahame, N. J. (2000). Selected lines and inbred strains. Tools in the hunt for the genes involved in alcoholism. *Alcohol Research and Health: the Journal of the National Institute on Alcohol Abuse and Alcoholism, 24*, 159–163.

Greeley, J., & Oei, T. (1999). Alcohol and tension reduction. In K. E. Leonard & H. T. Blane (Eds.), *Psychological theories of drinking and alcoholism, 2nd ed.* (pp. 14–53). New York: Guilford.

Guillemin, R., Vargo, T., Rossier, J., Minick, S., Ling, N., Rivier, C., Vale, W., & Bloom, F. (1977). β-Endorphin and adrenocorticotropin are secreted concomitantly by the pituitary gland. *Science, 197*, 1367–1369.

Heath, A. C., & Nelson, E. C. (2002). Effects of the interaction between genotype and environment. Research into the genetic epidemiology of alcohol dependence. *Alcohol Research and Health: the Journal of the National Institute on Alcohol Abuse and Alcoholism, 26*, 193–201.

Higley, J. D., Hasert, M. F., Suomi, S. J., & Linnoila, M. (1991). Nonhuman primate model of alcohol abuse: Effects of early experience, personality, and stress on alcohol consumption. *Proceedings of the National Academy of Sciences of the United States of America, 88*, 7261–7265.

Hilton, M. E. (1987). Drinking patterns and drinking problems in 1984: Results from a general population survey. *Alcoholism: Clinical and Experimental Research, 11*, 167–175.

Holmes, M. C., Antoni, F. A., Aguilera, G., & Catt, K. J. (1986). Magnocellular axons in passage through the median eminence release vasopressin. *Nature, 319*, 326–329.

Hull, J. G. (1981). A self-awareness model of the causes and effects of alcohol consumption. *Journal of Abnormal Psychology, 90*, 586–600.

Huot, R. L., Thrivikraman, K. V., Meaney, M. J., & Plotsky, P. M. (2001). Development of adult ethanol preference and anxiety as a consequence of neonatal maternal separation in Long Evans rats and reversal with antidepressant treatment. *Psychopharmacology, 158*, 366–373.

Ida, Y., Tsujimaru, S., Nakamaura, K., Shirao, I., Mukasa, H., Egami, H., & Nakazawa, Y. (1992). Effects of acute and repeated alcohol ingestion on hypothalamic–pituitary–gonadal and hypothalamic–pituitary–adrenal functioning in normal males. *Drug and Alcohol Dependence, 31*, 57–64.

Inder, W. J., Joyce, P. R., Wells, J. E., Evans, M. J., Ellis, M. J., Mattioli, L., & Donald, R. A. (1995). The acute effects of oral ethanol on the hypothalamic-pituitary-adrenal axis in normal human subjects. *Clinical Endocrinology, 42*, 65–71.

Iranmanesh, A., Veldhuis, J. D., Johnson, M. L., & Lizarralde, G. (1989). 24-Hour pulsatile and circadian patterns of cortisol secretion in alcoholic men. *Journal of Andrology, 10*, 54–63.

Kakihana, R., Butte, J. C., & Moore, J. A. (1980). Endocrine effects of maternal alcoholization: Plasma and brain testosterone, dihydrotestosterone, estradiol, and corticosterone. *Alcoholism: Clinical and Experimental Research, 4*, 57–61.

Kendler, K. S., Prescott, C. A., Neale, M. C., & Pedersen, N. L. (1997). Temperance board registration for alcohol abuse in a national sample of Swedish male twins, born 1902 to 1949. *Archives of General Psychiatry, 54*, 178–184.

Khachaturian, H., Lewis, M. E., Schafer, M. K. H., & Watson, S. J. (1985). Anatomy of the CNS opioid systems. *Trends in Neurosciences, 8*, 111–119.

Kim, C. K., Osborn, J. A., & Weinberg, J. (1996). Stress reactivity in fetal alcohol syndrome. In E. Abel (Ed.), *Fetal alcohol syndrome: From mechanism to behavior* (pp. 215–235). Boca Raton, FL: CRC.

Kim, C. K., Giberson, P. K., Yu, W., Zoeller, R. T., & Weinberg, J. (1999). Effects of prenatal ethanol exposure on hypothalamic–pituitary–adrenal responses to chronic cold stress in rats. *Alcoholism: Clinical and Experimental Research, 23*, 301–310.

Knych, E. T., & Prohaska, J. R. (1981). Effect of chronic intoxication and naloxone on the ethanol-induced increase in plasma corticosterone. *Life Sciences, 28*, 1987–1994.

Koob, G. F. (1992). Drugs of abuse: Anatomy, pharmacology and function of reward pathways. *Trends in Pharmacological Sciences, 13*, 177–184.

Koob, G. F.(2003). Alcoholism: Allostasis and beyond. *Alcoholism: Clinical and Experimental Research, 27*, 232–243.

Kraemer, G. W., & McKinney, W. T. (1985). Social separation increases alcohol consumption in rhesus monkeys. *Psychopharmacology, 86*, 182–189.

Laszlo, F. A., Varga, C., Pavo, I., Gardi, J., Vecsernyes, M., Galfi, M., Morschl, E., Laszlo, F., & Makara, G. B. (2001). Vasopressin pressor receptor-mediated activation of HPA axis by acute ethanol stress in rats. *American Journal of Physiology–Regulatory Integrative and Comparative Physiology, 280*, R458–465.

Lee, S., & Rivier, C. (1996). Gender differences in the effect of prenatal alcohol exposure on the hypothalamic–pituitary–adrenal axis response to immune signals. *Psychoneuroendocrinology, 21*, 145–155.

Lee, S., Imaki, T., Vale, W., & Rivier, C. (1990). Effect of prenatal exposure to ethanol on the activity of the hypothalamic-pituitary-adrenal axis of the offspring: Importance of the time of exposure to ethanol and possible modulating mechanisms. *Molecular and Cellular Neurosciences, 1*, 168–177.

Lee, S., Schmidt, D., Tilders, F., Cole, M., Smith, A., & Rivier, C. (2000a). Prolonged exposure to intermittent alcohol vapors blunts hypothalamic responsiveness to immune and non-immune signals. *Alcoholism: Clinical and Experimental Research, 24*, 110–122.

Lee, S., Schmidt, D., Tilders, F., & Rivier, C. (2000b). Increased activity of the hypothalamic–pituitary–adrenal axis of rats exposed to alcohol in utero: Role of altered pituitary and hypothalamic function. *Molecular and Cellular Neurosciences, 16*, 515–528.

Lee, S., Schmidt, D., Tilders, F. J. H., & Rivier, C. (2001). Effect of repeated exposure to alcohol on the response of the hypothalamic–pituitary–adrenal axis of the rat: I. Role of changes in hypothalamic neuronal activity. *Alcoholism: Clinical and Experimental Research, 25*, 98–105.

Leo, J. M., Glavas, M. M., Yu, W. K., Ellis, L., & Weinberg, J. (2002). Prenatal ethanol exposure differentially alters HPA regulation in male and female rats. *Society for Neuroscience Abstracts, 32*.

Levenson, R. W., Sher, K. J., Grossman, L. M., Newman, J., & Newlin, D. B. (1980). Alcohol and stress response dampening: Pharmacological effects, expectancy, and tension reduction. *Journal of Abnormal Psychology, 89*, 528–538.

Levenson, R. W., Oyama, O. N., & Meek, P. S. (1987). Greater reinforcement from alcohol for those at risk: parental risk, personality risk, and sex. *Journal of Abnormal Psychology, 96*, 242–253.

Li, T.-K., Lumeng, L., Doolittle, D. P., McBride, W. J., Murphy, J. M., Froehlich, J. C., & Morzorati, S. (1988). Behavioral and neurochemical associations of alcohol-seeking behavior. In K. Kuriyama, A. Takada, & H. Ishii (Eds.), *Biomedical and social aspects of alcohol and alcoholism.* (pp. 435–438). Amsterdam: Elsevier.

Lumeng, L., Hawkins, T. D., & Li, T.-K. (1977). New strains of rats with alcohol preference and nonpreference. In R. G. Thurman, J. R. Williamson, H. R. Drott, & B. Chance (Eds.), *Alcohol and aldehyde metabolizing systems* (Vol. 3, pp. 537–544). New York: Academic.

Lynch, W. J., Kushner, M. G., Rawleigh, J. M., Fiszdon, J., & Carroll, M. E. (1999). The effects of restraint stress on voluntary ethanol consumption in rats. *Experimental and Clinical Psychopharmacology, 7*, 318–323.

Matthews, S. G. (2002). Early programming of the hypothalamic–pituitary–adrenal axis. *Trends in Endocrinology and Metabolism, 13*, 373–380.

McClearn, G. E., & Rodgers, D. A. (1959). Differences in alcohol preference among inbred strains of mice. *Quarterly Journal of Studies on Alcohol, 20*, 691–695.

McEwen, B. S. (1998). Stress, adaptation, and disease. Allostasis and allostatic load. *Annals of the New York Academy of Sciences, 840*, 33–44.

McEwen, B. S., & Stellar, E. (1993). Stress and the individual. Mechanisms leading to disease. *Archives of Internal Medicine, 153*, 2093–2101.

Miller, P. M., Hersen, M., Eisler, R. M., & Hilsman, G. (1974). Effects of social stress on operant drinking of alcoholics and social drinkers. *Behaviour Research and Therapy, 12*, 67–72.

Mills, K. C., Bean, J. W., & Hutcheson, J. S. (1977). Shock induced ethanol consumption in rats. *Pharmacology, Biochemistry, and Behavior, 6*, 107–115.

Myers, R. D., Borg, S., & Mossberg, R. (1986). Antagonism by naltrexone of voluntary alcohol selection in the chronically drinking macaque monkey. *Alcohol, 3*, 383–388.

Nash, J. F. Jr., & Maickel, R. P. (1985). Stress-induced consumption of ethanol by rats. *Life Sciences, 37*, 757–765.

Nelson, L. R., Taylor, A. N., Lewis, J. W., Poland, R. E., Redei, E., & Branch, B. J. (1986). Pituitary-adrenal responses to morphine and footshock stress are enhanced following prenatal alcohol exposure. *Alcoholism: Clinical and Experimental Research, 10*, 397–402.

O'Doherty, F. (1991). Is drug use a response to stress? *Drug and Alcohol Dependence, 29*, 97–106.

Ogilvie, K. M., Lee, S., & Rivier, C. (1997a). Role of arginine vasopressin and corticotropin-releasing factor in mediating alcohol-induced adrenocorticotropin and vasopressin secretion in male rats bearing lesions of the paraventricular nuclei. *Brain Research, 744*, 83–95.

Ogilvie, K., Lee, S., & Rivier, C. (1997b). Effect of three different modes of alcohol administration on the activity of the rat hypothalamic–pituitary–adrenal axis. *Alcoholism: Clinical and Experimental Research, 21*, 467–476.

Ogilvie, K. M., & Rivier, C. (1996). Gender difference in alcohol-evoked hypothalamic–pituitary–adrenal activity in the rat: Ontogeny and role of neonatal steroids. *Alcoholism: Clinical and Experimental Research, 20*, 255–261.

Ogilvie, K. M., & Rivier, C. (1997). Gender difference in hypothalamic–pituitary–adrenal axis response to alcohol in the rat: Activational role of gonadal steroids. *Brain Research, 766*, 19–28.

O'Malley, S. S. (1996). Opioid antagonists in the treatment of alcohol dependence: Clinical efficacy and prevention of relapse. *Alcohol and Alcoholism, 31*, 77–81.

O'Regan, D., Welberg, L. L., Holmes, M. C., & Seckl, J. R. (2001). Glucocorticoid programming of pituitary-adrenal function: mechanisms and physiological consequences. *Seminars in Neonatology, 6*, 319–329.

Pacak, K., & Palkovits, M. (2001). Stressor specificity of central neuroendocrine responses: Implications for stress-related disorders. *Endocrine Reviews, 22*, 502–548.

Peterson, J. B., & Pihl, R. O., Seguin, J. R., Finn, P. R., & Stewart, S. H. (1993). Heart-rate reactivity and alcohol consumption among sons of male alcoholics and sons of nonalcoholics. *Journal of Psychiatry and Neuroscience, 18*, 190–198.

Piazza, N. J., Vrbka, J. L., & Yeager, R. D. (1989). Telescoping of alcoholism in women alcoholics. *International Journal of the Addictions, 24*, 19–28.

Pohorecky, L. A. (1981). The interaction of alcohol and stress: A review. *Neuroscience and Biobehavioral Reviews, 5*, 209–229.

Pohorecky, L. A. (1990). Interaction of ethanol and stress: Research with experimental animals—an update. *Alcohol and Alcoholism, 25*, 263–276.

Pohorecky, L. A. (1991). Stress and alcohol interaction: An update of human research. *Alcoholism: Clinical and Experimental Research, 15*, 438–459.

Pohorecky, L. A., Rassi, E., Weiss, J. M., & Michalak, V. (1980). Biochemical evidence for an interaction of ethanol and stress: Preliminary studies. *Alcoholism: Clinical and Experimental Research, 4*, 423–426.

Powers, R. J., & Kutash, I. L. (1985). Stress and alcohol. *International Journal of the Addictions, 20*, 461–482.

Prescott, C. A., & Kendler, K. S. (1999). Genetic and environmental contributions to alcohol abuse and dependence in a population-based sample of male twins. *American Journal of Psychiatry, 156*, 34–40.

Raber, J. (1998). Detrimental effects of chronic hypothalamic–pituitary–adrenal axis activation. From obesity to memory deficits. *Molecular Neurobiology, 18*, 1–22.

Randall, C. L., Roberts, J. S., Del Boca, F. K., Carroll, K. M., Connors, G. J., & Mattson, M. E. (1999). Telescoping of landmark events associated with drinking: A gender comparison. *Journal of Studies on Alcohol, 60*, 252–260.

Rasmussen, D. D., Boldt, B. M., Bryant, C. A., Mitton, D. R., Larsen, S. A., & Wilkinson, C. W. (2000). Chronic daily ethanol and withdrawal: 1. Long-term changes in the hypothalamo–pituitary–adrenal axis. *Alcoholism: Clinical and Experimental Research, 24*, 1836–1849.

Rees, L. H., Besser, G. M., Jeffcoate, W. J., Goldie, D. J., & Marks, V. (1977). Alcohol-induced pseudo-Cushing's syndrome. *Lancet, 1*, 726–728.

Rivest, S., & Rivier, C. (1994). Lesions of hypothalamic PVN partially attenuate stimulatory action of alcohol on ACTH secretion in rats. *American Journal of Physiology, 266*, R553–558.

Rivier, C., Bruhn, T., & Vale, W. (1984). Effect of ethanol on the hypothalamic–pituitary–adrenal axis in the rat: Role of corticotropin-releasing factor (CRF). *Journal of Pharmacology and Experimental Therapeutics, 229*, 127–131.

Rivier, C., Imaki, T., & Vale, W. (1990). Prolonged exposure to alcohol: Effect on CRF mRNA levels, and CRF- and stress-induced ACTH secretion in the rat. *Brain Research, 520*, 1–5.

Rivier, C., & Lee, S. (1996). Acute alcohol administration stimulates the activity of hypothalamic neurons that express corticotropin-releasing factor and vasopressin. *Brain Research, 726*, 1–10.

Rivier, C., Rivier, J., & Lee, S. (1996). Importance of pituitary and brain receptors for corticotrophin-releasing factor in modulating alcohol-induced ACTH secretion in the rat. *Brain Research, 721*, 83–90.

Rivier, C., & Vale, W. (1988). Interaction between ethanol and stress on ACTH and beta-endorphin secretion. *Alcoholism: Clinical and Experimental Research, 12*, 206–210.

Robins, L. N., Helzer, J. E., Weissman, M. M., Orvaschel, H., Gruenberg, E., Burke, J. D., & Regier, D. A. (1984). Lifetime prevalence of specific psychiatric disorders in three sites. *Archives of General Psychiatry, 41*, 949–958.

Roy, A., Mittal, N., Zhang, H., & Pandey, S. C. (2002). Modulation of cellular expression of glucocorticoid receptor and glucocorticoid response element-DNA binding in rat brain during alcohol drinking and withdrawal. *Journal of Pharmacology and Experimental Therapeutics, 301*, 774–784.

Sayette, M. A. (1993). An appraisal-disruption model of alcohol's effects on stress responses in social drinkers. *Psychological Bulletin, 114*, 459–476.

Sayette, M. A., Breslin, F. C., Wilson, G. T., & Rosenblum, G. D. (1994). Parental history of alcohol abuse and the effects of alcohol and expectations of intoxication on social stress. *Journal of Studies on Alcohol, 55*, 214–223.

Schuckit, M. A. (1998). Biological, psychological, and environmental predictors of the alcoholism risk: A longitudinal study. *Journal of Studies on Alcohol, 59*, 485–494.

Schuckit, M. A. (2000). Genetics of the risk for alcoholism. *American Journal on Addictions, 9*, 103–112.

Schuckit, M. A., Gold, E., & Risch, C. (1987). Plasma cortisol levels following ethanol in sons of alcoholics and controls. *Archives of General Psychiatry, 44*, 942–945.

Schuckit, M. A., Tsuang, J. W., Anthenelli, R. M., Tipp, J. E., & Nurnberger, J. I. (1996). Alcohol challenges in young men from alcoholic pedigrees and control families: A report from the COGA project. *Journal of Studies on Alcohol, 57*, 368–377.

Seeman, T. E., McEwen, B. S., Rowe, J. W., & Singer, B. H. (2001). Allostatic load as a marker of cumulative biological risk: MacArthur studies of successful aging. *Proceedings of the National Academy of Sciences of the United States of America, 98*, 4770–4775.

Selye, H. (1936). A syndrome produced by diverse nocuous agents. *Nature, 138*, 32.

Selye, H. (1974.) *Stress without distress*. Toronto: McClelland and Stewart Ltd.

Sher, K. J. (1987). Stress-response dampening. In H. T. Blane & K. E. Leonard (Eds.), *Psychological theories of drinking and alcoholism* (pp. 131–178). New York: Guilford.

Sher, K. J., & Levenson, R. W. (1982). Risk for alcoholism and individual differences in the stress-response-dampening effect of alcohol. *Journal of Abnormal Psychology, 91*, 350–367.

Sher, K. J., & Walitzer, K. S. (1986). Individual differences in the stress-response-dampening effect on alcohol: A dose-response study. *Journal of Abnormal Psychology, 95*, 159–167.

Silva, S. M., Paula-Barbosa, M. M., & Madeira, M. D. (2002). Prolonged alcohol intake leads to reversible depression of corticotropin-releasing hormone and vasopressin immunoreactivity and mRNA levels in the parvocellular neurons of the paraventricular nucleus. *Brain Research, 954*, 82–93.

Spanagel, R. (2000). Recent animal models of alcoholism. *Alcohol Research and Health: The Journal of the National Institute on Alcohol Abuse and Alcoholism, 24*, 124–131.

Spencer, R. L., & McEwen, B. S. (1990). Adaptation of the hypothalamic–pituitary–adrenal axis to chronic ethanol stress. *Neuroendocrinology, 52*, 481–489.

Steele, C. M., & Josephs, R. A. (1988). Drinking your troubles away II: An attention-allocation model of alcohol's effect on psychological stress. *Journal of Abnormal Psychology, 97*, 196–205.

Sterling, P., & Eyer, J. (1988). Allostasis: A new paradigm to explain arousal pathology. In J. Fisher & J. Reason (Eds.), *Handbook of life stress, cognition, and health* (pp. 629–649). New York: John Wiley & Sons.

Stewart, S. H., Finn, P. R., & Pihl, R. O. (1992). The effects of alcohol on the cardiovascular stress response in men at high risk for alcoholism: A dose response study. *Journal of Studies on Alcohol, 53*, 499–506.

Stott, D. J., Ball, S. G., Inglis, G. C., Davies, D. L., Fraser, R., Murray, G. D., & McInnes, G. T. (1987). Effects of a single moderate dose of alcohol on blood pressure, heart rate and associated metabolic and endocrine changes. *Clinical Science, 73*, 411–416.

Tabakoff, B., Jafee, R. C., & Ritzmann, R. F. (1978). Corticosterone concentrations in mice during ethanol drinking and withdrawal. *Journal of Pharmacy and Pharmacology, 30*, 371–374.

Taylor, A. N., Branch, B. J., Kokka, N., & Poland, R. E. (1983). Neonatal and long-term neuroendocrine effects of fetal alcohol exposure. *Monographs in Neural Sciences, 9*, 140–152.

Taylor, A. N., Branch, B. J., Liu, S. H., & Kokka, N. (1982). Long-term effects of fetal ethanol exposure on pituitary–adrenal response to stress. *Pharmacology, Biochemistry, and Behavior, 16*, 585–589.

Taylor, A. N., Branch, B. J., Liu, S. H., Wiechmann, A. F., Hill, M. A., & Kokka, N. (1981). Fetal exposure to ethanol enhances pituitary-adrenal and temperature responses to ethanol in adult rats. *Alcoholism: Clinical and Experimental Research, 5*, 237–246.

Taylor, A. N., Branch, B. J., Nelson, L. R., Lane, L. A., & Poland, R. E. (1986). Prenatal ethanol and ontogeny of pituitary–adrenal responses to ethanol and morphine. *Alcohol, 3*, 255–259.

Taylor, A. N., Branch, B. J., van Zuylen, J. E., & Redei, E. (1988). Maternal alcohol consumption and stress responsiveness in offspring. In G. P. Chrousos, D. L. Loriaux, & P. W. Gold (Eds.), *Mechanisms of physical and emotional stress. Advances in experimental medicine and biology* (Vol. 245, pp. 311–317). New York: Plenum.

Timmer, S. G., Veroff, J., & Colten, M. E. (1985). Life stress, helplessness, and the use of alcohol and drugs to cope: An analysis of national survey data. In S. Shiffman & T. Ashby Wills (Eds.), *Coping and substance use* (pp. 171–199). New York: Academic.

Veldman, R. G., & Meinders, A. E. (1996). On the mechanism of alcohol-induced pseudo-Cushing's syndrome. *Endocrine Reviews, 17*, 262–268.

Vescovi, P. P., DiGennaro, C., & Coiro, V. (1997). Hormonal (ACTH, cortisol, beta-endorphin, and met-enkephalin) and cardiovascular responses to hyperthermic stress in chronic alcoholics. *Alcoholism: Clinical and Experimental Research, 21*, 1195–1198.

Volpicelli, J. R. (1987). Uncontrollable events and alcohol drinking. *British Journal of Addiction, 82*, 381–392.

Waltman, C., Blevins, L. S., Boyd, G., & Wand, G. S. (1993). The effects of mild ethanol intoxication on the hypothalamic–pituitary–adrenal axis in nonalcoholic men. *Journal of Clinical Endocrinology and Metabolism, 77*, 518–522

Waltman, C., McCaul, M. E., & Wand, G. S. (1994). Adrenocorticotropin responses following administration of ethanol and ovine corticotropin-releasing hormone in the sons of alcoholics and control subjects. *Alcoholism: Clinical and Experimental Research, 18*, 826–830.

Wand, G. S. (1993). Alcohol, the hypothalamic-pituitary-adrenal axis, and hormonal tolerance. In S. Zakhari (Ed.), *Alcohol and the endocrine system* (pp. 251–270). Bethesda, MD: National Institutes of Health.

Wand, G. S., & Dobs, A. S. (1991). Alterations in the hypothalamic–pituitary–adrenal axis in actively drinking alcoholics. *Journal of Clinical Endocrinology and Metabolism, 72*, 1290–1295.

Wand, G. S., Mangold, D., Ali, M., & Giggey, P. (1999). Adrenocortical responses and family history of alcoholism. *Alcoholism: Clinical and Experimental Research, 23*, 1185–1190.

Weinberg, J. (1985). Effects of ethanol and maternal nutritional status on fetal development. *Alcoholism: Clinical and Experimental Research, 9*, 49–55.

Weinberg, J. (1987). Effects of early experience on responsiveness to ethanol: A preliminary report. *Physiology and Behavior, 40*, 401–406.

Weinberg, J. (1988). Hyperresponsiveness to stress: Differential effects of prenatal ethanol on males and females. *Alcoholism: Clinical and Experimental Research, 12*, 647–652.

Weinberg, J. (1989). Prenatal ethanol exposure alters adrenocortical development of offspring. *Alcoholism: Clinical and Experimental Research, 13*, 73–83.

Weinberg, J. (1992). Prenatal ethanol effects: Sex differences in offspring stress responsiveness. *Alcohol, 9*, 219–223.

Weinberg, J. (1993). Neuroendocrine effects of prenatal alcohol exposure. *Annals of the New York Academy of Sciences, 697*, 86–96.

Weinberg, J., & Gallo, P. V. (1982). Prenatal ethanol exposure: Pituitary-adrenal activity in pregnant dams and offspring. *Neurobehavioral Toxicology and Teratology, 4*, 515–520.

Weinberg, J., Taylor, A. N., & Gianoulakis, C. (1996). Fetal ethanol exposure: Hypothalamic–pituitary–adrenal and beta-endorphin responses to repeated stress. *Alcoholism: Clinical and Experimental Research, 20*, 122–131.

Williams, T. A., Calhoun, G., & Ackoff, R. L. (1982). Stress, alcoholism and personality. *Human Relations, 35*, 491–510.

Wilson, G. T., Abrams, D. B., & Lipscomb, T. R. (1980). Effects of intoxication levels and drinking pattern on social anxiety in men. *Journal of Studies on Alcohol, 41*, 250–264.

Zhou, Y., Franck, J., Spangler, R., Maggos, C. E., Ho, A., & Kreek, M. J. (2000). Reduced hypothalamic POMC and anterior pituitary CRF1 receptor mRNA levels after acute, but not chronic, daily "binge" intragastric alcohol administration. *Alcoholism: Clinical and Experimental Research, 24*, 1575–1582.

11 Influences on Diet and Stress Across Space and Time

A Contextual Perspective

Daniel Kim and Ichiro Kawachi

KEY POINTS

- Diet and stress are potentially influenced by spatial and temporal contexts.
- Spatial contexts may matter because of place-specific variations in exposures to risks and protective factors, such as social norms, institutions, and policies, and features of the physical environment.
- Relevant levels of spatial contexts may be entire countries and within countries, states, communities, and neighborhoods and school and work environments.
- Multilevel evidence exists that state-level income inequality is associated with individual health and may be mediated by stress resulting from social comparisons.
- Examples of factors at the neighborhood level impacting on diet and stress include residential segregation (e.g., by influencing access to supermarkets) and social capital (e.g., by affecting individuals' levels of social support).
- The availability of soft drinks through vending machines and subsidized school lunch programs may shape dietary intakes at schools, and job strain and effort-reward imbalance may determine levels of stress in the workplace.
- Temporal contexts exist at the population level (e.g., through changes in political, economic, socio-cultural factors over time), and at the individual level over the life course (e.g., through early life exposures, the formation of lifelong dietary habits).
- Future investigations should address methodological issues, such as through combined multilevel and longitudinal study design approaches, to enhance the validity for estimating the effects of spatial and temporal contexts on diet and stress.

1. INTRODUCTION

Health behaviors may be significantly influenced by contexts across both space and time. In the case of temporal context, for example, in 1977–1978 the average caloric intake in Americans aged 2 yr and older was estimated at 1791 kcal/d after adjusting for age group, sex, education level, race/ethnicity, household size, region, urban classification, and % poverty. By 1994–1996, the same statistic had grown to 1985 kcal/d, with

From: *Nutrients, Stress, and Medical Disorders*
Edited by: S. Yehuda and D. I. Mostofsky © Humana Press Inc., Totowa, NJ

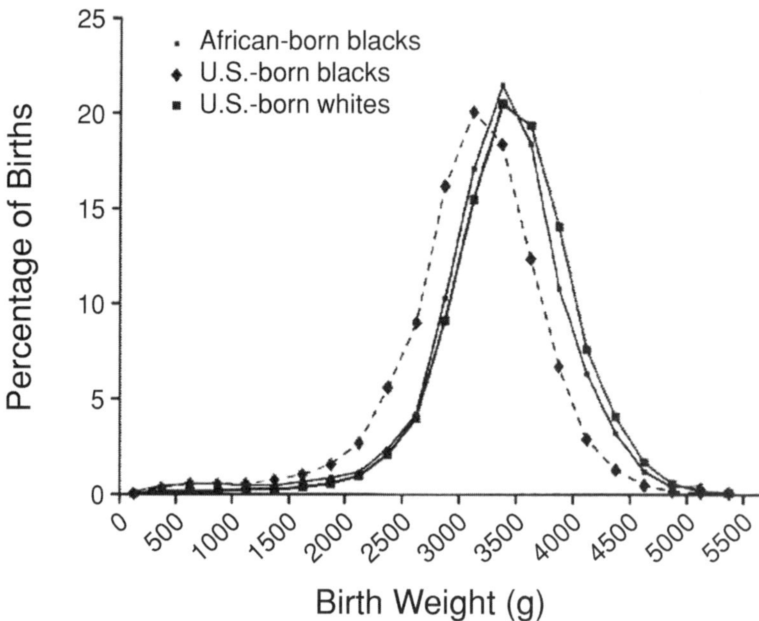

Fig. 1. Distribution of birthweights among infants of U.S.-born white and black women and African-born black women in Illinois, 1980–1995. The calculation of frequencies was based on all singleton births in Illinois. The study population included the infants of 3135 black women born in sub-Saharan Africa, 43,322 black women born in the United States (a sample that included 7.5% of the total number of black women giving birth in Illinois), and 44,046 US-born white women (2.5% of the total number of white women giving birth in Illinois). (From David & Collins, 1997).

significant increases in caloric intakes being observed across all age groups (Nielsen, Siega-Riz, & Popkin, 2002). Spatial context also appears to matter for health outcomes. For instance, the prevalence of low birthweight varies dramatically according to place of residence, even among genetically similar populations. The distribution of birthweights among infants of US-born black women has been shown to differ significantly (i.e., with a significantly lower mean and higher prevalences of low-birthweight babies) from the distributions for African-born black women and US-born white women (Fig. 1). Such marked variations within population subgroups suggest the presence of the effects of physical and/or social contexts on individual health over pure genetic/biological explanations.

Dietary intakes and levels of stress may be mediating factors along the pathways by which physical and social environments affect the health of individuals. The relationships between various dietary constituents and health are well established—numerous epidemiologic studies have demonstrated significant associations between the dietary intakes of macro- and micronutrients with the risks of developing cardiovascular disease, hypertension, and certain forms of cancer (US Department of Agriculture & US Department of Health and Human Services, 2000). Stress has also been proposed as a means by which external social conditions "get inside" the body (Kubzansky & Kawachi, 2000). Furthermore, emotions, including the negative emotions of anxiety and depression, may be considered as products of stress as well as potential mediators of its health effects (Kubzansky & Kawachi, 2000; Spielberger & Sarason, 1978).

This chapter highlights the relevance of various spatial and temporal contexts of dietary intakes and levels of stress to the health of individuals and populations. We describe evidence that such contexts matter while identifying gaps in the empirical data, including the role of population composition and "selection" explanations. Drawing primarily from US examples—with considerations of several key spatial contexts (states, communities and neighborhoods, and school and work environments) and temporal contexts at the population level and across the life course of individuals—this chapter will provide a general framework that should assist in conceptualizing and designing future clinical and epidemiologic studies and thereby in developing more effective interventions that target dietary intakes, levels of stress, and the incidence of medical disorders.

2. COUNTRY-LEVEL SPATIAL CONTEXTS

Differences in geographic context at the country level have long been recognized as associated with variations in dietary intakes and in health. In the 1950s, Ancel Keys initiated the Seven Countries Study to examine the relationships between diet and cardiovascular disease within and across 16 cohorts of approx 13,000 men (aged 40–59 yr) in the countries of Finland, Greece, Italy, Japan, the Netherlands, the United States, and Yugoslavia (Keys et al., 1967). Using dietary records, food consumption was estimated in these cohorts, and marked variations in dietary intakes and consumption patterns between countries were discovered (Kromhout et al., 1989). For example, dietary intakes of milk, potatoes, fats, and sugar products were very high in Finland, although meat, fruit, and vegetable consumption was high in the United States. In Italy, cereal and alcoholic drink consumption was prevalent, whereas Greece was characterized by high intakes of olive oil and fruits. In Japan, consumption of fish, rice, and soy products was high. These differences in food consumption were also observed to narrow over subsequent decades of follow-up, as countries underwent epidemiological transitions in dietary practices and associated patterns of morbidity (Kromhout et al., 1989).

According to the epidemiologist Geoffrey Rose (1985), the causes of *cases* of disease within a population need to be distinguished from the causes of the *incidence rate* of disease because the latter may vary considerably in type and in magnitude between populations. Rose provided the example of the population distributions of serum cholesterol levels in Japan, a country in which coronary heart disease is uncommon, and in eastern Finland, in which the incidence rate is relatively high. In these two countries, individuals with relative hypercholesterolemia (i.e., high cholesterol levels relative to the population mean) may account in part for some of the incident cases of disease within each country. However, the mean cholesterol level in Finland would be considered highly abnormal in Japan because the entire population distribution of cholesterol in Finland is shifted to the right compared to the distribution in Japan. From a population perspective, therefore, the majority of the population in Finland could be considered hyperlipidemic compared to the Japanese population (thereby explaining the much higher rates of cardiovascular disease in Finland as compared to Japan). In other words, considering only the abnormal tail of the distribution within any given context cannot adequately explain the population incidence rates of diseases in that population. Critically, it is only through comparisons of the population means (and through consideration of the determinants of population means of cholesterol) that such large differences in coronary heart disease incidence between the populations can be understood.

The differences in the population distributions of risk factors for disease may in turn be driven by socio-cultural and other factors operating at the societal level. But to what extent are these variations truly and fully contextually determined? It is plausible that these discrepancies in dietary intake and heart disease primarily or exclusively reflect differences in the characteristics and choices of individuals between countries that are not independently determined by context, i.e., they may be wholly related to the compositional characteristics of populations.

In this regard, migrant studies provide some clues in support of the influence of socio-cultural context on diet and stress, since these differences arise from members of the same racial/ethnic group. Japanese populations in Japan, Hawaii, and San Francisco were previously observed to have saturated fat intakes of 7, 23, and 26%, respectively (Kato, Tillotson, Nichaman, Rhoads, & Hamilton, 1973). Serum cholesterol, body weight, and age-adjusted coronary heart disease rates were also respectively higher with closer proximity to the mainland United States (Kato et al., 1973). These patterns are consistent with an effect of social context on dietary intake (since genetic factors would be relatively homogeneous across these populations of Japanese descent). It is also possible that migrant studies are affected by selection bias, i.e., those who migrate tend to be more healthy or less healthy than those who stay behind. However, this bias is unlikely to have accounted for the substantially higher heart disease risks observed among Japanese who migrated to the United States.

To give a further example, rates of suicide have been observed to vary considerably between countries and within countries over time. Using data from 50 countries covered by the World Values Survey (Aguir et al., 2000) and the European Values Survey (Halman, 2001) in the last two decades of the 20th century, Helliwell (2003) found marked variations in suicide rates between countries. Suicide rates in Iceland, Great Britain, southern European countries, Scandinavian countries (with the exception of Finland), and Latin American Catholic countries were considerably lower than in other industrial countries. Meanwhile, suicide rates in the former Soviet Union fell greatly in the 1980s but then increased dramatically in the 1990s, and are now more than double the rates found in countries in western Europe (Helliwell, 2003). In Sweden and Denmark between 1980 and 2000, suicide rates fell by one-third and one-half, respectively (Helliwell, 2003). These patterns are consistent with, although they cannot decisively establish, the existence of substantial country-specific contextual effects on stress.

3. WITHIN-COUNTRY SPATIAL CONTEXTS

Within countries, spatial contexts at different levels (e.g., states, counties, communities/neighborhoods, and school, and work environments) may influence nutrient intakes and levels of stress because of place-specific variations in exposures to risks and protective factors, such as social norms, cultural practices, institutions, and policies. In the United States, geographic scales can be conceptualized, from largest to smallest, as states, counties, municipalities and cities, census tracts, census tract blocks, and households. Figure 2 shows some of these spatial units, with communities and neighborhoods being defined at the county, census tract, and census block-group level, and school and work environments being physically located within these communities and neighborhoods. Of note, an individual may reside in a neighborhood and work and/or go to school in the same or a different neighborhood. Hence, an individual may be exposed to different

Country-level contexts:
e.g., socio-cultural influences on diet, attitudes towards work and leisure

Within-country spatial contexts:

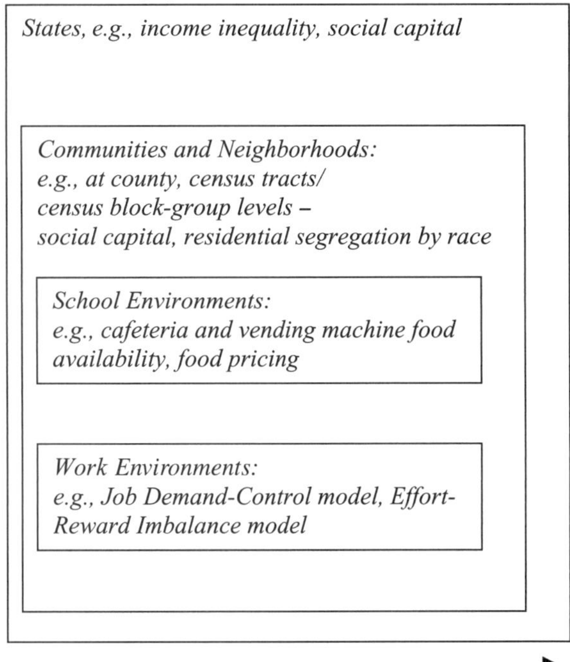

TIME/TEMPORAL CONTEXT (historical in populations; lifecourse in individuals)
e.g., technological changes in food production, food marketing; dietary/stress exposures during fetal critical periods

Fig. 2. Levels of spatial and temporal contexts and their potential influences on dietary intakes and stress.

physical and social contexts simultaneously. The temporal context also enters the picture because all of these spatial contexts are dynamic and changing over time and because these contexts and changes may produce effects at the same population and/or individual level at future points in time (Fig. 2).

Multilevel studies that incorporate at least one of these higher spatial levels along with individual-level measures have been conducted to separate the independent effects of spatial context and of population composition on individual health behaviors and outcomes. A "compositional" explanation for between-area differences would be that areas contain different types of individuals and that the differences between these individuals account for observed area-level differences. By contrast, a "contextual" explanation would implicate features of the physical or social environment that produce an effect in addition to or in interaction with individual characteristics (Macintyre & Ellaway, 2000). Although most investigators in this field have raised issues such as unmeasured individual characteristics, measurement error, and model misspecification as potential sources of bias, contextual effects are viewed as likely real phenomena and not simply statistical artifacts (Macintyre & Ellaway, 2000).

3.1. States

A growing body of empirical evidence supports a relationship between higher income inequality at the U.S. state level and higher all-cause and cause-specific mortality among individuals (e.g., Kaplan, Pamuk, Lynch, Cohen, & Balfour, 1996; Kennedy, Kawachi, & Prothrow-Stith, 1996). Additionally, the contextual effects of state-level income inequality may differ by population characteristics. One study observed that the significant relationship between state-level income inequality and health was limited to the non elderly (Daly, Duncan, Kaplan, & Lynch, 1998). In another study, high-income individuals reported better health status in states where income inequality was relatively high rather than low (Subramanian, Kawachi, & Kennedy, 2001).

Stress resulting from social comparisons has been hypothesized to be a potential mechanism that links income inequality to health outcomes (Kawachi, Levine, Miller, Lasch, & Amick, 1994; Wilkinson, 1996). Support for the impact of feelings of relative deprivation on stress, as hypothesized in high-income-inequality contexts, has emerged from research by the anthropologist William Dressler. He coined the term "cultural consonance in lifestyle," referring to the degree to which individuals succeed in achieving the normative lifestyle as defined by their culture. Even after controlling for other predictors of blood pressure, including age, gender, skin color, anthropometric measures, and socioeconomic status, and psychosocial variables, Dressler found that closer approximations to cultural consonance were associated with more favorable levels of arterial blood pressure, depressive symptoms, and globally perceived stress among individuals (Dressler, 1996; Dressler, Balieiro, & Dos Santos, 1998, 1999).

Furthermore, subjective social status, a novel single-item measure of where individuals place themselves on the social hierarchy, has been associated with levels of stress. In a sample of healthy white women in the United States, this measure was significantly and inversely related to self-reported measures of chronic stress and was marginally associated with cortisol habituation, each after adjusting for measures of objective socioeconomic status (education, household income, and occupation) (Adler, Epel, Castellazzo, & Ickovies, 2000). In adolescents, subjective social status has further been found to be significantly related to depressive symptoms along with the risk of overweight and obesity (Goodman et al., 2001). These studies suggest that perceptions of relative position, which are in part a product of social context, are linked to stress and potentially also to dietary intakes.

Variations in nutrient and food intakes by US state can be observed in state-level data from the Continuing Survey of Food Intakes by Individuals (CSFII) in 1994–96 (for prevalences by state, see the interactive community nutrition map at http://www.barc.usda.gov/bhnrc/cnrg/cnmapfr.htm). For instance, five states including Oregon, Florida, and Iowa had a high prevalence (≥45%) of their state populations that met the dietary guideline for limiting saturated fat intakes to <10% of total calories. Meanwhile, six states including Arkansas and Georgia were characterized by relatively low prevalences (<35%) of meeting this guideline. For the dietary recommendation of at least three daily servings of vegetables (US Department of Agriculture & US Department of Health and Human Services, 2000), four states including Arkansas, Georgia, and Florida were found to have relatively low prevalences (<45%) of meeting the recommendation, while eight states including Michigan and Iowa had relatively high prevalences (≥55%). Although these variations in nutrient and food intakes would suggest the effects of state contextual factors, population compositional factors and/or within-state contextual factors may have contributed to these between-state discrepancies. Multilevel analytic approaches are therefore needed to truly specify the level of contextual explanations and disentangle them from compositional ones.

3.2. Communities and Neighborhoods

Residential segregation by race/ethnicity, such as for black non-Hispanics and Hispanic populations, refers to the differentiation of these from other racial groups along subunits of a residential area. The "sorting" of these groups into different neighborhood contexts from whites (Acevedo-Garcia & Lochner, 2003) as a result of racial/ethnic prejudice and/or population group preferences can lead to greater economic deprivation and a greater likelihood of individual members living in a poor neighborhood (i.e., an area-level context of low socioeconomic position). In turn, the availability of inexpensive, low-fat, and nutritious food options has been shown to be lower in poor neighborhoods (e.g., Morland, Wing, & Diez Roux, 2002a; Morland, Wing, Diez Roux, & Poole, 2002b; Sooman, Macintyre, & Anderson, 1993). Morland et al. (2002b) found significantly more supermarkets in wealthier neighborhoods, and another study (Morland et al., 2002a) determined that fruit and vegetable intakes were 32% and 11% higher for each additional supermarket in the census tract for black and white Americans, respectively. These associations were relatively unchanged after controlling for individual-level income and education. Another multilevel analysis showed that low neighborhood socioeconomic status was associated with less favorable dietary intakes and patterns, although the associations with different dietary intakes were often not statistically significant, and individual-level income was a more consistent predictor of intakes (Diez Roux et al., 1999). In addition, low-income neighborhoods may be characterized by higher crime rates. Negative perceptions of the local environment, including levels of amenities and crime, have been shown to be significantly associated with anxiety (Sooman & Macintyre, 1995). The targeting and saturation of low-income African-American and other minority neighborhoods with fast food restaurants would also be anticipated to contribute to poorer eating habits and higher fat consumption (LaPoint, 2003). In fact, eating calorie-dense fast foods may serve a functional value for individuals under conditions of economic and environmental stress, as empirical evidence has suggested for smoking (Emmons, 2000; Romano, Bloom, & Syme, 1991). Furthermore, institutional and interpersonal racial discrimination within segregated neighborhoods may have the effect of chronically activating the hypothalamic–pituitary–adrenal (HPA) axis, thereby contributing to higher levels of allostatic load (a summary biological measure reflecting the cumulative physiological burden on the body through attempts to adapt to life's demands) (McEwan & Stellar, 1993). Higher allostatic load scores have been linked to higher risks of all-cause mortality and cardiovascular disease (Seeman, McEwan, Rowe, & Singer, 2001).

Differences between urban and rural contexts may also influence dietary intakes. In a multivariable logistic regression analysis based on the Kansas Behavioral Risk Factor Surveillance System (1992–1995), Adrian and Wilkinson (2000) found that adult Kansan men who resided in rural counties were nearly twice as likely to eat the recommended number of fruits and vegetables than those residing in urban counties after controlling for household income, health care coverage, and other socioeconomic variables at the county level. In the same analysis, county median household income was significantly associated with higher fruit and vegetable consumption (Adrian & Wilkinson, 2000).

Apart from physical resources and amenities as captured through area-level socioeconomic measures, it has furthermore been hypothesized that social capital and social cohesion play an important role in disease development and health promotion. Higher levels of social cohesion have been defined as the presence of relatively lower levels of social conflict and the presence of relatively strong social bonds (levels of interpersonal trust and reciprocity, i.e., social capital) (Kawachi & Berkman, 2000). Several multilevel analyses have found significant associations between social capital at the state level and health outcomes, including age-adjusted mortality rates and levels of self-rated health (Kawachi, Kennedy, & Glass, 1999; Kawachi, Kennedy, Lochner, & Prothrow-Stith, 1997; see Kawachi et al., 2004, for a more comprehensive review). In spite of the relative consistency of the findings, a limitation of the majority of these studies has been their cross-sectional design, which weakens the ability to demonstrate causal relationships. Adding a longitudinal dimension (e.g., by prospectively following individuals within a cohort) to future multilevel studies would potentially yield stronger evidence for the effects of social capital on health.

Possible mechanisms by which social cohesion/capital may be linked to health include influences on health-enhancing behaviors, the promotion of access to local services and amenities, access to resources and material goods, and psychosocial processes, which provide affective support and mutual respect (Kawachi & Berkman, 2000; Lin, 2001; Wilkinson, 1996). Each of these mechanisms plausibly has an impact on dietary intakes and stress levels. First, in the theory of diffusion of innovations, Rogers (1995) suggested that innovative behaviors diffuse much faster in communities that are cohesive and high in trust. Individuals within high-social-capital neighborhoods where healthy eating and leisure activity behaviors are prevalent may thus be more likely to adopt such behaviors. Informal social control may also exert influence over health behaviors (Sampson, 2003). Second, in social cognitive theory (Bandura, 1991), the belief in collective agency is linked to the efficacy of a group in meeting its needs. Thus, a neighborhood high in social capital and trust would be expected to effectively work together in lobbying for local services that may be relevant to levels of stress and dietary intake, such as adequate numbers of green spaces and supermarkets. The availability of green spaces may be associated with lower levels of stress (e.g., by offering places for exercise and leisure with family members), although supporting empirical evidence is sparse to date. One survey among county residents in North Carolina showed a positive association between neighborhood access to trails and other public spaces and engagement in any leisure physical activity (Huston, Evenson, Bors, & Gizlice, 2003). Third, the social resources theory (Lin, 2001) proposes that access to and use of social resources can lead to improved socioeconomic status. In turn, socioeconomic gains in individuals would be anticipated to improve mental and physical health. Lastly, psychosocial processes including high levels of social support and trust may moderate the deleterious effects of stress or may have independent direct effects on mental and physical health (Stansfeld, 1999).

3.3. School Environments

Given the large proportion of time spent in school environments and the presence of cafeterias and vending machines, schools represent potentially critical contexts during childhood and adolescence for the formation of dietary habits. An example is the National School Lunch Program in the United States, which subsidizes lunches for 28 million children in 98,000 public and nonprofit private schools. The program has been criticized by some nutrition experts for offering lower quality foods to its participants, many of whom come from low-income households with otherwise limited choices. Moreover, the American Academy of Pediatrics Committee on School Health in the United States (2004) recently published a policy statement recommending the reduced consumption and advertising of soft drinks in schools due to their nutritional implications. Soft drinks and fruit drinks are sold in school vending machines and at school events, with as much as 56–85% of children in school drinking at least one soft drink daily and 20% of these consuming four or more servings daily (Gleason & Suitor, 2001). With the high prevalence of soft drink consumption at schools, public health concerns have been raised because soft drink consumption tends to displace milk consumption (an important source of calcium and other nutrients at critical periods of peak bone mass formation in adolescence) (Lytle, Seifert, Greenstein, & McGovern, 2000). There is also evidence that such consumption may be displacing key nutrients within the subsidized school lunch program (Johnson, Panely, & Wang, 1998). Sweetened drinks have further been associated with overweight and obesity (Bellisle & Rolland-Cachera, 2001; Tordoff & Alleva, 1990), which may in part be fueling the ongoing obesity epidemic.

"Pouring-rights" contracts offer large lump-sum payments to school districts in exchange for exclusive sales of one company's products at schools. Among the list of recommendations made by the Committee on School Health was that school districts should invite public discussions prior to any decision to create soft drink contracts (American Academy of Pediatrics Committee on School Health, 2004). In this regard, social capital at the local level could potentially play a pivotal role in ultimately influencing soft drink consumption and thereby nutrient intakes at a young age. In theory, social capital could influence the collective resistance to state-level taxes on foods that could have subsequent consumption effects. For instance, around 1993 Louisiana and Maryland repealed their state soda and snack food taxes, respectively. For high school students surveyed through the U.S. Youth Risk Behavior Survey in 1999, Louisiana had the third highest prevalence of overweight among 33 surveyed states (Maryland was not one of the surveyed states, and obesity prevalences were not determined through this survey) (Kann et al., 2000). Among adults in 1998, these two states had the third and ninth highest prevalences of obesity out of 45 surveyed states (Critser, 2003), and Maryland had the fifth highest relative increase in the prevalence of adult obesity between 1991 and 1998 (Mokdad et al., 1999). Related to this impact of food taxes on consumption, results from several school-based experimental studies are consistent with consumption effects of food costs in the school environment (French et al., 2001; French et al., 1997).

3.4. Work Environments

The workplace context may play a significant role in determining levels of stress, dietary behaviors, and medical disorders. Two classic theoretical models relating to the psychosocial work environment have been established. One, the psychological demand-decision latitude model (or job demand-control [JD-C] model), was formulated by the sociologist Robert Karasek (1979) and consists of two dimensions: (a) qualitative emotional and quantitative psychological demands and (b) decision latitude, referring to the degree of control of an employee over decisions relating to work tasks. Based upon conceptualized interactions between these two dimensions (each dichotomized as high or low), four quadrants of combinations may be obtained for a worker (Fig. 3). In the quadrant of high psychological demands and low decision latitude, job strain is said to

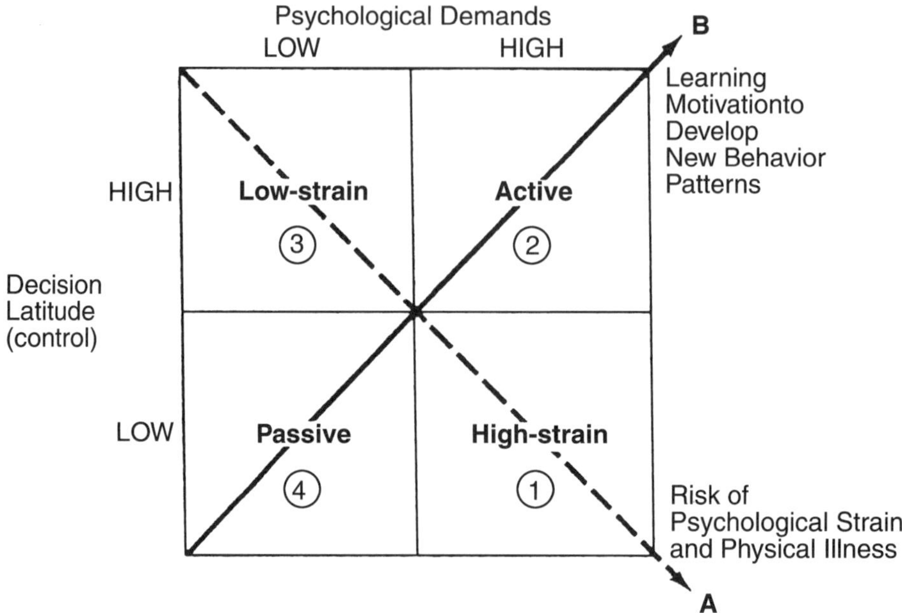

Fig. 3. Psychological demand–decision latitude model. (From Karasek, 1979).

occur. Job strain has been found to be an independent risk factor for the development of coronary heart disease in both men and women (Hammar, Alfredsson, & Johnson, 1998; Kuper & Marmot, 2003), although the findings from one study investigating job strain and coronary heart disease in women were null (Lee, Colditz, Berkman, & Kawachi, 2002).

Under conditions of job strain, Karasek hypothesized that the sympathoadrenal system is excessively activated while the body's ability to repair tissues is diminished, ultimately leading to illness (Karasek, 1979; Theorell, 2000). The elevated levels of catecholamines found in bus drivers in inner-city areas, for example, may be a physiological sequela of job strain (Evans & Carrere, 1991). More recently, this two-dimensional model has been modified to include a third dimension of social support at work, with jobs of low demand, low decision latitude, and low social support being expected to produce the highest level of job strain (Siegrist, 2002). Furthermore, in the Whitehall II Study, a longitudinal study of British civil servants, both women and men with low perceived control at work or at home had increased risks of developing anxiety and depression and these risks varied significantly by individual socioeconomic position (Griffin, Fuhrer, Stansfeld, & Marmot, 2002).

A second model of the psychosocial work environment, developed by the sociologist Johannes Siegrist (1996), is referred to as the effort-reward imbalance (ERI) model and concerns the degree to which workers are rewarded for their efforts. When a high degree of effort is not met with a high degree of reward, emotional stress and the risks of illnesses are predicted to increase (Theorell, 2000). Rewards can be in the form of financial compensation, self-esteem, and social control. Thus, in workplaces that allow for generous salaries, promotions, and appreciation in proportion to employees' efforts, workers are hypothesized to have lower levels of stress and better health status than similarly skilled employees in workplaces lacking these characteristics (Theorell, 2000).

Meanwhile, there is growing evidence for the capacity of the work environment to influence dietary intakes. For instance, in the WellWorks Study conducted in 24 worksites in eastern and central Massachusetts, members of worksite pairs (matched on the basis of the presence of a cafeteria, worksite size, type of smoking policy, company type, distribution by sex, distribution of blue-collar and white-collar jobs, and response rate to the baseline survey to assure comparability between worksite groups regarding these factors) were randomized to intervention and control groups (Sorensen et al., 1998). The intervention consisted of three key elements to promote healthy dietary changes and smoking cessation: joint worker–management participation in program planning and implementation, consultation with management on worksite environmental changes, and health education programs.

On average, workers in the intervention sites reduced their fat consumption significantly more (by 0.8 percentage points) than did workers in the control worksites. For fiber consumption, a statistically significant interaction between job category and intervention was observed, whereby changes in fiber intake were similar between the intervention and control groups for office workers and for professionals and managers, whereas fiber consumption among skilled and unskilled laborers in the intervention group increased 7 percentage points more than for similar workers in the control group (Sorensen et al., 1998). Workers in the intervention sites also increased their daily consumption of fruits and vegetables significantly more than did workers in the control sites. Overall, while the changes in the levels of behavioral risk factors among blue-collar workers ranged from 2% for fat consumption to 7% for fiber consumption, on a populationwide scale such changes could have substantial impacts on the prevention of cancer-related and coronary heart disease outcomes (Sorensen et al., 1998). Several other randomized worksite intervention studies to promote healthier eating have shown similarly favorable and significant results (Emmons, Linnan, Shadel, Marcus, & Abrams, 1999; Sorensen et al., 1999), whereas one study did not observe significant differences between treatment and control worksite groups (Sorensen et al., 2002).

4. TEMPORAL CONTEXTS AND THE LIFE COURSE

Changes over time, both at the population level (e.g., changes in political, economic, and socio-cultural factors) and at the individual level (e.g., stressful life events, early life exposures), across one's life course are also critical when considering the effects of context on nutrient intake and stress. These changes are important because they have the capacity to explain marked changes in the incidence of disease for populations and/or in the risks of disease for individuals over time.

At the population level, the mass preparation of food has been identified as a particularly strong driving force for the marked increase in calories consumed in recent decades internationally and the emergence of the obesity epidemic (Cutler, Glaeser, & Shapiro, 2003). Since 1970, technological innovations including vacuum-packing, better preservation, deep-freezing, and microwave ovens, have allowed food manufacturers to cook food centrally and to get it to consumers more efficiently for consumption in the home and in fast food restaurants. This transition from individual to mass preparation led to increases in the quantity and variety of foods consumed. In the United States, other important changes in the food industry (which has evolved from small farms to large corporations over the course of the 20th century) have altered dietary intakes. Nestle

(2003) identified a number of different marketing imperatives of the food industry designed to encourage Americans to consume more for profit maximization. These include taste ("make foods sweet, fat, and salty"), cost ("add value but keep costs low"), convenience ("make eating fast"), confusion ("keep the public puzzled"), advertising (with food and food service companies spending more than $11 billion annually on direct media advertising, nearly 70% of which is for convenience foods, candy and snacks, alcoholic beverages, soft drinks, and desserts, and only 2.2% of which is for fruits, vegetables, grains, and beans), introducing new products, and serving larger portions ("supersizing") (Nestle, 2003). With the conglomeration of food corporations and their move towards increasingly greater economic efficiency, specialization, and food manufacturing in recent years, each of these marketing imperatives is considered to have become stronger (Nestle, 2003).

The surge over the last century in the proportion of the US workforce made up by women (30% in 1952, nearly 50% by 1999) has created time pressures conducive to families eating out, along with a greater individual susceptibility to food industry wants. Food advertising on television has been increasingly targeted to children, particularly for inexpensive, fat- and sugar-loaded processed foods. Between 1992 and 2000, spending on marketing to children by food corporations in the United States nearly doubled (Center for Media Education, 2003). Such advertising has implications for health outcomes over the life course into adulthood through lifelong dietary habits (including brand loyalties) and possible biological setpoints established in early life. Contextual factors (e.g., residence in a low-income neighborhood) could have further health implications for the offspring of individuals through the mediating factors of nutrition and experiences of stress/affective states in mothers during fetal critical periods, whereby exposures during critical periods of fetal development could have latent effects on health and disease that only become apparent later in life (Barker, 1992; Ben-Shlomo & Kuh, 2002).

Epidemiologic studies following the terrorist attacks on September 11, 2001, in New York City provide evidence for the potential simultaneous health impacts of spatial and temporal context at the population and individual levels. For example, among adult survey respondents living in the immediate vicinity of the World Trade Center, the prevalences of post-traumatic stress disorder and of depression 5–8 wk after the attacks were substantially higher than for respondents living further away in Manhattan, even after adjusting for other significant predictors including an individual's sociodemographic characteristics (Galea et al., 2002). These findings serve to illustrate the significant health impact of an event that occurred within a specific spatial and temporal context.

5. CONCLUSIONS

Drawing on prior conceptual and empirical work, this chapter has highlighted the potential influences of different spatial and temporal contexts on dietary intakes and stress. Several theories are particularly relevant in discussing the mechanisms by which contextual factors such as income inequality, social capital, and the psychosocial work environment may produce health behaviors and health effects in individuals. At the country level, and to a greater degree within countries as at the levels of states, communities and neighborhoods, and school and work environments, empirical evidence for the presence of contextual effects is accumulating. The evidence suggests that area-level factors account at least in part for variations in dietary behaviors, stress, and health outcomes.

Nevertheless, the validity of making causal inferences from studies should be tempered with these studies' methodological limitations. Multilevel statistical models are needed to truly distinguish contextual effects from compositional ones. In addition, the combination of multilevel with longitudinal study designs in future studies would lend stronger credence to causal relationships. Contextual effects may also vary by population subgroups (e.g., as defined by race/ethnicity, socioeconomic position) and should be explored in future studies through the testing of cross-level interactions (i.e., interactions between contextual and individual-level factors). A further limitation in the empirical work to date is the lack of consideration of multiple contextual factors simultaneously, be they economic, cultural, political, or institutional factors (O'Campo, 2003). Such consideration would not only reduce potential bias in the contextual effect of interest, but would also facilitate a better understanding of the mechanisms involved. Finally, in relation to the latter, qualitative work such as ethnographic approaches would serve as a useful adjunct to quantitative methods by yielding insights and observations that may "elude statistical measurement" (Kawachi & Berkman, 2003).

By addressing these limitations, future investigations may help to more validly estimate the effects of specific spatial and temporal contexts on nutrition and stress in individuals, and thereby help to identify more fundamental or root causes of disease (Link & Phelan, 1995). In so doing, subsequent public health interventions and policies may be developed that should more effectively improve dietary intakes and levels of stress. Ultimately, by specifying, identifying, and intervening in relevant contextual influences of dietary intakes and stress, greater gains in the levels of population and individual health may be achieved.

ACKNOWLEDGMENTS

Daniel Kim is the recipient of a Postdoctoral Fellowship through the Canadian Institutes of Health Research.

REFERENCES

Acevedo-Garcia, D., & Lochner, K. A. (2003). Residential Segregation and Health. In I. Kawachi, & L. F. Berkman (Eds.), *Neighborhoods and health* (pp. 265–287). New York: Oxford University Press.

Adler, N. E., Epel, E. S., Castellazzo, G., & Ickovics, J. R. (2000). Relationship of subjective and objective social status with psychological and physiological functioning: Preliminary data in healthy white women. *Health Psychology, 19*, 586–592.

Adrian, M., & Wilkinson, A. (2000). The social context of smoking, nutrition, and sedentary health behavior in Kansas. In A. R. Tarlov & R. F. St. Peter (Eds.), *The society and population health reader: A state and community perspective* (pp. 161–177). New York: The New Press.

Aguir, C., Ahmad, A. H., Aliev, A., Alishauskiene, R., Andreyenkov, V., Arocena, J., Auh, S. Y., Bacevic, L., Balakireva, D., Barjaba, K., Barker, D., Basanez, M., Bashkirova, E., Benitez-Nazano, J., Black, A., Boguszak, M., Cauzani, A., Carballo de Cilley, M., Chen, P. C., Chhiber, P., et al. (2000). World values surveys and European values surveys, 1981–1984, 1990–1993, and 1995–1997 (computer file) ICPSR version. Ann Arbor, MI: Interuniversity Consortium for Political and Social Research.

American Academy of Pediatrics Committee on School Health in the United States. (2004). Soft drinks in schools. *Pediatrics, 113*, 152–154.

Bandura, A. (1991). Social cognitive theory of moral thought and action. In W. M. Kurtines & J. L. Gerwitz (Eds.), *Handbook of moral behavior and development* (pp. 45–103). Hillsdale, NJ: Erlbaum.

Barker, D. J. P. (1992). *Fetal and infant origins of adult disease.* London: British Medical Journal.Barker, D. J. P. (1992). *Fetal and infant origins of adult disease.* London: British Medical Journal.

Bellisle, F., & Rolland-Cachera, M. -F. (2001). How sugar-containing drinks might increase adiposity in children. *Lancet, 357*, 490–491.

Ben-Shlomo, Y., & Kuh, D. (2002). A life course approach to chronic disease epidemiology: Conceptual models, empirical challenges and interdisciplinary perspectives. *International Journal of Epidemiology, 31*, 285–293.

Center for Media Education. Marketing to children harmful: Experts urge candidate to lead nation in setting limits. Press Release. Available online: www.cme.org.press/001018pr.html. Accessed December 10, 2003.

Critser, G. (2003). *Fatland: How Americans became the fattest people in the world.* New York: Houghton Mifflin Co.

Cutler, D. M., Glaeser, E. L., & Shapiro, J. M. (2003). Why have Americans become more obese? *Journal of Economic Perspectives, 17*, 93–118.

David, R. J., & Collins, J. W. (1997). Differing birthweight among infants of U.S.-born blacks, African-born blacks, and U.S.-born whites. *New England Journal of Medicine, 337*, 1209–1214.

Daly, M. C., Duncan, G. J., Kaplan, G. A., & Lynch, J. W. (1998). Macro-to-micro links in the relation between income inequality and mortality. *Milbank Quarterly, 76*, 303–304, 315–339.

Diez Roux, A. V., Nieto, F. J., Caulfield, L., Tyroler, H. A., Watson, R. L., & Szklo, M. (1999). Neighborhood differences in diet: The Atherosclerosis Risk in Communities (ARIC) study. *Journal of Epidemiology and Community Health, 53*, 55–63.

Dressler, W. W. (1996). Culture and blood pressure: Using consensus analysis to create a measurement. *Cultural Anthropology Methods, 8*, 6–8.

Dressler W. W., Balieiro, M. C., & Dos Santos, J. E. (1998). Culture, socioeconomic status, and physical and mental health in Brazil. *Medical Anthropology Quarterly, 12*, 424–446.

Dressler, W. W., Balieiro, M. C., & Dos Santos, J. E. (1999). Culture, skin color, and arterial blood pressure in Brazil. *American Journal of Human Biology, 11*, 49–59.

Emmons, K. M. (2000). Health behaviors in a social context. In L. F. Berkman and I. Kawachi (Eds.), *Social epidemiology* (pp. 242–266). New York: Oxford University Press.

Emmons, K. M., Linnan, L. A., Shadel, W. G., Marcus, B., & Abrams, D. B. (1999). The Working Healthy Project: A worksite health-promotion trial targeting physical activity, diet, and smoking. *Journal of Occupational and Environmental Medicine, 41*, 545–555.

Evans, G., & Carrere, S. (1991). Traffic congestion, perceived control and psychophysiological stress among urban bus drivers. *Journal of Applied Psychology, 76*, 658–663.

French, S. A., Jeffery, R. W., Story, M., Breitlow, K. K., Baxter, J. S., Hannan, P., & Snyder, M. P. (2001). Pricing and promotion effects on low-fat vending snack purchases: The CHIPS Study. *American Journal of Public Health, 91*, 112–117.

French, S. A., Story, M., Jeffery, R. W., Snyder, P., Eisenberg, M., Sidebottom, A., & Murray, D. (1997). Pricing strategy to promote fruit and vegetable purchase in high school cafeterias. *Journal of the American Dietetic Association, 97*, 1008–1010.

Galea, S., Ahern, J., Resnick, H., Kilpatrick, D., Bucuvalas, M., Gold, J., & Vlahov, D. (2002). Psychological sequelae of the September 11 terrorist attacks in New York City. *New England Journal of Medicine, 346*, 982–987.

Gleason, P., & Suitor, C. (2001). *Children's diets in the mid-1990s: Dietary intake and its relationship with school meal participation.* Alexandria, VA: U.S. Department of Agriculture, Food and Nutrition Service, Office of Analysis, Nutrition and Evaluation.

Goodman, E., Adler, N. E., Kawachi, I., Frazier, A. L., Huang, B., & Colditz, G. A. (2001). Adolescents' perceptions of social status: Development and evaluation of a new indicator. *Pediatrics, 108*, E31.

Griffin, J. M., Fuhrer, R., Stansfeld, S. A., & Marmot, M. (2002). The importance of low control at work and home on depression and anxiety: Do these effects vary by gender and social class? *Social Science and Medicine, 54*, 783–798.

Halman, L. (2001). The European Values study: A third wave. Tilburg, the Netherlands: Work and Organization Research Centre.

Hammar, N., Alfredsson, L., & Johnson, J. V. (1998). Job strain, social support at work, and incidence of myocardial infarction. *Occupational and Environmental Medicine, 55*, 548–553.

Helliwell, J. F. Well-being and social capital: Does suicide pose a puzzle? http://www.wcfia.harvard.edu/conferences/socialcapital/Happiness%20Readings/Helliwell_2003.pdf. Accessed on November 5, 2003.

Huston, S. L., Evenson, K. R., Bors, P., & Gizlice, Z. (2003). Neighborhood environment, access to places for activity, and leisure-time physical activity in a diverse North Carolina population. *American Journal of Health Promotion, 18*, 58–69.

Johnson, R. K., Panely, C., & Wang, M. Q. (1998). The association between noon beverage consumption and the diet quality of school-age children. *Journal of Child Nutrition and Management, 22*, 95–100.

Kann, L., Kinchen, S. A., Williams, B. I., Ross, J. G., Lowry, R., Grumbaum, J. A., & Kolbe, L. J.; State and local YRBSS Coordinators. Youth Risk Behavior Surveillance System. (2000). Youth risk behavior surveillance—United States, 1999. *Morbidity and Mortality Weekly Report Centers for Disease Control Surveillance Summary, 49*, 1–32.

Kaplan, G. A., Pamuk, E. R., Lynch, J. W., Cohen, R. D., & Balfour, J. L. (1996). Inequality in income and mortality in the United States: Analysis of mortality and potential pathways. *British Medical Journal, 312*, 999–1003.

Karasek, R. A. (1979). Job demands, job decision latitude, and mental strain: Implications for job redesign. *Administrative Science Quarterly, 24*, 285–307.

Kato, H., Tillotson, J., Nichaman, M. Z., Rhoads, G. G., & Hamilton, H. B. (1973). Epidemiologic studies of coronary heart disease and stroke in Japanese men living in Japan, Hawaii and California. *American Journal of Epidemiology, 97*, 372–385.

Kawachi, I., & Berkman, L. F. (2000). Social cohesion, social capital, and health. In L. F. Berkman & I. Kawachi (Eds.), *Social epidemiology* (pp. 174–190). New York: Oxford University Press.

Kawachi, I., & Berkman, L. F. (2003). Introduction. In I. Kawachi & L. F. Berkman (Eds.), *Neighborhoods and health* (pp. 1–19). New York: Oxford University Press.

Kawachi, I., Kennedy, B. P., and Glass, R. (1999) Social capital and self-rated health: A contextual analysis. *American Journal of Public Health, 89*, 1187–1193.

Kawachi, I., Kennedy, B. P., Lochner, K., and Prothrow-Stith, D. (1997). Social capital, income inequality, and mortality. *American Journal of Public Health, 87*, 1491–1498.

Kawachi, I., Kim, D., Coutts, A., & Subramanian, S. V. (2004). Reconciling the three accounts of social capital: Commentary on "Health by association? Social capital, social theory and the political economy of public health." *International Journal of Epidemiology, 33*, 682–690.

Kawachi, I., Levine, S., Miller, S. M., Lasch, K., and Amick, B. C. III. (1994). *Income inequality and life expectancy: Theory, research, and policy.* Boston: The Health Institute, New England Medical Center.

Kennedy, B. P., Kawachi, I., and Prothrow-Stith, D. (1996). Income distribution and mortality: Cross sectional ecological study of the Robin Hood index in the United States. *British Medical Journal, 312*, 1004–1007. Erratum 312, 1194.

Keys, A., Aravanis, C., Blackburn, H. W., Van Buchenn, F. S. P., Buzina, R., Pjordjevic, B. S., Dontas, A. S., Fidanza, F., Karvonen, M. J., Kimura, N., Lekos, D., Monti, M., Puddu, V., & Taylor, H. L. (1967). Epidemiologic studies related to coronary heart disease: Characteristics of men aged 40–59 in seven countries. *Acta Medica Scandinavica, 460* (Suppl.), 1–392.

Kromhout, D., Keys, A., Aravanis, C., Buzina, R., Fidanza, F., Giampaoli, S., Jansen, A., Menotti, A., Nedeljkovic, S., & Pekkarinen, M. (1989). Food consumption patterns in the 1960s in seven countries. *Journal of Clinical Nutrition, 49*, 889–894.

Kubzansky, L., & Kawachi, I. (2000). Affective states and health. In L. F. Berkman & I. Kawachi (Eds.), *Social epidemiology* (pp. 213–241). New York: Oxford University Press.

Kuper, H., & Marmot, M. (2003). Job strain, job demands, decision latitude, and risk of coronary heart disease within the Whitehall II study. *Journal of Epidemiology and Community Health, 57*, 147–153.

Lapoint, V. African American perspectives on marketing fast food to children. http://www.commercialexploitation.com/articles/african_american_perspectives.htm. Accessed on December 6, 2003.

Lee, S., Colditz, G., Berkman, L., & Kawachi, I. (2002). A prospective study of job strain and coronary heart disease in US women. *International Journal of Epidemiology, 31*, 1147–1153.

Lin, N. (2001). *Social capital: A theory of social structure and action.* New York: Cambridge University Press.

Link, B. G., & Phelan, J. (1995). Social conditions as fundamental causes of disease. *Journal of Health and Social Behavior*, Spec No., 80–94.

Lytle L. A., Seifert, S., Greenstein, J., & McGovern, P. (2000). How do children's eating patterns and food choices change over time? Results from a cohort study. *American Journal of Health Promotion, 14*, 222–228.

Macintyre, S., & Ellaway, A. (2000) Ecological approaches: Rediscovering the role of the physical and social environment. In L. F. Berkman & I. Kawachi (Eds.), *Social epidemiology* (pp. 213–241). New York: Oxford University Press.
McEwan, B. S., & Stellar, E. (1993). Stress and the individual: Mechanisms leading to disease. *Archives of Internal Medicine, 153*, 2093–2101.
Mokdad, A. H., Serdula, M. K., Dietz, W. H., Bowman, B. A., Marks, J. S., & Koplan, J. P. (1999). The spread of the obesity epidemic in the United States, 1991–1998. *Journal of the American Medical Association, 282*, 1519–1522.
Morland, K., Wing, S., & Diez Roux, A. (2002a). The contextual effect of the local food environment on residents' diets: The atherosclerosis risk in communities study. *American Journal of Public Health, 92*, 1761–1767.
Morland, K., Wing, S., Diez Roux, A., & Poole, C. (2002b). Neighborhood characteristics associated with the location of food stores and food service places. *American Journal of Preventive Medicine, 22*, 23–29.
Nestle, M. (2003). *Food politics.* Los Angeles: University of California Press.
Nielsen, S. J., Siega-Riz, A. M., & Popkin, B. M. (2002). Trends in energy intake in U.S. between 1977 and 1996: Similar shifts seen across age groups. *Obesity Research, 10*, 370–378.
O'Campo, P. (2003). Invited commentary: Advancing theory and methods for multilevel methods of residential neighborhoods and health. *American Journal of Epidemiology, 157*, 9–13.
Rogers, E. (1995). *Diffusion of innovations.* New York: The Free Press.
Rose G. (1985). Sick individuals and sick populations. *International Journal of Epidemiology, 14,* 32–38.
Romano, P. S., Bloom, J., & Syme, L. (1991). Smoking, social support, and hassles in an urban African-American community. *American Journal of Public Health, 81*, 1415–1422.
Sampson, R. J. (2003). Neighborhood-level context and health: Lessons from sociology. In I. Kawachi & L. F. Berkman (Eds.), *Neighborhoods and health* (pp. 132–146). New York: Oxford University Press.
Seeman, T. E., McEwan, B. S., Rowe, J. W., & Singer, B. H. (2001). Allostatic load as a marker of cumulative biological risk: MacArthur studies of successful aging. *Proceedings of the National Academy of Sciences, 98*, 4770–4775.
Siegrist, J. (1996). Adverse health effects of high effort/low reward conditions. *Journal of Occupational Health Psychology, 1*, 27–41.
Siegrist J. (2002). Reducing social inequalities in health: Work-related strategies. *Scandinavian Journal of Public Health, 30*, 49–53.
Sooman, A., Macintyre, S., & Anderson, A. (1993). Scotland's health: A more difficult challenge for some? The price and availability of healthy foods in socially contrasting localities in the West of Scotland. *Health Bulletin, 51*, 276–284.
Sooman, A., & Macintyre, S. (1995). Health and perceptions of the local environment in socially contrasting neighborhoods in Glasgow. *Health and Place, 1*, 15–26.
Sorensen, G., Stoddard, A., Hunt, M. K., Hebert, J. R., Ockene, J. K., Avrunin J. S., Himmelstein, J., & Hammond, S. K. (1998). The effects of a health promotion-health protection intervention on behavior change: The WellWorks study. *American Journal of Public Health, 88*, 1685–1690.
Sorensen, G., Stoddard, A. M., LaMontagne, A. D., Emmons, K., Hunt, M. K., Youngstrom, R., McLellan, D., & Christiani, D. C. (2002). A comprehensive worksite cancer prevention intervention: Behavior change results from a randomized controlled trial (United States). *Cancer Causes and Control, 13*, 493–502.
Sorensen, G., Stoddard, A., Peterson, K., Cohen, N., Hunt, M. K., Stein, E., Palombo, R., & Lederman, R. (1999). Increasing fruit and vegetable consumption through worksites and families in the Treatwell 5-a-Day study. *American Journal of Public Health, 89*, 54–60.
Spielberger, C. D., & Sarason, J. G. (1978). *Stress and anxiety.* Washington, DC: Hemisphere.
Stansfeld, S. A. (1999). Social support and social cohesion. In M. Marmot, M. & R. G. Wilkinson (Eds.), *Social determinants of health* (pp. 155–178). New York: Oxford University Press.
Subramanian, S. V., Kawachi, I., & Kennedy, B. P. (2001). Does the state you live in make a difference? Multi-level analysis of self-rated health in the U.S. *Social Science and Medicine, 53*, 9–19.
Theorell, T. (2000). Social cohesion, social capital, and health. In L. F. Berkman & I. Kawachi (Eds.), *Social epidemiology* (pp. 95–117). New York: Oxford University Press.
Tordoff, M. G., & Alleva, A. M. (1990). Effect of drinking soda sweetened with aspartame or high-fructose corn syrup on food intake and body weight. *American Journal of Clinical Nutrition, 51*, 963–969.

U.S. Department of Agriculture & U.S. Department of Health and Human Services. (2000). *Report of the Dietary Guidelines Advisory Committee on the Dietary Guidelines for Americans, 2000.* Washington, DC: Government Printing Office.

Wilkinson, R.G. (1996). *Unhealthy societies: The afflictions of inequality*. London: Routledge.

III Health, Mental Health, and Cognitive Functions

12 Nutrition and Stress and the Developing Fetus

Rinat Armony-Sivan and Arthur I. Eidelman

KEY POINTS

- Prenatal maternal nutrition and maternal stress have a major impact on the growth and development of the fetus.
- Specific macro- and micronutrient deficits impact on the normal growth and development of the fetus.
- Prenatal maternal nutrition and maternal stress have an impact on intrauterine growth and development, postnatal infant medical outcome, infant and child neurobehavioral and cognitive development, and programs for adult cardiac, metabolic and mental health function.
- The effect of prenatal maternal nutrition and maternal stress on the fetus may be explained, to a degree, by common underlying mechanisms.
- Disturbances in both the adult and fetal hypothalamic–pituitary–adrenal axis result from maternal nutritional deficits and stress.

1. INTRODUCTION

The most dramatic events in the growth and development of an infant occur before birth and result from the dynamic interplay of the fetus's genetic potential and appropriate environmental stimuli, a process termed epigenetics (Kelly & Trasler, 2004). While this process may be viewed as a progressive unfolding and continuum, it now recognized that fetal life is characterized by "critical" or "sensitive" periods wherein exposure to specific environmental stimuli is required for the normal sequence of development of both anatomical structures and their subsequent functioning. Thus, the previously held concept that the fetus is safe from the vagaries of the maternal state and is functionally the equivalent of an obligatory parasite is no longer tenable. In particular, it is clear that the nutritional state of the mother, both quantitatively and qualitatively, has a major effect on fetal growth and development. This is best exemplified by the now understood role of folic acid in the development of the neural tube. Mothers who delivered infants with defects such as anencephaly and spina bifida were noted to have lower serum levels of folic acid. Conversely, women who took supplementary folic acid at the time of conception through the first trimester were substantially less likely, as compared to women who

From: *Nutrients, Stress, and Medical Disorders*
Edited by: S. Yehuda and D. I. Mostofsky © Humana Press Inc., Totowa, NJ

did not take folic acid, to deliver a fetus with neural tube defects. The protective advantage of supplementary folic acid was even more dramatic in those mothers who had already delivered an infant with a neural tube defect. Such results clearly confirm the critical importance of timing and the interplay with genetic predisposition when discussing nutritional factors as related to development (American Academy of Pediatrics Committee on Genetics, 1999; Czeizel & Dudas, 1992).

No less important are the recent observations that the environment of the developing fetus during these sensitive periods of development may also "program" for ultimate function, way beyond infancy. The concept that *in utero* environmental factors act early in fetal life and can permanently imprint physiological systems is known as prenatal programming. The concern is that if at critical windows of time during intrauterine existence there is an absence of the proper stimulus or the presence of an adverse stimulus, individual tissues and/or whole organ systems can be inappropriately programmed with deleterious consequences for later life.

The biological purpose of early life programming is not known. The present understanding is that the prenatal plasticity of the physiological systems allows for the organism to tolerate a less than ideal intrauterine environment wherein suboptimal maternal nutrition, stress, and/or disease exists. This is accomplished by altering the setpoint of the organ systems and/or its tissue functions. Resetting, perhaps better termed downregulating, various biochemical or physiological processes in turn increases the offspring's chance for survival under these adverse conditions. However, this survival advantage is at the price of a subsequent postnatal functional disadvantage in the now more optimal extrauterine environment (Lucas, 1998; Singhal, Wells, Cole, Fewtrell, & Lucas, 2003).

Human epidemiological and experimental animal studies have tested the nutritional programming hypothesis, and the consensus is that humans, like other species, have sensitive periods for nutrition in relation to later outcomes (Lucas, 1998). For example, impaired intrauterine growth caused by maternal suboptimal nutrition or placental insufficiency has been found to be associated with an increase incidence of cardiovascular and endocrine disease in adulthood (Barker, 1998). The fetal programming hypothesis has been tested experimentally in a number of species using a variety of techniques to impair fetal growth. The range and types of reported postnatal physiological disorders in these experimental animal models were similar to those seen in human populations. Several structural and functional mechanisms underlying these associations have been suggested, such as disproportionately large reductions in the growth of some fetal organs and tissues, impaired cellular development, or deficiency of and/or impaired hormonal regulation (Barker, 1998; Fowden & Forhead, 2004). Of particular interest are the experimental studies of intrauterine growth retardation (IUGR) that have demonstrated a reduction in cerebral cellularity and dendritic branching, particularly in the hippocampus and dentate gyrus (Mallard, Rees, Stringer, Cock, & Harding, 1998; Rees & Harding, 1988).

One of the most interesting findings of these animal models of induced IUGR is an altered functioning of the adult and fetal hypothalamic–pituitary–adrenal (HPA) axis (Economides, Nicolaides, & Campbell, 1991; Goland et al., 1993). Normally this axis mediates the release of glucocorticoids in response to diurnal cues and stress. Glucocorticoids, in turn, regulate their own secretion by negative feedback to the hypothalamus and the pituitary, inhibiting the synthesis and/or release of corticotropin-releasing hormone (CRH), arginine, vasopressin, and adrenocorticotropic hormone (ACTH), thus

Table 1
Maternal Prenatal Status and Short- and Long-Term Outcomes

Fetal growth
Fetal development
Postnatal medical outcome
Infant and child neurobehavioral and cognitive outcome
Child and adult mental health outcome

modulating the stress response. Further control of HPA activity takes place at extrahypothalamic sites, notably the hippocampus and the amygdala (Fowden & Forhead, 2004). This apparent programming of the HPA axis by events in fetal life in experimental models raises the question as to what degree there is a link in humans between the fetal experience and later neurobehavioral development, including cognitive, motor, and emotional outcomes.

Fetal nutrition and stress, two fundamental environmental factors of early life, have been studied separately in relation to adult health. This chapter focuses on the degree to which these factors can affect growth and development in the broadest sense. In particular, the possible interrelationship of these factors during the fetal period and the long-term implications of an altered intrauterine environment are emphasized. Conceptually, the effects of prenatal maternal nutritional and psychosocial status on short- and long-term development can be categorized using five different parameters (Table 1). Although each of these parameters can be addressed as an independent outcome variable, it is clear that there is a complex interrelationship between them, and this chapter presents a unifying hypothesis that underlies this presumed relationship.

2. MATERNAL NUTRITION

It has long been recognized that both quantitative and specific qualitative maternal nutritional factors have a vital role in guaranteeing normal fetal growth as well as the structural and functional development of particular tissues and organ systems. The nutritional requirements of the pregnant woman can be divided into (a) macronutrients: protein (including specific essential amino acids such as carnitine and taurine), fat (including specific essential fatty acids such as linolenic and linoleic acid), and carbohydrates, and (b) the mineral and vitamin micronutrients. The actual increase in major macro- and micronutrient requirements during pregnancy as compared to the prepregnancy state are summarized in Table 2 (Eidelman, 2001). In general, macronutrients provide for the fetus's basic energy needs, maintenance, and growth, whereas specific micronutrients are essential for the molecular and cellular development in a range of fetal organs (Table 3) (Ashworth & Antipatis, 2001). Thus, it is clear that the fetus is critically dependent on the basic nutritional status of the pregnant mother for normal growth and development.

3. MATERNAL NUTRITION AND FETAL GROWTH

The first trimester and the major part of the second trimester of the pregnancy reflect the phase of cellular hyperplasia and hypertrophy, whereas the third trimester is primarily

Table 2
Increased Maternal Nutritional Requirements During Pregnancy

Element	*Additional daily requirement*
Calories (kcal)	300
Protein (g)	15
Calcium (mg)	250
Iron (mg)	30
Zinc (mg)	15–25
Copper (mg)	2
Folate (μg)	400

Source: Adapted from Eidelman, 2001.

Table 3
Micronutrients That Play a Role in the Normal Development of Function of Fetal and Neonatal Organs

Organ	*Mineral*	*Vitamin*
Liver	Fe, Se, Cu, Zn, Cd	A, B_{12}, choline, folic acid
Heart	Cu, Zn	A, D
Kidney	Fe, Cd, Zn, Pb	A
Brain	Fe, Cu, Zn, I	A, B_6, B_{12}, folic acid, biotin
Lung	Cu, Zn, Cd	A
Bone	Ca, Mg	D, E, C

Source: Adapted from Ashworth & Antipatis, 2001.

one of fetal growth that reflects cellular hypertrophy. Thus, if the mother does not provide adequate macronutrient substrate to the fetus during the first and second trimesters of gestation, there is a uniform decrease in the number of cells and cell size, leading to symmetrical IUGR. Inadequate nutrition in the third trimester, especially in the last 2 mo of the pregnancy, will lead to a nonuniform decrease in cell size and a minimal decrease in cell number. This process leads to a clinical entity called asymmetrical intrauterine growth retardation with relative brain sparing (Eidelman, 2001), a situation classically noted in toxemia of pregnancy. Most likely, the pathophysiology of this condition is a disruption in placental perfusion that interferes with the transfer of nutrients even in an otherwise well-nourished mother. It should be emphasized, though, that when severe maternal vascular disturbances occur that result in placental trophoblast and hormonal dysfunction occur early in gestation, growth restriction may be associated with abnormal brain growth, symmetrical IUGR, and even microcephaly. This has been confirmed by Tolsa et al. (2004), who studied such IUGR preterm infants with magnetic resonance imaging (MRI) brain scans and noted decreased brain volume and cerebral cortical gray matter.

From a human population point of view, two historical disasters, the siege of Leningrad (1941–1944) (Antonov, 1947) and the Dutch winter famine (1944–1945) (Stein, Susser, Saengler, & Marolla, 1975), provided a unique opportunity to study the effect of severe/ extreme maternal malnutrition in a previously and presumably otherwise healthy population. The Leningrad study noted that the greatest effect on birthweight (i.e., a reduction of 600 g) occurred when mothers conceived while in a malnourished state and continued to be malnourished throughout the pregnancy. If the mothers were malnourished only during the first trimester, there was an increase in the spontaneous abortion rate, but subsequent birthweight was minimally affected. Malnutrition in the second trimester, providing that nutrition was adequate in the third trimester had essentially no effect on growth. Third-trimester malnutrition, such as occurred in the Amsterdam population, resulted in average birthweight reduction of 300 g.

The results of other observational studies of human mothers with poor nutrition in populations from developing and developed societies have varied. In general, mothers in developing countries suffer from a degree of chronic malnutrition and have lower preconception birthweight (Ceesay et al., 1997). This itself leads to lower infant birthweight. When coupled with a pattern of high-energy expenditure, typical of the chronically malnourished woman in undeveloped countries, birthweight is on average 300–400 g less, and the incidence of low birthweight is nearly twice that of infants born to well-nourished women from developed countries. To what degree the malnourished woman in developing countries is also subject to increased caloric expenditure and stressful situations is difficult to assess, let alone quantitate. In contrast, observational studies in populations from developed countries have resulted in inconsistent findings at best and, essentially, have not documented any gross correlation between maternal nutritional state *per se* and birthweight (Matthews, Yudkin, & Neil, 1999).

Of interest is the observation that low maternal levels of the noncaloric micronutrients, such as iron (Felt & Lozoff, 1996), zinc (Scholl, Hediger, Schall, Fischer, & Khoo, 1993), and folic acid (Scholl, Hediger, Schall, Khoo, & Fischer, 1996), have also been correlated with growth restriction of the fetus. Furthermore, deficiencies in fetal levels of long-chain polyunsaturated fatty acids (LCPUFAs), especially docosahexaenoic acid (DHA) and arachadonic acid (AA), have been noted in intrauterine growth-restricted fetuses (Cetin et al., 2002)

4. MATERNAL NUTRITION AND FETAL DEVELOPMENT

In addition to the global effects of prenatal nutrition on fetal growth and survival, prenatal nutrition is associated with structural and/or functional impairments of fetal organs and tissues, such as thymus, liver, spleen, kidney, and thyroid, in addition to the effect on the central nervous system. Impaired fetal development is related to exposure of the pregnant mother to a low-protein diet or micronutrient deficiencies (Fowden & Forhead, 2004; Langley-Evans, Langley-Evans, & Marchand, 2003; Osada et al., 2002;). It is important to note that the vulnerability of different organs to suboptimal nutritional status is also determined by the sensitive periods of development (Rhind, Rae, & Brooks, 2001, 2003). For instance, the period when the kidney and brain are most vulnerable is very early in development, when both organs are in an extremely primitive state of development (Wintour et al., 2003).

Increasing concern has been expressed regarding the adequacy of maternal dietary levels of DHA, an ω-3 LCPUFA. DHA is the primary structural fatty acid of neural tissue, and the brain level of DHA correlates with neurodevelopment outcome and visual function (Koletzko et al., 2001). In the third trimester the DHA content of the cerebral cortex increases fivefold and is dependant on the preferential placental transfer of DHA from the mother to the fetus. The fetus, in contrast to the term infant, cannot synthesize DHA from the normal dietary essential fatty acid precursor (α-linolenic acid) and thus is totally dependant on the maternal DHA level. A recent study, which noted that infants whose mothers supplemented their diet with DHA-rich cod liver oil from the 18th week of gestation to 3 mo had improved cognitive function at 4 yr, further supports the conclusion regarding the effect of perinatal nutrition on long-term neurodevelopmental outcome (Helland, Smith, Saarem, Saugstad, & Drevon, 2003).

Other micronutrient deficiencies during fetal life are known to affect relative organ growth and can have profound and sometimes persistent effects on the molecular, cellular, immunological, and morphological development of a range of fetal tissues, including the nervous system. In addition to folic acid, the minerals zinc, iron, and copper and the antioxidant vitamins A and E are of particular importance (Osada et al., 2002). The beneficial effects of folic acid are not confined to events in early pregnancy and the prevention of neural tube defects. Low concentrations of folic acid throughout gestation impair cellular growth and replication. Zinc deficiency is teratogenic in all species examined (Golub, Takeuchi, Keen, Hendrickx, & Gershwin, 1996; Rogers, Keen, & Hurley, 1985). Experimental animal studies have shown that maternal vitamin A deficiency during pregnancy is associated with inappropriate growth and functioning of fetal lung, kidney, heart, and liver. In addition, dysfunction of the developing nervous system was affected by suboptimal maternal vitamin A status (Ashworth & Antipatis, 2001). Maternal iron deficiency during pregnancy was found to be associated with larger hearts and smaller kidneys and spleens (Gambling et al., 2003). Other animal model studies have demonstrated a direct effect of iron deficiency during pregnancy on the developing central nervous system. In such models decreases in brain iron content have been associated with electrophysiological alterations, impaired dopaminergic function, decreased cytochrome *c* oxidase activity, abnormal dendritic morphology, and impaired myelin production (Connor & Menzies, 1996; deUngria et al., 2000; Jorgenson, Wobken, & Georgieff, 2003; Rao, Tkac, Townsend, Gruetter, & Georgieff, 2003; Yehuda & Youdim, 1989; Yu, Steinkirchner, Rao, & Larkin, 1986).

5. MATERNAL NUTRITION AND LONG-TERM MEDICAL OUTCOMES

A large body of epidemiological studies in diverse human populations has shown that suboptimal maternal nutrition is associated with an increased incidence of cardiovascular, metabolic, and other diseases in later life. This programming occurs across the normal range of birthweights and has the worst prognosis at the extreme ends of the birthweight spectrum. Low birthweight has been linked to hypertension, ischemic heart disease, glucose intolerance, insulin resistance, type II diabetes, hyperlipidemia, hypercortisolemia, obesity, obstructive pulmonary disease, renal failure, and reproductive disorders in the adult. Nutritional programming has been described in populations of different age, sex, and ethnic origin and occurs independently of the adult level of obesity or exercise (Barker, 1998; Rhind et al., 2001). Evidence in several animal species for programming has been demonstrated by studies in which prenatal macro- or micronutrient manipulation leads to postnatal hypertension, glucose intolerance, insulin insensitivity, and alterations in the functioning of the adult HPA axis (Bloomfield et al. 2003; Gambling et al., 2003; Langley-Evans, 2001; Woodall, Breier, Johnston, & Gluckman, 1996; Woodall, Johnston, Breier, & Gluckman, 1996).

A recent study by Roseboom et al. (2001) of the Dutch famine cohort reported that there is a correlation between an increased risk of adult-onset disease with the gestational age at the time of famine exposure. It was shown that individuals who had been exposed to famine in late or mid-gestation had reduced glucose tolerance, whereas individuals who were exposed to famine in early gestation had a more atherogenic lipid profile. Animal studies have also shown that timing during pregnancy is an important determinant of the pattern of fetal growth and of specific postnatal outcomes. For example, in rats, caloric restriction during pregnancy leads to hypertension in the adult when it occurs throughout gestation, but not when it is confined solely to the second half of pregnancy (Holemans et al., 1999).

Recently, a number of studies have reported that rapid growth velocity after birth, and not birthweight *per se*, is strongly associated with risk for adult conditions such as type II diabetes and cardiovascular disease (Adair & Cole, 2003; Singhal et al., 2003). These data suggest that birthweight, representing the end product of intrauterine growth, is not sufficient in of its self to increase the risk for adult disease. The risk for adult disease increases when intrauterine growth restriction is associated with an increased rate of weight gain after birth. In an attempt to provide a conceptual and mechanistic framework to explain these findings, the thrifty phenotype hypothesis was proposed by Hales and Barker (1992). The term "thrifty" was derived from an earlier hypothesis, the thrifty genotype hypothesis of Neel (1962), who proposed that a natural evolutionary selection process operated during thousands of years of poor and intermittent nutrition and selected for genes that conferred a thrifty metabolic state that would aid survival in such adverse conditions. Diabetes, for example, occurs only when the availability of nutrients became excessive in relation to energy expenditure, leading to obesity. When fetal nutrition is poor, an adaptive response develops so as to optimize the growth of certain organs, such as the brain, to the detriment of other organs, such as those of the viscera. According to this hypothesis, these adaptations serve to improve the chances of fetal survival and also lead to an altered postnatal metabolism, which serves the purpose of enhancing postnatal survival under conditions of intermittent and poor nutrition. It is proposed that these adaptations only become detrimental when nutrition is overabundant and obesity results. Despite the fact that low birthweight is common in many populations worldwide, in those countries where adult low-calorie, high-energy-expenditure lifestyles are maintained there is a very low prevalence of diabetes. If such individuals are exposed postnatally to a calorie-rich diet coupled with a relatively sedentary lifestyle, their downregulated systems cannot adjust to an excessive nutritional load and an increase in the risk for diabetes ensues (Hales & Barker, 2001). In vivo and in vitro animal studies of protein-restricted pregnancies have provided findings showing remarkable parallels with the human conditions including permanent changes in the expression of regulatory proteins (Desai et al., 1997; Ozanne et al., 2003; Petry, Dorling, Pawlak, Ozanne, & Hales, 2001)

6. MATERNAL NUTRITION AND LATER NEUROCOGNITIVE FUNCTION

Considerable effort has been invested in testing the hypothesis, supported by animal studies, that suboptimal prenatal nutrition at a vulnerable stage in brain development has permanent effects on cognitive function. Epidemiological studies, mostly conducted in developing countries, found associations between malnutrition and reduced cognitive performance. However, these findings might not be causal, considering potential confounders such as poverty, poor social circumstances, and lack of stimulation, all of which might explain the adverse outcomes (Lucas, 1998). Similarly, while repeated studies have noted the correlation of IUGR with poor neurovedelopmental function (Hutton, Pharoah, Cooke, & Stevenson, 1997; McCarton, Wallace, Divon, & Vaughan, 1996; van Beek, Hopkins, Hoeksma, & Samsom, 1994), attributing such outcomes to nutrition *per se* is confounded by variables such as prematurity, multiple gestation, poor placental function, and/or underlying systemic maternal disease.

There is a growing body of research on the association between prenatal deficiency of specific micronutrients, such as iron (Armony-Sivan, Eidelman, Lanir, Sredni, & Yehuda, 2004; Siddappa et al., 2004; Tamura et al., 2002) and zinc (Black, 2003), with short- and/or long-term neurobehavioral outcomes. For example, Tamura et al. (2002) reported that cord serum ferritin concentrations in term human newborn infants correlated with ultimate cognitive function at 5 yr of age. Siddappa and colleagues (2004) reported that term and near-term infants of diabetic mothers who were born with low cord ferritin concentrations had altered auditory recognition memory in the immediate neonatal period and significantly lower psychomotor development score at 1 yr. Although such correlations do not confirm the causal relationship, given the multiple confounders in such study populations (as noted by Beard & Connor, 2003, and Fleming, 2002), these data suggest that the developing brain might be vulnerable to prenatal iron deficiency. The recently reported DHA supplemental study supports the conclusion that specific nutrients and timing of exposure are critical to normal neurodevelopmental outcome (Helland, Smith, Saarem, Saugstad, & Drevon, 2003).

7. MATERNAL NUTRITION AND LATER PSYCHOPATHOLOGY

Susser et al. (1996) addressed the hypothesis that prenatal malnutrition may be a risk factor for schizophrenia by studying children born after the Dutch famine of 1944–1945. They reported that severe food deprivation during the first trimester was correlated to a substantial increase in hospitalization for schizophrenia. In an experimental rat study, prenatal protein deprivation induced changes in prepulse inhibition and striatal *N*-methyl-D-aspartate (NMDA) receptor binding, neurodevelopmental changes associated with schizophrenia in humans (Palmer, Printz, Butler, Dulawa, & Printz, 2004). Because micronutrients such as zinc, essential fatty acids, and vitamin E serve as crucial cofactors in brain development, it has been suggested that prenatal micronutrient deficiencies may be involved in later mental and developmental disorders, such as schizophrenia, Parkinson's disease, epilepsy, and autism (Johnson, 2001). Koenig, Kirkpatrick, & Lee (2002) proposed that nutritional deprivation is just one of many types of stress that may occur during gestation and that the negative impact on the fetus occurs through the final common pathway of hypercortisolinemia. In particular, they suggested that such prenatal hyperglucocorticoid exposure increases the risk for the development of schizophrenia.

8. GLUCOCORTICOIDS, PRENATAL STRESS, AND PROGRAMMING

For most of gestation, fetal glucocorticoid levels are low and reflect maternal endogenous production and placental transfer. This transplacental concentration gradient is regulated, in part, by placental enzyme (11βHSD2), which converts active glucocorticoids from the mother to their inactive metabolites. This enzyme is, therefore, a key factor in limiting fetal exposure to maternal glucocorticoids. Fetal excess exposure to glucocorticoid may occur under various conditions, such as decreased placental 11βHSD2 activity, increased maternal cortisol levels, such as when the mother is subjected to a variety of stresses, or when there is increased cortisol secretion by the fetal adrenal itself. Such increased fetal cortisol levels have been documented in IUGR infants (Economides et al., 1991; Goland et al., 1993)

The potential effects of high levels of glucocorticoids on fetal growth and development have been examined in several animal models by treating the pregnant dams with synthetic glucocorticoids or by inducing stress responses in the dams with excessive light or noise. Such stress situations induce elevation of maternal cortisol levels and in turn increase fetal cortisol levels. Fetal overexposure to steroids has been found to be related to decreased fetal growth in both animal and human studies (Bloom, Sheffield, McIntire, & Leveno, 2001; Cleasby, Kelly, Walker, & Seckl, 2003; O'Regan, Kenyon, Seckl, & Holmes, et al., 2004). Moreover, glucocorticoids have major effects on the differentiation of a wide range of tissues, including lungs, liver, kidney, muscle, fat, and gut (*see* Fowden & Forhead, 1998). Thus, it is not surprising that excess exposure to glucocorticoids permanently programs cardiovascular and metabolic physiology in adult offspring (O'Regan et al., 2004).

There are several pathways by which excess exposure to glucocorticoids affects long-term health. Glucocorticoids stimulate morphological and functional changes in the tissues and activate many biochemical processes that have little or no function *in utero* but that are essential for survival postnatally (Fowden & Forhead, 1998). At a cellular level, glucocorticoid exposure *in utero* alters receptors, enzymes, ion channels, and transporters in a wide range of different cell types. They also change the expression of various growth factors, cytoarchitectural proteins, binding proteins, and components of the intracellular signaling pathways (Antonow-Schlorke, Schwab, & Nathanielsz, 2003; Breed, Margraf, Alcorn, & Mendelson, 1997; Chinoy et al., 1998; Hai, Sadowska, Francois, & Stonestreet, 2002). At the molecular level, glucocorticoids affect a number of different processes, which include impact on transcription, mRNA stability, translation, and/or posttranslation processing of the protein product. Several genes are known to be regulated by glucocorticoids (Li, Saunders, Fowden, Dauncey, & Gilmour, 1998).

The pioneering work of Liggins and Howie (1972) led to the widespread use of maternally administered synthetic glucocorticoids (betamethasone) to stimulate the fetal lung to synthesize surface-active lung phospholipids (surfactant). This acceleration of the maturation of the lungs significantly reduces both the incidence and the severity of the respiratory distress syndrome in preterm infants and thus has improved survival rates dramatically in the <1500-g infant (for a review, *see* Kay, Bird, Coe, & Dudley, 2000). As a result, since the 1994 National Institutes of Health Consensus Development Conference it has been recommended that prenatal steroid treatment be offered to all women at risk of preterm delivery between 24 and 34 wk of gestation. However, increasing concern has been voiced as to the trade-off between lung maturation and the adverse effect on growth (birthweight), lung size, and, most importantly, brain (Walfisch, Hallak, & Mazor, 2001) when such routine antenatal steroid treatment is used.

Beyond the concern that steroid-induced lung maturation arrests growth is the concern about its effect on the HPA axis, which is central to the normal integration of the endocrine and behavioral response to stress. A number of animal studies have shown that excessive glucocorticoids *in utero* result in programming the HPA regulation in adult offspring. Excessive prenatal glucocorticoid exposure leads to a decrease in type I and type II glucocorticoid receptors in the hippocampus (Koehl et al., 1999) and a diminished ability to modulate subsequent stress-induced glucocorticoid secretion. Within the developing brain, the limbic system (primarily the hippocampus) is particularly sensitive to endogenous and exogenous glucocorticoids, which may have implications for behavior (Banjanin, Kapoor, & Matthews, 2004; Welberg, Seckl, & Holmes, 2001). Indeed, several studies have shown that prenatal stress induces a phase advance in the circadian rhythm of locomotor activity and an increase in the paradoxical sleep in adult rats (Koehl, Barbazanges, Le Moal, & Maccari, 1997; Koehl et al., 1999). A recent study by Canlon et al. (2003) found that prenatal exposure to excessive glucocorticoids increases the susceptibility of the inner ear to acoustic noise trauma in adult life.

Relatively few studies have addressed the effects of prenatal stress on cognitive function. Studies in rats have shown that both acute and repeated maternal stress reduces learning by adult offspring in an operant discrimination task and alters their behavior in water maze (Weller, Glaubman, Yehuda, Caspy, & Ben-Uria, 1988). Lemaire, Koehl, Le Moal, and Abrous (2000) studied prenatally stressed rats and noted decreased neurogenesis in the hippocampal region and subsequent disturbances in their capacity for spatial memory. In a series of studies in pregnant rhesus monkeys exposed to repeated periods of loud noise, it was shown that such animals bear offspring with reduced attention span and neuromotor capabilities. Under conditions of challenge, prenatally stressed monkeys showed more disturbance behaviors and reduced exploration (Schneider, Moore, & Kraemer, 2004; Schneider, Moore, Kraemer, Roberts, & DeJesus, 2002). In general, the prenatal stress that occurs early in pregnancy is associated with programming of the central nervous system. More specifically, such early prenatal stress is related to hippocampal damage and impaired hippocampal-related behaviors, such as working memory. Tolsa et al. (2004) reported that IUGR infants suffered from increased disorganization of their autonomic state and attention interaction with their surroundings (Tolsa et al., 2004). It is important to note that although most studies have reported a significant relationship between prenatal stress and behavioral impairments there are reports of no effect or even beneficial ones. For example, Fujioka and colleagues showed that mild stress has been observed to benefit later learning in rats (Fujioka et al., 2001). Therefore, more research is needed in humans to explore the impact of specific prenatal stressors on later development and the possibility of a dose-related phenomenon.

Prenatal stress has also been studied in relation to emotional behavior. Fride and Weinstock (1988) found that prenatally stressed adult rats were often described as having a higher degree of "emotionality." For example, when exposed to an open field, prenatally stressed rats typically show decreased locomotion and increased defecation. Avoidance of anxiogenic locations in adult prenatally stressed animals has also been shown. In contrast, Ordyan and Pivina (2003) found that prenatal stress results in a significant decrease in the level of anxiety and an increase in movement activity among adult male rats.

Several factors make it difficult to generalize from the results on prenatal stress in animal studies to humans. First, the nature of prenatal stress in humans and animals is very different. In animal models, stressors are external events that are controlled in terms of frequency, intensity, and duration. However, most studies on prenatal stress in humans focus on maternal emotional responses to daily circumstances in their life. Maternal anxiety and depression may reflect an emotional response to stressful events;

however, they also represent inherent personality characteristics. Women who are psychologically stressed during pregnancy are most likely to be stressed after pregnancy. However, even after taking into account the multiple confounders in human studies, which limit our ability to confirm a causal relationship, the available data support the hypothesis that the developing fetus is vulnerable to maternal stress and may suffer from a wide range of neurobehavioral abnormalities as a result of this prenatal exposure.

In humans, maternal anxiety during pregnancy has been noted to be associated with growth delays and higher levels of activity in the fetus. In addition, neurobehavioral outcomes after birth, such as greater relative right frontal electroencephalogram activation, lower vagal tone, changes in sleep and wake states, and less than optimal performance on the Brazelton Neonatal Behavior Assessment Scale have been reported (Field et al., 2003; Niederhofer & Reiter, 2004). Maternal stress during pregnancy was also found to be related to long-term neurobehavioral development, such as motor development, temperament, and attention in infancy, behavioral disorders and negative emotionality at preschool age, and school marks at the age of 6 yr (Buitelaar, Huizink, Mulder, de Medina, & Visser, 2003; Huizink, de Medina, Mulder, Visser, & Buitelaar, 2002; Huizink, Robles de Medina, Mulder, Visser, & Buitelaar, 2003; Niederhofer & Reiter, 2004; O'Connor, Heron, Golding, Beveridge, & Glover, 2002; O'Connor, Heron, Golding, Glover, & the ALSPAC Study Team, 2003). It is important to note that in addition to the correlation between self-report measures of maternal stress during pregnancy and infant development, maternal physiological measures such as morning saliva cortisol levels in late pregnancy were also negatively related to both mental and motor development at 3 and 8 mo of age (Buitelaar et al., 2003). The mechanism for maternal-stress-induced behavioral changes may not be limited to the effect of glucocorticoid, in that abnormalities in neurotransmitter activity have also been noted in experimental models (Takahashi, Turner, & Kalin, 1992). Maternal anxiety is also associated with reduced cerebral blood flow in the fetus (Sjostrom, Valentin, Thelin, & Marsal, 1997), indicating that the effect on the fetus may be more global.

A recent study of the effect of a natural disaster (the January 1998 ice storm in Quebec, Canada) enabled researchers to examine the effect of an external acute severe stress on pregnant women and their offspring. Researchers studying the children at 2 yr of age noted that the level of prenatal stress exposure accounted for a significant proportion of the variance in the dependent variables, above and beyond that already accounted for by non-ice storm-related factors. The researchers noted that high levels of prenatal stress exposure, particularly early in the pregnancy, negatively affected the brain development of the fetus and was reflected in lower general intellectual and language abilities in toddlers (Laplante et al., 2004).

9. CONCLUSIONS

Reviewing the literature about the role of prenatal nutrition and stress on growth and development emphasizes how critical are the events during the prenatal period to our well-being throughout life. This chapter gave us the opportunity to review two prenatal environmental factors that have extensive impact on both neurobehavioral development and physical and mental health. Traditionally, prenatal nutrition and stress have been studied separately, but the data presented in this chapter indicate that both may be explained by the same mechanisms and have comparable effects on both fetal and adult life. Moreover, it is clear that suboptimal nutrition is related to stress situations and vise versa. For example, historical disasters in Leningrad and Amsterdam were characterized by increased levels of stress, not only severe nutritional deprivation. On the other hand, stressful situations may result in appetite and eating disturbances. Thus, future studies of the interrelationships between prenatal nutrition, stress in fetal growth and development, and life-long neurobehavioral outcomes are urgently needed.

REFERENCES

Adair, L. S., & Cole, T. J. (2003). Rapid child growth raises blood pressure in adolescent boys who were thin at birth. *Hypertension, 41*, 451–456.

American Academy of Pediatrics Committee on Genetics. (1999). Folic acid for the prevention of neural tube defects. *Pediatrics, 104*, 325–327.

Antonov, A. N. (1947). Children born during the siege of Leningrad in 1942. *Journal of Pediatrics, 30*, 250.

Antonow-Schlorke, I., Schwab, M., Li, C., & Nathanielsz, P. W. (2003). Glucocorticoid exposure at the dose used clinically alters cytoskeletal proteins and presynaptic terminals in the fetal baboon brain. *Journal of Physiology, 547*, 117–123.

Armony-Sivan, R., Eidelman, A. I., Lanir, A., Sredni, D., & Yehuda, S. (2004). Iron status and neurobehavioral development of premature infants. *Journal of Perinatology, 24*, 757–762.

Ashworth, C. J., & Antipatis, C. (2001). Micronutrient programming of development throughout gestation. *Reproduction, 122*, 527–535.

Banjanin, S., Kapoor, A., & Matthews, S. G. (2004). Prenatal glucocorticoid exposure alters hypothalamic-pituitary-adrenal function and blood pressure in mature male guinea pigs. *Journal of Physiology, 558*, 305–318.

Barker, D. J. P. (1998). *In utero* programming of chronic disease. *Clinical Science, 95*, 115–128.

Barker, D. J. P. (2002). Fetal programming of coronary heart disease. *Trends in Endocrinology and Metabolism, 13*, 364–368.

Beard, J. L., & Connor, J. R. (2003). Iron status and neural functioning. *Annual Review of Nutrition, 23*, 41–58.

Black, M. M. (2003). The evidence linking zinc deficiency with children's cognitive and motor functioning. *Journal of Nutrition, 133*, 1473S–1476S.

Bloom, S. L., Sheffield, J. S., McIntire, D. D., & Leveno, K. J. (2001). Antenatal dexamethasone and decreased birthweight. *Obstetrics and Gynecology, 97*, 485–490.

Bloomfield, F. H., Oliver, M. H., Giannoulias, C. D., Gluckman, P. D., Harding, J. E., & Challis, J. R. (2003). Brief undernutrition in late-gestation sheep programs the hypothalamic–pituitary–adrenal axis in adult offspring. *Endocrinology, 144*, 2933–2940.

Breed, D. R., Margraf, L. R., Alcorn, J. L., & Mendelson, C. R. (1997). Transcription factor C/EBPdelta in fetal lung: Developmental regulation and effects of cyclic adenosine 3',5'-monophosphate and glucocorticoids. *Endocrinology, 138*, 5527–5534.

Buitelaar, J. K., Huizink, A. C., Mulder, E. J., de Medina, P. G., & Visser, G. H. (2003). Prenatal stress and cognitive development and temperament in infants. *Neurobiology of Aging, 24*, S53–S60.

Canlon, B., Erichsen, S., Nemlander, E., Chen, M., Hossain, A., Celsi, G., & Ceccatelli, S. (2003). Alteration in the intrauterine environment by glucocorticoids modifies the developmental programme of the auditory system. *European Journal of Neuroscience, 17*, 2035–2041.

Ceesay, S. M., Prentice, A. M., Cole, T. J., Foord, F., Weaver, L. T., Poskitt, E. M., & Whitehead, R. G. (1997). Effects on birthweight and perinatal mortality of maternal dietary supplements in rural Gambia: 5 year randomised controlled trial. *British Medical Journal, 315*, 786–790.

Cetin, I., Giovannini, N., Alvino, G., Agostoni, C., Riva, E., Giovannini, M., & Pardi, G. (2002). Intrauterine growth restriction is associated with changes in polyunsaturated fatty acid fetal-maternal relationships. *Pediatric Research, 52*, 750–755.

Chinoy, M. R., Volpe, M. V., Cilley, R. E., Zgleszewski, S. E., Vosatka, R. J., Martin, A., Nielsen, H. C., & Krummel, T. M. (1998). Growth factors and dexamethasone regulate Hoxb5 protein in cultured murine fetal lungs. *American Journal of Physiology Lung Cellular and Molecular Physiology, 274*, L610–L620.

Cleasby, M. E., Kelly, P. A., Walker, B. R., & Seckl, J. R. (2003). Programming of rat muscle and fat metabolism by *in utero* overexposure to glucocorticoids. *Endocrinology, 144*, 999–1007.

Connor, J. R., & Menzies, S. L. (1996). Relationship of iron to oligodendrocytes and myelination. *Glia, 17*, 83–93.

Czeizel, A. E., & Dudas, I. (1992). Prevention of the first occurrence of neural-tube defects by periconceptional vitamin supplementation. *New England Journal of Medicine, 327*, 1832–1835.

Desai, M., Byrne, C. D., Meeran, K., Martenz, N. D., Bloom, S. R., & Hales, C. N. (1997). Regulation of hepatic enzymes and insulin levels in offspring of rat dams fed a reduced-protein diet. *American Journal of Physiology Gastrointestinal and Liver Physiology, 273*, G899–G904.

deUngria, M., Rao, R., Wobken, J. D., Luciana, M., Nelson, C. A., & Georgieff, M. K. (2000). Perinatal iron deficiency decreases cytochrome c oxidase (CytOx) activity in selected regions of neonatal rat brain. *Pediatric Research, 48*, 169–176.

Economides, D. L., Nicolaides, K. H., & Campbell, S. (1991). Metabolic and endocrine findings in appropriate and small for gestational age fetuses. *Journal of Perinatal Medicine, 19*, 97–105.

Eidelman, A. I. (2001). The relationship of maternal nutrition to fetal growth and outcome. In E. Lebenthal and N. Shapira (Eds.), *Nutrition in the female life cycle* (pp. 71–82). Jerusalem: ISAS International Seminars Ltd.

Felt, B. T., & Lozzof, B. (1996). Brain iron and behavior of rats are not normalized by treatment of iron deficiency anemia during early development. *Journal of Nutrition, 126*, 693–701.

Field, T., Diego, M., Hernandez-Reif, M., Schanberg, S., Kuhn, C., Yando, R., & Bendell, D. (2003). Pregnancy anxiety and comorbid depression and anger: Effects on the fetus and neonate. *Depression and Anxiety, 17*, 140–151.

Fleming, R. E. (2002). Cord serum ferritin levels, fetal iron status, and neurodevelopmental outcomes: Correlations and confounding variables. *Journal of Pediatrics, 140*, 145–148.

Fride, E., & Weinstock, M. (1988). Prenatal stress increases anxiety related behavior and alters cerebral lateralization of dopamine activity. *Life Sciences, 42*, 1059–1065.

Fowden, A. L., & Forhead, A. J. (2004). Endocrine mechanisms of intrauterine programming. *Reproduction, 127*, 515–526.

Fowden, A. L., Li, J., & Forhead, A. J. (1998). Glucocorticoids and the preparation for life after birth: Are there long-term consequences of the life insurance? *Proceedings of the Nutrition Society, 57*, 113–122.

Fujioka, T., Fujioka, A., Tan, N., Chowdhury, G. M., Mouri, H., Sakata, Y., & Nakamura, S. (2001). Mild prenatal stress enhances learning performance in the non-adopted rat offspring. *Neuroscience, 103*, 301–307.

Gambling, L., Dunford, S., Wallace, D. I., Zuur, G., Solanky, N., Srai, S. K., & McArdle, H. J. (2003). Iron deficiency during pregnancy affects postnatal blood pressure in the rat. *Journal of Physiology, 552*, 603–610.

Goland, R. S., Jozak, S., Warren, W. B., Conwell, I. M., Stark, R. I., & Tropper, P. J. (1993). Elevated levels of umbilical cord plasma corticotropin-releasing hormone in growth-retarded fetuses. *Journal of Clinical Endocrinology and Metabolism, 77*, 1174–1179.

Golub, M. S., Takeuchi, P. T., Keen, C. L., Hendrickx, A. G., & Gershwin, M. E. (1996). Activity and attention in zinc-deprived adolescent monkeys. *American Journal of Clinical Nutrition, 64*, 908–915.

Hai, C. M., Sadowska, G., Francois, L., & Stonestreet, B. S. (2002). Maternal dexamethasone treatment alters myosin isoform expression and contractile dynamics in fetal arteries. *American Journal of Physiology Heart and Circulatory Physiology, 283*, H1743–H1749.

Hales, C. N., & Barker, D. J. P. (1992). Type 2 (non-insulin-dependent) diabetes mellitus: The thrifty phenotype hypothesis. *Diabetologia, 35*, 595–601

Hales, C. N., & Barker, D. J. P. (2001). The thrifty phenotype hypothesis. *British Medical Bulletin, 60*, 5–20.

Helland, I. B., Smith, L., Saarem, K., Saugstad, O. D., & Drevon, C. A. (2003). Maternal supplementation with very-long-chain n-3 fatty acids during pregnancy and lactation augments children's IQ at 4 years of age. *Pediatrics, 111*, e39–44.

Holemans, K., Gerber, R., Meurrens, K., De Clerck, F., Poston, L., & Van Assche, F. A. (1999). Maternal food restriction in the second half of pregnancy affects vascular function but not blood pressure of rat female offspring. *British Journal of Nutrition, 81*, 73–79.

Huizink, A. C., de Medina, P. G., Mulder, E. J., Visser, G. H., & Buitelaar, J. K. (2002). Psychological measures of prenatal stress as predictors of infant temperament. *Journal of the American Academy of Child and Adolescent Psychiatry, 41*, 1078–1085.

Huizink, A. C., Robles de Medina, P. G., Mulder. E. J., Visser, G. H., & Buitelaar, J. K. (2003). Stress during pregnancy is associated with developmental outcome in infancy. *Journal of Child Psychology and Psychiatry and Allied Disciplines, 44*, 810–818.

Hutton, J. L., Pharoah, P. O., Cooke, R. W., & Stevenson, R. C. (1997). Differential effects of preterm birth and small gestational age on cognitive and motor development. *Archives of Disease in Childhood Fetal and Neonatal Edition, 76*, F75–F81.

Johnson, S. (2001). Micronutrient accumulation and depletion in schizophrenia, epilepsy, autism and Parkinson's disease? *Medical Hypotheses, 56*, 641–645.

Jorgenson, L. A., Wobken, J. D., & Georgieff, M. K. (2003). Perinatal iron deficiency alters apical dendritic growth in hippocampal CA1 pyramidal neurons. *Developmental Neuroscience, 25*, 412–420.

Kay, H. H., Bird, I. M., Coe, C. L., & Dudley, D. J. (2000). Antenatal steroid treatment and adverse fetal effects: What is the evidence? *Journal of the Society for Gynecologic Investigation, 7*, 269–278.

Kelly, T. L., & Trasler, J. M. (2004). Reproductive epigenetics. *Clinical Genetics, 65*(4), 247–260.

Koehl, M., Barbazanges, A., Le Moal, M., & Maccari, S. (1997). Prenatal stress induces a phase advance of circadian corticosterone rhythm in adult rats which is prevented by postnatal stress. *Brain Research, 759*, 317–320.

Koehl, M., Darnaudery, M., Dulluc, J., Van Reeth, O., Le Moal, M., & Maccari, S. (1999). Prenatal stress alters circadian activity of hypothalamo–pituitary–adrenal axis and hippocampal corticosteroid receptors in adult rats of both gender. *Journal of Neurobiology, 40*, 302–315.

Koenig, J. I., Kirkpatrick, B., & Lee, P. (2002). Glucocorticoid hormones and early brain development in schizophrenia. *Neuropsychopharmacology, 27*, 309–318.

Koletzko, B., Agostoni, C., Carlson, S.E., Clandinim, T., Hornstrag, G., Neuringer, M., Uauy, R., Yamashiro, Y., & Willatts, P. (2001). Long chain polyunsaturated fatty acid—LCPUFA and perinatal development. *ACTA Pediatrica, 90*, 460–464.

Langley-Evans, S. C. (2001). Fetal programming of cardiovascular function through exposure to maternal undernutrition. *Proceedings of the Nutrition Society, 60*, 505–513.

Langley-Evans, S. C., Langley-Evans, A. J., & Marchand, M. C. (2003). Nutritional programming of blood pressure and renal morphology. *Archives of Physiology and Biochemistry, 111*, 8–16.

Laplante, D. P., Barr, R. G., Brunet, A., Galbaud Du Fort, G., Meaney, M., Saucier, J. F., Zelazo, P. R., & King, S. (2004). Stress during pregnancy affects general intellectual and language functioning in human toddlers. *Pediatric Research, 56*, 400–410.

Lemaire, V., Koehl, M., Le Moal, M., & Abrous, D. N. (2000). Prenatal stress produces learning deficits associated with an inhibition of neurogenesis in the hippocampus. *Proceedings of the National Academy of Sciences of the United States of America, 97*, 11,032–11,037.

Li, J., Saunders, J. C., Fowden, A. L., Dauncey, M. J., & Gilmour, R. S. (1998). Transcriptional regulation of insulin-like growth factor-II gene expression by cortisol in fetal sheep during late gestation. *Journal of Biological Chemistry, 273*, 10,586–10,593.

Liggins, G. C., & Howie, R. N. (1972). A controlled trial of antepartum glucocorticoid treatment for prevention of the respiratory distress syndrome in premature infants. *Pediatrics, 50*, 515–525.

Lucas, A. (1998). Programming by early nutrition: An experimental approach. *Journal of Nutrition, 128*, 401S–406S.

Mallard, E. C., Rees, S., Stringer, M., Cock, M. L., & Harding, R. (1998). Effects of chronic placental insufficiency on brain development in fetal sheep. *Pediatric Research, 43*, 262–270.

Matthews, F., Yudkin, P., & Neil, A. (1999). Influence of maternal nutrition on outcome of pregnancy: Prospective cohort study. *British Medical Journal, 319*, 339–343.

McCarton, C. M., Wallace, I. F., Divon, M., & Vaughan, H. G. Jr. (1996). Cognitive and neurologic development of the premature, small for gestational age infant through age 6: Comparison by birthweight and gestational age. *Pediatrics, 98*, 1167–1178.

Neel, J. V. (1962). Diabetes mellitus: A "thrifty" genotype rendered detrimental by "progress?" *American Journal of Human Genetics, 14*, 353–362.

Niederhofer, H., & Reiter, A. (2004). Prenatal maternal stress, prenatal fetal movements and perinatal temperament factors influence behavior and school marks at the age of 6 years. *Fetal Diagnosis and Therapy, 19*, 160–162.

O'Connor, T. G., Heron, J., Golding, J., Beveridge, M., & Glover, V. (2002). Maternal antenatal anxiety and children's behavioural/emotional problems at 4 years. Report from the Avon Longitudinal Study of Parents and Children. *British Journal of Psychiatry, 180*, 502–508.

O'Connor, T. G., Heron, J., Golding, J., Glover, V., & the ALSPAC Study Team. (2003). Maternal antenatal anxiety and behavioural/emotional problems in children: A test of a programming hypothesis. *Journal of Child Psychology and Psychiatry and Allied Disciplines, 44*, 1025–1036.

Ordyan, N. E., & Pivina, S. G. (2003). Anxiety levels and neurosteroid synthesis in the brains of prenatally stressed male rats. *Neuroscience and Behavioral Physiology, 33*, 899–903.

O'Regan, D., Kenyon, C. J., Seckl, J. R., & Holmes, M. C. (2004). Glucocorticoid exposure in late gestation in the rat permanently programmes gender specific differences in adult cardiovascular and metabolic physiology. *American Journal of Physiology Endocrinology and Metabolism, 287*, e863–870.

Osada, H., Watanabe, Y., Nishimura, Y., Yukawa, M., Seki, K., & Sekiya, S. (2002). Profile of trace element concentrations in the feto-placental unit in relation to fetal growth. *ACTA Obstetricia et Gynecologica Scandinavica, 81*, 931–937.

Ozanne, S. E., Olsen, G. S., Hansen, L. L., Tingey, K. J., Nave, B. T., Wang, C. L., Hartil, K., Petry, C. J., Buckley, A. J., & Mosthaf-Seedorf, L. (2003). Early growth restriction leads to down regulation of protein kinase C zeta and insulin resistance in skeletal muscle. *Journal of Endocrinology, 177*, 235–241.

Palmer, A. A., Printz, D. J., Butler, P. D., Dulawa, S. C., & Printz, M. P. (2004). Prenatal protein deprivation in rats induces changes in prepulse inhibition and NMDA receptor binding. *Brain Research, 996*, 193–201.

Petry, C. J., Dorling, M. W., Pawlak, D. B., Ozanne, S. E., & Hales, C. N. (2001). Diabetes in old male offspring of rat dams fed a reduced protein diet. *International Journal of Experimental Diabetes Research, 2*, 139–143.

Rao, R., Tkac, I., Townsend, E. L., Gruetter, R., & Georgieff, M. K. (2003). Perinatal iron deficiency alters the neurochemical profile of the developing rat hippocampus. *Journal of Nutrition, 133*, 3215–3221.

Rees, S., & Harding, R. (1988). The effects of intrauterine growth retardation on the development of the Purkinje cell dendritic tree in the cerebellar cortex of fetal sheep: A note on the ontogeny of the Purkinje cell. *International Journal of Developmental Neuroscience, 6*, 461–469.

Rhind, S. M., Rae, M. T., & Brooks, A. N. (2001). Effects of nutrition and environmental factors on the fetal programming of the reproductive axis. *Reproduction, 122*, 205–214.

Rhind, S. M., Rae, M. T., & Brooks, A. N. (2003). Environmental influences on the fetus and neonate—timing, mechanisms of action and effects on subsequent adult function. *Domestic Animal Endocrinology, 25*, 3–11.

Rogers, J. M., Keen, C. L., & Hurley, L. S. (1985). Zinc deficiency in pregnant Long-Evans hooded rats: Teratogenicity and tissue trace elements. *Teratology, 31*, 89–100.

Roseboom, T. J., van der Meulen, J. H., Ravelli, A. C., Osmend, C., Barker, D. J., & Bleker, O. P. (2001). Effects of prenatal exposure to the Dutch famine on adult disease in later life: An overview. *Twin Research, 4*, 293–298.

Schneider, M. L., Moore, C. F., & Kraemer, G. W. (2004). Moderate level alcohol during pregnancy, prenatal stress, or both and limbic–hypothalamic–pituitary–adrenocortical axis response to stress in rhesus monkeys. *Child Development, 75*, 96–109.

Schneider, M. L., Moore, C. F., Kraemer, G. W., Roberts, A. D., & DeJesus, O. T. (2002). The impact of prenatal stress, fetal alcohol exposure, or both on development: Perspectives from a primate model. *Psychoneuroendocrinology, 27*, 285–298.

Scholl, T. O., Hediger, M. L., Schall, J. I., Fischer, R. L., & Khoo, C. S. (1993). Low zinc intake during pregnancy: Its association with preterm and very preterm delivery. *American Journal of Epidemiology, 137*, 1115–1124.

Scholl, T. O., Hediger, M. L., Schall, J. I., Khoo, C. S., & Fischer, R. L. (1996). Dietary and serum folate: Their influence on the outcome of pregnancy. *American Journal of Clinical Nutrition, 63*, 520–525.

Siddappa, A. M., Georgieff, M. K., Wewerka, S., Worwa, C., Nelson, C. A., & Deregnier, R. A. (2004). Iron deficiency alters auditory recognition memory in newborn infants of diabetic mothers. *Pediatric Research, 55*, 1034–1041.

Singhal, A., Wells, J., Cole, T. J., Fewtrell, M., & Lucas, A. (2003). Programming of lean body mass: A link between birthweight, obesity, and cardiovascular disease? *American Journal of Clinical Nutrition, 77*, 726–730.

Sjostrom, K., Valentin, L., Thelin, T., & Marsal, K. (1997). Maternal anxiety in late pregnancy and fetal hemodynamics. *European Journal of Obstetrics, Gynecology, and Reproductive Biology, 74*, 149–155.

Stein, Z., Susser, M., Saengler, G., & Marolla, F. (1975). *Famine and human development. The Dutch hunger winter of 1944–1945*. New York: Oxford University Press.

Susser, E., Neugebauer, R., Hoek, H. W., Brown, A. S., Lin, S., Labovitz, D., & Gorman, J. M. (1996). Schizophrenia after prenatal famine. Further evidence. *Archives of General Psychiatry, 53*, 25–31.

Takahashi, L. K., Turner, J. G., & Kalin, N. H. (1992). Prenatal stress alters brain catecholaminergic activity and potentiates stress-induced behavior in adult rats. *Brain Research, 574*, 131–137.

Tamura, T., Goldenberg, R. L., Hou, J., Johnston, K. E., Cliver, S. P., Ramey, S. L., & Nelson, K. G. (2002). Cord serum ferritin concentrations and mental and psychomotor development of children at five years of age. *Journal of Pediatrics, 140*, 165–170.

Tolsa, C.B., Zimine, S., Warfield, S.K., Freschi, M., Sancho Rossignol, A., Lazeyras, F., Hanquinet, S., Pfizenmaier, M., & Huppi, P. S. (2004). Early alteration of structural and functional brain development in premature infants born with intrauterine growth restriction. *Pediatric Research, 56*, 132–138.

van Beek, Y., Hopkins, B., Hoeksma, J. B., & Samsom, J. F. (1994). Prematurity, posture and the development of looking behaviour during early communication. *Journal of Child Psychology and Psychiatry and Allied Disciplines, 35*, 1093–1107.

Walfisch, A., Hallak, M., & Mazor, M. (2001). Multiple courses of antenatal steroids: Risks and benefits. *Obstetrics and Gynecology, 98*, 491–497.

Welberg, L. A., Seckl, J. R., & Holmes, M. C. (2001). Prenatal glucocorticoid programming of brain corticosteroid receptors and corticotrophin-releasing hormone: Possible implications for behaviour. *Neuroscience, 104*, 71–79.

Weller, A., Glaubman, H., Yehuda, S., Caspy, T., & Ben-Uria, Y. (1988). Acute and repeated gestational stress affect offspring learning and activity in rats. *Physiology and Behavior, 43*, 139–143.

Wintour, E. M., Johnson, K., Koukoulas, I., Moritz, K., Tersteeg, M., & Dodic, M. (2003). Programming the cardiovascular system, kidney and the brain—a review. *Placenta, 24*, S65–S71.

Woodall, S. M., Breier, B. H., Johnston, B. M., & Gluckman, P. D. (1996). A model of intrauterine growth retardation caused by chronic maternal undernutrition in the rat: Effects on the somatotrophic axis and postnatal growth. *Journal of Endocrinology, 150*, 231–242.

Woodall, S. M., Johnston, B. M., Breier, B. H., & Gluckman, P. D. (1996). Chronic maternal undernutrition in the rat leads to delayed postnatal growth and elevated blood pressure of offspring. *Pediatric Research, 40*, 438–443.

Yehuda, S., & Youdin, M. B. H. (1989). Brain iron: A lesson from animal models. *American Journal of Clinical Nutrition, 50*, 618–629.

Yu, G. S. M., Steinkirchner, T. M., Rao, G. A., & Larkin, E. C. (1986). Effect of prenatal iron deficiency on myelination in rat pups. *American Journal of Pathology, 125*, 620–624.

13 Lipids and Depression

Basant K. Puri

KEY POINTS

- Epidemiological evidence points to an inverse relationship between the consumption of *n*-3 long-chain polyunsaturated fatty acids and the incidence of both depression and suicide.
- Biochemical evidence points to changes in levels of *n*-3 long-chain polyunsaturated fatty acids in peripheral measures of fatty acid metabolism including erythrocyte membrane and plasma levels.
- The first trial of ultra-pure eicosapentaenoic acid in a severe case of treatment-resistant depression showed marked benefits clinically and in terms of structural neuroanatomy and neurospectroscopic measures of cerebral fatty acid metabolism.
- Subsequent randomized double-blind placebo-controlled clinical trials of eicosapentaenoic acid as an adjunctive therapy in depression, including treatment-resistant depression, have shown significant antidepressant actions of this *n*-3 long-chain polyunsaturated fatty acid.
- The evidence thus far suggests that ultra-pure eicosapentaenoic acid is an effective antidepressant that lacks the adverse side-effect profile of traditional antidepressants.

1. INTRODUCTION

Depression is a cause of increasing concern worldwide. During the 20th century, striking changes occurred in the epidemiology of major depression, including a marked increase in lifetime risk (Cross-National Collaborative Group, 1992) and a decreased age of onset (Klerman, 1988; Klerman & Weissman, 1988). This has coincided with well-documented similarly striking changes in dietary fatty acid intake, particularly in the western world, including a move to more highly saturated fats than polyunsaturated fats and, within the polyunsaturated fat intake, a move away from *n*-3 fatty acids to *n*-6 fatty acids (particularly linoleic acid) (Eaton & Kanner, 1985; Lands, 1992).

Curiously, in a major cross-national 10-country epidemiological study of major depression published in the 1990s, the annual prevalence of major depression was found to show a sixfold variation between different countries, from 0.8 cases per 100 adults in Taiwan to 5.8 cases per 100 adults in New Zealand (Weissman et al., 1993). This pattern is similar to that found for mortality from coronary artery disease, suggesting that dietary

From: *Nutrients, Stress, and Medical Disorders*
Edited by: S. Yehuda and D. I. Mostofsky © Humana Press Inc., Totowa, NJ

factors might be of importance (Hibbeln, 1998). In the first part of this chapter, evidence is put forward that the dietary intake of lipids, in particular *n*-3 long-chain polyunsaturated fatty acids, is associated with depression. The second part of the chapter then describes the therapeutic use of *n*-3 long-chain polyunsaturated fatty acids, particularly eicosapentaenoic acid, in this disorder. Finally, some putative mechanisms for the antidepressant action of eicosapentaenoic acid are briefly discussed.

2. EVIDENCE FOR THE INVOLVEMENT OF LIPIDS IN DEPRESSION

2.1. Epidemiology

Data for nine countries comparing the annual prevalence of major depression with the annual apparent fish consumption (calculated by fish catch plus imports minus exports) was found to be significantly negatively correlated ($p < 0.005$) (Hibbeln, 1998). On the one hand, countries such as New Zealand, West Germany (before the fall of the Berlin Wall), and Canada were found to have high annual prevalences of major depression of around 5–6 cases per 100 adults, but low apparent fish consumption of less than 50 pounds per person. On the other hand, Japan was found to have an annual prevalence of major depression of less than 0.13 cases per 100 adults, but a high apparent fish consumption of almost 150 pounds per person.

In depressed patients, a seasonal variation has been reported in the severity of depressive symptomatology. In one study carried out in the mid-1980s, the Zung Depression (self-rated) Scale scores were recorded from 104 consecutively admitted depressed patients. Peaks were observed in April–May and troughs in August–September (Maes, Meltzer, Suy, & De Meyer, 1993b). The same group also analyzed the national data on suicide, violent suicide, nonviolent suicide, and homicide (categorized according to ICD-9) for Belgium for the period 1979–1987 using spectral analyses (Maes, Cosyns, Meltzer, De Meyer, & Peeters, 1993a). A seasonal variation was found in violent suicide only (not in nonviolent suicide), with more deaths occurring in spring and summer than in winter and autumn (fall).

In a further Belgian study of *n*-3 and *n*-6 polyunsaturated fatty acids in 23 healthy volunteers, carried out between December 11, 1991 and December 25, 1992, a significant seasonal variation was found in just the cases of arachidonic acid, eicosapentaenoic acid, and docosahexaenoic acid (De Vriese, Christophe, & Maes, 2004). Arachidonic acid was lowest in winter (defined as December 21 to March 20, inclusive). Eicosapentaenoic acid was lower in winter and spring (defined as March 21 to June 20, inclusive) than in summer (June 21 to September 20, inclusive). Docosahexaenoic acid was lowest in the winter season. All the polyunsaturated fatty acid data for these 23 controls were then compared with the weekly number of deaths from violent and nonviolent suicide in Belgium for 1979–1987 described previously. Simple regression analyses revealed no significant correlations. Changes in certain fatty acid levels over the previous 2 wk showed significant correlations, however. By defining $\delta(x)$ as

$$\delta(x) = (\text{value of } x \text{ 2 wk earlier}) - (\text{current value of } x)$$

it was found that δ-arachidonic acid, δ-eicosapentaenoic acid, and δ-docosahexaenoic acid were significantly and negatively correlated with the rate of violent, but not nonviolent, suicide. Multiple regression showed that δ-eicosapentaenoic acid was the single best variable correlating with violent suicide (De Vriese et al., 2004).

2.2. Biochemistry

There is strong and consistent evidence that the levels of *n*-3 long-chain polyunsaturated fatty acids, particularly eicosapentaenoic acid, are reduced in the plasma and erythrocyte membranes of depressed patients (Peet and Bennett, 2003).

Maes et al. (1996) carried out assays of serum phospholipids in the postfasting (12-h) blood samples of 36 patients with *Diagnostic and Statistical Manual of Mental Disorders* (DSM-III-R) (American Psychiatric Association, 1987) major depression (with or without melancholia) and 14 patients with DSM-III-R adjustment disorder with depressed mood and dysthymia. These were compared with blood samples taken from 24 normal subjects. All the patients were Caucasian and of Flemish origin. Compared with the other two groups, the patients with major depression had significantly higher ratios of arachidonic acid to eicosapentaenoic acid in both serum cholesteryl esters and phospholipids and a significantly increased ratio of *n*-6 to *n*-3 polyunsaturated fatty acids in the cholesteryl ester fraction. Compared with the normal controls, the major depression patients had a significantly lower level of α-linolenic acid (18:3 *n*-6) in cholesteryl esters. Also, compared with the other two groups, the patients with major depression had significantly lower levels of eicosapentaenoic acid in serum cholesteryl esters and phospholipids.

Adams, Lawson, Sanigorski, and Sinclair (1996) studied 20 moderately to severely depressed patients. A significant correlation was found between the ratio of erythrocyte phospholipid arachidonic acid to eicosapentaenoic acid and the severity of depression as rated by both the 21-item Hamilton Depression Rating Scale and a second linear rating scale of severity of depressive symptoms that omitted anxiety symptoms. There was also a significant negative correlation between erythrocyte eicosapentaenoic acid and the linear rating scale. The ratio of plasma phospholipid arachidonic acid to eicosapentaenoic acid was also significantly correlated with the severity of depression measured by the linear rating scale, as was the ratio of erythrocyte *n*-6 to *n*-3 long-chain (C20 and C22 carbon) polyunsaturated fatty acids.

Peet, Murphy, Shay, and Horrobin (1998) measured erythrocyte membrane fatty acid phospholipid composition in 15 patients suffering from DSM-IV (American Psychiatric Association, 1994) major depressive episodes and 15 age- and sex-matched normal controls. The patients' psychotropic medication was stopped at least 1 wk before blood was taken for this study. In comparison with the controls, the depressed patients had significantly reduced values for total *n*-3 fatty acids, docosapentaenoic acid (*n*-3), docosahexaenoic acid, total *n*-6 fatty acids, linoleic acid, and dihomo-γ-linolenic acid. The depressed patients were found to have higher levels of oleic acid (18:1 *n*-9), palmitic acid (16:0), and stearic acid (18:0).

In a further study by Malcolm Peet's group (Edwards, Peet, Shay, & Horrobin, 1998), erythrocyte membrane phospholipid levels and dietary intake of polyunsaturated fatty acids were measured in 10 patients suffering from DSM-IV major depressive episodes and 14 age- and sex-matched normal controls. A significant depletion was found in erythrocyte membrane *n*-3 polyunsaturated fatty acids in the depressed patients, which was not the result of reduced caloric intake. Moreover, both the erythrocyte membrane and dietary intake of *n*-3 polyunsaturated fatty acids showed a significant negative correlation with the severity of depression as measured using the Beck Depression Inventory (Beck, Ward, Mendelson, Mock, & Erbaugh, 1981).

These findings, taken as a whole, raised the possibility that depressive symptoms may be alleviated by *n*-3 polyunsaturated fatty acid supplementation (Edwards et al., 1998).

3. TREATMENT WITH EICOSAPENTAENOIC ACID

3.1. The First Case: Treatment-Resistant Depression

3.1.1. Clinical Details

A detailed case report (Puri, Counsell, Hamilton, Richardson, & Horrobin, 2001; Counsell, Richardson, & Horrobin, 2002a) presenting the first case of the use of eicosapentaenoic acid in depression has been published. The case concerned a 21-yr-old male student with a 7-yr history of unremitting, treatment-resistant depressive symptoms.

At the age of 19 yr pharmacotherapy was started because of increasing illness severity with prominent low self-esteem, insomnia, sadness, inner tension, poor appetite, poor concentration, increasing social phobia, lethargy, pessimistic thoughts, and suicidal thoughts. Over the following year, the patient failed to respond to a variety of antidepressant, hypnotic, and antipsychotic medication; in fact, his clinical condition continued to deteriorate. He was close to the point of having to give up his studies at college. A 2-mo trial involving the addition of lithium carbonate to his antidepressant treatment was also unsuccessful.

At this stage, the patient was referred to the author. At this time the patient was actively suicidal in spite of ongoing treatment with the selective serotonin reuptake inhibitor paroxetine (20–30 mg daily) for 10 mo, and his symptoms met the DSM-IV-TR (American Psychiatric Association, 2000) criteria for major depressive disorder, recurrent.

The addition of purified ethyl eicosapentaenoate at a dose of 4 g daily led to rapid improvement, including cessation of the previously unremitting severe suicidal ideation, within 1 mo. The patient's social phobia also improved dramatically. There was a progressive benefit, and after 9 mo, his symptoms had disappeared altogether. No adverse side effects from the eicosapentaenoic acid preparation were reported.

3.1.2. Investigations

A number of investigations were carried out at both baseline and 9-mo follow-up. The patient underwent formal depression ratings, the niacin skin flush test, three-dimensional (3D) high-resolution cerebral magnetic resonance imaging (MRI), and cerebral 31-phosphorus magnetic resonance spectroscopy (^{31}P-MRS). The results of these are now described.

3.1.3. Depression Ratings

Ratings of the patient's symptoms of depression were carried out at baseline and at 9-mo follow-up using the Montgomery-Åsberg Depression Rating Scale (Montgomery and Åsberg, 1979). The baseline score on this scale was 32, which is consistent with a severe degree of depression. At 9-mo follow-up, the score had fallen to zero; there were no symptoms remaining at all.

3.1.4. Niacin Skin Flush Test

At both time points, the standardized niacin skin flush test (Ward, Sutherland, Glen, & Glen, 1998) was carried out and the volumetric niacin response (Puri, 2003; Puri, Hirsch, Easton, & Richardson, 2002b) calculated. At baseline, the volumetric niacin response was 20 mol s/L, which is a relatively low value. However, by the time of the 9-mo follow-up, it had risen by 30% to 26 mol s/L.

3.1.5. MRI, Image Segmentation and Subvoxel Registration

Sagittal 3D T_1-weighted rf spoiled images (TR = 30 ms, TE = 3 ms, flip angle = 30°, 156 × 256 × 114 image matrix, 1.6 mm section thickness, 25 cm field of view) were acquired on a 1.5 T Picker Eclipse scanner (Marconi Medical Systems, Cleveland, OH) at each examination. Phantom measurements were taken to confirm that no changes in magnetic gradient strength had occurred.

The volume scans were accurately registered (Bydder, 1995), and subtraction images were obtained to demonstrate changes between baseline images and the accurately registered follow-up images (Bydder and Hajnal, 1997a, 1997b; Puri, 2004). The registered anatomical and subtraction images were then reformatted into the transverse plane with isotropic voxels measuring 0.977^3 mm^3.

The subtraction images showed that during the 9-mo period of treatment with eicosapentaenoic acid, complex structural changes occurred in the brain. These included changes in the cerebral cortex and ventricular system, including an overall reduction in the lateral ventricular volume.

3.1.6. Cerebral ^{31}P-MRS

^{31}P-MRS data were obtained at the same sessions as the 3D MRI data acquisitions using a birdcage quadrature head coil double-tuned to protons (^{1}H, 64 MHz) and 31-phosphorus (26 MHz). Spectra were obtained using an image-selected in vivo spectroscopy sequence with a TR of 10 s with 64 signal averages localized on a 70 × 70 × 70 mm^3 voxel. These data were analyzed using the Advanced Method for Accurate, Robust, and Efficient Spectral fitting (AMARES) algorithm to yield relative peak areas for the phosphomonoesters (PMEs), inorganic phosphate (Pi), phosphodiesters (PDEs), phosphocreatine (PCr), and α-, β-, and γ-nucleotide triphosphate (α-, β-, and γNTP) resonances; the PME:PDE, PME:βNTP and PDE:βNTP ratios were also calculated.

The values of the resonance peak areas and the PME:PDE, PME:βNTP, and PDE:βNTP ratios at baseline and follow-up are shown in Table 1. In particular, over the 9-mo period there occurred a 53% increase in cerebral relative PME concentration, a 10% decrease in cerebral relative PDE concentration, and a 79% increase in the cerebral PME:PDE ratio.

3.1.7. Discussion

Supplementation with ultra-pure eicosapentaenoic acid (as ethyl eicosapentaenoate) was associated with remission of all the symptoms and signs of depressive illness in this actively suicidal young patient with increasingly severe depression, who had previously failed to respond to any single or combination pharmacological intervention. The patient's social phobia also improved during this time.

Given that the PME and PDE peaks can be used to index membrane phospholipid synthesis and breakdown, respectively (Pettegrew et al., 1991), the 30% improvement in the volumetric niacin response, the 53% increase in cerebral relative PME concentration, the 10% decrease in cerebral relative PDE concentration, and the 79% increase in the cerebral PME:PDE ratio all indicate that the eicosapentaenoic acid supplementation was associated with reduced neuronal phospholipid turnover, a large increase in cerebral phospholipid biosynthesis, and some decrease in phospholipid breakdown. Moreover, since phospholipids are important in the formation and remodeling of dendrites and synapses, these relatively large changes are likely to be causally linked to the structural cerebral changes observed.

Table 1
Relative Concentrations of Cerebral Metabolites and PME:βNTP, PDE:βNTP, and PME:PDE Ratios Determined by ^{31}P-MRS

	Baseline	*9-Mo follow-up*
%PME	9.23	14.11
%Pi	3.81	4.22
%PDE	46.60	41.99
%PCr	10.19	10.37
%γNTP	9.65	9.38
%αNTP	11.59	12.32
%βNTP	8.93	7.60
PME: βNTP	1.034	1.856
PDE: βNTP	5.221	5.523
PME:PDE	0.198	0.336

PME, phosphomonoester; NTP, nucleotide triphosphate; PDE, phosphodiester; PCr, phosphocreatine. Source: Modified from Puri et al., 2001.

3.2. Double-Blind Trials in Depression

The first double-blind trial of eicosapentaenoic acid in depression to be carried out was that of Peet and Horrobin (2002). In this study 70 patients with depression (scoring at least 15 on the 17-item Hamilton Depression Rating Scale [Hamilton, 1960]) that was persistent in spite of ongoing treatment with a standard antidepressant at an adequate dosage were randomized on a double-blind basis to receive one of the following doses of eicosapentaenoic acid (as ethyl eicosapentaenoate) for 12 wk in addition to unchanged background medication: 0 (placebo group), 1, 2, or 4 g daily. Patients underwent assessment using the 17-item Hamilton Depression Rating Scale, the Montgomery-Åsberg Depression Rating Scale, and the Beck Depression Inventory. The 1 g/d group showed a significantly better outcome than the placebo group on all three rating scales. In the intention-to-treat group, 5 (29%) of 17 patients receiving placebo and 9 (53%) of 17 patients receiving 1 g/d of ethyl eicosapentaenoate achieved a 50% reduction on the Hamilton Depression Rating Scale score. In the per-protocol group, the corresponding figures were 3 (25%) of 12 patients for placebo and 9 (69%) of 13 patients for the 1 g/d group. The 2 g/d group showed little evidence of efficacy, whereas the 4 g/d group showed nonsignificant trends toward improvement. All the individual items on all three rating scales improved with the 1 g/d dosage compared with the placebo, with strong beneficial effects on items rating depression, anxiety, sleep, lassitude, libido, and suicidality.

The second double-blind trial was that of Nehmets, Stahl, and Belmaker (2002). Nineteen patients with a diagnosis of DSM-IV major depressive disorder took part in a 4-wk, parallel-group, double-blind addition of either placebo or 2 g/d ethyl eicosapentaenoate to ongoing antidepressant therapy. Patients continued their current antidepressant treatment at the same dose they were receiving when they entered the study, which they had been receiving for at least 3 wk at a therapeutic dose. The patients' baseline scores on the 24-item Hamilton Depression Rating Scale were at least 18. Treatment and time showed a statistically significant interaction; the eicosapentaenoic acid group was significantly different from the placebo group at wk 2, 3, and 4. Over the 4-wk period the mean reduction of Hamilton Depression Rating Scale score in patients receiving the eicosapentaenoic acid was 12.4, compared with 1.6 in the placebo group.

Su, Huang, Chiu, and Shen (2003) randomized 28 outpatients with a DSM-IV diagnosis of major depressive disorder and a score of over 18 on the 21-item Hamilton Depression Rating Scale to receive adjunctive treatment with either *n*-3 long-chain polyunsaturated fatty acids or a placebo for 8 wk. The active treatment consisted of a daily dose of 2.2 g of eicosapentaenoic acid and 1.1 g of docosahexaenoic acid. Six patients dropped out before the end of the study; of these, two were in the active group and four in the placebo group. Compared with the placebo group, the active group showed significant improvements in the Hamilton Depression Rating Scale scores from wk 4 onwards.

4. CONCLUSIONS

In contrast to the existing families of antidepressant drugs, eicosapentaenoic acid is a safe treatment with almost no adverse side effects; indeed, the side effects of this agent are generally beneficial. In the case report discussed, although a spontaneous remission or a placebo response cannot be ruled out, in view of the findings and the protracted nature of the patient's illness and the fact that his illness had previously been worsening, it seems likely that the dramatic improvement was associated with the supplementation with ethyl eicosapentaenoate. This conclusion is supported by the positive results of the first three randomized double-blind, placebo-controlled trials of eicosapentaenoic acid supplementation in depression.

Three potential mechanisms of action of eicosapentaenoic acid in depression will now be discussed briefly.

First, it is known that cell membrane fatty acid composition affects cell membrane fluidity, which in turn influences the physicochemical properties of membrane receptors and enzyme such as adenylate cyclase (Horrobin & Bennett, 2003). For instance, it has been shown that membrane fluidity can be modulated by linoleic acid and that in turn membrane fluidity markedly modulates the binding of serotonin to mouse brain membranes (Heron, Shinitzky, Hershkowitz, & Samuel, 1980).

Second, a broad meta-analysis of the relation of depression to immunological assays carried out by Zorrilla et al. (2001) showed the following immunological correlates for depression: an overall leukocytosis, manifesting as a relative neutrophilia and lymphenia; increased CD4/CD8 ratios; increased circulating haptoglobin, prostaglandin E_2 (PGE2), and interleukin (IL)-6 levels; reduced natural-killer-cell cytotoxicity; and reduced lymphocyte proliferative response to mitogen. Plasma levels of IL-12, which plays a key role in promoting Th1 responses and subsequent cell-mediated immunity have also been found to be increased in depression (Kim et al., 2002). These results are consistent with a general immunoactivation occurring in depression. Thus, eicosapentaenoic acid may be acting as an antidepressant via its immunomodulatory actions.

Finally, it has been reported that changes in sleep and body mass in depression may be related to reports of resistance to dexamethasone suppression of the hypothalamic–pituitary–adrenocortical axis (Carroll, 1982; Rush et al., 1996). Access of the endogenous glucocorticoids corticosterone and cortisol to the brain are regulated by ABCB1-type P-glycoproteins in vivo, and ABCB1-type P-glycoprotein function has indeed found to modulate the activity of the hypothalamic–pituitary–adrenocortical system (Muller et al., 1993). Thus, another mechanism for the action of eicosapentaenoic acid might be via its inhibition of the biosynthesis of PGE2, since PGE2 induces P-glycoprotein expression (Ratnasinghe et al., 2001; Ziemann, Schafer, Rudell, Kahl, & Hirsch-Ernst, 2002).

REFERENCES

Adams, P. B., Lawson, S., Sanigorski, A. & Sinclair, A. J. (1996). Arachidonic acid to eicosapentaenoic acid ratio in blood correlates positively with clinical symptoms of depression. *Lipids, 31 (Suppl)*, S157–S161.

American Psychiatric Association. (1987). *Diagnostic and statistical manual of mental disorders* (3rd ed., Rev.) (DSM-III-R), Washington, DC: American Psychiatric Association.

American Psychiatric Association. (1994). *Diagnostic and statistical manual of mental disorders* (4th ed.) (DSM-IV), Washington, DC: American Psychiatric Association.

American Psychiatric Association. (2000). *Diagnostic and statistical manual of mental disorders* (4th ed., Text Rev.) (DSM-IV-TR), Washington, DC: American Psychiatric Association.

Beck, A. T., Ward, C. H., Mendelson, M., Mock, J., & Erbaugh, J. (1981). An inventory for measuring depression. *Archives of General Psychiatry, 38*, 147–150.

Bydder, G. M. (1995). The Mackenzie Davidson Memorial Lecture: Detection of small changes to the brain with serial magnetic resonance imaging. *British Journal of Radiology, 68*, 1271–1295.

Bydder, G. M., & Hajnal, J. V. (1997a). Registration and subtraction of serial MRI—Part 2: Image interpretation. In W. G. Bradley & G. M. Bydder (Eds.) *Advanced MR imaging techniques* (pp. 239–258). London: Martin Dunitz.

Bydder, G. M., & Hajnal, J. V. (1997b). Registration and subtraction of serial MRI—Part 3: Applications. In W. G. Bradley & G. M. Bydder (Eds.) *Advanced MR imaging techniques* (pp. 259–280). London: Martin Dunitz.

Carroll, B. J. (1982). The dexamethasone suppression test for melancholia. *British Journal of Psychiatry, 140*, 292–304.

Cross-National Collaborative Group. (1992). The changing rate of major depression. *Journal of the American Medical Association, 268*, 3098–3105.

De Vriese, S. R., Christophe, A. B., & Maes, M. (2004). In humans, the seasonal variation in poly-unsaturated fatty acids is related to the seasonal variation in violent suicide and serotonergic markers of violent suicide. *Prostaglandins, Leukotrienes and Essential Fatty Acids, 71*, 13–18.

Eaton, S. B., & Kanner, M. (1985). Paleolithic nutrition. *New England Journal of Medicine, 312*, 283–289.

Edwards, R., Peet, M., Shay, J., & Horrobin, D. (1998). Omega-3 polyunsaturated fatty acid levels in the diet and in red blood cell membranes of depressed patients. *Journal of Affective Disorders, 48*, 149–155.

Hamilton, M. (1960). A rating scale for depression. *Journal of Neurology, Neurosurgery and Psychiatry, 23*, 56–62.

Heron, D. S., Shinitzky, M., Hershkowitz, M., & Samuel, D. (1980). Lipid fluidity markedly modulates the binding of serotonin to mouse brain membranes. *Proceedings of the National Academy of Sciences of the USA, 77*, 7463–7467.

Hibbeln, J.R. (1998). Fish consumption and major depression. *Lancet, 351*, 1213.

Horrobin, D. F., & Bennett, C. N. (2003) Phospholipid metabolism and the pathophysiology of psychiatric and neurological disorders. In M. Peet, I. Glen, & D. F. Horrobin (Eds.), *Phospholipid spectrum disorder in psychiatry and neurology*, (2nd ed., pp. 3–47). Carnforth, Lancashire: Marius.

Kim, Y. K., Suh, I. B., Kim, H., Han, C. S., Lim, C. S., Choi, S. H., & Licinio, J. (2002). The plasma levels of interleukin-12 in schizophrenia, major depression, and bipolar mania: Effects of psychotropic drugs. *Molecular Psychiatry, 7*, 1107–1114.

Klerman, G. L. (1988). The current age of youthful melancholia. *British Journal of Psychiatry, 152*, 4–14.

Klerman, G. L., & Weissman, M. M. (1988). Increasing rates of depression. *Journal of the American Medical Association, 261*, 2229–2235.

Lands, W. E. (1992). Biochemistry and physiology of n-3 fatty acids. *Federation of American Societies for Experimental Biology Journal, 6*, 2530–2536.

Maes, M., Cosyns, P., Meltzer, H. Y., De Meyer, F, & Peeters, D. (1993a). Seasonality in violent suicide but not in nonviolent suicide or homicide. *American Journal of Psychiatry, 150*, 1380–1385.

Maes, M., Meltzer, H. Y., Suy, E., & De Meyer, F. (1993b). Seasonality in severity of depression: Relationships to suicide and homicide occurrence. *Acta Psychiatrica Scandinavica, 88*, 156–161.

Maes, M., Smith, R., Christophe, A., Cosyns, P., Desnyder, R., & Meltzer, H. (1996). Fatty acid composition in major depression: Decreased omega 3 fractions in cholesteryl esters and increased C20: 4 omega 6/ C20:5 omega 3 ratio in cholesteryl esters and phospholipids. *Journal of Affective Disorders, 38*, 35–46.

Montgomery, S. A., & Åsberg, M. (1979). A new depression scale designed to be sensitive to change. *British Journal of Psychiatry, 134*, 382–389.

Muller, M. B., Keck, M. E., Binder, E. B., Kresse, A. E., Hagemeyer, T. P., Landgraf, R., Holsboer, F., & Uhr, M. (1993). ABCB1 (MDR1)-type P-glycoproteins at the blood-brain barrier modulate the activity of the hypothalamic–pituitary–adrenocortical system: Implications for affective disorder. *Neuropsychopharmacology, 28*, 1991–1999.

Nemets, B., Stahl, Z., & Belmaker, R.H. (2002). Addition of omega-3 fatty acid to maintenance medication treatment for recurrent unipolar depressive disorder. *American Journal of Psychiatry, 159*, 477–479.

Peet, M., & Bennett, C. N. (2003). Relationship between brain lipids, depression and suicide. In M. Peet, I. Glen, & P. F. Horrobin (Eds.), *Phospholipid spectrum disorder in psychiatry and neurology* (2nd ed., pp. 403–408). Carnforth, Lancashire: Marius.

Peet, M., & Horrobin, D. F. (2002). A dose-ranging study of the effects of ethyl-eicosapentaenoate in patients with ongoing depression despite apparently adequate treatment with standard drugs. *Archives of General Psychiatry, 59*, 913–919.

Peet, M., Murphy, B., Shay, J., & Horrobin, D. (1998). Depletion of omega-3 fatty acid levels in red blood cell membranes of depressive patients. *Biological Psychiatry, 43*, 315–319.

Pettegrew, J. W., Keshavan, M. S., Panchalingam, K., Strychor, S., Kaplan, D. B., Tretta, M. G., & Allen, M. (1991). Alterations in brain high-energy phosphate and membrane phospholipid metabolism in first-episode, drug-naive schizophrenics. A pilot study of the dorsal prefrontal cortex by in vivo phosphorus 31 nuclear magnetic resonance spectroscopy. *Archives of General Psychiatry, 48*, 563–568.

Puri, B. K. (2003). Niacin testing in other psychiatric and neurological disorders. In *Phospholipid spectrum disorder in psychiatry and neurology* (2nd ed., pp. 353–356). Carnforth, Lancashire: Marius.

Puri, B. K. (2004). Monomodal rigid-body registration and applications to the investigation of the effects of eicosapentaenoic acid intervention in neuropsychiatric disorders. *Prostaglandins, Leukotrienes and Essential Fatty Acids, 71*, 177–179.

Puri, B. K., Counsell, S. J., Hamilton, G., Richardson, A. J., & Horrobin, D. F. (2001). Eicosapentaenoic acid in treatment-resistant depression associated with symptom remission, structural brain changes and reduced neuronal phospholipid turnover. *International Journal of Clinical Practice, 55*, 560–563.

Puri, B. K., Counsell, S. J., Richardson, A. J., & Horrobin, D. F. (2002a). Eicosapentaenoic acid in treatment-resistant depression. *Archives of General Psychiatry, 59*, 91–92.

Puri, B. K., Hirsch, S. R., Easton, T., & Richardson, A. J. (2002b). A volumetric biochemical niacin flush-based index that noninvasively detects fatty acid deficiency in schizophrenia. *Progress in Neuropsychopharmacology and Biological Psychiatry, 26*, 49–52.

Ratnasinghe, D., Daschner, P. J., Anver, M. R., Kasprzak, B. H., Taylor, P. R., Yeh, G. C., & Tangrea, J. A. (2001). Cyclooxygenase-2, P-glycoprotein-170 and drug resistance; is chemoprevention against multidrug resistance possible? *Anticancer Research, 21*, 2141–2147.

Rush, A. J., Giles, D. E., Schlesser, M. A., Orsulak, P. J., Parker, C. R. Jr, Weissenburger, J. E., Crowley, G. T., Khatami, M., & Vasavada, N. (1996). The dexamethasone suppression test in patients with mood disorders. *Journal of Clinical Psychiatry, 57*, 470–484.

Su, K. P., Huang, S. Y., Chiu, C. C., & Shen, W. W. (2003). Omega-3 fatty acids in major depressive disorder. A preliminary double-blind, placebo-controlled trial. *European Neuropsychopharmacology, 13*, 267–271.

Ward, P. E., Sutherland, J., Glen, E. M., & Glen, A. I. (1998). Niacin skin flush in schizophrenia: A preliminary report. *Schizophrenia Research, 29*, 269–274.

Weissman, M. M., Bland, R. C., Canino, G. J., Faravelli, C., Greenwald, S., Hwu, H. G., Joyce, P. R., Karam, E. G., Lee, C. K., Lellouch, J., Lepine, J. P., Newman, S. C., Rubio-Stipec, M., Wells, J. E., Wickramaratne, P. J., Wittchen, H., & Yeh, E. K. (1993). Cross-national epidemiology of major depression and bipolar disorder. *Journal of the American Medical Association, 276*, 293–299.

Ziemann, C., Schafer, D., Rudell, G., Kahl, G. F., & Hirsch-Ernst, K. I. (2002). The cyclooxygenase system participates in functional mdr1b overexpression in primary rat hepatocyte cultures. *Hepatology, 35*, 579–588.

Zorrilla, E. P., Luborsky, L., McKay, J. R., Rosenthal, R., Houldin, A., Tax, A., McCorkle, R., Seligman, D. A., & Schmidt, K. (2001). The relationship of depression and stressors to immunological assays: A meta-analytic review. *Brain, Behavior, and Immunity, 15*, 199–226.

14 Nicotine, Sleep, and Depression

Javier Velázquez-Moctezuma
and René Drucker-Colín

KEY POINTS

- Nicotine receptors are widely distributed in the brain.
- Nicotine interacts with γ-aminobutyric acid, noradrenaline, serotonin, and glutamate.
- Nicotine has been shown to have an antidepressant effect in a variety of animal models.
- Nicotine similarly has an antidepressant effect in nonsmoking depressed patients. This effect may be related to serotoninergic stimulation.
- Data suggest that addicted smokers may be self-medicating against depression.

1. INTRODUCTION

Since the classical experiments of Otto Loewi, it has been known that acetylcholine acts as a neurotransmitter. The actions of acetylcholine are exerted on its receptors, and these receptors are subdivided according to pharmacological sensitivity to two alkaloids of natural origin—muscarine and nicotine. Although the effects of nicotine on the nervous system have been known for a number of years, research on nicotinic receptors focused mainly on the neuromuscular junction and in the neuro-neuronal synapsis in the autonomic ganglia. The actions of nicotine on the central nervous system (CNS) were largely ignored for years. In the last two decades, however, research on the effects of nicotine on the CNS has greatly increased. Recent results have revealed that there is a complex network of nicotine receptor subtypes, closely related to several neurotransmitter systems, that are able to regulate their function. This influence seems to be particularly important in the recently discovered reciprocal relationship between depression and the alterations of sleep often observed in this psychiatric disease. In this chapter we will review the current knowledge of the effects of nicotine and how it influences depression and concurrent sleep alterations.

2. BACKGROUND

Nicotine is an alkaloid of vegetable origin. It is the main component of tobacco leaves, and it has been assumed for years that nicotine is the component responsible for the addiction to tobacco smoking. Because smoking is an ancient, widespread, and lethal addiction of human beings, nicotine has been considered a noxious substance that facili-

From: *Nutrients, Stress, and Medical Disorders*
Edited by: S. Yehuda and D. I. Mostofsky © Humana Press Inc., Totowa, NJ

tates the appearance of lung cancer or emphysema. However, as research on smoking has progressed, it has become clear that many additional substances underlie the pathological effects of tobacco smoking. There is also increasing evidence of the therapeutic effects of nicotine alone on neurological diseases such as Parkinson's disease, Alzheimer's disease and Gilles de la Tourette's syndrome (Mihailescu & Drucker-Colín, 2000).

In 1979 Gilbert reviewed evidence as to the beneficial effects of nicotine on mood and other subjective experiences (Gilbert, 1979). Since then, two main areas of research on this issue have evolved. One has shown evidence that the effects of nicotine on mood are limited to amelioration of the negative symptoms that appear after deprivation of nicotine in dependent smokers. However, it has also been shown that nicotine alone is capable of improving mood even in the absence of deprivation of negative symptoms (Kalman, 2002). Because nicotine exerts its action on brain structures and neurotransmitters systems involved in the regulation of mood, it has been suggested that tobacco smoking addiction could be a form of self-medication to relieve the negative symptomatology linked to depression (Markou, Kosten, & Koob, 1998).

A number of studies have suggested a close relationship between smoking and depression (Glassman, 1993). Epidemiological results indicate a high incidence of cigarette smoking among depressed individuals (Covey, 1999). Furthermore, individuals with a history of depression were less likely to quit smoking than nondepressed individuals, presumably owing to the occurrence of severe withdrawal symptoms (Tsoh et al., 2000). The negative symptoms were reversed by resumption of smoking or antidepressant treatment (Lief, 1996). Moreover, major depression is often observed in individuals trying to quit smoking (Killen, Fortmann, Schatzberg, Hayward, & Varady, 2003). We have recently observed that subjects abstaining from tobacco smoking show a 50% increase in the Hamilton Depression Rating Scale score (Moreno, Calderón, & Drucker-Colín, 2005).

Alterations of sleep architecture have been observed in psychiatric disorders, particularly in depression (Benca, Obermayer, Thised, & Gillin, 1992). The most conspicuous association between sleep and depression is the reduction of rapid eye movement (REM) sleep latency, although an increased latency to sleep is often observed when insomnia is present (Giles, Jarret, Roffward, & Rush, 1987). Pharmacological antidepressant treatment induces, besides the reversion of depressive symptoms, the normalization of the altered sleep architecture (Gillin, Lardon, Ruiz, & Golshan, 1997; Hendrickse et al., 1994). In addition, cholinergic participation in sleep regulation has been repeatedly demonstrated (Velázquez-Moctezuma, Shiromani, & Gillin, 1990). However, the participation of acetylcholine in depression does not have similar support from experimental evidence. David Janowsky and colleagues put forth the hypothesis that depression and mania are linked to the equilibrium between cholinergic and monoaminergic tone. When the cholinergic component increases, the monoaminergic component decreases, resulting in depression. On the contrary, when the monoaminergic tone increases and the cholinergic tone decreases, the results are a picture of mania (Janowsky, El-Yousef, Davis, & Sekerke, 1972). According to this hypothesis, acetylcholine could be the common substrate that explains the alterations of sleep observed in most depressive states.

Recent studies have shown that nicotine improves both mood and sleep alterations in depressed nonsmoking patients after prolonged administration (Haro-Valencia & Drucker-Colín, 2004; Mihailescu & Drucker-Colín, 2000). Furthermore, recent studies show that chronic administration of nicotine has a significant beneficial effect on mood and sleep. Depressed subjects with increased sleep latency and decreased REM sleep latency were treated with transdermal administration of nicotine for 8 mo. Since the first month a significant correlation was observed between the improvement in Hamilton Depression Rating Scale scores and the normalization of both sleep and REM sleep latencies. Most of the subjects reached normal values and maintained these values for months after the end of nicotine administration (Haro-Valencia & Drucker-Colín, 2004). Thus, the cholinergic system and, in particular, nicotinic receptors could be involved in the comorbidity often observed in depression and sleep disorders.

3. NICOTINE AND THE REWARD SYSTEM

Tobacco smoking is an ancient and widespread addiction of the human population. The main component of tobacco leaves that leads to addiction is nicotine, which, like other addictive drugs, seems to have an effect on the so-called reward system. The regulation of the reward system involves the participation of several neurotransmitters, chiefly dopamine (DA). Thus, the interactions of nicotine with neurotransmitters involved in the reward system deserve special analysis.

During the 1990s, it became clear that dopaminergic neurons located in the ventral tegmental area (VTA) and projecting to the nucleus accumbens (NAC) are a critical component of the reward system. Lesion of VTA dopaminergic neurons leads to a decrease in self-administered drugs, including nicotine (Louis & Clarke, 1998; Vezina, Herve, Glowinski, & Tassin, 1994). In addition, the administration of dopaminergic antagonists by microperfusion directly into the NAC elicits a similar reduction in self-administered addictive drugs, including nicotine (Corrigall & Coen, 1991). Imperato and colleagues (DiChiara & Imperato, 1988; Imperato, 1986) showed that a single systemic injection of nicotine is capable of inducing an increase in DA release in the NAC, which can be observed for almost an hour. Furthermore, when the nicotine antagonist mecamylamine (MeC) was been infused directly into the VTA, nicotine administration did not increase DA release in the NAC. When MeC was directly infused into the NAC, the release of DA consecutive to nicotine administration was not blocked (Nisell, Nomikos, & Svensson, 1994).

It is conceivable that the pleasurable effects of smoking are mediated by a direct action of nicotine on the dopaminergic neurons of the VTA that projects to the NAC. This notion is further supported by experiments in which nicotine antagonists were infused both in the VTA and in the NAC. When dehydro-β-erytroidine (DHBE), a nicotine antagonist, was infused into the VTA of rats, nicotine self-administration diminished, while when DHBE was infused into the NAC, nicotine self-administration was not affected (Corrigal, Coen, & Adamson, 1994).

Because experimental evidence suggests that VTA dopaminergic neurons are involved in self-administration of addictive drugs, attention must be focused on the factors affecting VTA excitability. It has been shown that dopaminergic VTA neurons receive afferents arising from different regions and containing different neurotransmitters. The most relevant excitatory influence on VTA dopaminergic neurons comes from the glutamatergic neurons located in the prefrontal cortex (Carr & Sesack, 2000; Kalivas, Duffy, & Barow, 1989). The most important inhibitory influence on VTA dopaminergic neurons comes from γ-aminobutyric acid (GABA)ergic neurons located in the NAC and in the ventral pallidum (Kalivas, Churchhill, & Klitenick, 1993). The main cholinergic influence comes

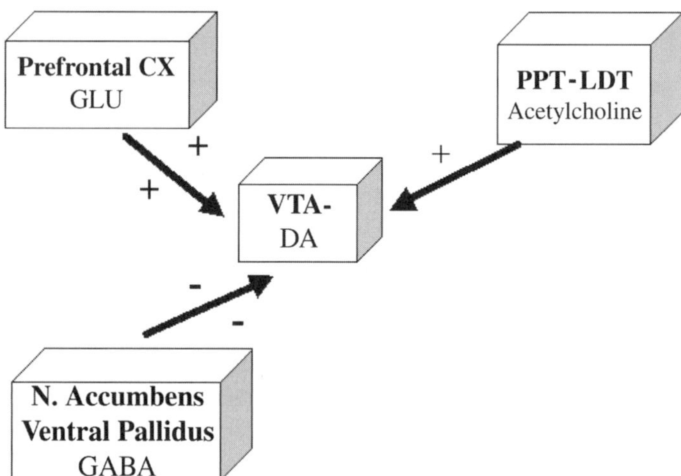

Fig. 1. Schematic representation of the main influences on the dopaminergic neurons located in the VTA.

from the cholinergic nucleus located in the brainstem, the pedunculo-pontine tegmental nucleus (PPT), and the lateral dorsal tegmental (LDT) nucleus (Garzon, Vaughan, Uhl, Kuhar, & Pickel, 1999). Other neurotransmitters, such as noradrenaline and serotonin, may also participate in the regulation of these neurons (Tzschentke, 2001) (Fig. 1).

Several nicotine receptor subtypes have been located in neurons of the VTA, mainly in dopaminergic and GABAergic neurons as well as in presynaptic terminals of glutamatergic neurons that make contact with dopaminergic neurons. The mechanisms by which nicotine causes the release of DA in the NAC could be the result of a direct action on dopaminergic neurons regulating both inhibitory as well as excitatory influences.

Dopaminergic neurons located in the VTA have been shown to express mRNAs for a number of nicotine receptor subunits. Although significant differences in this expression have been identified within the population of dopaminergic neurons, it has become clear that α-subunits 2–7 and β-subunits 2–4 are all expressed (Klink, Kerchove, Zoli, & Changeux, 2001). Using pharmacological tools it has been possible to identify three different subtypes of nicotinic receptor. One has been shown to have an α-7 subunit, whereas the other two show some evidence of a lack of the α-7 subunit and have been called non-α-7 receptors (Klink et al., 2001; Pidoplichco, DeBiasi, Williams, & Dani, 1997). The same authors reported that the non-α-7 nicotine receptors are located in most dopaminergic neurons, whereas those nicotine receptors expressing the α-7 subunit are located in fewer than half of the dopaminergic neurons.

The expression of mRNA for different nicotine receptor subunits shows important differences when compared to the dopaminergic neurons. Most nicotine receptors located in GABAergic neurons seem to be linked to the α-4 and β-2 subunits. The α-2 subunit is completely absent, and less than 25% of the GABAergic neurons express mRNA for α-subunits 5 and 6 and β-subunits 3 and 4. As in the case of nicotine receptor subtypes located in the dopaminergic neurons, the nicotine receptor subtypes located in the GABAergic neurons can be readily blocked with MeC (Mansvelder, Keath, & McGehee, 2002).

4. NICOTINE, MOOD, AND SLEEP

Since the pioneering studies of Hernández-Peón in the 1960s it has been known that acetylcholine is involved in the regulation of sleep and emotional behavior (Hernández-Peón, Chavez-Ibarra, Morgane, & Timo-Iaria, 1963). However, for a number of years the research on sleep regulation focused on the participation of the muscarinic receptors, for which pharmacological tools were available (Velázquez-Moctezuma, Shiromani, & Gillin, 1990). The effects of nicotine on sleep were controversial mainly owing to the different methodologies used. George, Haslett, and Jenden (1964) reported that nicotine had no behavioral or polygraphic effect when administered directly into the Giant Tegmental Cells. Moreover, intravenous administration of nicotine to narcoleptic dogs did not increase food-induced cataplexy (Delashaw, Foutz, Guilleminault, & Dement, 1979). On the other hand, it has been reported that small doses of nicotine given intravenously to freely behaving cats significantly increased REM sleep, which effect could be blocked by previous administration of MeC (Domino & Yamamoto, 1965). These results were replicated after subcutaneous administration of nicotine (Jewett & Norton, 1986). A similar increase in REM sleep was obtained after microinjection of nicotine in the Giant Tegmental Cells. Chronically implanted cats injected with a small dose of nicotine showed an increase of approx 50% in total REM sleep duration. This increase was accompanied by a decrease in wakefulness, with no significant variation in slow-wave sleep. These effects of nicotine administration were different from the effects observed after muscarinic stimulation in the same region. Although both muscarinic and nicotinic stimulation induced a significant increase in REM sleep, muscarinic stimulation also induces a decrease in slow-wave sleep, while nicotinic stimulation decreased wakefulness (Velázquez-Moctezuma, Shalauta, Gillin, & Shiromani, 1990).

Salín-Pascual, Moro Lopez, González Sánchez, and Blanco Centurión (1999) reported the effects of both acute and chronic administration of several doses of nicotine on sleep architecture in rats. Acute administration decreased REM and slow-wave sleep and increased wakefulness in a dose-dependent fashion. After 3 d of nicotine administration an increase in REM sleep was observed, whereas chronic administration of high doses induced a decrease of REM sleep. The authors concluded that the effects of nicotine on sleep largely depend on the dose, route, and time of administration.

Studies on humans have contributed to the controversy about the effects of nicotine on sleep, mainly owing to methodological differences. Few studies have been performed in normal nonsmoking volunteers. Thus, it was reported that nicotine patches in nonsmoking adults decrease total sleep time, sleep efficiency, and REM sleep (Davila, Hurt, Offard, Harris, & Shepard, 1994). Simultaneously, Gillin, Lardon, Ruiz, and Golshan (1994) reported that nicotine in healthy normal nonsmoking volunteers induced a dose-dependent decrease in total sleep time and in the percentage of REM sleep.

Most studies on the effects of nicotine on sleep in humans have been done in psychiatric patients, mainly in depressed adults. Salín-Pascual, De la Fuente, Galicia Polo, and Drucker-Colín (1995) reported the effects of nicotine patches on sleep and mood in healthy nonsmoking volunteers and nonsmoking patients with major depression. The results indicated that the acute administration of nicotine to depressed patients increased REM sleep and induced a short-term improvement of mood without any changes in other sleep parameters, whereas the control volunteers showed sleep fragmentation and a reduction in REM sleep time. A similar experiment was repeated later by the same group using the same administration but for 4 d. Results showed that both the control and experimental groups displayed a significant increase in REM sleep time. In addition, depressed subjects showed a significant improvement of mood, assessed through the Hamilton Depression Rating Scale score (Salín-Pascual & Drucker-Colín, 1998). More recently, similar effects were shown after several months of nicotine administration (Haro-Valencia & Drucker-Colín, 2004). Nicotine's antidepressant action may be related to its effect on the stimulation of raphe dorsalis neurons and concurrent serotonin release (Mihailescu, Palomero-Rivero, Meade-Huerta, Maza-Flores, & Drucker-Colín, 1998).

David Kalman (2002) reviewed and analyzed the methodological issues that prevent us from arriving at solid conclusions. In most of the studies, subjects were smokers who were deprived of nicotine for 2 h or for a night. A number of studies used former smokers, never-smokers, occasional smokers, and even current smokers. As would be expected, the results observed after the administration of nicotine in these subjects were diverse. The second methodological aspect that seems to induce great variation is dosing and method of administration. The pharmacokinetics of nicotine varies depending on whether it is administered by nasal spray, dermal patch, intravenously, subcutaneously, or, of course, through tobacco smoking. Finally, the third methodological issue involves the method by which the improvement of mood or the other effects of nicotine have been assessed. Despite the great amount of controversial information, some positive correlations indicate that the effects of nicotine on mood are influenced by individual differences and situational contingencies.

5. SUBTYPES AND DISTRIBUTION OF NICOTINE RECEPTORS

As mentioned above, research on the nicotinic acetylcholine receptors (nACrs) focused on receptors located at the neuromuscular junction or those of the electric eel organ. These tissues contain many receptors on which it was possible to perform experiments aimed at their biochemical characterization. Thus, it was possible during the 1970s to define nACrs as a glycoprotein of 290 kDa. This protein was later subdivided into four subunits named α, β, γ, and δ, according to molecular weight. Thereafter the subunits were designated by numbers according to the presence of a cysteine doublet (Itier & Bertrand, 2001). It has been reported that there are at least 11 genes in vertebrates encoding for nicotine receptor subunits. Nicotine receptors located in the central nervous system are, like the receptors in the neuromuscular junction, five units assembled in a pentamer, but unlike peripheral receptors, central receptors seems to contain only α- and β-subunits. Cloning experiments have revealed the presence of at least nine α- (2–10) and three β- (2–4) subunits forming the neuronal nicotinic receptors.

This structural conformation of the nicotinic receptors suggests the possible existence of a large number of receptor subtypes. Currently only a few have been identified. Experiments using radioactive nicotine have detected the presence of receptors containing the combination of subunits α-4/β-2 subunits in approx 90% of the nicotine receptors in the brain (Whiting & Lindstrom, 1986). In addition, it has been reported that the binding site for acetylcholine is located at the interface between two adjacent subunits. Thus, the binding-site properties depend largely on the contribution of each subunit. Experiments in nicotinic receptors from oocytes injected with different combinations of cDNA showed that the exchange of the α- and β-subunits modifies the sensitivity to acetylcholine (Corringer, Le Novere, & Changeux, 2000). Therefore, the combinations

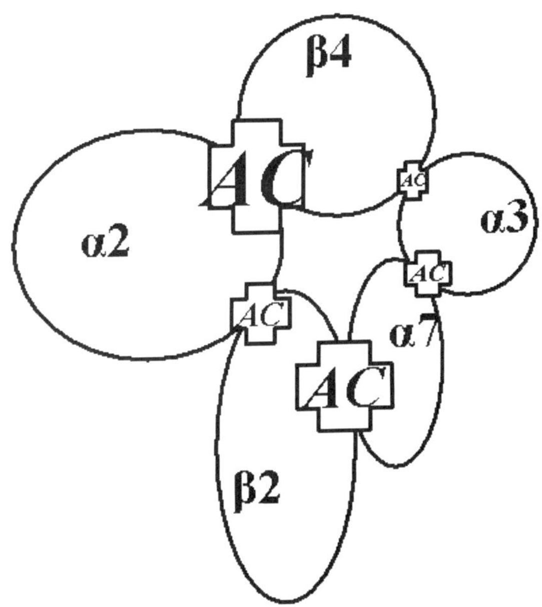

Fig. 2. Schematic representation of nicotinic receptor. The interaction with acetylcholine (*AC*) will depend on the subunits forming the pentameric receptor.

of subunits in this pentameric receptor will result in widely different sensitivities to acetylcholine, which could be a suitable mechanism for the regulation of excitability of the postsynaptic neuron (Fig. 2).

Early experiments performed on the nicotinic receptors of the neuromuscular junction revealed the existence of populations of receptors subtypes. Similar to other receptors' subtypes, the first subdivision was based on the differential pharmacological sensitivity to one drug, the snake toxin α-bungarotoxin (Ascher, Large, & Rang, 1979). In the last decade, a number of specific agonists and antagonists of the nicotine receptor has emerged, confirming the existence of a large number of nicotine receptor subtypes. Besides acetylcholine and nicotine, the classical agonists of the nicotinic receptor, other specific agonists have been developed with special affinities for specific receptor subunits. One of these, SIB-1508Y, is remarkably important because its high affinity for those receptors containing the α-2/β-4 subunits, which, as mentioned above, represent nearly 90% of the total nicotinic receptors in the brain (Sacaan et al., 1997). There are a number of specific antagonists for nicotinic receptors, among which MeC seems to be the most potent because it is able to block all types of nicotinic receptors, although with great differences in inhibition potency (Chávez-Noriega et al., 1997).

The generation of genetically manipulated strains of mice has shed light on the importance of the nicotinic receptor subunits in the normal functioning of the cholinergic system and its regulation of other neurotransmitter systems. It has been shown that the addiction to nicotine is significantly lower in β-2 knockout mice compared to their normal siblings (Picciotto et al., 1998). This elegant work indicates that only one subunit is critical for the development of the addiction to nicotine and suggests that individual differences in the presence of this subunit could explain the differences between subjects concerning their susceptibility to addiction.

Studies using immunocytochemical localization techniques have shown that both the α- and β-subunits are widely distributed in the brain, although with remarkable differences (Mihailescu & Drucker-Colín, 2000). The α-4 and β-2 subunits are present in large numbers compared with other α- and β-subunits. β-2 Subunits can be found throughout the brain, whereas α-4 subunits are not present in the hippocampus or cerebellum (Wada et al., 1989; Hill, Zoli, Burgeois, & Changeux, 1993).

6. NICOTINE–NEUROTRANSMITTER INTERACTIONS

As mentioned above, a great amount of evidence exists demonstrating the interactions of nicotine with the dopaminergic system. Nicotine receptors are predominantly located in the presynaptic membrane, and, therefore, nicotine could participate in the release of neurotransmitters such as GABA, noradrenaline, serotonin, glutamate, and, of course, acetylcholine. Nicotine receptors can also be found in the varicosities of the axon terminals that do not make synaptic contact (Vizi & Lendvai, 1999). The functional meaning of this location has been linked to the liberation of other neurotransmitters in a nonsynaptic fashion. These transmitters will exert their action at a distant target after reaching it through diffusion.

The septohippocampal cholinergic pathway, one of the major cholinergic pathways of the nervous system, is involved in memory and cognitive functions. However, only7 % of cholinergic varicosities make synaptic contact in the hippocampus, suggesting that the major release of acetylcholine occurs at a nonsynaptic location. Nicotine presynaptic receptors have a positive-feedback effect on acetylcholine release. It has been suggested that this extrasynaptic release of acetylcholine influences, after a diffusion process, the release of other neurotransmitters such as GABA, glutamate, noradrenaline, and serotonin (Vizi & Lendvai, 1999). Furthermore, it has been reported that nicotine can improve memory and attention deficits in Alzheimer's disease patients. Thus, it is possible that the high-affinity nicotine receptors located presynaptically influence the release not only of acetylcholine but also of other neurotransmitters involved in memory and attention deficits. This release of acetylcholine takes place not only at synaptic locations but also at extrasynaptic ones.

It has been suggested that nicotine receptors located at nonsynaptic sites must have higher affinity than those located at a synaptic level. The concentration of acetylcholine at synaptic sites is around the milimolar range, whereas nicotine at a concentration of 300 nM can induce upregulation of the α-4/β-2 nicotine receptor subtype (Ke, Eisenhow, Bencherif, & Lukas, 1998). Vizi and Lendvai (1999) have suggested that substances released from the nerve terminals act as tonic modulators and can communicate with other neurons without having any synaptic contact. Thus, a nonsynaptically released ligand diffuses away from its origin and acts at a remote cell with highly sensitive receptors that can discriminate among a variety of available diffusible signals. In the hippocampus nearly 90% of the cholinergic, noradrenergic, and serotonergic varicosities make no synaptic contact, but they are capable of releasing transmitters (Umbriaco, Garcia, Beaulieu, & Descarries, 1995; Vizi & Labos, 1991). The location of nicotine receptors in these presynaptic varicosities strongly suggests that nicotine plays an important regulatory role in the release of other transmitters, promoting volume transmission (Fig. 3).

As mentioned above, only 7% of cholinergic varicosities in the hippocampus make synaptic contact. Thus, the modulatory actions of nicotine on the release of other neu-

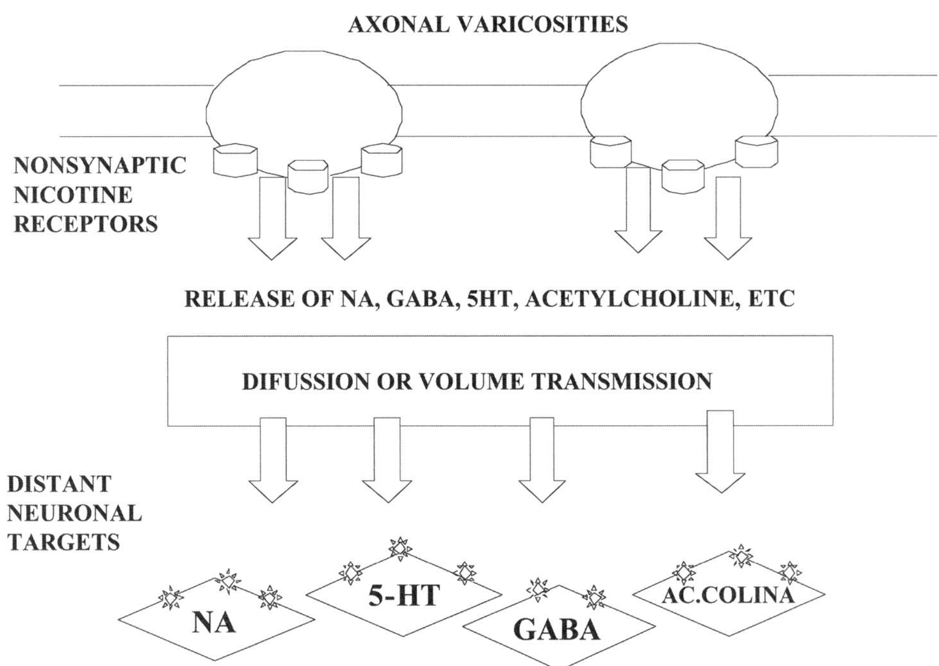

Fig. 3. The nicotinic nonsynaptic receptors located in the axonal varicosities promote the release of several neurotransmitters, which in turn exert their effects on a distant target through volume transmission.

rotransmitters seem to be performed mainly by its presynaptic action at nonsynaptic sites. The released transmitters diffuse and establish presynaptic contacts at synaptic sites establishing a tonic modulation of the synaptic transmission. It has been suggested that this is the main mechanism by which nicotine regulates the release of other transmitters (Vizi & Lendvai, 1999). Nicotine receptors can be found in the presynaptic terminals of cholinergic neurons, regulating the release of acetylcholine in the dorsal hippocampus. Furthermore, it has been suggested that the nicotinic receptor involved in this action does not contain the α-7 subunit (Vizi & Kiss, 1998).

It has been reported that nicotine receptors can be found in the presynaptic fibers of GABAergic fibers in several brain regions (Wonnacott, 1997). Furthermore, the nicotine receptors seem to involve an α-7 subunit that induces the release of GABA, leading to the inhibition of the main glutamatergic cells in the hippocampus (Alkondon, Rocha, Maelicke, & Alburquerque, 1993). Iontophoretic application of nicotine in the septum elicits significant inhibition of the septal neurons. This effect is mediated by the release of GABA as a result of the action of nicotinic receptors located in the presynaptic membrane of GABAergic neurons (Yang, Criswell, & Breese, 1996). In addition, it has been shown that nicotine increases the release of glutamate in the somatosensory cortex, and this action is mediated by a presynaptic nicotine α-7 nicotine receptor subtype (Aramakis & Metherate, 1998).

A recent paper demonstrated the permissive role of nicotine presynaptic receptors in the release of several neurotransmitters in the prefrontal cortex (Tao, Correa, Adams, Santori, & Sacaan, 2003). These authors analyzed the release of acetylcholine, noradrenaline, dopamine, and serotonin in prefrontal cortical slices after the administration of nicotine and nicotine agonists. The results indicate that all the neurotransmitters analyzed displayed an increase in release, but with some particularities that suggest the involvement of several nicotine receptor subtypes in the mediation of this effect. Taking into account the fact that the prefrontal cortex participates in higher brain functions such as cognition, these data could shed some light on the mechanisms by which nicotine exerts beneficial effects in Alzheimer's disease patients.

7. NICOTINE AS AN ANTIDEPRESSANT IN ANIMAL MODELS

According to the DSM-IV (1995), depression has two main symptoms, dysphoria and anhedonia, often accompanied by one or more secondary symptoms such as alteration in appetite, sleep, motor activity, attention, suicidal ideas, or excessive guilt. Some of these symptoms can be replicated in laboratory animals (Willner, 1991). Recently experimental evidence supporting the antidepressant activity of nicotine in animal models has been published.

The forced swim test developed by Roger Porsolt is widely accepted as a screening test for antidepressant activity (Porsolt, Le Pichon, & Jalfre, 1977; Borsini & Meli, 1988). Administration of nicotine to intact Wistar rats, both acutely and chronically, induced a decrease in immobility in the forced swim test. This result supports the notion that nicotine has an antidepressant activity (Vázquez-Palacios, Bonilla-Jaime, & Velázquez-Moctezuma, 2004). Similar results were reported by Tizabi et al. (1999), who administered nicotine in the Flinders Sensitive line of rats. This strain of rat has been selectively bred for cholinergic hypersensitivity, and it is a widely accepted animal model of depression (Overstreet, 1986). In this strain nicotine showed antidepressant activity when it was orally administered (Djuric, Dunn, Overstreet, Dragomir, & Steiner, 1999). Another widely accepted animal model of depression is the "learned helplessness" paradigm. Semba, Mataki, Yamada, Nankai, and Toru (1998) tested nicotine in this model and reported a decrease in the number of escape failures, which supports the idea that nicotine has an antidepressant activity.

Moreover, neonatal treatment with clomipramine in rats induced a depressive-like behavior during adulthood, and, thus, this procedure has been proposed as an animal model of depression (Vogel, Hartley, Neill, Hagler, Kors, 1990). Martínez-González, Prospéro-García, Mihailescu, and Drucker-Colín (2002) reported that chronic administration of nicotine results in a significant decrease in alcohol intake in rats neonatally treated with clomipramine, which suggests an antidepressant action. Using the same paradigm, Vázquez-Palacios et al. (2005) found that both acute and chronic administration of nicotine induced an antidepressant-like effect when rats neonatally treated with clomipramine underwent the forced swim test during adulthood.

8. CONCLUSIONS

The evidence to date on the effects of nicotine on mood and sleep in both animals and human subjects supports the notion that some beneficial antidepressant effects can be obtained. It must be emphasized that tobacco addiction is a condition quite different from the picture observed following the administration of nicotine alone. The nocuous effects of tobacco smoking could be derived from several substances besides nicotine that enter the organism through tobacco smoke. Evidence of the beneficial effects of nicotine administration on altered mental processes supports the need for more research in order to explain the inconsistencies reported in the various publications.

REFERENCES

Alkondon, M., Rocha, E. S., Maelicke, A., & Alburquerque, E. X. (1993) Diversity of nicotinic acetylcholine receptors in rat brain: V. Alpha-bungarotoxin-sensitive nicotinic receptors in olfactory bulb neurons and presynaptic modulation of glutamate release. *Journal of Pharmacology and Experimental Therapeutics, 265*, 1455–1473.

Aramakis, V. B., & Metherate, R. (1998). Nicotine selectively enhances NMDA receptor-mediated synaptic transmission during postnatal development in sensory neocortex. *Journal of Neuroscience, 18*, 8485–8495.

Ascher, P., Large, W. A., & Rang, H. P. (1979). Studies on the mechanism of action of acetylcholine antagonists on rat parasympathetic ganglion cells. *Journal of Physiology, 295*, 139–170.

Benca, R. M., Obermayer, W. H., Thisted, R. A., & Gillin, J. C. (1992). Sleep and psychiatric disorders; a meta-analysis. *Archives of Genetic Psychiatry, 49*, 651–668.

Borsini, F., & Meli, A. (1988) Is the forced swimming test a suitable model for revealing antidepressant activity? *Psychopharmacology, 94*, 147–160.

Carr, D. B., & Sesack, S. R. (2000) Projections from the rat prefrontal cortex to the ventral tegmental area: Target specificity in the synaptic associations with mesoaccumbens and mesocortical neurons. *Journal of Neuroscience, 20*, 3864–3873.

Chávez-Noriega, L. E., Corona, J. H., Washburn, M. S., Urrutia, A., Elliot, K. J., & Johnson, E. C. (1997). Pharmacological characterization of recombinant human neuronal nicotinic acetylcholine receptors h alpha2 beta2, h alpha2-beta4, h alpha3-beta2, h alpha 3-beta 4, h alpha4-beta2, h alpha4-beta4 and h alpha7 expressed in xenopus oocytes. *Journal of Pharmacology and Experimental Therapeutics, 280*, 346.

Corrigall, W. A., & Coen, K. M. (1991). Selective dopamine antagonists reduce nicotine self-administration. *Psychopharmacology, 104*, 171–176.

Corrigall, W. A., Coen, K. M., & Adamson, K. L. (1994). Self-administered nicotine activates the mesolimbic dopamine system through the ventral tegmental area. *Brain Research, 653*, 274–278.

Corringer, P. J., Le Novere, N., & Changeux, J. P. (2000). Nicotinic receptors at the amino acid level. *Annual Review of Pharmacology and Toxicology, 40*, 431–458.

Covey, L. S. (1999). Tobacco cessation among patients with depression. *Primary Care, 26,* 691–706.

Davila, D. G., Hurt, R. D., Offord, K. P., Harris, C. D., & Shepard, J. W., Jr. (1994). Acute effects of transdermal nicotine on sleep architecture, snoring, and sleep-disordered breathing in nonsmokers. *American Journal of Respiratory and Critical Care Medicine, 150*, 469–474.

Delashaw, J. B., Foutz, A. S., Guilleminault, C., & Dement, W. C. (1979) Cholinergic mechanisms and narcolepsy in dogs. *Experimental Neurology, 66*, 745–757.

Diagnostic and Statistical Manual of Mental Disorders: DSM-IV. (1995). American Psychiatric Association. Washington, DC.

DiChiara, G., & Imperato, A. (1988). Drugs abused by humans preferentially increase synaptic dopamine concentrations in the mesolimbic system of freely moving rats. *Proceedings of the National Academy of Science USA, 85*, 5274–5278.

Djuríc, V. J., Dunn, E., Overstreet, D. H., Dragomir, A., & Steiner, M. (1999). Antidepressant effect of ingested nicotine in female rats of Flinders resistant and sensitive lines. *Physiology Behavior, 67*, 533–537.

Domino, E., & Yamamoto, K. (1965). Nicotine: Effect on the sleep cycle of the cat. *Science, 150*, 637–638.

Garzon, M., Vaughan, R. A., Uhl, G. R., Kuhar, M. J., & Pickel, V. M. (1999). Cholinergic axon terminals in the ventral tegmental area target a subpopulation of neurons expressing low levels of the dopamine transporter. *Journal of Comparative and Neurology, 410*, 197–210.

George, R., Haslett, E. L., & Jenden, D. J. (1964). A cholinergic mechanism in the brain stem reticular formation: Induction of paradoxical sleep. *International Journal of Neuropharmacology, 3*, 541–552.

Gilbert, D. G. (1979). Paradoxical tranquilizing and emotion-reducing effects of nicotine. *Psychological Bulletin, 86*, 643–661.

Giles, D. E., Jarret, R. B., Roffwarg, H. P., & Rush, A. J. (1987) Reduced rapid eye movement latency. A predictor of recurrence in depression. *Neuropsychopharmacoogy, 1*, 51–59.

Gillin, J. C., Lardon, M., Ruiz, C., & Golshan, S. (1994). Dose-dependent effects of transdermal nicotine on early morning awakening and rapid eye movement sleep time in nonsmoking normal volunteers. *Journal of Psychopharmacology, 14*, 264–267.

Gillin, J. C., Rapaport, M., Erman, M. K., Winocur, A., & Albala, B. J. (1997). A comparision of nefazodone and fluoxetine on mood and on objective, subjective, and clinician rated measures of sleep in depressed patients: A double-blind, 8-week clinical trial. *Journal of Clinical and Psychiatry, 58*, 185–192.

Glassman, A. H. (1993). Cigarette smoking: Implications for psychiatric illness. *American Journal of Psychiatry, 150*, 546–553.

Haro-Valencia, R., & Drucker-Colín, R. R. (2004). A two-year study on the effects of nicotine and its withdrawal on mood and sleep. *Pharmacopsychiatry, 37*, 221–227.

Hendrickse, W. A., Roffwarg, H. P., Grannemann, B. D., Orsulak, P. J., Armitage, R., Cain, J. W., Battaglia, J., Debus, J. R., & Rush, A. J. (1994). The effects of fluoxetine on the polysomnogram of depressed outpatients: A pilot study. *Neuropsychopharmacology, 10*, 85–91.

Hernández-Peón, R., Chavez-Ibarra, G., Morgane, P. J., & Timo-Iaria, C. (1963). Limbic cholinergic pathways involved in sleep and emotional behavior. *Experimental Neurology, 8*, 93–111.

Hill, J. A., Zoli, M., Burgeois, J. P., & Changeux, J. P. (1993). Immunocytochemical localization of a neuronal nicotinic receptor: The beta 2 subunit. *Journal of Neuroscience, 13*, 1551–1568.

Imperato, A., Mulas, A., & Di Chiara, G. (1986). Nicotine preferentially stimulates dopamine release in the limbic system of freely moving rats. *European Journal of Pharmacology, 132*, 337–338.

Itier, V., & Bertrand, D. (2001). Neuronal nicotinic receptors: From protein structure to function. *FEBS Letters, 504*, 125–128.

Janowsky, D. S., El-Yousef, M. K., Davis, J. M., & Sekerke, H. J. (1972). A cholinergic-adrenergic hypothesis of mania and depression. *Lancet, 2*, 632–635.

Jewett, R. E., & Norton, S. (1986). Effect of some stimulant and depressant drugs on sleep cycles of cats. *Experimental Neurology, 15*, 463–474.

Kalivas, P. W., Churchill, L., & Klitenick, M. A. (1993). GABA and enkephalin projection from the nucleus accumbens and ventral pallidum to the ventral tegmental area. *Neuroscience, 57*, 1047–1060.

Kalivas, P. W., Duffy, P., & Barrow, J. (1989). Regulation of the mesocorticolimbic dopamine system by glutamic acid receptor subtypes. *Journal of Pharmacology and Experimental Therapeutics, 251*, 378–387.

Kalman, D. (2002). The subjective effects of nicotine: Methodological issues, a review of experimental studies, and recommendations for future research. *Nicotine and Tobacco Research, 4*, 25–70.

Ke, L., Eisenhow, C. M., Bencherif, M., & Lukas, R. J. (1998). Effects of chronic nicotine treatment on expression of diverse nicotinic acetylcholine receptor subtype: 1. Dose- and time-dependant effects of nicotine treatment *Journal of Pharmacology and Experimental Therapeutics, 286*, 825–840.

Killen, J. D., Fortmann, S. P., Schatzberg, A., Hayward, C., & Varady, A. (2003). Onset of major depression during treatment for nicotine dependence. *Addictive Behaviors, 28*, 461–470.

Klink, R., de Kerchove, D. A., Zoli, M., & Changeux, J. P. (2001). Molecular and physiological diversity of nicotine acetylcholine receptor in the midbrain dopaminergic nuclei. *Journal of Neuroscience, 21*, 1452–1463.

Lief, H. I. (1996). Bupropion treatment of depression to assist smoking cessation. *American Journal of Psychiatry, 153*(3), 442.

Louis, M., & Clarke, P. B. (1998). Effect of ventral tegmental 6-hydroxydopamine lesions on the locomotor stimulant action of nicotine in rats. *Neuropharmacology, 37*(12), 1503–1513.

Mansvelder, H. D., Keath, J. R., & McGehee, D. S. (2002). Synaptic mechanisms underlie nicotine-induced excitability of brain reward areas. *Neuron, 33*, 905–919.

Markou, A. Kosten, T. R., & Koob, G. F. (1998). Neurobiological similarities in depression and drug dependence: A self-medication hypothesis. *Neuropsychopharmacology, 18*, 135–174.

Martínez-González, D., Prospéro-García, O., Mihailescu, S., & Drucker-Colín, R. (2002). Effects of nicotine on alcohol intake in a rat model of depression. *Pharmacology, Biochemistry and Behavior, 72*, 355–364.

Mihailescu, S. & Drucker-Colín, R. R. (2000). Nicotine, brain nicotine receptors and neuropsychiatric disorders. *Archives of Medical Research, 31*, 131–144.

Mihailescu, S., Palomero-Rivero, M., Meade-Huerta, P., Maza-Flores, A., & Drucker-Colín, R. (1998). Effects of nicotine and mecamylamine on rat dorsal raphe neurons. *European Journal of Pharmacology, 360*, 31–36.

Moreno, A., Calderón, M. C., & Drucker-Colín, R. (2005). Long-term study of mood and sleep of chronic smokers during abstinence. *Addiction* (submitted).

Nisell, M., Nomikos, G. G., & Svensson, T. H. (1994). Systemic nicotine-induced dopamine release in the rat nucleus accumbens is regulated by nicotinic receptors in the ventral tegmental area. *Synapse, 16,* 36–44.

Overstreet, D. H. (1986). Selective breeding for increased cholinergic function: Development of a new model of depression. *Biology Psychiatry, 21*, 49–58.

Picciotto, M. R., Solí, M., Rimondini, R., Lena, C., Marubio, L. M., Pich, E. M., Fuxe, K., & Changeux, J. P. (1998). Acetylcholine receptors containing the beta2 subunit are involved in reinforcing properties of nicotine. *Nature, 391*, 173–177.

Pidoplichco, V. I., DeBiasi, M., Williams, J. T., & Dani, J. A. (1997). Nicotine activates and desensitizes midbrain dopamine neurons. *Nature, 390*, 401–404.

Porsolt, R., Le Pichon, M., & Jalfre, M. (1977). Depression: A new animal model sensitive to antidepressant treatmenta. *Nature, 266*, 730–732.

Sacaan, A. I., Reid, R. T., Santori, E. M., Adams, P., Correa, L. D., Mahaffy, L. S., Bleicher, L., Oxford, N. D., Stauderman, K. A., McDonald, I. A., Rao, T. S., & Lloyd, G. K. (1997). Pharmacological characterization of SIB-1765F: A novel cholinergic ion channel agonist. *Journal of Pharmacology and Experimental Therapeutics, 280*, 373.

Salín-Pascual, R. J., De la Fuente, J. R., Galicia Polo, L., & Drucker-Colín, R. R. (1995). Effects of transdermal nicotine on mood and sleep in nonsmoking major depressed patients. *Psychopharmacology, 121*, 476–479.

Salín-Pascual, R. J., & Drucker-Colín, R. R. (1998). A novel effect of nicotine on mood and sleep in major depression. *Neuroreport, 9*, 57–60.

Salín-Pascual, R. J., Moro Lopez, M. L., González Sánchez, H., & Blanco Centurión, C. (1999). Changes in sleep after acute and repeated administration of nicotine in the rat. *Psychopharmacology, 145*, 133–138.

Semba, J., Mataki, C., Yamada, S., Nankai, M., & Toru, M. (1998). Antidepressant-like effects of chronic nicotine on learned helplessness paradigm in rats. *Biology Psychiatry, 43*, 389–391.

Tao, T. S., Correa, L. D., Adams, P., Santori, E. M., & Sacaan, A. I.(2003). Pharmacological characterization of dopamine, norepinephrine and serotonin in the rat prefrontal cortex by neuronal nicotinic acetylcholine receptor agonists. *Brain Research, 990*, 203–208.

Tsoh, J. Y., Humfleet, G. L., Munoz, R. F., Reus, V. I., Hartz, D. T., & Hall, S. M. (2000). Development of major depression after treatment for smoking cessation. *American Journal of Psychiatry 157*(3), 368–374.

Tzschentke, T. M. (2001). Pharmacology and behavioral pharmacology of the mesocortical dopamine system. *Progress in Neurobiology, 63*(3), 241–320.

Umbriaco, D., Garcia, S., Beaulieu, C., & Descarries, L. (1995). Relational features of acetylcholine, noradrenaline, serotonion and GABA axon terminal in the striatum radiatum of adult rat hippocampus (CA1). *Hippocampus, 5*, 605–620.

Vázquez-Palacios, G., Bonilla-Jaime, H., & Velázquez-Moctezuma, J. (2004). Antidepressant-like effects of the acute and chronic administration of nicotine in the rat forced swimming test and its interaction with flouxetine. *Pharmacology, Biochemistry and Behavior, 78*, 165–169.

Vázquez-Palacios, G., Bonilla-Jaime, H., & Velázquez-Moctezuma, J. (2005). Antidepressant effects of nicotine and fluoxetine in an animal model of depression induced by neonatal treatment with clomipramine. *Progress in Neuropsychopharmacology and Biological Psychiatry, 29*, 39–46.

Velázquez-Moctezuma, J., Shalauta, M. D., Gillin, J. C., & Shiromani, P. J. (1990) Microinjection of nicotine in the medial pontine reticular formation elicits REM sleep. *Neuroscience Letters, 115*, 265-268.

Velázquez-Moctezuma, J., Shiromani, P. J. & Gillin, J. C. (1990). Acetylcholine and acetylcholine receptor subtypes in REM sleep generation. *Progress in Brain Research, 84*, 407–413.

Vezina, P., Herve, D., Glowinski, J., & Tassin, J. P. (1994). Injections of 6-OHDA into the ventral tegmental area destroy mesocorticolimbic dopamine neurons but spare the locomotor activating effects of nicotine. *Neuroscience Letters, 168*, 11–114.

Vizi, E. S., & Kiss, J. P. (1998). Neurochemistry and pharmacology of the major hippocampal transmitter systems: Synaptic and nonsynaptic interactions. *Hippocampus, 8*, 566–607.

Vizi, E. S., & Labos, E. (1991). Nonsynaptic interactions at presynaptic level. *Progress in Neurobiology, 37*, 145–163.

Vizi, E. S., & Lendvai, B. (1999). Modulatory role of presynaptic nicotinic receptors in synaptic and nonsynaptic chemical communication in the central nervous system. *Brain Research Reviews, 30*, 219–235.

Vogel, G., Hartley, P., Neill, D., Hagler, M., & Kors, D. (1990). A new animal model of endogenous depression: A summary of present finding. *Neuroscience Biobehavior Review, 14*, 85–91.

Wada, E., Wada, K., Boulter, J., Deneris, E., Heinemann, S., Patrick, J., & Swanson, L. W. (1989). Distribution of alpha2, alpha3, alpha 4 and beta 2 nicotinic receptor subunit mRNAs in the central nervous system: A hybridization histochemical study in the rat. *Journal of Comparative Neurology, 284*, 314.

Whiting, P., & Lindstrom, J. (1986). Pharmacological properties of immuno-isolated neuronal acetylcholine receptors. *Journal of Neuroscience, 6*, 3061.

Willner, P. (1991). *Behavioral models in psychopharmacology*. Cambridge, UK:Cambridge University Press.

Wonnacott, S. (1997). Presynaptic nicotinic Ach receptors. *Trends in Neuroscience, 20*, 92–98.

Yang, X., Criswell, H. E., & Breese, G. R. (1996). Nicotine-induced inhibition in medial septum involves activation of presynaptic nicotinic cholinergic receptors on gamma-aminobutyric acid-containing neurons. *Journal of Pharmacology and Experimental Therapeutics, 276*, 482–489.

15 Aggression, Fish Oil, and Noradrenergic Activity

Tomohito Hamazaki

KEY POINTS

- Fish oil reduces aggression in young adults, female schoolchildren, and children with attention-deficit/hyperactivity disorder.
- Attention-related symptoms of attention deficit/hyperactivity disorder are improved by learning but not following docosahexaenoic acid.
- The effects of docosahexaenoic acid could be explained by depression of central noradrenergic activity rather than enhancement of central serotonergic activity.
- Central nonadrenergic activity could explain fish oil's preventive effects against sudden cardiac death (lethal arrhythmias).

1. INTRODUCTION

Fish oil is known to exert an influence on behavior and mood. We have been studying the effects of fish oil, especially docosahexaenoic acid (DHA), a major active component of fish oil, on aggression in double-blind trials (*see* below). Cross-national association of economy-related seafood consumption with the incidence of major depression (Hibbeln, 1998) and bipolar disorders (Noaghiul & Hibbeln, 2003) suggest that greater seafood consumption predicts lower lifetime prevalence rates of those psychiatric disorders. Stoll et al. (1999) reported a preliminary interventional trial of patients with bipolar disorder in which symptoms were reduced in the fish oil group. A few double-blind studies (Nemets, Stahl, & Belmaker, 2002; Peet & Horrobin, 2002) aimed at major depression with eicosapentaenoic acid (EPA), another major active fish oil component, were also successful. We recently performed a case-control study of suicide attempt in China and found that EPA and DHA in the red blood cells of suicide attempters (n = 100) were significantly lower than in controls (n = 100) (Huan et al., 2004).

These studies all imply that fish oil may activate the central serotonergic system. However, our other recent studies seem to support a hypothesis that the central noradrenergic system may be depressed by fish oil administration. This chapter discusses the relationship of aggression and fish oil from a new point of view, namely, the central adrenergic system.

From: *Nutrients, Stress, and Medical Disorders*
Edited by: S. Yehuda and D. I. Mostofsky © Humana Press Inc., Totowa, NJ

2. THE AGGRESSION-CONTROLLING EFFECTS OF FISH OIL

About 10 yr ago we performed a double-blind study using students as subjects. Forty-one students were allocated to either a control (n = 22) or a DHA group (n = 19) in a double-blind manner. Subjects of the DHA group were asked to take 10–12 capsules containing DHA-rich fish oil (1.5–1.8g DHA/d) for 3 mo. Those in the control group took a soybean-based control oil. At the start and end of the study, aggression of the subjects was measured with the Picture-Frustration (PF) Study (Rosenzweig, 1978). This psychological test consisted of 24 pictures illustrating frustration. Subjects were asked to look at pictures and describe their first reactions. Their reactions were regarded as aggression if their comments were against others. The degree of aggression was calculated as 100 × total aggressive comments/24. There was a stressor component at the end of the study. A few days after the second (last) PF Study, either the final or most important term exams started for all the subjects. Therefore, subjects were likely stressed while busy preparing for the exams around the last PF Study. Aggression in the control group increased (from 35 to 45; $p < 0.002$) because of the presence of the stressor, but it stayed unchanged (at 31) in the DHA group. There were highly significant differences in changes in aggression between the two groups ($p < 0.003$). This study indicated a possibility that stressor-enhanced aggression might be controlled by prior administration of DHA (Hamazaki et al., 1996). When there was no stressor, DHA supplementation did not decrease aggression, but might even have increased it with marginal significance (Hamazaki et al., 1998).

Several groups of investigators have reported relationships between fish oil and aggression or hostility. Gesch, Hammond, Hampson, Eves, and Crowder (2002) performed a placebo-controlled, double-blind, randomized trial of nutritional supplements (including essential fatty acids) on 231 young adult prisoners for a minimum of 2 wk, and found that, compared with those receiving placebos, those receiving the active capsules committed significantly fewer offenses. The amounts of fatty acids provided to the experimental group were so small—80 mg EPA and 44 mg DHA—that it is difficult to determine if those n-3 fatty acids contributed to reducing the offenses. However, this study is in line with the idea that n-3 fatty acids are able to control aggressive behavior.

Very recently a relationship between DHA and hostility was also found in a large-scale epidemiological study. Iribarren et al. (2004) reported a cross-sectional observational study as part of an ongoing cohort study, the Coronary Artery Risk Development in Young Adults (CARDIA) study. The multivariate odds ratios of scoring in the upper quartile of hostility measure using the Cook-Medley scale were significantly lower by 10% with one standard deviation higher DHA intake.

In one of our recent DHA-supplementation studies, 166 schoolchildren 9–12 yr of age (81 boys and 85 girls) were in a placebo-controlled, double-blind trial (Itomura et al., 2005). Subjects in the DHA group took DHA-fortified foods (3.6 g of DHA + 0.84 g of EPA/wk) for 3 mo. Impulsivity in girls assessed by their parents was significantly decreased in the DHA group compared with the control group. This effect of DHA was not observed in boys. Impulsivity is also related to serotonin function (Krakowski, 2003).

3. DHA, THE SEROTONERGIC SYSTEM, AND AGGRESSION

An inverse relationship between a lifelong aggression history and concentrations of 5-hydroxyindolacetic acid (5-HIAA), the major metabolite of serotonin, in the cerebrospinal fluid (CSF) was shown in a group of 26 age-similar military men with no history of major psychiatric illness (Brown, Goodwin, Bellenger, Goyer, & Major, 1979). Since then, the association between low concentrations of CSF 5-HIAA and aggressive behavior has been pointed out in other studies (Higley et al., 1996; Virkkunen et al., 1994). The relationship between central serotonin and aggressive behavior is further strengthened by intervention studies controlling central serotonin functions. Pihl et al. (1995) administered to normal males amino acid mixtures designed to raise or lower tryptophan availability and thus to raise or lower brain serotonin synthesis; they also administered alcoholic or nonalcoholic drinks. Lowered tryptophan levels and ingestion of alcohol were associated with increased aggression. There are quite a few interventional studies using selective serotonin reuptake inhibitors (SSRIs); impulsive aggressive behavior was reduced with fluoxetine, an SSRI, in patients with personality disorders (Coccaro, Astill, Herbert, & Schut, 1990).

Of particular interest is a finding by Knutson et al. (1998) that an SSRI reduced hostility of normal volunteers in a double-blind trial. They administered paroxetine, an SSRI, or placebo and found that hostility was reduced as early as after 1 wk of treatment. Consequently, central serotonin concentrations may be related to hostility even in people without baseline clinical depression or other psychological disorders. Although there is a complex interplay among various factors like impulse control, affect regulation, substance abuse, and social functioning (Krakowski, 2003), serotonin function is generally believed to affect aggressive behavior, as shown above.

On the other hand, there are associations between DHA and the serotonergic system. In observational studies Hibbeln, Linnoila, et al. (1998) found that higher plasma concentrations of DHA and arachidonic acid predicted higher concentrations of CSF 5-HIAA among healthy volunteers, but plasma concentrations of DHA were inversely correlated with CSF 5-HIAA concentrations among early-onset alcoholics, who are at risk for aggressive behavior. It was also reported that violent subjects had significantly lower concentrations of CSF 5-HIAA than nonviolent subjects matched for their severity of alcohol dependence and that plasma DHA concentrations were inversely correlated with CSF 5-HIAA among those violent subjects (Hibbeln, Umhau, et al., 1998). Consequently, the relationship between plasma DHA levels and CSF 5-HIAA might be different depending on whether study subjects are healthy or early-onset alcoholic, or normal or violent.

From these considerations, the serotonergic system in the frontal cortex seems to link DHA and hostility in healthy humans. However, another hypothesis has developed from an interventional study with children of attention-deficit/hyperactivity disorder (AD/HD), as shown below.

4. TREATMENT OF AD/HD CHILDREN WITH DHA-CONTAINING FOODS

We performed a placebo-controlled, double-blind study to investigate whether DHA supplementation was able to ameliorate AD/HD symptoms in children (Hirayama, Hamazaki, & Terasawa, 2004). The study included 40 AD/HD children 6–12 yr of age who were mostly without medication. Subjects in the DHA group (n = 20) took active foods fortified with fish oil (fermented soybean milk, bread rolls, and steamed bread; 3.6 g DHA/wk from these foods) for 2 mo, whereas those in the control group (n = 20) took indistinguishable control foods without fish oil fortification. The following items were measured at the start and end of the study:

1. Attention deficit, hyperactivity, and impulsivity (AD/HD-related symptoms according to DSM-IV criteria)
2. Aggression assessed by both parents and teachers (counted only if answers of both parents and teachers were the same)
3. Visual perception (finding symbols out of a table)
4. Visual and auditory short-term memory
5. Development of visual-motor integration
6. Continuous performance
7. Impatience

Results were rather unexpected. Changes in tests 1, 2, 3, 5, and 7 over time did not significantly differ between the two groups. However, visual short-term memory and errors of commission (continuous performance) significantly improved in the control group compared with the changes over time in the DHA group (intergroup differences at $p = 0.02$ and 0.001, respectively). Improvement of visual short-term memory and continuous performance in the control group was probably owing to learning effects. These results suggested that DHA supplementation may have canceled the learning effect. Later reassessment (Hamazaki & Hirayama, 2004) revealed that aggression was significantly decreased in the DHA group, if the scores of parents and teachers were combined, even when their assessment did not agree. Aggression is not the primary symptom of AD/HD, but AD/HD subjects are quite often aggressive because of interpersonal stress.

Our findings that DHA administration canceled the learning effect are similar to the results of an intervention study with AD/HD children performed by Voigt et al. (2001). They administered 345 mg DHA/d for 4 mo in a placebo-controlled, double-blind study. Errors of omission (a simple measure of inattention of the test of variables of attention performed in their study) were significantly increased in their DHA group, although there were no significant differences between the DHA and control groups (Voigt et al., 2001).

Deterioration of attention compared with the control group cannot be explained by enhanced serotonergic function in the DHA group. The reasons why attention deteriorated in the DHA group were not clear, but the noradrenergic system might be the key point. The main mechanism of psychostimulants, which are often used to ameliorate the symptoms of AD/HD, likely depends on enhancing release of noradrenaline from sympathetic nerve endings and chromaffin cells (Cooper, Bloom, & Roth, 2003; Rothman et al., 2001) and on activation of the noradrenergic system in the brain, which in turn modulates higher cortical functions including attention (Biederman & Spencer, 1999). DHA administration seems to have exerted the exactly opposite influence. Thus, we propose a new hypothesis: DHA suppresses the noradrenergic system. This hypothesis also agrees with aggression-control effects shown in students (Hamazaki et al., 1996) and AD/HD children (Hamazaki & Hirayama, 2004), because aggression is intimately related with stimulation of the noradrenergic system (Haller, Makara, & Kruk, 1998).

5. OTHER CIRCUMSTANTIAL EVIDENCE INDICATING THAT DHA DECREASES CENTRAL NORADRENERGIC ACTIVITY

We performed two intervention studies using young adults as subjects to investigate the effects of fish oil administration on peripheral noradrenaline concentrations. The first study was done with medical students who were under the chronic stress of term exams for more than 2 mo. The study started just before the exams and ended during the exams. During that period, DHA-rich fish oil (1500 mg DHA + 170 mg EPA/d) or placebo capsules were administered in a double-blind fashion. Fasting blood samples after a 30-min rest with a catheter in a forearm vein were obtained at the start and end of the study for catecholamine measurements. In the DHA group, the plasma ratio of adrenaline to noradrenaline at rest was significantly increased in both intra- and intergroup comparison (Sawazaki, Hamazaki, Yazawa, & Kobayashi, 1999). Plasma noradrenaline concentrations were significantly decreased in the DHA group, but intergroup comparison showed a tendency toward significance.

In the second double-blind study (Hamazaki et al., in press), students were used as subjects again, but the study period did not occur during any term exams. In the fish oil group, 760 mg of EPA + DHA administered daily for 2 mo. Plasma noradrenaline concentrations were significantly decreased in the fish oil group compared with the control group.

The baseline plasma noradrenaline concentrations in the second study were markedly lower than those of the first study, reflecting the fact that subjects in the second study were not under serious psychological stress, as in the case of the first study. The effect of fish oil on lowering plasma noradrenaline was observed irrespective of whether study subjects were under chronic stress or not. Although peripheral noradrenaline values do not directly reflect its central activity, both peripheral and central noradrenergic activities often vary together (Peskind et al., 1995; Svensson, 1987). Therefore, the central noradrenergic system seemed depressed with fish oil administration.

Plasma noradrenaline values at rest did not vary after fish oil administration in other studies with healthy subjects. Hughes et al. (1991) performed a double-blind crossover trial and found that fish oil-treated, normotensive, or hypertensive groups had similar changes in blood pressure, plasma catecholamine levels, and β-endorphins during the cold pressor test. Mills, Mah, Ward, Morris, and Floras (1990) performed a randomized, double-blind trial to investigate the effects of dietary fatty acids on cardiovascular responses to lower-body negative pressure. They found that fish oil increased forearm blood flow after forearm ischemia, but no difference in plasma noradrenaline values was observed. The administration period of 1 mo employed in these two studies (Hughes et al., 1991; Mills et al., 1990) might be too short for *n*-3 fatty acids to affect the peripheral noradrenaline value.

6. EFFECT OF DHA OR FISH OIL ON BEHAVIOR THROUGH SEROTONERGIC AND NORADRENERGIC FUNCTIONS

Figure 1 shows the effects of DHA on behavior described in this chapter. If the central noradrenergic activity is downregulated by DHA or fish oil, what is the mechanism? Does enhanced central serotonergic activity have something to do the central noradrenergic system? Although the inhibitory action of peripheral serotonin and related drugs on neurotransmitter release from postganglionic sympathetic nerves has been repeatedly confirmed with many different models (Saxena & Villalón, 1990), the SSRI fluvoxamine increases endogenous noradrenaline release in the locus ceruleus in rat brain slices (Palij & Stamford, 1994). In addition, the serotonin releaser and uptake inhibitor fenfluramine increases noradrenergic activity in the locus ceruleus (Clement, Gemsa, & Wesemann, 1992). Therefore, it is not likely that the decrease in plasma noradrenaline levels by DHA

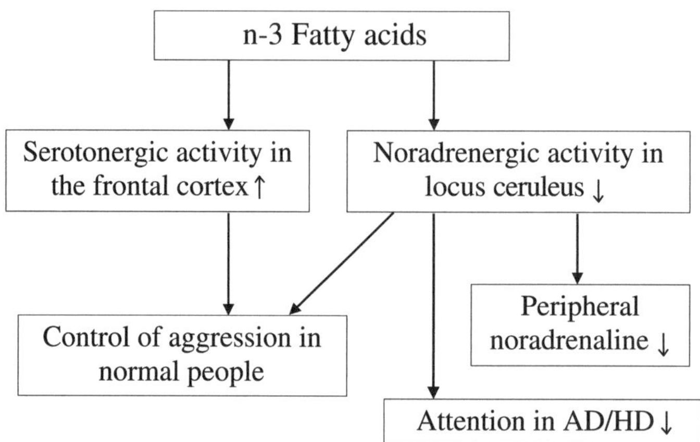

Fig. 1. Proposed effects of *n*-3 fatty acids on serotonergic and noradrenergic activity.

administration observed in our studies is through changes in central serotonergic neuronal activity. Inhibition of corticotropin-releasing factor (CRF) activity may reduce plasma noradrenaline levels, but reduction in CRF by DHA administration has not been reported. Further investigations are necessary.

7. CONCLUSIONS

Prior administration of fish oil diminished enhancement of aggression during times of mental stress in healthy young students. A large-scale epidemiological study (the CARDIA study) indicated that eating fish was related to lower hostility. Impulsivity of girls (9–12 yr of age) rated by their parents was significantly reduced after DHA-fortified food supplementation in a double-blind study. Aggressive behavior of children with AD/HD was also reduced during the fish-oil-administration period. These effects of fish oil are reasonably attributed to the enhancement of serotonin function by the DHA or *n*-3 fatty acids contained in fish oil. However, in the trial with AD/HD children we found that the scores of attention-related tests improved in the control group during the intervention period of 2 mo, probably owing to a learning effect. Subjects in the DHA showed no improvement. This nonbeneficial effect of DHA on attention might be explained more easily through depression of the central noradrenergic system than the serotonergic system. Actually, plasma noradrenaline concentrations were significantly reduced in our two intervention studies with fish oil. Central noradrenergic function may become another key issue when behavior, mood, or stress is discussed in the context of fatty acid nutrition. Our recent studies indicate that fish oil may depress central noradrenergic activity. This hypothesis may help to explain the effects of fish oil on behavior, including stress-associated aggression, but further investigations are necessary.

REFERENCES

Biederman, J., & Spencer, T. (1999). Attention-deficit/hyperactivity disorder (ADHD) as a noradrenergic disorder. *Biological Psychiatry, 46*, 1234–1242.

Brown, G. L., Goodwin, F. K., Ballenger, J. C., Goyer, P. F., & Major, L. F. (1979). Aggression in humans correlates with cerebrospinal fluid amine metabolites. *Psychiatry Research, 1*, 131–139.

Clement, H. W., Gemsa, D., & Wesemann, W. (1992). Serotonin-norepinephrine interactions: A voltametric study on the effect of serotonin receptor stimulation followed in the n. raphe dorsalis and the locus coeruleus of the rat. *Journal of Neural Transmission (General Section), 88*, 11–23.

Coccaro, E. F., Astill, J. L., Herbert, J. L., & Schut, A. G. (1990). Fluoxetine Treatment of Impulsive Aggression in DSM-III-R Personality Disorder Patients. *Journal of Clinical Psychopharmacology, 10*, 373–375.

Cooper, J. R., Bloom, F. E., & Roth, R. H. (2003). Noradrenaline and adrenaline. In *Biochemical Basis of Neuropharmacology* (8th ed., pp. 181–224). New York: Oxford University Press.

Gesch, C. B., Hammond, S. M., Hampson, S. E., Eves, A., & Crowder, M. J. (2002). Influence of supplementary vitamins, minerals and essential fatty acids on the antisocial behaviour of young adult prisoners. *British Journal of Psychiatry, 181*, 22–28.

Haller, J., Makara, G. B., & Kruk, M. R. (1998). Catecholaminergic involvement in the control of aggression: Hormones, the peripheral sympathetic, and central noradrenergic systems. *Neuroscience and Biobehavioral Reviews, 22*, 85–97.

Hamazaki, K., Itomura, M., Huan, M., Nishizawa, H., Sawazaki, S., Tanouchi, M., Watanabe, S., Hamazaki, T., Terasawa, K., & Yazawa, K. (2005, in press). The effect of ω-3 fatty acid-containing phospholipids on blood catecholamine concentrations in healthy volunteers: a randomized, placebo-controlled, double-blind trial. *Nutrition*.

Hamazaki, T., Sawazaki, S., Itomura, M., Asaoka, E., Nagao, Y., Nishimura, N., Yazawa, K., Kuwamori, T., & Kobayashi, M. (1996). The effect of docosahexaenoic acid on aggression in young adults. A placebo-controlled double-blind study. *Journal of Clinical Investigation, 97*, 1129–1133.

Hamazaki, T., Sawazaki, S., Nagao, Y., Kuwamori, T., Yazawa, K., Mizushima, Y., & Kobayashi, M. (1998). Docosahexaenoic acid does not affect aggression of normal volunteers under nonstressful conditions. A randomized, placebo-controlled, double-blind study. *Lipids, 33*, 663–667.

Hamazaki, T., & Hirayama S. (2004). Re: The effect of docosahexaenoic acid-containing food administration on symptoms of attention-deficit/hyperactivity disorder—a placebo-controlled double-blind study [letter to the editor]. *European Journal of Clinical Nutrition, 58*, 838.

Hibbeln, J. R. (1998). Fish Consumption and Major Depression. *Lancet, 351*, 1213.

Hibbeln, J. R., Linnoila, M., Umhau, J. C., Rawlings, R., George, D. T., & Salem, N., Jr. (1998). essential fatty acids predict metabolites of serotonin and dopamine in cerebrospinal fluid among healthy control subjects, and early- and late-onset alcoholics. *Biological Psychiatry, 44*, 235–242.

Hibbeln, J. R., Umhau, J. C., Linnoila, M., George, D. T., Ragan, P. W., Shoaf, S. E., Vaughan, M. R., Rawlings, R., & Salem, N., Jr. (1998). A replication study of violent and nonviolent subjects: Cerebrospinal fluid metabolites of serotonin and dopamine are predicted by plasma essential fatty acids. *Biological Psychiatry, 44*, 243–249.

Higley, J. D., Mehlman, P. T., Poland, R. E., Taub, D. M., Vickers, J., Suomi, S. J., & Linnoila, M. (1996). CSF testosterone and 5-HIM correlate with different types of aggressive behaviors. *Biological Psychiatry, 40*, 1067–1082.

Hirayama, S., Hamazaki, T., & Terasawa K. (2004). The effect of docosahexaenoic acid-containing food administration on symptoms of attention-deficit/hyperactivity disorder—a placebo-controlled double-blind study. *European Journal of Clinical Nutrition, 58*, 467–473.

Huan, M., Hamazaki, K., Sun, Y., Itomura, M., Liu, H., Kang, W., Watanabe, S., Terasawa, K., & Hamazaki, T. (2004). Suicide attempt and n-3 fatty acid levels in red blood cells: A case control study in China. *Biological Psychiatry, 56*, 490–496.

Hughes, G. S., Jr., Ringer, T. V., Francom, S. F., Caswell, K. C., DeLoof, M. J., & Spillers, C. R. (1991). Effects of fish oil and endorphins on the cold pressor test in hypertension. *Clinical Pharmacology and Therapeutics, 50*, 538–546.

Iribarren, C., Markovitz, J. H., Jacobs, D. R., Jr., Schreiner, P. J., Daviglus, M., & Hibbeln, J. R. (2004). Dietary intake of n-3, n-6 fatty acids and fish: Relationship with hostility in young adults—the CARDIA study. *European Journal of Clinical Nutrition, 58*, 24–31.

Itomura, M., Hamazaki, K., Sawazaki, S., Kobayashi, M., Terasawa, K., Watanabe, S., & Hamazaki, T. (2005). The effect of fish oil on physical aggression in schoolchildren—A randomized, double-blind, placebo-controlled trial. *Journal of Nutritional Biochemistry, 16*, 163–171.

Knutson, B., Wolkowitz, O. M., Cole, S. W., Chan, T., Moore, E. A., Johnson, R. C., Terpstra, J., Turner, R. A., & Reus, V. I. (1998). selective alteration of personality and social behavior by serotonergic intervention. *American Journal of Psychiatry, 155*, 373–379.

Krakowski, M. (2003). Violence and serotonin: Influence of impulse control, affect regulation, and social functioning. *Journal of Neuropsychiatry and Clinical Neurosciences, 15*, 294–305.

Mills, D. E., Mah, M., Ward, R. P., Morris, B. L., & Floras, J. S. (1990). Alteration of baroreflex control of forearm vascular resistance by dietary fatty acids. *American Journal of Physiology, 259*, R1164–1171.

Nemets, B., Stahl, Z., & Belmaker, R. H. (2002). Addition of omega-3 fatty acid to maintenance medication treatment for recurrent unipolar depressive disorder. *American Journal of Psychiatry, 159*, 477–479.

Noaghiul, S., & Hibbeln, J. R. (2003). Cross-national Comparisons of Seafood Consumption and Rates of Bipolar Disorders. *American Journal of Psychiatry, 160*, 2222–2227.

Palij, P., & Stamford, J. A. (1994). Real-time monitoring of endogenous noradrenaline release in rat brain slices using fast cyclic voltametry: 3. Selective detection of noradrenaline efflux in the locus coeruleus. *Brain Research, 634*, 275–282.

Peet, M., & Horrobin, D. F. (2002). A dose-ranging study of the effects of ethyl-eicosapentaenoate in patients with ongoing depression despite apparently adequate treatment with standard drugs. *Archives of General Psychiatry, 59*, 913–919.

Peskind, E. R., Wingerson, D., Murray, S., Pascualy, M., Dobie, D. J., Le Corre, P., Le Verge, R., Veith, R. C., & Raskind, M. A. (1995). Effects of Alzheimer's disease and normal aging on cerebrospinal fluid norepinephrine responses to yohimbine and clonidine. *Archives of General Psychiatry, 52*, 774–782.

Pihl, R. O., Young, S. N., Harden, P., Plotnick, S., Chamberlain, B., & Ervin, F. R. (1995). Acute effect of altered tryptophan levels and alcohol on aggression in normal human males. *Psychopharmacology, 119*, 353–360.

Rosenzweig, S. (1978). *Rosenzweig picture-frustration study: Basic manual.* St. Louis: Rana House.

Rothman, R. B., Baumann, M. H., Dersch, C. M., Romero, D. V., Rice, K. C., Carroll, F. I., & Partilla, J. S. (2001). Amphetamine-type central nervous system stimulants release noradrenaline more potently than they release dopamine and serotonin. *Synapse, 39*, 32–41.

Sawazaki, S., Hamazaki, T., Yazawa, K., & Kobayashi, M. (1999). The effect of docosahexaenoic acid on plasma catecholamine concentrations and glucose tolerance during long-lasting psychological stress: A double-blind placebo-controlled study. *Journal of Nutritional Science and Vitaminology, 45*, 655–665.

Saxena, P. R. & Villalón, C. M. (1990). cardiovascular effects of serotonin agonists and antagonists. *Journal of Cardiovascular Pharmacology, 15*(Suppl. 7), S17–S34.

Stoll, A. L., Severus, W. E., Freeman, M. P., Rueter, S., Zboyan, H. A., Diamond, E., Cress, K. K., & Marangell, L. B. (1999). Omega 3 fatty acids in bipolar disorder: A preliminary double-blind, placebo-controlled trial. *Archives of General Psychiatry, 56*, 407–412.

Svensson, T. H. (1987). Peripheral, autonomic regulation of locus coeruleus noradrenergic neurons in brain: Putative implications for psychiatry and psychopharmacology. *Psychopharmacology, 92*, 1–7.

Virkkunen, M., Rawlings, R., Tokola, R., Poland, R. E., Guidotti, A., Nemeroff, C., Bissette, G., Kalogeras, K., Karonen, S.-L., & Linnoila, M. (1994). CSF biochemistries, glucose metabolism, and diurnal activity rhythms in alcoholic, violent offenders, fire setters, and healthy volunteers. *Archives of General Psychiatry, 51*, 20–27.

Voigt, R. G., Llorente, A. M., Jensen, C. L., Fraley, J. K., Berretta, M. C., & Heird, W. C. (2001). A randomized, double-blind, placebo-controlled trial of docosahexaenoic acid supplementation in children with attention-deficit/hyperactivity disorder. *Journal of Pediatrics, 139*, 189–196.

16 Stress in the Pathogenesis of Eating Disorders and Obesity

Gal Dubnov and Elliot M. Berry

KEY POINTS

- Anorexia nervosa, bulimia nervosa, and obesity are multifactorial disease states caused by biological, psychological, and social factors acting on a genetic background.
- Mental stress may act as a powerful inhibitor or stimulator of food intake, depending on the circumstances.
- Various animal models combined with human studies identify the hypothalamic–pituitary–adrenal axis as the principal mechanism for stress-induced disordered eating.
- Attempting to reduce anxiety by overeating can be an important factor in perpetuating the current obesity epidemic.
- Understanding the mechanism of diseases with either extreme anorexia or increased appetite will aid in their prevention and treatment.

1. INTRODUCTION

Eating disorders and obesity are multifactorial disease conditions with several accompanying comorbidities, including a shortened life span. Entangled among their risk factors and within their intricate pathogenesis is mental stress. This power of the mind has been repeatedly shown to affect somatic illnesses, most commonly coronary artery disease (Iso et al., 2002; Krantz, Shaps, Carrey, & Natelson, 2000; Sheps et al., 2002), so mental stress may convincingly result in physical harm. The center of appetite regulation is in close proximity to areas that control the stress response in the hypothalamus, hence the connection between feeding regulation and stress seems not to be by chance. It should be noted that the topic is broad, and the interrelationships within and between biological, psychological, and social factors are complex. This chapter will present several key issues regarding the role of stress in the pathogenesis and etiology of eating disorders, chiefly anorexia nervosa (AN), bulimia nervosa (BN), and obesity.

2. STRESS IN ANOREXIA NERVOSA

AN is a complex disease condition in which a mental state and biological factors act on a genetic susceptibility and result in extreme thinness and its severe medical and psychological sequelae. According to the *Diagnostic and Statistical Manual of Mental*

From: *Nutrients, Stress, and Medical Disorders*
Edited by: S. Yehuda and D. I. Mostofsky © Humana Press Inc., Totowa, NJ

Table 1
DSM-IV Criteria for Anorexia Nervosa

1. Intense fear of becoming fat or gaining weight, even though underweight.
2. Refusal to maintain body weight at or above a minimally normal weight for age and height (i.e., weight loss leading to maintenance of body weight <85% of that expected or failure to make expected weight gain during period of growth, leading to body weight <85% of that expected).
3. Disturbed body image, undue influence of shape or weight on self-evaluation, or denial of the seriousness of the current low body weight.
4. Amenorrhea or absence of at least three consecutive menstrual cycles (those with periods only inducible after estrogen therapy are considered amenorrheic).

Source: American Psychiatric Association, 1994.

Disorders, Fourth Edition (DSM-IV) (American Psychiatric Association, 1994), AN is diagnosed when a subject has four of the diagnostic criteria presented in Table 1. Two types of AN are identified: a restrictive type, characterized by inhibition of food intake and no regular purging, and a binge-eating/purging type, where regular binging and purging occur. The pathogenesis of AN, like that of most diseases, includes genetic, biological, and environmental factors (Fairburn & Harrison, 2003). The genetic component is estimated to account for 48–76% of the risk, as inferred from twin studies. The biological component can be demonstrated by animal studies of neurotransmitter functions or by examples of eating disorders induced/maintained by intracranial lesions (Ward, Tiller, Treasure, & Russell, 2000). In this review of selected cases, several patients with intracranial lesions are presented, and additional similar reports are quoted. These examples underscore the importance of proper functioning of our feeding center in appetite regulation. The environmental factors affecting it act at several levels, including psychological, social, and familial elements. One of these environmental risk factors may be stress (Slade, 1982).

2.1. Animal Models of Stress-Induced Anorexia Nervosa

Although very useful in the laboratory setting, animal models for such complex and multifactorial disease processes will rarely equal the actual human illness. However, they provide important clues regarding constituents of the etiology. Several models of stress-induced anorexia exist, using mainly rodents and utilizing various stressors (Siegfried, Berry, Had, & Avraham, 2003). These include tail pinching, cold swimming, electric shock, noise, separation, immobilization, and others. In our laboratory we have used three models of stress-induced anorexia that mimic some of the aspects of the clinical picture of AN. These include separation, activity, or diet restriction (DR), all causing a weight loss of around 25% of initial weight. In the separation model, mice are held in a cage so that they can smell and see each other, yet physical contact is limited to meals only (van Leeuwen, Bonne, Avraham, & Berry, 1997). This model is easy and simple to perform, produces rapid weight loss, inflicts pure mental stress without the physical component of pain, and is one of the more ethical stress situations. Use of this model revealed that separation causes severe weight loss and impaired cognitive function through modification of acetylcholine and monoamine neurotransmitter actions (Hao, Avraham, Bonne, & Berry, 2001). The second model, increased activity, resembles the exaggerated physical activity performed by many AN patients together with reduced caloric intake. The activity model includes placing animals on a running wheel for several hours daily together with dietary restriction and results in a lower food intake, sometimes to the extreme of self-starvation and death. This model also induces amenorrhea, a prerequisite for the clinical diagnosis of AN. Once again, cholinergic, adrenergic, and serotonergic tones were altered with concomitant weight loss (Avraham, Hao, Mendelson, & Berry, 2001). It should be emphasized that in addition to the imposed dietary restriction, the mice displayed an additional voluntary decrease in food intake. The third model involves diet restriction alone, and once again neuroendocrine changes are demonstrated (Avraham, Bonne, & Berry, 1996; Avraham, Hao, Mendelson, Bonne, & Berry, 2001). Other stress–induced anorexia models also provide insight into this phenomenon. For example, in a study of chronic stress of varying intensities and duration, it was found that intensity was more important than duration (Marti, Marti, & Armario, 1994). Rats were exposed to increasing levels of stress, and it was found that food intake was unaffected by handling, slightly reduced by restraint, and significantly reduced by immobilization. This suggests a dose-dependent inhibition of food intake by stress, while the duration of the stressor seemed to have no effect. In a model of social stress brought about by dominance seeking among male rats, it was found that while the fight for dominance caused weight loss, it was much more so in the subordinate animals (Tamashiro et al., 2004). Further, when two males had to compete for dominance, the weight loss of the subordinate one was much larger than that of the three subordinate rats when four males were competing, also suggesting some form of dose dependency. The decreased weight of all competing animals was sustained throughout the 14-d experiment, as compared to that of control noncompeting rats.

Although chronic stress may play a central role in AN pathogenesis, studies have shown that even a single stressing event can reduce food intake (Alario, Gamallo, Beato, & Trancho, 1987; Ciccocioppo, Martin-Fardon, Weiss, & Massi, 2001), lasting for as long as 9 d (Valles, Marti, Garcia, & Armario, 2000). In this latter study, return to normal food intake following psychological stress induced by immobilization was even slower than that following the physical stress of lipopolysaccharide administration, even though lipopolysaccharide caused a larger decrease in food intake. The immobilized rats had a persistently lower body weight even 15 d after the 2-h stressing event. This suggests that in this matter, the power of the "mind"/memory may be stronger than that of the somatic body. Interestingly, not only the amount of food was affected by stress, but that of specific macronutrients as well: acute (2 h) and chronic (2 h daily for 5 d) stress resulted in lower carbohydrate and fat intake, with no change in protein intake. Hence food selection may also be altered by stress, and not only by its quantity. These data show that the stress does not have to be daily: even if a stressor acts every once in a while, it may have a lasting effect on food intake.

Given the biopsychosocial hypotheses for developing eating disorders, animal models that provide a combination of genetics and environment are even more promising. The two genetic models, Crhr2-deficient and CB1-deficient mice, show a disordered feeding phenotype only while temporary food restriction is forced (Bale et al., 2000; Di Marzo et al., 2001). These mutant mice showed a lower increase in food consumption following food restriction, as compared to normal mice. This resembles the clinical picture of eating disorders, where an apparently healthy adolescent (yet with a supposedly pathological genetic and/or biological background) is driven into a state of voluntary reduced eating.

2.2. Human Studies of Stress-Induced Anorexia Nervosa

Although interventional trials of stress induction may be performed in laboratory animals, these are harder to apply in human volunteers, mainly owing to ethical reasons. Therefore, the use of observational studies—with their large risk of bias in such a population—is more frequent. It is commonly believed that stress plays a factor in eating disorders (Slade, 1982), and this was shown in several studies. A stressing event prior to disease onset was reported by two-thirds of anorectic patients (Schmidt, Tiller, Blanchara, Andrews, & Treasure, 1997), while hospitalized anorectics report more negative life events than healthy controls or patients with other psychiatric states (Horesh et al., 1995). In cross sectional analyses, stress and anorexia are found to coincide (Ball & Lee, 2002). Another study conducted among female teenagers again found that increased levels of stressors were related to eating disorders, the relationship partly mediated by low self-esteem (Fryer, Waller, & Kroese, 1997).

Three longitudinal studies (Ball & Lee, 2002; Patton, Johnson-Sabine, Wood, Mann, & Wakeling, 1990; Rosen, Compas, & Tacy, 1993) did not find a strong relationship between stress and later eating disorders. Although eating disorders were related to stress in the cross-sectional analysis at the beginning of follow-up, stress did not predict future eating disorders (Ball & Lee, 2002; Rosen, Compas, & Tacy, 1993). In one study the opposite was found—that eating disorders at baseline predicted future stress (Rosen, Compas, & Tacy, 1993). This shows the importance of longitudinal studies in search of risk factors for such complex disease processes. However, these data cannot prove that stress has no role in AN pathogenesis. As seen in the animal studies described above, the initial stressful episode/period causes a *transient* reduction of food intake, even though it may last for several days. It is not truly expected that a single stress situation alone will initiate clinical AN, although most AN patients describe a severe event or a marked difficulty in the year prior to their illness onset (Schmidt et al., 1997). Further, the reproducible connection between stress and AN in cross-sectional studies perhaps suggests that stress *maintains* the eating disorder. Thus, perhaps a stressful event initiated the disease, but current stress continues to maintain it. Some authors propose that AN patients use the feeling of control to alleviate their feeling of stress (Slade, 1982).

In summary, data from animal studies and cross-sectional ones strongly suggest a role for stress in initiating eating disorders, yet higher-quality follow-up studies suggest that a transient stressful period does not necessarily result in an eating disorder. It is possible that chronic stress acting throughout the disease helps to sustain the eating disorder to the point where biological changes take effect and control is lost. A large body of research is therefore needed in order to untangle the numerous risk factors of such a multifactorial disease and elucidate the role of stress. Better methodology should always be pursued so as to minimize the several types of bias associated with questionnaire use among patients with psychopathologies.

3. STRESS IN BULIMIA NERVOSA

In BN, the individual engages in recurrent bouts of overeating (binging episodes) after which a catharsis is sought in the form of vomiting, laxative or diuretic use, fasting, or exercising—all methods to compensate for the overeating bout and maintain body image and weight. According to the DSM-IV (American Psychiatric Association, 1994), BN is

Table 2
DSM-IV Criteria for Bulimia Nervosa

1. Recurrent episodes of binge eating, characterized by:
   a. Eating a substantially larger amount of food in a discrete period of time (i.e., 2 h) than would be eaten by most people in similar circumstances during that same time period.
   b. A sense of lack of control over eating during the binge.
2. Recurrent inappropriate compensatory behavior to prevent weight gain; i.e., self-induced vomiting, use of laxatives, diuretics, fasting, or hyperexercising.
3. Binges or inappropriate compensatory behaviors occuring, on average, at least twice weekly for at least 3 mo.
4. Self-evaluation unduly influenced by body shape or weight.
5. The disturbance does not occur exclusively during episodes of anorexia nervosa.

Source: American Psychiatric Association, 1994.

diagnosed when a subject has the diagnostic criteria presented in Table 2. As seen in AN, mental state, biological factors, and genetic susceptibility combine to form the disease (Fairburn & Harrison, 2003). The genetic part is believed to account for 30–80% of the disease, as may be seen in several studies performed to date. Once again, environmental factors are assumed to drive the person into the obsession of weight control and maintaining the disordered eating.

Stress from various sources can play a role in the emergence of BN (Fairburn, Welch, Doll, Davies, & O'Connor, 1997), just as was found for AN. The similarity between the eating behavior in BN and that in the binging and purging type of AN suggests a similarity in their pathogenesis and relation to stress. The more interesting issue is how stress induces a restriction in food intake in one individual but a binging or bulimic phenotype in another. In a study designed to assess changes in food amount and selection, a similar proportion of subjects reported overeating (~40%) or decreased eating (~40%) during stress, whereas the remaining 20% reported that their food intake was unchanged following stress (Oliver & Wardle, 1999). The fact that a large number of healthy adults change their food intake during stress highlights the feasible role of stress in initiating and maintaining eating disorders. In addition, most subjects reported an increased intake of snacks during stress, including subjects reporting overall decreased food consumption. An interventional study by these researchers confirmed the preference for sweet foods following mental stress (Oliver, Wardle, & Gibson 2000); hence, stress also brings about a change in food selection.

There is no explanation at this point in time as to why some people decrease and some increase food intake under stress. One possibility involves study methodology: we tend to group different causes of stress, disregarding their impact on emotion. In their review, Canetti, Bachar, and Berry (2002) summarized how different emotions bring about different changes in food intake. For example, boredom, depression, fatigue, anger, or joy may bring about higher food intake, but fear, tension, pain, or sadness may result in lower intake. Perhaps certain subtypes of stressful events in a susceptible person favor developing AN, and others increase the chance for BN. Several studies demonstrate the role of stress in binge eating and BN. Recent work in our laboratory has shown that binging/purging behavior may have a different genetic background than the restrictive behavior involving the cannabinoid system (Siegfried et al., 2004).

3.1. Animal Models in Stress-Induced Binge Eating

The animal models used for the study of BN, binging-type AN, or binge-eating disorder are those that engage in binging episodes. We are unaware of laboratory animals who engage in voluntary purging, whether vomiting or exercising excessively in order to lose weight. One of the more interesting models only recently presented is that of a rat that, following a period of dietary restriction and electric shock (= stress) will eat significantly more when exposed to palatable food (Hagan, Chandler, Wauford, Rybak, & Oswald, 2003; Hagan et al., 2002). There are precise requirements for the diet–shock–palatable food combination in order to produce the hyperphagia: it does not occur after stress alone, after diet restriction alone, if they are far apart, or if the food offered is normal chow. These prerequisites somewhat resemble the multifactorial origin of eating disorders and highlight the complexity of the process. Another model of stress-induced eating, without a painful physical stressor, involves use of white noise (Krebs, Weyers, Macht, Weijers, & Janke, 1997). Here, rats exposed to the noise consumed their meals faster than their peer controls, clearly resembling a binging episode. These animal models will certainly allow for a better understanding of binge-eating episodes, yet more research is needed to create additional models of such overeating.

3.2. Human Studies of Stress-Induced Binge Eating

Studies have shown that continuous stressful life events predispose to binge eating and to BN (Fairburn et al., 1997, 1998). These include negative self-evaluation, adverse childhood experiences, and repeated comments about body shape, weight, or eating. The stress of adapting to new cultural surroundings, termed acculturative stress, has also been found to correlate with bulimic symptoms (Perez, Voelz, Pettit, & Joiner, 2002). In a study conducted among women who engaged in binge eating, it was found that daily problems—another form of continuous stress—resulted in an increase in energy intake, despite no effect on the number of binge episodes (Crowther, Sanftner, Bonifazi, & Sheperd, 2001). It is noteworthy that while daily problems did not differ between the patients and controls, they were perceived as more stressful, suggesting impaired coping among women with the eating disorder. Hence, stress did not bring about more binge episodes, but did increase food intake eventually. These examples of studies regarding various stressors indicate that various types of stress act as factors in the spectrum of disorders of binge eating.

4. THE BIOLOGICAL MECHANISM OF STRESS-INDUCED EATING DISORDERS

It is quite apparent that the mechanism of mental stress-induced anorexia involves the hypothalamic–pituitary–adrenal (HPA) axis. This comes from studies where food intake was reduced by both mental stress and stress hormone administration, such as adrenocorticotropic hormone (ACTH), dexamaethasone, and corticotropin-releasing factor (CRF) (Alario et al., 1987; Ciccocioppo et al., 2001; Glowa & Gold, 1991). Another important link between mental stress and CRF comes from the administration of an endogenous ligand to the opioid receptor-like 1 (nociceptin/orphanin FQ): intraventricular injection of this compound obliterated the anorexigenic effect of either electric footshock, immobilization, or CRF administration (Ciccocioppo et al., 2001). This provides sound evidence that both CRF-induced and mental stress-induced anorexia share the same pathway. A comprehensive review of the etiology of AN suggests stress as a central factor in this illness (Connan, 2003). It is suggested that both genetic factors and early life experiences, as early as the first prenatal trimester, generate a hypersensitive HPA axis. A persistently elevated CRF level leads to the nutritional imbalance, as observed in animal studies. CRF has an interrelationship with serotonin activity, another factor in appetite regulation, known to be altered in AN patients. It also inhibits synthesis of neuropeptide Y, a hormone acting to increase food intake. An acute stressor that acts upon this hypersensitive stress system may trap the patient in chronic stress, similarly to an allergen acting on the hyperreactive airways of an asthma patient. Later in the disease course, the chronic stress of the AN patient may maintain the increased activation of the HPA axis.

Another interesting finding is that 74% of patients with AN and/or BN had antibodies against rat pituitary cells, directed against melanocyte-stimulating hormone (MSH) or ACTH (Fetissov et al., 2002). This suggests another mechanism connecting the stress axis and eating disorders, an immunological one, although much more study is needed to explain this finding. The authors hypothesized several pathways connecting these autoantibodies with eating disorders and appetite, including neuropeptide Y (a major peptide-stimulating food intake), the melanocortin receptor MC4, inflammatory cytokines, or serotonin—all of which are connected with appetite regulation. Further, an MC4 receptor antagonist has been shown to lessen stress-induced anorexia in rats, yet without having a direct effect on food intake without stress (Chaki, Ogawa, Toda, Funakoshi, & Okuyama, 2003). MSH itself is also connected with appetite, as its administration was previously found to reduce food intake in rats (Oohara, Negishi, Shimizu, Sato, & Mori, 1993), yet interfered with the anorexigenic effect of CRF. Hence, a complex and interrelated pathway of hypothalamic and pituitary stress hormones can affect appetite and food intake, including human AN and BN states.

5. STRESS IN OBESITY

Although not a formal eating disorder, obesity cannot occur without an increased energy intake in relation to the body's energy expenditure. In addition, it has been shown that overweight girls may exhibit some behaviors similar to those with eating disorders, such as concern with weight, shape, eating, dieting, low self-esteem, and more depression (Burrows & Cooper, 2002). These behaviors, in addition to childhood obesity, are recognized risk factors for eating disorders. Among the reasons for the current epidemic of obesity, the unhealthy western lifestyle tops the list: energy intake is increased owing to the appealing deals and increased caloric density, whereas energy output is decreased as a result of staircases, elevators, transportation, television, and computer games. In addition, a stressful lifestyle may also contribute to increased energy intake if one finds comfort in food. For example, one study showed that stress-eaters had a slightly higher body mass index (BMI, in kg/m^2, a measure of adiposity), were more likely to be overweight, and consumed more fast food and energy-dense foods when compared with those not overeating under stress (Laitinen, Ek, & Sovio, 2002). Among women, higher eating during stress was associated with an increased chance of becoming obese.

It has been suggested that stress is a large contributor to modern-day obesity (Bjorntorp, 2001; Dallman et al., 2003; Drapeau, Therrien, Richard, & Tremblay, 2003). Combining data from in vitro studies in animals and in humans, these authors provide evidence that

that is the case. A chronic elevation of cortisol is brought about by longstanding stress, which activates the HPA axis. Cortisol then acts to induce accumulation of visceral fat in addition to a possible increase in food intake. This is seen also in Cushing's syndrome and chronic corticosteroid treatment, suggesting that this effect is indeed related to cortisol. The elevated visceral fat, the increased actions of cortisol, or both may then act to induce insulin resistance and its accompanying metabolic syndrome (Rosmond, 2003). The mechanism suggested is that of chronic resistance to leptin, an appetite-depressing hormone secreted by adipose tissue, with a concomitant increase in the actions of neuropeptide Y, an appetite-stimulating factor. In addition, glucocorticosteroids act centrally in the brain to induce the ingestion of comfort food under stress. Although most of these data emerge from animal studies, the stress effect has also been demonstrated in humans. Among women who reacted to stress by high cortisol secretion, an increase in food intake, especially in high-fat sweet food, was noted when compared with low secretors (Epel, Lapidus, McEwen, & Brownell, 2001). In a large study, stress-related cortisol secretion was related to increased visceral adiposity, a worse lipid profile, higher insulin and glucose levels, and higher blood pressure (Rosmon, Dallman, & Bjorntorp, 1998).

Several theories as to emotion-induced overeating exist (Canetti, Bachar, & Berry, 2002). One is that anxiety results in overeating, which is intended to decrease anxiety. The mechanism may involve an attempt to increase tryptophan delivery to neurons affecting mood, with a resulting elevation in serotonin levels. Serotonin is known to have a role in mood regulation, as its reuptake inhibition is the prime mechanism of a large variety of antidepressant drugs—the selective serotonin reuptake inhibitors (SSRIs). A second mechanism may include modulation of endogenous opioid activity, well known for its rewarding and addictive properties (Yeomans & Gray, 2002). Another explanation for emotion-derived hunger is that the learning process of the hungry feeling has gone wrong, confusing it with other feelings of discomfort. A biological explanation may be that a slowing of gastric contractions under stress results in decreased eating in normal weight individuals, but not in the obese, in whom eating continues. Whatever the mechanism, overeating during stress is a common finding among the obese. Understanding this mechanism is essential in the fight to control the obesity epidemic.

6. CONCLUSION

Mental stress has a role among additional genetic, biological, and psychological factors in initiating and maintaining eating disorders and obesity. The mechanism is believed to involve hyperactivation of the HPA axis, and both animal and human studies allow for a rough explanation for these disorders in which appetite regulation is found. More research is needed to further elucidate the precise mechanisms of over- or undereating during stress, so that psychological and drug therapy may be better tolerated.

REFERENCES

Alario, P., Gamallo, A., Beato, M. J., & Trancho, G. (1987). Body weight gain, food intake and adrenal development in chronic noise stressed rats. *Physiology and Behavior, 40*, 29–32.

American Psychiatric Association. (1994). *Diagnostic and statistical manual of mental disorders: DSM-IV.* Washington, DC: American Psychiatric Association.

Avraham, Y., Bonne, O., & Berry, E. M. (1996). Behavioral and neurochemical alterations caused by diet restriction—the effect of tyrosine administration in mice. *Brain Research, 732*, 133–144.

Avraham, Y., Hao, S. Z., Mendelson, S., & Berry, E. M. (2001). Tyrosine improves appetite, cognition, and exercise tolerance in activity anorexia. *Medicine and Science in Sports and Exercise, 33*, 2104–2110.

Avraham, Y., Hao, S., Mendelson, S., Bonne, O., & Berry, E. M. (2001). Diet restriction in mice causes a decrease in hippocampal choline uptake and muscarinic receptors that is restored by administration of tyrosine: Interaction between cholinergic and adrenergic receptors influencing cognitive function. *Nutritional Neuroscience, 4*, 153–167.

Bale, T. L., Contarino, A. B., Smith, G. W., Chan, R., Gold, L. H., Sawchenko, P. E., Koob, G. F., Vale, W. W., & Lee, K. F. (2000). Mice deficient for corticotropinreleasing hormone receptor-2 display anxiety-like behaviour and are hypersensitive to stress. *Nature Genetics, 24*, 410–404.

Ball, K., & Lee, C. (2002). Psychological stress, coping, and symptoms of disordered eating in a community sample of young Australian women. *International Journal of Eating Disorders, 31*, 71–81.

Bjorntorp, P. (2001). Do stress reactions cause abdominal obesity and comorbidities? *Obesity Reviews, 2*, 73–86.

Burrows, A., & Cooper, M. (2002). Possible risk factors in the development of eating disorders in overweight pre-adolescent girls. *International Journal of Obesity and Relatated Metabolic Disorders, 26*, 1268–1273.

Canetti, L., Bachar, E., & Berry, E. M. (2002). Food and emotion. *Behavioural Processes, 60*, 157–164.

Chaki, S., Ogawa, S., Toda, Y., Funakoshi, T., & Okuyama, S. (2003). Involvement of the melanocortin MC4 receptor in stress-related behavior in rodents. *European Journal of Pharmacology, 474*, 95–101.

Ciccocioppo, R., Martin-Fardon, R., Weiss, F., & Massi, M. (2001). Nociceptin/orphanin FQ inhibits stress- and CRF-induced anorexia in rats. *Neuroreport, 12*, 1145–1149.

Connan, F., Campbell, I. C., Katzman, M., Lightman, S. L., & Treasure, J. (2003). A neurodevelopmental model for anorexia nervosa. *Physiology and Behavior, 79*, 13–24.

Crowther, J. H., Sanftner, J., Bonifazi, D. Z., & Sheperd, K. L. (2001). The role of daily hassles in binge eating. *International Journal of Eating Disorders, 29*, 449–454.

Dallman, M. F., Pecoraro, N., Akana, S. F., La Fleur, S. E., Gomez, F., Houshyar, H., Bell, M. E., Bhatnagar, S., Laugero, K. D., & Manalo, S. (2003). Chronic stress and obesity: A new view of "comfort food." *Proceedings of the National Academy of Sciences of the United States of America, 100*, 11,696–11,701.

Di Marzo, V., Goparaju, S. K., Wang, L., Liu, J., Batkai, S., Jarai, Z., Fezza, F., Miura, G. I., Palmiter, R. D., Sugiura, T., & Kunos, G. (2001). Leptin-regulated endocannabinoids are involved in maintaining food intake. *Nature, 410*, 822–825.

Drapeau, V., Therrien, F., Richard, D., & Tremblay, A. (2003). Is visceral obesity a physiological adaptation to stress? *Panminerva Medica, 45*, 189–195.

Epel, E., Lapidus, R., McEwen, B., & Brownell, K. (2001). Stress may add bite to appetite in women: A laboratory study of stress-induced cortisol and eating behavior. *Psychoneuroendocrinology, 26*, 37–49.

Fairburn, C. G., Doll, H. A., Welch, S. L., Hay, P. J., Davies, B. A., & O'Connor, M. E. (1998). Risk factors for binge eating disorder: A community-based, case-control study. *Archives of General Psychiatry, 55*, 425–432.

Fairburn, C. G., & Harrison, P. J. (2003). Eating disorders. *Lancet, 361*, 407–416.

Fairburn, C. G., Welch, S. L., Doll, H. A., Davies, B. A., & O'Connor, M. E. (1997). Risk factors for bulimia nervosa. A community-based case-control study. *Archives of General Psychiatry, 54*, 509–517.

Fetissov, S. O., Hallman, J., Oreland, L., Af Klinteberg, B., Grenback, E., Hulting, A. L., & Hokfelt, T. (2002). Autoantibodies against alpha-MSH, ACTH, and LHRH in anorexia and bulimia nervosa patients. *Proceedings of the National Academy of Sciences of the United States of America, 99*, 17,155–17,160.

Fryer, S., Waller, G., & Kroese, B. S. (1997). Stress, coping, and disturbed eating attitudes in teenage girls. *International Journal of Eating Disorders, 22*, 427–436.

Glowa, J. R., & Gold, P. W. (1991). Corticotropin releasing hormone produces profound anorexigenic effects in the rhesus monkey. *Neuropeptides,18*, 55–61.

Hagan, M. M., Chandler, P. C., Wauford, P. K., Rybak, R. J., & Oswald, K. D. (2003). The role of palatable food and hunger as trigger factors in an animal model of stress induced binge eating. *International Journal of Eating Disorders, 34*, 183–197.

Hagan, M.M., Wauford, P.K., Chandler, P.C., Jarrett, L.A., Rybak, R.J., & Blackburn, K. (2002). A new animal model of binge eating: Key synergistic role of past caloric restriction and stress. *Physiology and Behavior, 77*, 45–54.

Hao, S. Z., Avraham, Y., Bonne, O., & Berry, E. M. (2001). Separation-induced body weight loss, impairment in alternation behavior, and autonomic tone: Effects of tyrosine. *Pharmacology, Biochemistry, and Behavior, 68*, 273–281.

Horesh, N., Apter, A., Lepkifker, E., Ratzoni, G., Weizmann, R., & Tyano, S. (1995). Life events and severe anorexia nervosa in adolescence. *Acta Psychiatrica Scandinavica, 9*, 15–19.

Iso, H., Date, C., Yamamoto, A., Toyoshima, H., Tanabe, N., Kikuchi, S., Kondo, T., Watanabe, Y., Wada, Y., Ishibashi, T., Suzuki, H., Koizumi, A., Inaba, Y., Tamakoshi, A., & Ohno, Y. (2002). Perceived mental stress and mortality from cardiovascular disease among Japanese men and women: The Japan Collaborative Cohort Study for Evaluation of Cancer Risk Sponsored by Monbusho (JACC Study). *Circulation, 106*, 1229–1236.

Krantz, D. S., Sheps, D. S., Carney, R. M., & Natelson, B. H. (2000). Effects of mental stress in patients with coronary artery disease: Evidence and clinical implications. *Journal of the American Medical Association, 283*, 1800–1802.

Krebs, H., Weyers, P., Macht, M., Weijers, H. G., & Janke, W. (1997). Scanning behavior of rats during eating under stressful noise. *Physiology and Behavior, 62*, 151–154.

Laitinen, J., Ek, E., & Sovio, U. (2002). Stress-related eating and drinking behavior and body mass index and predictors of this behavior. *Preventive Medicine, 3*, 429–439.

Martı, O., Martı, J., & Armario, A. (1994). Effects of chronic stress on food intake in rats: Influence of stressor intensity and duration of daily exposure. *Physiology and Behavior, 55*, 747–753.

Oliver, G., & Wardle, J. (1999). Perceived effects of stress on food choice. *Physiology and Behavior, 66*, 511–515.

Oliver, G., Wardle, J., & Gibson, E. L. (2000). Stress and food choice: A laboratory study. *Psychosomatic Medicine, 62*, 853–865.

Oohara, M., Negishi, M., Shimizu, H., Sato, N., & Mori, M. (1993). Alpha-melanocyte stimulating hormone (MSH) antagonizes the anorexia by corticotropin releasing factor (CRF). *Life Sciences, 53*, 1473–1477.

Patton, G. C., Johnson-Sabine, E., Wood, K., Mann, A. H., & Wakeling, A. (1990). Abnormal eating attitudes in London schoolgirls—a prospective epidemiological study: Outcome at twelve month follow-up. *Psychological Medicine, 20*, 383–394.

Perez, M., Voelz, Z. R., Pettit, J. W., & Joiner, T. E., Jr. (2002). The role of acculturative stress and body dissatisfaction in predicting bulimic symptomatology across ethnic groups. *International Journal of Eating Disorders, 31*, 442–454.

Rosen, J. C., Compas, B. E., & Tacy, B. (1993). The relation among stress, psychological symptoms, and eating disorder symptoms: A prospective analysis. *International Journal of Eating Disorders, 14*, 153–162.

Rosmond, R. (2003). Stress induced disturbances of the HPA axis: A pathway to Type 2 diabetes? *Medical Science Monitor: International Medical Journal of Experimental and Clinical Research, 9*,, RA35–39.

Rosmond, R., Dallman, M. F., & Bjorntorp, P. (1998). Stress-related cortisol secretion in men: relationships with abdominal obesity and endocrine, metabolic and hemodynamic abnormalities. *The Journal of Clinical Endocrinology and Metabolism, 83*, 1853–1859.

Schmidt, U., Tiller, J., Blanchard, M., Andrews, B., & Treasure, J. (1997). Is there a specific trauma precipitating anorexia nervosa? *Psychological Medicine, 27*, 523–530.

Sheps, D. S., McMahon, R. P., Becker, L., Carney, R. M., Freedland, K. E., Cohen, J. D., Sheffield, D., Goldberg, A. D., Ketterer, M. W., Pepine, C. J., Raczynski, J. M., Light, K., Krantz, D. S., Stone, P. H., Knatterud, G. L., & Kaufmann, P. G. (2002). Mental stress-induced ischemia and all-cause mortality in patients with coronary artery disease: Results from the Psychophysiological Investigations of Myocardial Ischemia study. *Circulation, 105*, 1780–1784.

Siegfried, Z., Berry, E. M., Hao, S., & Avraham, Y. (2003). Animal models in the investigation of anorexia. *Physiology and Behavior, 79*, 39–45.

Siegfried, Z., Kanyas, K., Latzer, Y., Karni, O., Bloch, M., Lerer, B., & Berry, E. M. (2004). Association study of cannabinoid receptor gene (CNR1) alleles and anorexia nervosa: Differences between restricting and binging/purging subtypes. *American Journal of Medical Genetics, 125B*, 126–130.

Slade, P. (1982). Towards a functional analysis of anorexia nervosa and bulimia nervosa. *British Journal of Clinical Psychology, 21*(Pt. 3), 167–179.

Tamashiro, K. L., Nguyen, M. M., Fujikawa, T., Xu, T., Yun Ma, L., Woods, S. C., & Sakai, R. R. (2004). Metabolic and endocrine consequences of social stress in a visible burrow system. *Physiology and Behavior, 80*, 683–693.

Valles, A., Marti, O., Garcia, A., & Armario, A. (2000). Single exposure to stressors causes long-lasting, stress-dependent reduction of food intake in rats. *American Journal of Physiology—Regulatory, Integrative and Comparative Physiology, 279*, R1138–1144.

van Leeuwen, S. D., Bonne, O., Avraham, Y., & Berry, E. M. (1997). Separation as a new animal model for self-induced weight loss. *Physiology and Behavior, 62*, 77–81.

Ward, A., Tiller, J., Treasure, J., & Russell, G. (2000). Eating disorders: Psyche or soma? *International Journal of Eating Disorders, 27*, 279–287.

Yeomans, M. R., & Gray, R. W. (2002). Opioid peptides and the control of human ingestive behaviour. *Neuroscience and Biobehavioral Reviews, 26*, 713–728.

IV

Chronic Disorders and Inflammation

17 Effect of Dietary Hypercholesteremia on Host Immune Response

Roger M. Loria

KEY POINTS

- Once the cell membrane capacity to incorporate cholesterol is exceeded, dietary hypercholesteremia leads to the formation of lipid vacuoles in lymphocytes, monocytes, and neutrophils. This is associated with impaired general defense reactions such as inflammation in accordance with Selye's description of the wear-and-tear phenomeneon.
- Excessive dietary cholesterol causes impairment in leukocyte and Kupffer cell functions, as evidenced by reduced clearance of viral and bacterial agents and inability to reject tumor cells. Dietary hypercholesteremia also increases host susceptibility to infections.
- Dietary hypercholesteremia suppresses cell-mediated immunity after its induction.

1. INTRODUCTION

Although the concept of immunonutrition as a subject area and its use (Calder & Kew, 2002) is a relatively recent one, Hippocrates recognized a linkage between nutrition and good health in the following: "If we could give every individual the right amount of nourishment, and exercise, not too little and not too much, we would have found the safest way to health." Many have documented the specific connection between nutrition host resistance and immunity (Field, 2000; Field, Johnson, & Schley, 2002).

The scientific recognition that dietary fat as well as the effects of long-chain polyunsaturated fatty acids (PUFAs), eicosapentaenoic acid (EPA), and docosahexaenoic acid (DHA) have independent effects on immune functions has been subsequently documented (Field et al., 2002; Miles, Allen, & Calder, 2002; Miles, Aston, & Calder, 2003) and therefore will not be discussed here. Elevated dietary cholesterol levels have a particularly significant effect on the immune response (Feo, Canuto, Torrielli, Garcea, & Dianzani, 1976; Loria, Kibrick, & Madge, 1976; Minick, Murphy, & Campbell, 1966) and will be the focus of this chapter.

Evidence that increased stress suppresses host immunity is extensive (Knoflach, Mayrl, Mayerl, Sedivy, & Wick, 2003; Sheridan et al., 1998; Sheridan, Stark, Avitsur, & Padgett, 2000), and it has been reported to influence cholesterol levels (Agarwal, Gupta, Singhal, & Bajpai, 1997; Bianca de Juarez, Iglesias, Scoppa, Agnelli, & Gauna, 2000). Indeed, a positive correlation between lower serum cholesterol levels and perceived lower psycho-

From: *Nutrients, Stress, and Medical Disorders*
Edited by: S. Yehuda and D. I. Mostofsky © Humana Press Inc., Totowa, NJ

logical stress was reported (Thomas, Goodwin, & Goodwin, 1985) in a study of 256 healthy elderly adults who also had higher indices of immune function.

Animal experiments showed that stressed animals had higher levels of total cholesterol and that activation of macrophage with nonspecific activators resulted in lowering of serum cholesterol fraction (Brennan, Fleshner, Watkins, & Maier, 1996). Indeed, our results as well as others show that excessive dietary cholesterol causes impairment in leukocyte and Kupffer cell function, as evidenced by reduced clearance of viral and bacterial agents and an inability to reject tumor cells, even though recognition of the antigen(s) and activation of effector cells have taken place.

Dietary hypercholesteremia does not impair humoral immunity, but suppresses cell-mediated immunity after its induction. The formation of lipid-laden leukocytes/lipophages and their persistence is consistent with the phenomenon of wear-and-tear, resulting in an impaired general defense reactions such as inflammation in accordance with Selye's descriptions (Selye, 1936).

By suppressing host immunity, dietary hypercholesteremia also impairs the host's ability to cope with stress, thereby becoming an independent stress factor.

2. CHOLESTEROL EFFECT LYMPHOCYTES AND MACROPHAGES FUNCTIONS

Cholesterol is an integral part of the cell membrane and of lymphocyte and macrophage membrane domains. It is dispersed throughout the membrane, forming elements called lipid rafts (Edidin, 2003; Kwik et al., 2003). These lipid rafts are composed of high-melting sphingolipids packed with cholesterol and generate a liquid-gel-ordered phase unit.

Data show that the cholesterol content of the lipid rafts determines the ability of the cell to recruit proteins required in the initial steps of T-lymphocyte signaling (Alonso & Millan, 2001; Larbi, Douziech, Dupuis, et al. 2004; Larbi, Douziech, Khalil, et al. 2004; Millan, Montoya, Sanch, Sanchez-Madrid, & Alonso, 2002). In lymphocytes, these lipid raft domains are shown to function in receptor-mediated signaling, pathogen entry and exit, expression of surface-associated molecules, enzymatic activities, cellular activation, signal transduction, and other membrane functions (Calder, 2003). Indeed, the class I human major histocompatibility molecules (HLA) required for antigen presentation for CD8 + effector T lymphocytes show a clustered lateral distribution (homoassociation) at the surface of activated human T and B lymphocytes, as well as virus-transformed T and B lymphoblasts, in contrast to a disperse distribution on resting human peripheral blood lymphocytes (Bene et al., 1994)

Cholesterol enrichment of the plasma membrane increased membrane fluidity and reduced the expression of heavy- and light-chain determinants of HLA-I molecules and free heavy chains.

The concentration and total amount of cholesterol and lipid in the plasma membrane of lymphoblastoid cells appear to be implicated in the regulation of the lateral organization of the membrane, which determines the efficiency of HLA-I molecule presentation (Bodnar, Jenei, Bene, Damjanovich, & Matko, 1996; Bodnar et al., 2003). In humans, membrane cholesterol and phospholipid levels correlate with serum high-density lipoprotein (HDL) concentrations. The results also show that this correlation extends to the

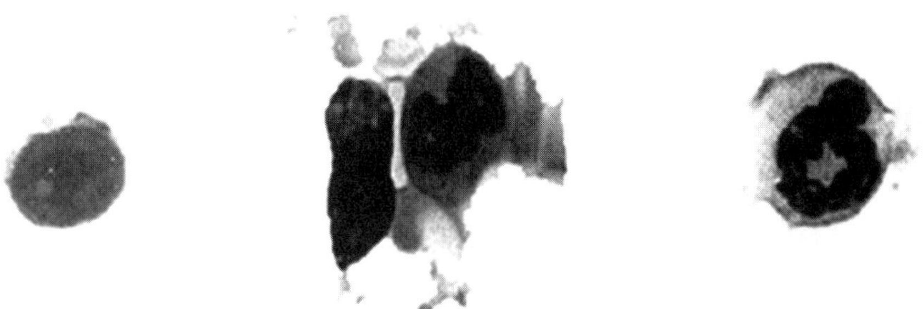

Fig. 1. Intracytoplasmic vacuoles from the peripheral blood of hypercholesteremic CD-1 male mice. Stained for lipids with Oil–Red O/Giemsa stain. ×1000 magnification.
Left, lymphocyte; middle, monocytes; right, neutrophil. The intracytoplasmic vacuoles stained red for lipid deposition appear as light gray inclusions indicated by arrows. (From Sniezek & Loria, unpublished data.)

lipid composition of peripheral blood mononuclear cells (PBMCs) of individuals with high or low serum HDL. This difference was reported to lead to a greater pro-inflammatory response in individuals with high HDL, as illustrated by an increase in the levels of interleukin (IL)-1b , IL-6, macrophages and chemokines, inflammatory protein-1 α, and growth-related peptide α (GROα). (Eggesbo, Hjermann, Joo, Orstebo, & Kierulf, 1995; Eggesbo et al., 1994, 1996). A link between Alzheimer's disease (AD) and cell membrane cholesterol is also evident (Sparks, Kuo, Roher, Martin, & Lukas, 2000). Indeed, cholesterol interacts with the amyloid β proteins 40 and 42 in a reciprocal manner (Gibson Wood, Eckert, Gavboa, Urule Muller, & Walker, 2003). Amyloid β 42 was not visualized directly on cholesterol-depleted bilayers. With the use of fluorescence anisotropy and fluorimetry procedures, amyloid β 42 appeared to induce membrane changes governed by composition and interaction with lipid bilayers (Yip, Darabie, & McLaurin, 2002). It was concluded that modification of the transbilayer distribution of cholesterol, and not the total amount of cholesterol, provides a cooperative environment for amyloid β synthesis and its accumulation in cell membranes, leading to cell dysfunction (McLaurin, Darabie, & Morrison, 2003).

3. EFFECTS OF DIETARY HYPERCHOLESTEREMIA ON LEUKOCYTES

In addition to membrane effects, once the cell membrane is saturated, cholesterol accumulates in cytoplasmic vacuoles, turning leukocytes into lipophages. Experiments in this laboratory showed that high cholesterol intake results in lipid-stained vacuoles within leukocytes (Fig. 1). In outbred CD-1 (Crl:CD-1® [ICR]BR) mice and inbred C57BL/6J male mice fed the same hypercholesteremic diet, the percent of leukocytes containing Oil-Red O staining vacuoles varied significantly. Hypercholesteremic, outbred CD-1 mice lipophage counts were as follows: monocytes, 40%; lymphocytes, 7%; and neutrophils, 7%. In inbred C57BL/6J mice lipophage counts were as follows: monocytes, 62%; lymphocytes, 3%; and neutrophils, 14%. Except for rare cases, no lipid vacuoles were evident in control normocholesteremic animals (Sniezek & Loria, unpublished data). Accumulation of cholesterol in leukocytes may be one of the significant factors leading to reticuloendothelial blockade.

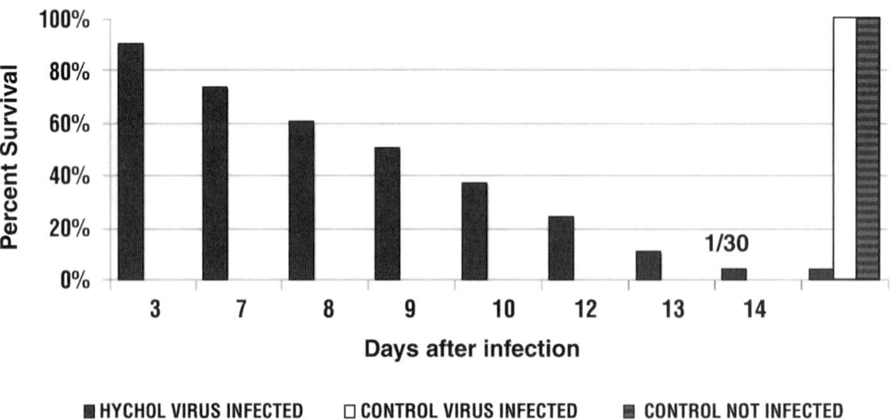

Fig. 2. Dietary hypercholesteremia increases susceptibility to viral infection. CD-1 male mice fed a hypercholesteremic diet were challenged with 3×10^6 coxsackievirus B5 infectious units. Hypercholesteremic animals infected with virus ■; control normal mice infected with same virus dose □; control normal mice not infected ▦. (Adapted from Loria et al., 1976.)

4. EFFECTS OF DIETARY HYPERCHOLESTEREMIA ON HOST RESISTANCE TO INFECTIONS AND IMMUNITY

Loria et al. (1976) reported that dietary hypercholesteremia was associated with a significant reduction of host resistance leading to an increased susceptibility to infection by a human cardiotropic virus (Loria, Kos, Campbell, & Madge, 1979). As illustrated in Fig. 2, outbred CD-1 mice fed a hypercholesteremic diet and infected with a dose of 3×10^6 coxsackievirus B5 infectious unit exhibited 97% mortality, with only 1 out of 30 animals (3%) surviving at 14 d. No mortality was observed in normocholesteremic animals infected with an identical dose. Similarly, control inbred C57BL/6J male mice were resistant to a challenge of 4×10^8 infectious units of coxsackievirus B5, whereas 50% of hypercholesteremic animals died following a challenge of 2.4×10^5 infectious units, a 3 order of magnitude increase in susceptibility (Sneizek & Loria, unpublished data). One hallmark of viral infection is an inflammatory response, as evident by mononuclear cell infiltration of the infected target tissues. This ability of mononuclear cells to respond and clear infectious agents from infected tissues is significantly diminished in hypercholesteremic animals. Consequently, a marked augmentation of coxsackievirus-B5-mediated cardiopathy and cardiomyolysis was observed (Fig. 3). Evidence of virus localization, greater replication, and persistence in the aorta was obtained (Campbell, Loria, & Madge, 1978). Atherosclerotic changes in the aorta became evident several months after acute infection of animals fed the high-cholesterol diet. Such pathology was not evident in virus-infected normocholesteremic animals (Figs. 4–6). The effects of dietary hypercholesteremia extended to an increase in susceptibility to bacterial infections. Indeed, the dose that causes a 50% mortality in normal C57BL/6L animals is 1.5×10^7 colony-forming unit of *Listeria monocytogenes*, which is reduced 40-fold to 3.7×10^5 colony-forming units in hypercholesteremic animals. Hepatic titers of *L. monocytogenes* decreased rapidly after 6 d of infection in normal animals but persisted in hypercholesteremic animals (Kos, Kos, & Kaplan, 1984). The ability of the host to reject a tumor was markedly diminished in hypercholesteremic animals (Table 1). Consequently, the effects

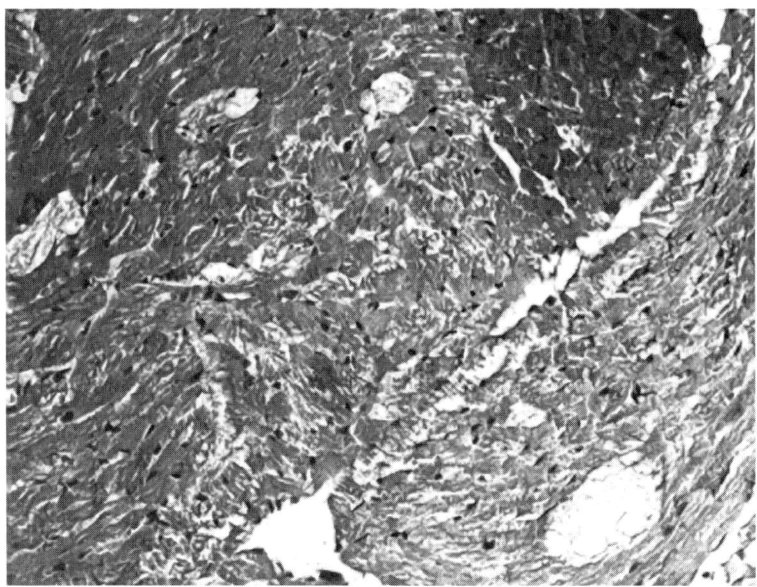

Fig. 3. Heart section from hypercholesteremic coxsackievirus-infected CD-1 mouse. Focal areas of myocytolysis. Inflammatory cellular infiltration is absent. Hematoxylin & eosin stain ×720 (From Campbell, Loria, & Madge, 1976.)

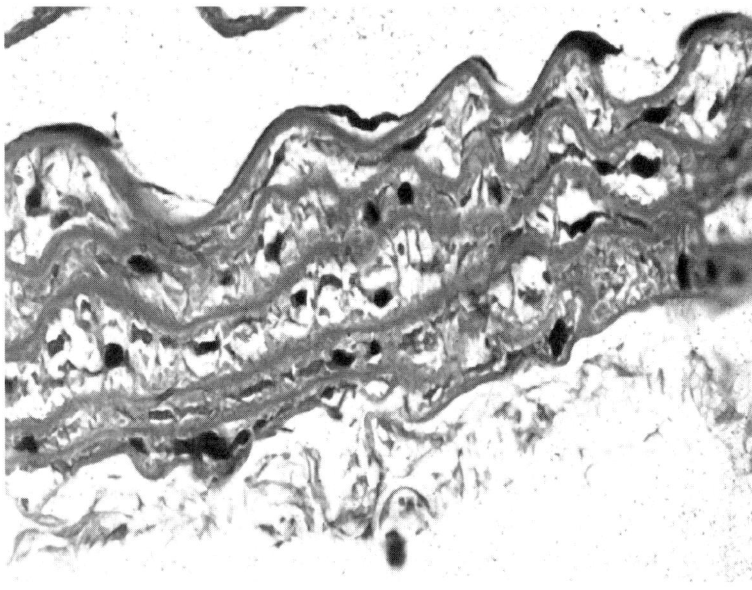

Fig. 4. Aorta from 5 mo post infected hypercholesteremic CD-1 mouse . A marked distruption of the media smooth muscle cells. Hematoxylin & eosin stain ×720. (From Campbell, et al., 1978.)

on macrophage activation were examined using two different criteria to identify the locus of immune impairment. Both the expression of new surface antigen associated with macrophage activation of peritoneal exudate (Kaplan, Bear, Kirk, Cummins, & Mohanakumar, 1978) and their cytotoxic activity against tumor cells in vitro were tested.

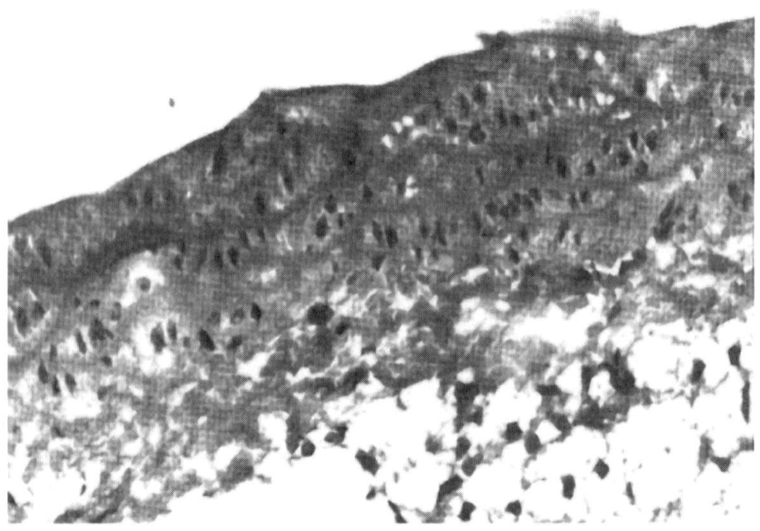

Fig. 5. Aorta from uninfented hypercholesteremic CD-1 mouse . No evidence of cellular changes. Hematoxylin & eosin stain ×720. (From Campbell et al., 1978)

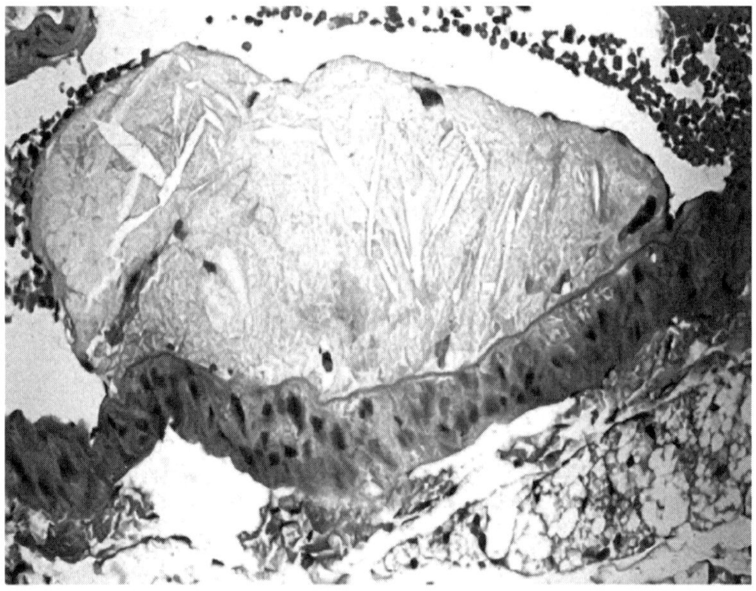

Fig. 6. Hypercholesteremic CD-1 mouse 10 mo after infection with a coxsackievirus B5. Note cholesterol clefts in atherosclerotic plaque adhering to aorta wall. Unifected hypercholesteremic animals or infected normal animals did not develop plaques. (From Loria, 1986.)

No significant difference between the hypercholesteremic and normal groups was observed (Kos et al., 1979). These findings suggested that in vivo elevated cholesterol did not appear to impair antigen recognition but impaired the effector function of activated macrophages to reject tumors.

Table 1
Effects of Hypercholesteremia on Tumor Regression

Host	*Macrophage attractant* (C. parvum)[a]	*Tumor rejection*[b]	*Animals protected from tumor killing (%)*
Normal	No	0	
Normal	Yes	5	50
Hypercholesteremic	No	1	0
Hypercholesteremic	Yes	1	0

[a]*C. parvum* is a heat-killed vaccine preparation, which functions as a macrophage attractant; 17.5 mg/kg were injected into the lession on d 3 of the experiment.

[b]Number of rejections out of 10 animals per group. C57BL/6J were inoculated with 5×10^4 methyl cholanthrene-induced fibrosarcoma 2182 tumor cell.

Source: Kos, 1979.

Table 2
Hepatic Effects of Dietary Hypercholesteremia[a]

Diet	*Total cholesterol (mg/g liver*[b]*)*	*Total protein (mg/g liver*[c]*)*	*Liver weight (% total body weight)*
Hypercholesteremic	8.5 ± 0.7	84.0 ± 4.3	10. 2 ± 0.8
Control	4.1 ± 1.0	155.0 ± 22.5	4.7 ± 0.4
Ratio	2.07	0.54	2.17

[a]C57BL/6J male mice were on the hypercholesteremic diet for 10 wk.

[b]Data are average of four livers.

[c]Data are average of nine livers.

Source:Adapted from Campbell, 1982.

Elevated cholesterol levels were associated with physiological changes, particularly the accumulation of intrahepatic cholesterol leading to gross focal necrosis in virus-infected animals (Fig. 7). The increased susceptibility to infection reached a plateau after 10 wk on the hypercholesteremic diet. This coincided with a twofold increase in the ratio of hepatic total cholesterol and a twofold reduction of protein (Table 2). Substitution of the hypercholesteremic diet with a normal control diet led to fast restoration of hepatic protein concentration and host resistance. There was a significant correlation between the increase in virus-mediated mortality and total cholesterol levels (r = 0.96) when liver total cholesterol was expressed as a percentage of control values. Similarly, the reduction in hepatic protein per gram of tissue also showed a positive correlation (r = 0.833) with increased susceptibility.

It is apparent that one of the determinant factors reducing host resistance is the ratio of hepatic cholesterol to protein. This metabolic imbalance led to reduced virus clearance from the blood and liver. In these experiments, 3×10^8 infectious units of coxsackievirus were injected into the intraperitoneal cavity, and virus titers were measured at 15 and 30 min and hourly from 1 to 4 h. The average virus clearance from the blood and the liver, respectively, was lower in hypercholesteremic animals by 0.89–0.75 log at each of the five time points. Tabulation of the reduced clearance over the 4-h time span, as a crude

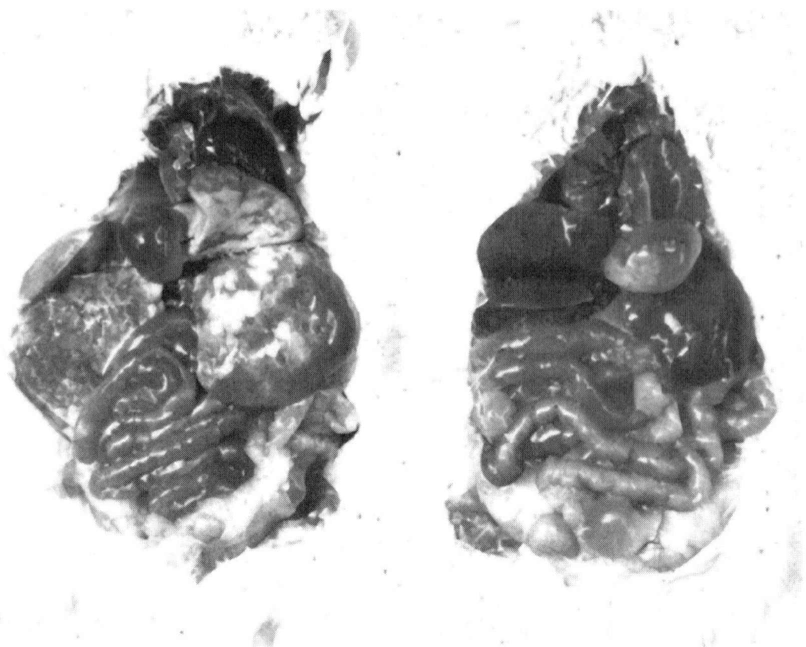

Fig. 7. Enlarged patchy and mottled liver of hypercholesteremic mouse infected with coxsackievirus B5 (left) that contrasts with homogeneous appearance of liver from uninfected hypercholesteremic animal (right). (Adapted from Loria et al., 1976.)

Table 3
Effects of Dietary Cholesterol Elevation on Antibody Response

	Antibody titers (units/mL)[b]	
Days postinfection[a]	*Control diet*	*Hypercholesteremic diet*
1	<20	<20
3	<20	<20
5	100 ± 36	300 ± 142
7	288 ± 134	368 ± 22*
14	6860 ± 2860	10,659 ± 2860

[a]Infected with 1×10^5 infectious units of coxsackievirus B5.

[b]One unit/mL neutralizes one-half HeLa cell monolayers culture infected with 100 tissue culture infectious dose 50 of coxsackievirus B5.

*Statistically significant $p < 0.05$ by student's t-test.

Source: Campbell, Loria, Madge, & Kaplan, 1982.

indicator, amounted to 5.3–4.5 log of infectious virus from the blood and liver, respectively (Campbell, Loria, Madge, & Kaplan, 1982).

In order to determine whether elevated cholesterol mediated a suppression of the humoral immune response, the level of antibodies against a human coxsackievirus was tested in both normal and hypercholesteremic animals. The results presented in Table 3 show that antibody synthesis, levels, and rates were not affected by the high-cholesterol diet. In order to establish that elevated cholesterol levels did not interfere with antibody binding, passive immunization was carried out. Hyperimmune sera injected into hypercholesteremic animals infected with coxsackievirus B5 effectively protected animals, as evident from a 92% survival as compared to no survival in nonimmunized hypercholesteremic controls (Campbell et al., 1982).

The results show that excess cholesterol intake induces an hepatic blockade and Kupffer cell inhibition. In addition, evidence of impairment in cell-mediated immune functions, but not humoral immunity, is apparent. Experiments that transferred immune spleen cells against *L. monocytogenes* from normal donors to hypercholesteremic recipients showed a diminished function in the recipients, which indicates that the hypercholesteremic "environment" is contributing to the immune impairment. Reverse experiments, transferring immune spleen cells from hypercholesteremic animals to normal animals, resulted in significant protection. This led to the conclusion that immune T lymphocytes are generated in the hypercholesteremic host and that the immune impairment occurs at a later stage (Kos et al., 1984).

Confirmation of these observations was provided by Pereira, Steffan, Koehren, Douglas, and Kirn (1987), who reported that normal A/J mice that are fully resistant to mouse hepatitis type 3 become susceptible to this virus after dietary-induced hypercholesterolemia. Accordingly, a direct relationship was found between the high levels of plasma and hepatic cholesterol and the mortality from mouse hepatitis virus. The loss of host resistance was correlated with an impairment of Kupffer cell activation. Since the liver is the target organ for mouse hepatitis virus, this model unmasks the hepatic pathology mediated by hypercholesteremia to this organ.

The fundamental basis of these observations is also supported by Ludewig et al. (2001), who reported similar effects of genetically induced hypercholesterolemia on cellular immunity.

Apolipoprotein-E-deficient and low-density-lipoprotein-receptor-deficient mice had aggravated virus-induced immunopathology a deficient virus clearance from spleen and nonlymphoid organs, including liver. Activation of antiviral cytotoxic T lymphocytes (CTLs), measured by ex vivo cytotoxicity and interferon (IFN)-γproduction, and recruitment of specific CTLs into blood and liver were impaired in hypercholesteremic mice. These investigators conclude that hypercholesterolemia had a significant suppressive effect on cellular immunity and increases the susceptibility to acute or chronic infections as well as diseases with an immunopathological components such as atherosclerosis.

5. CONCLUSIONS

Among the many tasks leukocytes perform are phagocytosis, antigen presentation, and antibody synthesis. Similarly, Kupffer cells also carry out phagocytic functions.

The cholesterol content of the plasma membrane is a major determinant of the regulation of membrane fluidity and enables leukocytes to function and transmit signals across the cell membrane. The levels of cholesterol in the serum and tissues have a marked effect on the content and subsequent function of leukocytes. Excessive dietary cholesterol impairs the functions of leukocytes and Kupffer cells. This dysfunction is evident from reduced clearance of viral and bacterial agents and inability to reject tumor cells, even though recognition of the antigen(s) and activation of effector cells have taken place. The results show that dietary hypercholestremia does not impair humoral immunity, but suppresses cell-mediated immunity, and the impaired function appears to occur after its induction. Sustained dietary hypercholesteremia leads to formation of lipid-laden leukocytes with intracellular vacuoles containing lipids. This is an illustration of a biological insult caused by malnourishment. The formation of lipid-laden cells is consistent with the wear and tear phenomenon and results in impaired general defense reactions such as inflammation, as described by Selye (1936). By this definition, dietary-induced and maintained hypercholesteremia can be considered a nocuous agent or process. Dietary hypercholesteremia abrogates the host's ability to cope with stress and is clearly an independent stress factor.

REFERENCES

Agarwal, V., Gupta, B., Singhal, U., & Bajpai, S. K. (1997). Examination stress: Changes in serum cholesterol, triglycerides and total lipids. *Indian Journal of Physiolology and Pharmacology, 41*(4), 404–408.

Alonso, M. A. & Millan, J. (2001). The role of lipid rafts in signaling and membrane trafficking in T lymphocytes. *Journal of Cell Science 114*(Pt. 22), 3957–3965.

Bene, L., Balazs, M., Matko, J., Most, J., Dierich, M. P., Szollosi, J., & Damjanovich, S. (1994). Lateral organization of the ICAM-1 molecule at the surface of human lymphoblasts: A possible model for its co-distribution with the IL-2 receptor, class I and class II HLA molecules. *European Journal of Immunology, 24*(9), 2115–2123.

Bianca de Juarez, M., Iglesias, R., Scoppa, H. G., Agnelli, H., & Gauna, H. F. (2000). Cholesterolemia and arterial pressure levels. Relationship with different chronic stress configurations. *Revista de la Facultad de Ciencias Medicas de la Universidad Nacional. de Cordoba, 57*(2), 227–237.

Bodnar, A., Bacso, Z., Enei, A. Jovin, T. M., Edidin, M., Damjanovich, S., & Matko, J. (2003). Class I HLA oligomerization at the surface of B cells is controlled by exogenous beta(2)-microglobulin: Implications in activation of cytotoxic T lymphocytes. *International Immunology, 15*(3), 331–339.

Bodnar, A., Jenei, A., Bene, L., Damjanovich, S., & Matko, J. (1996). Modification of membrane cholesterol level affects expression and clustering of class I HLA molecules at the surface of JY human lymphoblasts. *Immunology Letters, 54*(2–3), 221–226.

Brennan, F. X., Jr., Fleshner, M., Watkins, L. R., & Maier, S. F. (1996). Macrophage stimulation reduces the cholesterol levels of stressed and unstressed rats. *Life Science, 58*(20), 1771–1776.

Calder, P. C. (2003). Immunonutrition. *British Medical Journal, 327*(7407), 117–118.

Calder, P. C., & Kew, S. (2002). The immune system: A target for functional foods? *The British Journal of Nutrition, 88* (Suppl 2.), S165–77.

Campbell, A. E., Loria, R. M., & Madge, G. E. (1976). Infection of hypercholesterolemic mice with coxsackievirus B. *Journal of Infectious Disease, 133*(6), 655–662.

Campbell, A. E., Loria, R. M., & Madge, G. E. (1978). Coxsackievirus B cardiopathy and angiopathy in the hypercholesteremic host. *Atherosclerosis 31*(3), 295–306.

Campbell, A. E., Loria, R. M., Madge, G. E., & Kaplan, A. M. (1982). Dietary hepatic cholesterol elevation: Effects on coxsackievirus B infection and inflammation." *Infection and Immunity, 37*(1), 307–317.

Edidin, M. (2003). The state of lipid rafts: From model membranes to cells. *Annual Review of Biophysics and Biomolecular Structure, 32,* 257–283.

Eggesbo, J. B., Hagve, T. A., Borsum, K., Hostmark, A. T., Hjermann, I., & Kierulf, P. (1996). Lipid composition of mononuclear cell membranes and serum from persons with high or low levels of serum HDL cholesterol. *Scandinavian Journal of Clinical and Laboratory Investigation, 56*(3), 199–210.

Eggesbo, J. B., Hjermann, I, Joo, G. B., Ovstebo, R., & Kierulf, P. (1995). LPS-induced release of EGF, GM-CSF, GRO alpha, LIF, MIP-1 alpha and PDGF-AB in PBMC from persons with high or low levels of HDL lipoprotein. *Cytokine, 7*(6), 562–567.

Eggesbo, J. B., Hjermann, I., Lund, P. K., Joo, G. B., Ovstebo, R., & Kierulf, P. (1994). LPS-induced release of IL-1 beta, IL-6, IL-8, TNF-alpha and sCD14 in whole blood and PBMC from persons with high or low levels of HDL-lipoprotein. *Cytokine, 6*(5), 521–529.

Feo, F., Canuto, R. A., Torrielli, M. V., Garcea, R., & Dianzani, M. U. (1976). Effect of a cholesterol-rich diet on cholesterol content and phagocytic activity of rat macrophages. *Agents Actions, 6*(1–3), 135–142.

Field, C. J. (2000). Use of T cell function to determine the effect of physiologically active food components. *American Journal of Clinical Nutrition, 71*(6 Suppl), 1720S–1727S.

Field, C. J., Johnson, I. R., & Schley, P. D. (2002). Nutrients and their role in host resistance to infection. *Journal of Leukocyte Biology, 71*(1), 16–32.

Gibson Wood, W., Eckert, G. P., Igbavboa, U., Muller, W. E., & Walter E. (2003). Amyloid beta-protein interactions with membranes and cholesterol: Causes or casualties of Alzheimer's disease. *Biochimica et Biophysica Acta, 1610*(2), 281–290.

Kaplan, A. M., Bear, H. D., Kirk, L., Cummins, C., & Mohanakumar, T. (1978). Relationship of expression of a cell-surface antigen on activated murine macrophages to tumor cell cytotoxicity." *Journal of Immunology, 120*(6), 2080–2085.

Knoflach, M., Mayrl, B., Mayerl, C., Sedivy, R., & Wick, G. (2003). Atherosclerosis as a paradigmatic disease of the elderly: Role of the immune system. *Immunology and Allergy Clinics of North America, 23*(1), 117–132.

Kos, W. L., Kos, K. A., & Kaplan, A. M. (1984). Impaired function of immune reactivity to Listeria monocytogenes in diet-fed mice. *Infection and Immunity, 43*(3), 1094–1096.

Kos, W. L., Loria, R. M., Snodgrass, M. J., Cohen, D., Thorpe, T. G., & Kaplan, A. M. (1979). Inhibition of host resistance by nutritional hypercholesteremia. *Infection and Immunity, 26*(2), 658–667.

Kwik, J., Boyle, S., Fooksman, D., Margolis, L., Sheetz, M. P., & Edidin, M. (2003). Membrane cholesterol, lateral mobility, and the phosphatidylinositol 4,5-bisphosphate-dependent organization of cell actin. *Proceedings of the National Academy of Sciences of the United States of America,100*(24), 13,964–13,969.

Larbi, A., Douziech, N., Dupuis, G., Khalil, A., Pelletier, H., Guerard, K. P., & Fulop, T., Jr. (2004). Age-associated alterations in the recruitment of signal-transduction proteins to lipid rafts in human T lymphocytes. *Journal of Leukocyte Biology, 75*(2), 373–381.

Larbi, A., Douziech, N., Khalil, A., Dupuis, G., Gherairi, S., Guerard, K. P., & Fulop, T., Jr. (2004). Effects of methyl-beta-cyclodextrin on T lymphocytes lipid rafts with aging. *Experimental Gerontology, 39*(4), 551–558.

Loria, R. M. (1986). Coxsackievirus B, lipids, and immunity as shared determinants in diabetes and atherosclerosis. In A. Szentivanyi & H. Friedman (Eds.), *Viruses, immunity, and immunodeficiency*. New York: Plenum.

Loria, R. M., Kibrick, S., & Madge, G. E. (1976). Infection of hypercholesterolemic mice with coxsackievirus B. *Journal of Infectious Diseases, 133*(6), 655–662.

Loria, R. M., Kos, W. L., Campbell, A. E., & Madge, G. E. (1979). Suppression of aortic elastic tissue autofluorescence for the detection of viral antigen. *Histochemistry, 61*(2), 151–155.

Ludewig, B., Jaggi, M., Dumrese, T., Brduscha-Riem, K., Odermatt, B., Hengartner, H., & Zinkernagel, R. M. (2001). Hypercholesterolemia exacerbates virus-induced immunopathologic liver disease via suppression of antiviral cytotoxic T cell responses. *Journal of Immunology, 166*(5), 3369–3376.

McLaurin, J., Darabie, A. A., & Morrison, M. R. (2003). Cholesterol, a modulator of membrane- associated Abeta-fibrillogenesis. *Pharmacopsychiatry, 36*(Suppl 2), S130–135.

Miles, E. A., Allen, E., & Calder, P. C. (2002). In vitro effects of eicosanoids derived from different 20-carbon Fatty acids on production of monocyte-derived cytokines in human whole blood cultures. *Cytokine, 20*(5), 215–223.

Miles, E. A., Aston, L., & Calder, P.C. (2003). In vitro effects of eicosanoids derived from different 20-carbon fatty acids on T helper type 1 and T helper type 2 cytokine production in human whole-blood cultures. *Clinical and Experimental Allergy : Journal of the British Society for Allergy and Clinical Immunology, 33*(5), 624–632.

Millan, J., Montoya, M. C., Sancho, D., Sanchez-Madrid, F., & Alonso, M. A. (2002). Lipid rafts mediate biosynthetic transport to the T lymphocyte uropod subdomain and are necessary for uropod integrity and function. *Blood, 99*(3), 978–984.

Minick, C. R., Murphy, G. E., & Campbell, W. G., Jr. (1966). Experimental induction of athero- arteriosclerosis by the synergy of allergic injury to arteries and lipid-rich diet. I. Effect of repeated injections of horse serum in rabbits fed a dietary cholesterol supplement. *The Journal of Experimental Medicine, 124*(4), 635–652.

Padgett, D. A., Loria, R. M., & Sheridan, J. F. (2000). Steroid hormone regulation of antiviral immunity. *Annals of the New York Academy of Sciences, 917*, 935–943.

Pereira, C. A., Steffan, A. M., Koehren, F., Douglas, C. R., & Kirn, A. (1987). Increased susceptibility of mice to MHV 3 infection induced by hypercholesterolemic diet: Impairment of Kupffer cell function. *Immunobiology, 174*(3), 253–265.

Selye, H. (1936). A syndrome produced by diverse nocuous agents. *Nature, 138*, 32.

Sheridan, J. F., Dobbs, C., Jung, J., Chu, X., Konstantinos, A., Padgett, D., & Glaser, R (1998). Stress-induced neuroendocrine modulation of viral pathogenesis and immunity. *Annals of the New York Academy of Sciences, 840*, 803–808.

Sheridan, J. F., Stark, J. L., Avitsur, R., & Padgett, D. A. (2000). Social disruption, immunity, and susceptibility to viral infection. Role of glucocorticoid insensitivity and NGF. *Annals of the New York Academy of Sciences, 917*, 894–905.

Sniezek, L. J., & Loria, R. M. (1977). Coxsackie B5 virus in the hypercholesteremic mouse. Virginia Commonwealth University, Masters dissertation.

Sparks, D. L., Kuo, Y. M., Roher, A., Martin, T., & Lukas, R. J. (2000). Alterations of Alzheimer's disease in the cholesterol-fed rabbit, including vascular inflammation. Preliminary observations. *Annals of the New York Academy of Sciences, 903*, 335–344.

Thomas, P. D., Goodwin, J. M., & Goodwin, J. S. (1985). Effect of social support on stress-related changes in cholesterol level, uric acid level, and immune function in an elderly sample. *American Journal of Psychiatry, 142*(6), 735–737.

Yip, C. M., Darabie, A. A., & McLaurin, J. (2002). Abeta42-peptide assembly on lipid bilayers. *Journal of Molecular Biology, 318*(1), 97–107.

18 Treatment of Huntington's Disease With Eicosapentaenoic Acid

Basant K. Puri

KEY POINTS

- There is strong evidence pointing to the involvement of lipids in the pathophysiology of Huntington's disease, perhaps through an as-yet-unidentified action of *huntingtin*.
- Single cases and trials utilizing long-chain polyunsaturated fatty acids show therapeutic benefit in Huntington's disease.
- The clinical benefit appears particularly strong in the case of ultra-pure eicosapentaenoic acid.
- Beneficial changes in neuropsychological functioning and in terms of structural brain changes also appear to accompany treatment with ultra-pure eicosapentaenoic acid.
- This treatment offers a new and potentially beneficial intervention for this otherwise intractable inherited disorder.

1. INTRODUCTION

Huntington's disease (or chorea) is a progressive, inherited neurodegenerative disease characterized by autosomal dominant transmission and the emergence of abnormal involuntary movements and cognitive deterioration, with progression to dementia and death over 10–20 yr; the gene responsible, *huntingtin*, is located on chromosome 4 (Harper, 1996; Huntington's Disease Collaborative Research Group, 1993). Until the studies using eicosapentaenoic acid, there was no evidence of effective treatment for this disorder.

Several lines of evidence pointed this author towards the possibility of a therapeutic role for long-chain polyunsaturated fatty acids in this disease. These included the original single-case studies of patients treated with long-chain polyunsaturated fatty acids by K. S. Vaddadi, membrane phospholipid metabolism in Huntington's disease, the demonstration of impaired phospholipid-related signal transduction in this disease, a study of the effects of long-chain polyunsaturated fatty acids on a transgenic mouse model of Huntington's disease, and the effects of eicosapentaenoate on the human brain in other neuropsychiatric disorders revealed by recently developed serial magnetic resonance imaging (MRI) registration techniques. Following a consideration of these background studies, this chapter contains an account of the results of direct treatment with eicosapentaenoic acid in Huntington's disease.

From: *Nutrients, Stress, and Medical Disorders*
Edited by: S. Yehuda and D. I. Mostofsky © Humana Press Inc., Totowa, NJ

2. BACKGROUND STUDIES

2.1. Two Single-Case Studies

In 1994, Vaddadi (2003) began treating a female patient in her early 80s with long-chain polyunsaturated fatty acids. In 1991, the patient had been noted to have short-term memory deficits, athetoid movements, and non-insulin-dependent diabetes mellitus. She was diagnosed as suffering from Huntington's disease the following year and treated until the end of 1993 with haloperidol. During this time her chorea, dysarthria, and depression worsened. Her cytosine-adenine-guanine (CAG) repeat numbers were 16 and 41 for two alleles. In April 1994, she was assessed by Vaddadi's team and commenced on Efamol™, a fatty acid preparation containing γ-linolenic acid. By September of that year there was a marked reduction in her abnormal involuntary movements and some improvement in her speech, memory, and general interactions. The clinical improvement was maintained until the time of her death in 1997.

Vaddadi's second open-trial case report (2003) was of a male Huntington's disease patient in his 60s who also showed improvements in his abnormal involuntary movements following treatment with Efamol and, in particular, with Efamol-Marine™, which contains γ-linolenic acid, docosahexaenoic acid, and a relatively small amount of eicosapentaenoic acid.

2.2. Membrane Phospholipid Metabolism

Based on the finding of reduced levels of phosphoethanolamine and ethanolamine in Huntington's disease, Ellison, Beal, and Martin (1987) proposed alterations in membrane phospholipid metabolism. This is consistent with the finding by Sakai et al. (1991) that the mean level of erythrocyte membrane docosahexaenoic acid in six patients with Huntington's disease was significantly lower than that in 14 matched normal controls. Docosahexaenoic acid is a component of ethanolamine glycerophospholipids, the metabolism of which is known to be disturbed in both Huntington's and Alzheimer's diseases (Ellison et al., 1987). Because docosahexaenoic acid levels are also lower in Alzheimer's disease, this suggests that a common mechanism of neuronal loss could be involved in both disorders.

2.3. Impaired Phospholipid-Related Signal Transduction

Puri (2001) measured the response to topical aqueous methyl nicotinate solution at 5-min intervals over 20 min in six inpatients with advanced (stage III) Huntington's disease and in 14 age- and sex-matched normal individuals with no history of this or any other major neurological disorder. The results were converted into the volumetric niacin response (VNR), which indexes phospholipid-related signal transduction (Puri, Hirsch, Easton, & Richardson, 2002). The mean VNR in the Huntington's disease patients, 16.3 (standard error 2.6) mol s/L, was significantly lower than that of 28.3 (standard error 2.1) mol s/L in the control group ($p = 0.004$), which is consistent with the conclusion that Huntington's disease may be associated with an abnormality of neuronal membrane fatty acid metabolism, possibly as a consequence of an as-yet-unidentified action of *huntingtin*.

2.4. Transgenic Mouse Studies

R6/1 mice are transgenic for a human genomic fragment containing promoter elements exon 1 and a portion of intron 2 of the *huntingtin* gene and display a progressive neurological phenotype; they carry an approximate CAG repeat expansion of 115. The R6/1 line has a relatively late age of onset and an insidious progression of phenotype, with subsequent seizures, bradykinesia, loss of body mass, and death, and it shows greater homology with the typical course of illness in the human disorder than does the R6/2 line (Davies et al., 1997; Mangiarini et al., 1996). Clifford et al. (2002) carried out a study in which R6/1 and normal mice were randomized to receive a mixture of essential fatty acids and long-chain polyunsaturated fatty acids or placebo on alternate days from conception. The active treatment included linoleic acid, γ-linolenic acid, eicosapentaenoic acid, and docosahexaenoic acid. Over mid-adulthood, topographical assessment of behavior showed that the transgenic mice had improved survival, progressive shortening of stride length, with progressive reductions in locomotion, elements of rearing, sniffing, sifting, and chewing and an increase in grooming, which were either not evident or materially diminished in those receiving essential fatty acids; the R6/1 mice also showed reductions in body mass and in brain dopamine D_1-like and D_2-like quantitative receptor autoradiography, which were unaltered by essential fatty acids. These findings indicate that early and sustained treatment with essential fatty acids and long-chain polyunsaturated fatty acids protected against motor deficits in transgenic R6/1 mice expressing exon 1 of the *huntingtin* gene and suggest that essential fatty acids may have therapeutic potential in Huntington's disease.

2.5. Cerebral Effects of Pure Eicosapentaenoic Acid in Other Neuropsychiatric Disorders

Use of a rigid-body monomodal subvoxel registration technique developed at Hammersmith Hospital, London, and based on the sinc interpolation function, allows highly accurate intrasubject registration of serial three-dimensional (3D) MRI brain scans (Bydder, 1995; Bydder & Hajnal, 1997). Ventricular changes detected using such techniques can now be quantified accurately (Puri, 2004; Saeed, Puri, Oatridge, Hajnal, & Young, 1998). These powerful imaging techniques have recently begun to be applied to the study of the effects of eicosapentaenoic acid intervention in neuropsychiatric disorders (Puri, 2004). The first such application, in a long-standing case of schizophrenia not being treated with conventional medication, showed that sustained remission of positive and negative symptoms associated with treatment with eicosapentaenoic acid (alone) was accompanied by a reversal of cerebral atrophy (Puri & Richardson, 1998; Puri et al., 2000). Similarly, the first case of treatment-resistant depression treated with eicosapentaenoic acid (as an adjunct treatment) was also accompanied by a reversal of cerebral atrophy (Puri, Counsell, Hamilton, Richardson, & Horrobin, 2001).

Furthermore, eicosapentaenoic acid inhibits phospholipase A_2; the phospholipase A_2 group of enzymes may play an important role in the generation of intracellular free radical enzymes and appears to be important in neurodegeneration (Klivenyi et al., 1998). Given the central importance of cerebral atrophy in Huntington's disease, this limited evidence gave further support to the potential benefits of eicosapentaenoic acid in this disease.

3. TREATMENT WITH EICOSAPENTAENOIC ACID

Given the above lines of evidence pointing to the potential therapeutic role of eicosapentaenoic acid in Huntington's disease, this hypothesis was directly tested in a study published by our group (Puri, Bydder, et al., 2002). Details of this study are now given.

3.1. Patients

The patients were recruited from a specialist center in London offering 24-h medical and nursing care for patients with cerebral damage. All of the patients suffered from end-stage (stage III) Huntington's disease, scoring 40 or below on the Independence Scale of the Unified Huntington's Disease Rating Scale (Huntington Study Group, 1996).

Initially, eight patients were blindly randomized into an active treatment group (four patients) with 2 g of ethyl eicosapentaenoic acid (LAX-101, Laxdale Ltd., Stirling, Scotland) daily or a matching placebo group (four patients). Unfortunately, before the trial began, one patient who was randomized to receive the active treatment died as a result of the Huntington's disease.

The two groups did not differ significantly with respect to age ($p = 0.27$) or sex ($p = 0.63$).

3.2. Treatments Administered

The active treatment of 2 g daily of ultra-pure ethyl eicosapentaenoic acid for 6 mo was provided in the form of soft gelatin capsules, each containing 500 mg ethyl eicosapentaenoic acid. The placebo consisted of identically appearing capsules containing inert liquid paraffin. For patients unable to swallow them, the capsules were broken by the nursing staff and the contents either mixed with drinks and swallowed or, where appropriate, mixed with feed and entered via a preexisting percutaneous endoscopic gastrostomy (PEG) tube.

At the end of the study, those nursing staff who had been involved in breaking open the capsules were interviewed; in all cases the staff incorrectly identified the treatment. Furthermore, none of the ratings used were carried out by the nursing staff.

3.3. Neuropsychological Ratings

All of the patients were evaluated at baseline and at 6-mo follow-up on the motor component of the Unified Huntington's Disease Rating Scale (Huntington Study Group, 1996).

Unfortunately, owing to the severity of the stage III Huntington's disease, it was found that the psychological ratings component of the Unified Huntington's Disease Rating Scale could only be fully carried out in five of the patients at baseline. It was therefore decided to repeat this component only in these five patients at 6-mo follow-up.

3.4. Magnetic Resonance Scanning Protocol

Sagittal 3D T_1-weighted rf spoiled images (TR = 30 ms, TE = 3 ms, flip angle = 30°, 156×256 image matrix, 114 slices, 1.6 mm slice thickness, 25 cm field of view) were acquired on a 1.5 T Eclipse (Marconi Medical Systems) scanner at each examination. Phantom measurements were taken to confirm that no changes in magnetic gradient strength had occurred. Because of the movement disorder, leading in turn to motion artefacts, only four patients underwent successful MRI at baseline and 6 mo.

3.5. Determination of Structural Cerebral Ventricular Change

The MRI cerebral volume scans for each patient were accurately registered using monomodal subvoxel rigid-body registration based on the sinc interpolation function (Puri, 2004). Using these registered images, subtraction images were obtained for each patient, and these registered anatomical and subtraction images were reformatted into the

Table 1
Baseline and 6-mo Follow-Up Scores for the Orofacial Motor and Other Motor Components of the Unified Huntington's Disease Rating Scale[a]

Orofacial movements		*Other movements*		*Total score*	
Baseline	*6 mo*	*Baseline*	*6 mo*	*Baseline*	*6 mo*
Patients on placebo:					
12	13	20	26	32	39
16	19	33	36	49	55
12	16	15	23	27	39
2	4	5	22	7	26
Patients on EPA:					
19	16	26	30	45	46
14	12	31	27	45	39
11	1	19	15	30	16

[a]Higher numbers indicate a worse state.
Source: Modified from Puri et al., 2002.

transverse plane with isotropic voxels of size 0.977^3 mm^3. They were used to evaluate the changes, if any, between the baseline and 6-mo follow-up images. Because of the high degree of cerebral atrophy in the stage III Huntington's disease patients, it was not possible to quantify the lateral ventricular volumes.

3.6. Motor Function

On the orofacial component of the Unified Huntington's Disease Rating Scale, three patients improved and four deteriorated. The former three patients were the ones in the active group who had received eicosapentaenoic acid, while all four patients who deteriorated had received the placebo ($p = 0.029$).

In terms of the other components of the motor scale of the Unified Huntington's Disease Rating Scale, two patients improved and five deteriorated. Both patients who improved were in the active treatment group and had received eicosapentaenoic acid. In spite of the small numbers of patients and controls, the change in the total movement score for the patients on eicosapentaenoic acid was significantly better than that for the patients on the placebo ($p = 0.019$). The motor function data for all the patients are shown in Table 1.

3.7. Psychological Function

Four of the five patients assessed both at baseline and at 6-mo follow-up showed little change with respect to the psychological ratings of the Unified Huntington's Disease Rating Scale. In the case of the fifth patient, however, there was a dramatic change. This patient had scored extremely poorly on the Stroop color ratings at baseline (18 errors). However, surprisingly for a stage III Huntington's disease patient, she was assessed to have a perfect score (no errors) on this task at the 6-mo follow-up test.

It turned out that only one of the five patients from whom psychology ratings had successfully been obtained had received the eicosapentaenoic acid, and this was the same patient who had shown the dramatic improvement in the color Stroop ratings. (Because of the small numbers involved, this was not a statistically significant result.) The changes in ratings on the Stroop test are shown in Table 2.

Table 2
Changes in Error Scores in the Components of the Stroop Test[a] for Patients on Placebo and Eicosapentaenoic Acid (EPA)[b]

Stroop color naming	*Stroop word reading*	*Stroop interference test*
Patients on placebo:		
0	5	4
0	0	0
−5	−5	7
−2	0	0
Patient on EPA:		
−18	0	−6

[a]6-mo error score minus baseline error score.

[b]It was not possible to obtain scores on both occasions from the remaining two patients. Note that negative changes in error scores correspond to improvement, and vice versa; zero changes correspond to no change.

Source:Modified from Puri et al., 2002.

3.8. Structural Cerebral Changes

Of the four patients who successfully underwent cerebral magnetic resonance scanning at baseline and 6-mo follow-up, it turned out that two were in the placebo group and two were in the active treatment group. Subtraction of the registered images showed that an increase in ventricular size had taken place in both patients on the placebo. A detailed manual inspection of the difference images, slice by contiguous slice, revealed that in the placebo group the sulci had generally widened and some of the gyri had thinned. These changes were consistent with a progression of the cerebral atrophy and were in line with expectations in end-stage Huntington's disease.

In contrast, the subtraction images from the two patients treated with eicosapentaenoic acid showed clear evidence of an overall decrease in ventricular size. In these patients, the difference images also showed evidence of some sulcal thinning. Thus, while the placebo was associated with progressive cerebral atrophy, the ethyl eicosapentaenoic acid was associated with a reverse process.

4. CONCLUSIONS

The results of the above randomized double-blind, placebo-controlled study showed that the administration of ultra-pure eicosapentaenoic acid is associated with improvements in both cerebral structure and function in the patients with end-stage Huntington's disease. (In comparison, the patients taking the placebo showed the expected deterioration in cerebral structure and functioning.) Thus, these results are consistent with the hypothesis proposed earlier, whereby Huntington's disease is considered to be a phospholipid spectrum disorder that may be amenable to treatment with essential fatty acids.

A similar study was carried out by Vaddadi, Soosai, Chiu, and Dingjan (2002) and published at the same time as the study by Puri, Bydder, et al. (2002). In their study, Vaddadi and colleagues found significant improvement in (non-end-stage) Huntington's disease following daily treatment with 560 mg of γ-linolenic acid, 280 mg of eicosapentaenoic acid, 160 mg of docosahexaenoic acid, 400 mg of α-lipoic acid, 240 mg of D-α-tocopheryl acetate, and linoleic acid.

As a result of the above studies, a larger multicenter trial of purified ethyl eicosapentaenoate (LAX-101, Laxdale Ltd., Stirling, Scotland) in 135 patients with stage I orrr stage II Huntington's disease has been carried out. At the time of writing the results of this study have not entered the public domain. Exploratory analysis has shown that a significantly higher number of patients in the per protocol cohort, treated with EPA, showed stable or improved motor function (Puri et al., 2005). Intriguingly, there also appeared to be a pharmacogenetic effect, with a significant interaction being found between treatment and a factor defining patients with high vs low CAG repeats (Puri et al., 2005)

REFERENCES

Bydder, G. M. (1995). The Mackenzie Davidson Memorial Lecture: Detection of small changes to the brain with serial magnetic resonance imaging. *British Journal of Radiology, 68*, 1271–1295.

Bydder, G. M., & Hajnal, J. V. (1997). Registration and subtraction of serial MRI—Part 2: Image interpretation. In W. G. Bradley & G. M. Bydder (Eds.), *Advanced MR imaging techniques* (pp. 239–258). London: Martin Dunitz.

Clifford, J. J., Drago, J., Natoli, A. L., Wong, J. Y., Kinsella, A., Waddington, J. L. & Vaddadi, K. S. (2002). Essential fatty acids given from conception prevent topographies of motor deficit in a transgenic model of Huntington's disease. *Neuroscience, 109*, 81–88.

Davies, S. W., Turmaine, M., Cozens, B. A., DiFiglia, M., Sharp, A. H., Ross, C. A., Scherzinger, E., Wanker, E. E., Mangiarini, L., & Bates, G. P. (1997). Formation of neuronal intranuclear inclusions underlies the neurological dysfunction in mice transgenic for the HD mutation. *Cell, 90*, 537–548.

Ellison, D. W., Beal, M. F., & Martin, J. B. (1987). Phosphoethanolamine and ethanolamine are decreased in Alzheimer's disease and Huntington's disease. *Brain Research, 417*, 389–392.

Harper, P. S., (Ed.). (1996). *Huntington's disease,* (2nd ed.). London: W. B. Saunders.

Huntington Study Group. (1996). Unified Huntington's Disease Rating Scale: Reliability and consistency. *Movement Disorders, 11*, 136–142.

Huntington's Disease Collaborative Research Group. (1993). A novel gene containing a trinucleotide repeat that is expanded and unstable on Huntington's disease chromosomes. *Cell, 72,* 971–983.

Klivenyi, P., Beal, M. F., Ferrante, R. J., Andreassen, O. A., Wermer, M., Chin, M. R., & Bonventre, J. V. (1998). Mice deficient in group IV cytosolic phospholipase A2 are resistant to MPTP neurotoxicity. *Journal of Neurochemistry, 71*, 2634–2637.

Mangiarini, L., Sathasivam, K., Seller, M., Cozens, B., Harper, A., Hetherington, C., Lawton, M., Trottier, Y., Lehrach, H., Davies, S. W., & Bates, G. P. (1996). Exon 1 of the HD gene with an expanded CAG repeat is sufficient to cause a progressive neurological phenotype in transgenic mice. *Cell, 87*, 493–506.

Puri, B. K. (2001). Impaired phospholipid-related signal transduction in advanced Huntington's disease. *Experimental Physiology, 86*, 683–685.

Puri, B. K. (2004). Monomodal rigid-body registration and applications to the investigation of the effects of eicosapentaenoic acid intervention in neuropsychiatric disorders. *Prostaglandins, Leukotrienes and Essential Fatty Acids, 71*, 177–179.

Puri, B. K., Bydder, G. M., Counsell, S. J., Corridan, B. J., Richardson, A. J., Hajnal, J. V., Appel, C., McKee, H. M., Vaddadi, K. S., & Horrobin, D. F. (2002). MRI and neuropsychological improvement in Huntington disease following ethyl-EPA treatment. *Neuroreport, 13*, 123–126.

Puri, B. K., Counsell, S. J., Hamilton, G., Richardson, A. J., & Horrobin, D. F. (2001). Eicosapentaenoic acid in treatment-resistant depression associated with symptom remission, structural brain changes and reduced neuronal phospholipid turnover. *International Journal of Clinical Practice, 55*, 560–563.

Puri, B. K., Hirsch, S. R., Easton, T., & Richardson, A. J. (2002). A volumetric biochemical niacin flush-based index that noninvasively detects fatty acid deficiency in schizophrenia. *Progress in Neuropsychopharmacology and Biological Psychiatry, 26*, 49–52.

Puri, B. K., Leavitt, B. R., Hayden, M. R., Ross, C. A., Rosenblatt, A., Greenamyre, J.. T., Hersch, S., Vaddadi, K. S., Sword, A., Horrobin, D. F., & Murck, H. (2005). Ethyl-EPA in Huntington's disease: A double-blind, randomized, placebo-controlled trial. *Neurology* (in press).

Puri, B. K., & Richardson, A. J. (1998). Sustained remission of positive and negative symptoms of schizophrenia following treatment with eicosapentaenoic acid. *Archives of General Psychiatry, 55*, 188–189.

Puri, B. K., Richardson, A. J., Horrobin, D. F., Easton, T., Saeed, N., Oatridge, A., Hajnal, J. V., & Bydder, G. M. (2000). Eicosapentaenoic acid treatment in schizophrenia associated with symptom remission, normalisation of blood fatty acids, reduced neuronal membrane phospholipid turnover and structural brain changes. *International Journal of Clinical Practice, 54*, 57–63.

Saeed, N., Puri, B. K., Oatridge, A., Hajnal, J. V., & Young, I. R. (1998). Two methods for semi-automated quantification of changes in ventricular volume and their use in schizophrenia. *Magnetic Resonance in Medicine, 16*, 1237–1247.

Sakai, T., Antoku, Y., Iwashita, H., Goto, I., Nagamatsu, K., & Shii, H. (1991). Chorea-acanthocytosis: Abnormal composition of covalently bound fatty acids of erythrocyte membrane proteins. *Annals of Neurology, 29*, 664–669.

Vaddadi, K. (2003). Essential fatty acids in the treatment of Huntington's disease. In M. Peet, I. Glen, & D. F. Horrobin (Eds.), *Phospholipid spectrum disorder in psychiatry and neurology* (2nd ed.). (pp. 565–574). Carnforth, Lancashire: Marius.

Vaddadi, K. S., Soosai, E., Chiu, E., & Dingjan, P. (2002). A randomised, placebo-controlled, double blind study of treatment of Huntington's disease with unsaturated fatty acids. *Neuroreport, 13*, 29–33.

19 Major Stressors in Women's Health

The Role of Nutrition

Adrianne Bendich and Ronit Zilberboim

KEY POINTS

- Women have higher rates of many serious diseases, including depression, autoimmune diseases, and osteoporosis, than do men.
- Women are affected by conditions linked to the menstrual cycle, including dysmenorrhea, amenorrhea, premenstrual syndrome, and polycystic ovarian syndrome.
- Caloric restriction can result in severe weight loss and cause or exacerbate amenorrhea, whereas weight loss in obese polycystic ovarian syndrome patients can result in significant lessening of symptoms and may reduce infertility.
- Menopause is a stressful period during which some symptoms can be lessened with dietary changes.
- Corticosteroids, used in the treatment of autoimmune diseases, significantly increase the risk of secondary osteoporosis.
- Postmenopausal bone loss as well as age-associated loss in bone mineral density (in both men and women) result in one-third of all women over 50 yr of age expected to fracture a bone during their lifetime.
- Calcium and vitamin D are critical in reducing the risk of osteoporotic fractures. Antiosteoporosis drug efficacy is predicated on adequate calcium and vitamin D status.

1. INTRODUCTION

The objectives of this chapter are to examine the differences in the causes of death and disability between men and women and determine if diet and/or nutritional status are factors contributing to these differences. We will examine the role of nutrition during several of the critical periods in a woman's life when stresses are increased. We will look at menstrual issues with emphasis on premenstrual syndrome (PMS), polycystic ovarian syndrome (PCOS), and pregnancy. Additionally, we will review two major diseases associated with female aging: autoimmune disease and osteoporosis.

1.1. Morbidity and Mortality Differences Between Men and Women and Women of Different Races/Ethnic Groups

Sex matters. Differences in prevalence and severity of diseases, disorders, and conditions exist between the sexes for many but not all diseases. These differences result in a

From: *Nutrients, Stress, and Medical Disorders*
Edited by: S. Yehuda and D. I. Mostofsky © Humana Press Inc., Totowa, NJ

Table 1
Leading Causes of Death for US Males and Females in 2000

	Males		*Females*	
	Rank	*% of total deaths*	*Rank*	*% of total deaths*
Heart disease	1	29	1	30
Cancer	2	24	2	22
Cerebrovascular disease	3	5	3	8
Accidents	4	5	8	3
Chronic respiratory disease	5	5	4	5
Diabetes	6	3	5	3
Influenza/pneumonia	7	2	6	3
Suicide	8	2		
Kidney disease	9	1.5	9	2
Liver disease	10	1.5		
Alzheimer's disease			7	3
Septicemia			10	1
All other causes		20		20

Source: National Vital Statistics, 2002.

life expectancy in the United States of 79.9 yr for women compared to 74.7 yr for men (National Vital Statistics, 2002). The 10 leading causes of death differ between women and men, as seen in Table 1. Health behaviors also differ between the sexes and may be related to mortality rates as well as the prevalence and severity of certain diseases. For instance, accidents are the fourth leading cause of death in men and only the eighth cause of mortality in women: the US Centers for Disease Control and Prevention (CDC) reported that about 30% of adult men had five or more alcoholic drinks in one day during the past year compared to about 11% of women. About the same percentage of men (25%) as women (21%) are current smokers, and about the same percentage are also obese. However, the percentage of black women who were obese was 35% compared to 20% in white women and only 6% in Asian women. Physical inactivity is slightly higher in women (41%) than in men (36%), and Hispanic women were the least active (55%). Hispanic women had very low rates of high alcohol consumption (7%) as well as smoking (12%). Significant differences between race/ethnic groups among women are also seen in the rates of maternal mortality. The average maternal mortality rate in 2001 was 9.9 deaths/ 100,000 live births. The rate in white women was 7.2/100,000 compared to the threefold higher rate of 24.7 deaths/100,000 in black women (National Vital Statistics, 2002). These data speak not only to the differences between the sexes, but also to the wider differences within the female population based on race/ethnicity .

The prevalence of depression also differs between the sexes. Of the approx 20 million Americans affected by depression, women are at least twice as likely as men to experience major depressive periods. Specifically 10–23% of US women of childbearing age (18–44 yr) experience symptoms of depression—twice the rate observed in men at matching ages. Major depression can impair social and physical functioning more than certain serious medical conditions that can be successfully identified and treated (Ahluwalia, Holtzman, Mack, & Mokdad, 2003; Mazure, Keita, & Blehar, 2002). The origin of these differences is attributed to hormones, stress, and several predispositions, including higher levels of physical and mental impairment. Women who are less educated and earn lower salaries or who are single have more frequent negative physical and mental health-related measurements than women at higher economic levels (Ahluwalia et al., 2003). (The potential role of nutrition in the development of depressive disease is reviewed in several chapters in this volume.)

There were some positive changes in the health behaviors of women between 1991 and 2001: about 76% of women over 40 yr of age had mammograms in 2001 compared to about 63% a decade earlier. Unfortunately, prevalence of high blood pressure in women 65 yr or older increased to about 55% compared to about 45% earlier. This could certainly be related to the increase in obesity seen in the same period—from about 12% to 21% (Mack & Ahluwalia, 2003). When adult women were asked to rate their overall health status from excellent to poor, 62% rated themselves as excellent or very good, about 25% rated themselves as good, and about 10% indicated that their health was fair or poor (Ahluwalia et al., 2003). Yet in the same survey, about 13% report frequent mental stress, about 20% reported feeling worried, tense, or anxious, and over 40% said they did not get enough sleep.

1.2. Vitamin Status and Chronic Disease

Fairfield and Fletcher (2002) reviewed the literature published from 1966 to 2001 that examined the association of vitamin status and chronic diseases. They identified nine vitamins that are central to the health of adults: folate, vitamins B_6, B_{12}, D, E, A, C, and K. They found that not only was low vitamin status associated with increased risk of diseases such as cardiovascular disease, cancer, and osteoporosis, but also that higher-than-recommended intake levels are often associated with reduced disease risk. Moreover, certain vitamins are associated with reduction in the risks of several diseases; for example, low folate status is associated with increased risk of coronary heart disease, colon and breast cancer, as well as neural tube birth defects. In some cases, such as vitamin C where the highest intakes are associated with the lowest risk of cancer of the breast, esophagus, stomach, and oral cavity, it is unclear if this association is attributable to the vitamin alone or rather to the fruits that contain high levels of it. Nevertheless, there is a growing appreciation among health professionals that dietary intake of optimal levels of essential micronutrients is often associated with chronic disease risk reduction (Bendich & Deckelbaum, 2001a, 2001b).

1.3. Use of Dietary Supplements

Some of the significant differences between the health statistics comparing men and women or women of different race/ethnic groups cited above may be owing in part to differences in dietary intakes of both macro- and micronutrients as well as the use of dietary supplements. Dietary supplements are used by about half of the US adult population and women use supplements more than men (44 vs 35%, respectively) (Patterson, Kristal, & Neuhouser, 2001). Age is also a factor, and as women age, their use of supplements increases (52–55% in women over 50 yr of age). For instance, in a cohort of over 16,000 postmenopausal women enrolled in the Women's Health Initiative (WHI), 44% took multivitamin supplements regularly prior to entry into the study, 53% took vitamin E, 53% took vitamin C, and 52% took calcium. These data are consistent with usage in the entire cohort from the WHI (over 68,000 in the clinical intervention trial as well as the more than 93,000 women in the observational study), where more than 55% took supplemental vitamin C from either a multivitamin or a single supplement; about 57% took supplemental vitamin E (Shikany, Patterson, Agurs-Collins, & Anderson, 2003). Data from the National Health and Nutrition Examination Survey (NHANES) I and II showed that more Caucasians than blacks used supplements and usage increased in both groups with age (Block et al., 1988; Koplan, Annest, Layde, & Rubin, 1986). Similarly, the 1987 National Health Interview Survey (NHIS) found that 60% of Caucasian vs 45% of black women consumed any type of supplement during the past year (Subar & Block, 1990). Only 15% of Caucasian women 17–24 yr of age reported daily supplement use, whereas 40% of those 55–64 yr used a supplement daily; the respective percentages in age-matched black women were 12% and 21%.

Frank, Bendich, and Denniston (2000) documented the dietary supplement use patterns as well as diets of a large cohort of US women physicians. Half of the women physicians took a multivitamin/mineral supplement, and one-third did so regularly (at least five times per week). However, with the exception of calcium, less than a third took any other supplement and less than 20% did so regularly. Regular vitamin/mineral use increased with age, and antioxidant intake was higher among those with known risks for heart disease. Female physicians with a personal history of osteoporosis were nearly three times as likely as those without such a history to take some supplemental calcium regularly. Those who took any supplement regularly also consumed more fruits and vegetables per day (3.4 servings) than non-supplement users. Regular users of any supplement also consumed less fat than non-supplement users. Additionally, those who regularly consumed any supplement were more likely to be vegetarian and to comply with dietary guidelines than were those who were nonusers.

More women physicians at risk for or suffering from chronic diseases used supplements than those not at such risk. For instance, 74% of those with breast cancer compared to 46% of those without used supplements, and 26% of those with high blood pressure and cholesterol took vitamin E supplements compared to about 16% of those without these risk factors. Lyle et al. also found that more women (24%) with a history of cancer used vitamin E supplements (>30 IU) than those who had not had cancer (7%) (Lyle et al., 1999). Regular use of nutritional supplements by women physicians increased with age. In the Nurse's Health Study supplement use also increased with age (Willett, Sampson, & Bain, 1981). Women physicians who were widowed had the highest percentage of regular vitamin users (57%) compared to those who were single or never married (41%). A national survey also showed that 40% of those widowed, separated, or divorced vs 34% of those never married used supplements, suggesting that this is not merely a function of age (Moss, Levy, Kim, & Park, 1989). Among nondrinking women physicians, 52% (compared to 45% of drinkers) regularly used supplements. Supplement use was also higher in the national survey in those with the lowest alcohol consumption (Subar & Block, 1990). More than 75% of osteoporotic women physicians took calcium supplements compared to 25% in those who did not have osteoporosis. Overall, 38% of the entire cohort took a calcium supplement (26% regularly), which is much higher than the data from NHANES III, which showed that about 2% of women took calcium during the previous month. Variations in supplement use also reflected variations in disease risk factors. About 35% of the women physicians reported a personal or family history of coronary heart disease (CHD). This may have increased use of both antioxidants and folic-acid-containing supplements, as these have been indicated as reducing CHD risk, and physicians may be particularly aware of the link between family history and risk of heart disease (Patterson et al., 2001). A recent prospective epidemiological study on supplement use and cancer risk reported that 57% of the more than 77,000 people enrolled 50–76 yr old were taking multivitamins (Satia-Abouta et al., 2003; White et al., 2004). About 52% were women, and they used multivitamins, vitamin C, and vitamin E supplements more frequently than men; women also took calcium supplements about five times more frequently than men.

2. FEMALE STRESSORS

Both mental and physical stress has been associated with the reproductive life of women from menarche (the first menstruation) through the monthly menstrual cycle to menopause (the end of menstruation). These biological functions are affected by various intrinsic and extrinsic factors, including genetic parameters, socioeconomic conditions, general health and lifestyle, as well as nutritional factors and physical activity (Thomas, Renaud, Benefice, de Meeus, & Guegan, 2001).

2.1. Menstruation

Dysmenorrhea is a common gynecological complaint consisting of painful cramps accompanying menstruation. In cases where there is no other major abnormality, it is known as primary dysmenorrhea (Marjoribanks, Proctor, & Farquhar, 2003). Balbi et al. (2000) has reported that approx 85% of adolescent girls experienced primary dysmenorrhea pain monthly. Early menarche increased the risk, whereas consumption of fish, eggs, and fruit decreased the risk. Fish and eggs are excellent dietary sources of long-chain ω-3 fatty acids that are associated with reduced levels of inflammatory prostaglandins. Research has shown that women with dysmenorrhea have high levels of prostaglandins known to cause cramping abdominal pain.

Weight loss also affects the menstrual cycle. McLean and Barr (2003) reported that female university students who deliberately reduced their caloric intakes had significantly more irregular menstrual cycles than women who were less restrained in their eating habits. Taken to the extreme, severe weight restriction can have serious adverse effects that go beyond alterations in the menstrual cycle. The female athlete triad consists of amenorrhea, disordered eating, and osteoporosis. The primary factor inducing reduction in bone mass in this disorder is considered to be estrogen deficiency (hypogonadism). The prevalence of amenorrhea was related to the intensity, duration, and type of exercise. Nutritional status was also an important determinant of the response of the reproductive system to physically powerful training. Exercise levels were directly related to induced amenorrhea and were also associated with reduced bone mineral density (BMD) despite the known positive effect of weight-bearing exercise on bone density (Miller, 2003). While the common theory associated insufficient fat storage with the disorders of the reproductive system, recent data support reduced energy availability as the regulating factor. Thus, reversal of such disorders may be possible with the aid of dietary supplementation combined with increased energy intake (Loucks, 2003).

Loss of BMD also occurs in females suffering from anorexia nervosa (AN) who have levels of estrogen deficiency similar to those found in females suffering from the female athlete triad. Unfortunately, in studies of AN subjects, estrogen therapy failed to restore bone mass (reviewed in Miller, 2003). It has been documented that severe under-nutrition directly affects bone mass and weight or body mass index (BMI) and can also be correlated with osteocalcin, a protein that is synthesized by bone-forming cells and is used as a marker of bone formation. Weight gain, especially if associated with regained menses, is highly correlated with increased bone density. It also has been suggested that nutritionally regulated hormones, such as insulin-like growth factor-1 (IGF-1), that are adversely affected by low protein intakes are important contributors to bone loss in AN cases (Miller, 2003). Because these disorders affect young women during the period of significant bone acquisition, there is an increased potential for osteoporotic bone disease in later life (Gordon, 2003).

2.2. PMS

The term premenstrual syndrome refers to a cluster of mood, physical, and cognitive symptoms that occur 1–2 wk prior to the start of menstrual bleeding and subside with the onset of menstruation. As many as 80% of women of reproductive age may experience premenstrual emotional and physical changes (American College of Obstetricians and Gynecologists [ACOG] Committee Opinion, 1995). Up to 40% of women of reproductive age experience premenstrual symptoms sufficient to affect their daily lives, and 5% experience severe impairment (Daugherty, 1998). Symptoms vary among individuals; the most common symptoms include fatigue, irritability, abdominal bloating, breast tenderness, labile mood with alternating sadness and anger, and depression (ACOG Committee Opinion, 1995).

Many types of dietary supplements have been advocated for the reduction of certain symptoms of PMS (Table 2). Limited data suggest that magnesium, vitamin E, and carbohydrate supplements might have positive effects on certain symptoms. Trials with vitamin B_6 supplementation have had conflicting results, and high doses of this vitamin taken for prolonged periods of time can cause neurological symptoms. Clinical studies of evening primrose oil have had conflicting results; the two most rigorous studies showed no evidence of benefit (Bendich, 2000).

There is a long history of scientific examination of the link between calcium status and the menstrual cycle. A 1930 study (Okey, Stewart, & Greenwood, 1930) showed that plasma calcium levels were lower in the premenstrual period compared to those seen in the week following menstruation. A preliminary dietary study (Penland & Johnson, 1993) demonstrated decreased symptoms of premenstrual and menstrual distress when women received diets containing 1336 mg/d of calcium, as opposed to 587 mg. A large US-based, multicenter clinical trial (Thys-Jacobs, Starkey, Bernstein, & Tian, 1998) involving 466 women with diagnosed PMS received 1200 mg/d of calcium or placebo for three menstrual cycles. The calcium-supplemented cohort showed an overall 48% reduction in symptoms as compared to a 30% reduction in the placebo group. All four symptom factor composite scores (negative affect, water retention, food cravings, and pain) were significantly improved in the calcium-supplemented group.

There is evidence that abnormalities in calcium and vitamin D regulation may contribute to the causation of PMS and that PMS may be linked to other disorders associated with inadequate calcium intake, such as osteoporosis. In a study that compared women with established vertebral osteoporosis to controls (Lee & Kanis, 1994), it was found that the risk of osteoporosis was higher among those with a history of PMS. Another study found evidence of reduced bone mass in women with PMS as compared to asymptomatic controls (Thys-Jacobs, Alvir, & Fratarcangelo, 1995). PMS may serve as a clinical marker of low calcium status, perhaps reflecting an underlying abnormality in calcium metabolism, and it may serve as an early warning sign to young women of a possible increased risk of osteoporosis.

A recent population-based, prospective study of women in the transition to menopause reported that 36–44% of women between 35 and 44 yr of age had PMS. Women with PMS had a twofold increased risk of hot flushes, a 2.3-fold increased risk of depressed mood, and 1.5-fold increased risk of decreased libido compared to the women without PMS. The study confirms earlier studies that found an increased prevalence of menopausal symptoms in women who had PMS before menopause (Freeman, Sammel, Rinaudo, & Sheng, 2004). At present no studies have reported an association between calcium intake and menopausal symptoms.

2.3. Polycystic Ovarian Syndrome

PCOS is classified as a metabolic disorder that affects approximately 6–10% of US women (Beers & Berklow, 1999b; Norman, Wu, & Stankiewicz, 2004). The syndrome is characterized by the finding of polycystic ovaries on ultrasound examination and lengthened menstrual cycles from 28–30 d to 45–60 d. In addition, there is often impaired glucose tolerance, hypercholesterolemia, excess body weight, hirsutism, persistent acne, alopecia, elevated serum testosterone, and infertility. Women who have a family history of diabetes are at increased risk for PCOS, and women with PCOS are at increased risk of developing type 2 diabetes (Dunaif & Lobo, 2002; Norman et al., 2004). In obese women with PCOS, moderate weight loss has been shown to reduce elevated insulin levels, normalize menstrual function, and increase fertility/pregnancy rates (Kiddy et al., 1992). A number of the signs of PCOS would predict a higher risk of cardiovascular disease. In fact, a recent study has shown an increased occurrence of coronary artery calcification in age- and weight-matched women with PCOS. Increased coronary artery calcification is an emerging non-invasive marker of increased cardiovascular risk (Christian et al., 2003).

Michelmore, Balen, and Dunger (2001) examined the association of eating disorders such as bulimia and PCOS in a cohort of young college women. They assessed symptoms of PCOS and eating disorders in 230 women using physical exams and questionnaires and found that having polycystic ovaries does not predispose women to develop eating disorders.

For many women with PCOS, the major stress is infertility. Thys-Jacobs, Donovan, Papadopoulos, Sarrel, and Bilezikian (1999) hypothesized that ovarian functions may be adversely affected by abnormal calcium homeostasis as well as insufficient dietary calcium and vitamin D in women with PCOS. The investigators have examined the effects of calcium supplementation in a pilot unblinded study in a small cohort of women with PCOS. For 6 mo 13 women were given 1500 mg of calcium daily and 50,000 units of ergocalciferol (vitamin D_2) weekly or biweekly to maintain a normal serum 25-hydroxyvitamin D level. Within 2 mo of initiating treatment, 7 of 9 women with abnormal menstrual cycles had regular cycles; the 4 with regular menstrual cycles continued to have normal cycles. Two women became pregnant during the study. Further well-con-

Table 2
Supplements Used to Treat PMS Symptoms

Supplement	*Rational*	*Study design*	*Outcomes*	*Conclusions and comments*	*Ref.*
Calcium	Plasma calcium levels linked to the menstrual cycle A similarity between PMS symptoms and those occurring during hypocalcemia	Randomized double-blind crossover 33 participants completed 1000 mg/d elemental calcium (as calcium carbonate)	Significant reduction in premenstrual symptoms after supplementation	Amounts of calcium are well within accepted safety limits Tolerable Upper Intake Level (UL) has been set at 2500 mg/d USDA's 1994 Continuing Survey of Food Intakes by Individuals showed that menstruating women consume far less than 1000 mg/d of calcium from food Calcium is safe even for women who may become pregnant Calcium supplementation is inexpensive	Douglas, 2002
		Controlled metabolic live-in dietary study for 10 women with normal menstrual cycles 1336 mg/d of calcium, as opposed to 587 mg/d (with 1 or 5.6 mg manganese)	Decreased symptoms of premenstrual and menstrual distress including pain, mood, and water retention	Dietary calcium and manganese may have a functional role in the manifestation of symptomatology typically associated with menstrual distress	Penland & Johnson, 1993
	Disturbances in calcium regulation may underlie the pathophysiologic characteristics of premenstrual syndrome Calcium supplementation may be an effective therapeutic approach	US-based, multicenter clinical trial with 466 healthy women completing the trial 1200 mg/d of elemental calcium (as calcium carbonate) or placebo Four symptom factors negative affect, water	Those receiving calcium showed an overall 48% reduction in total core symptom scores of 17 criteria from baseline, as compared to a 30% reduction in the placebo group	Calcium supplementation is a simple and effective treatment in premenstrual syndrome, resulting in a major reduction in overall luteal phase symptoms	Thys-Jacobs et al., 1998

		retention, food cravings, and pain) and 17 core symptoms were evaluated before and during treatment (prospectively documenting over 2 menstrual cycles followed by 3 menstrual cycles	All symptom factors were significantly reduced relative to prospective baseline		
		Review of the literature		Calcium supplementation should be considered a sound treatment option in women who experience PMS	Ward & Holimon, 1999
		Review of the literature		Calcium carbonate should be recommended as first-line therapy for women with mild to moderate PMS	Douglas, 2002
Manganese	Manganese levels vary with th menstrual cycle in humans Low manganese intakes are associated with disruption of reproduction in animals	In a metabolic ward study, 10 healthy women were assigned to diets high and low in manganese (5.6 vs 1.0 mg/d) for 39-day periods	Lower dietary manganese intake was associated with increased mood and pain symptoms during the premenstrual phase of the cycle	Lower intake level tested in this study was about 50% of typical manganese intake It is unclear whether the difference between the two levels of manganese represents a benefit of manganese supplementation or an adverse effect of manganese depletion	Penland & Johnson, 1993
Magnesium	Levels of magnesium in erythrocytes and leukocytes of women with PMS were lower than those in women without PMS Magnesium is involved in the activity of serotonin and other neurotransmitters	A trial involving 38 subjects with relatively mild premenstrual symptoms Randomized, double-blind, placebo-controlled, crossover study Daily supplement of 200 mg	Reduced symptoms related to fluid retention in the second but not the first month of use No significant effects on mood-related symptoms reported	Magnesium supplementation at doses used in trials described above is usually well tolerated	Walker et al., 1998

(continued)

Table 2
(continued)

Supplement	*Rational*	*Study design*	*Outcomes*	*Conclusions and comments*	*Ref.*
	Magnesium participates in vascular contraction, neuromuscular function, and cell membrane stability	magnesium (MgO) for two menstrual cycles Six symptom categories, including anxiety, craving, depression, hydration, were recorded			
		32 women with PMS Supplementation with 360 mg/d of magnesium (during second half of menstrual cycle)	Significantly reduced total PMS symptoms and specifically those symptoms related to mood changes		Facchinetti et al., 1991
		20 patients with premenstrual migraine Prophylactic supplementation with magnesium 360 mg/d or placebo during second half of menstrual cycle	Significantly reduced the number of days with headache		Facchinetti, Sances, Borella, Genazzani, & Nappi, 1991
Vitamin B_6	Vitamin B_6 is a cofactor in the synthesis of neurotransmitters	Placebo control 28 women with PMS 250 mg B_6 Nutritional counseling 1-mo intervention	No significant PMS benefit of B6 supplementation	Women with PMS who take vitamin B_6 supplements despite lack of clear evidence of efficacy need to be aware that high doses can cause sensory neuropathy	Bendich, 2000; Berman, Taylor, & Freeman, 1990; Diegoli, da Fonseca, Diegoli, & Pinotti, 1998
Vitamin E		Double-blind trial 41 women with PMS received 400 IU/dof vitamin E or placebo Three cycles	Significant improvements in some affective and physical symptoms observed in vitamin E group	Women with PMS were not biochemically deficient in vitamin E, and plasma vitamin E levels were not lower than those of women who do not have PMS (Mira, Stewart, & Abraham, 1988; Chuong, Dawson, & Smith, 1990)	Chuong, Dawson, & Smith, 1990; London, Murphy, Kitlowski, & Reynolds, 1987; Mira, Stewart, & Abraham, 1988

Combination supplements containing essential nutrients		Multivitamin/multimineral supplement high in magnesium and vitamin B_6 (Optivite) Double-blind, randomized study on 44 women with PMS to receive placebo, 6 or 12 tablets Baseline established for 1 mo followed by 3 menstrual cycles	Significantly more effective than placebo in relieving premenstrual symptoms	Recommended dose (6–12 tablets/d) provides 300–600 mg of vitamin B_6, well in excess of the UL of 100 mg/d (Institute of Medicine, 1998) Provides 12,500–25,000 IU of vitamin A as retinol, which is above the safety limit of 8000 IU/d for women of childbearing potential (Oakley & Erickson, 1995) Of components of Optivite, the one with the greatest evidence of efficacy is magnesium; a dose of 6–12 tablets/d of Optivite would provide 250–500 mg/d of this mineral, which is within the range associated with beneficial effects on PMS symptoms in studies of magnesium alone	Chakmakjian, Higgins, & Abraham, 1985; London, Bradley, & Chiamori, 1991; Oakley, 1998; Oakley & Erickson, 1995; Standing Committee on the Scientific Evaluation of Dietary Reference Intakes Food and Nutrition Board Institute of Medicine, 1997)
	Dietary approach to evaluate alleviating symptoms of premenstrual syndrome	Yeast-based, magnesium-containing combination supplement (Sillix Donna) Single double-blind study of 40 patients affected by mild to moderate premenstrual syndrome for up to 6 mo	No side effects observed Treatment significantly more effective at all times Significantly reduced premenstrual scores at 6 mo	Most likely beneficial ingredient in Sillix Donna is magnesium; the recommended dose (2 tablets twice a day) provides 400 mg Sillix Donna does not contain any components in quantities that exceed current safety limits	Facchinetti et al., 1997

trolled clinical studies are needed to fully understand the potential for calcium and vitamin D to affect certain aspects of PCOS.

2.4. Pregnancy

2.4.1. Pregnancy Outcomes: Birth Defect Prevention

Pregnancy is a time of increased stress for the mother-to-be. There are many fears concerning the health of the unborn child. Women often become aware of the two leading causes of infant mortality in the United States: birth defects and premature birth (Czeizel, 2001; Scholl, 2001). One of the most important discoveries of the 20th century was that folic acid, along with other micronutrients, could prevent many serious birth defects as well as reduce the risk of premature and low-birthweight birth outcomes. Many of the initial observations concerning the link between diet and serious birth defects were made in the United Kingdom. Smithells and colleagues noted that infants who were born with neural tube defects (NTDs) who either lacked a cranium and brain (anencephaly) or with a hole in their spines (spina bifida) often had mothers with poor dietary intakes and were from areas of poverty (Schorah & Smithells, 1991; Smithells et al., 1980). Of great concern was the fact that women with one affected pregnancy were at about a 10-fold increased risk of having a second infant with an NTD. Smithells and colleagues used a multivitamin that contained vitamin C and several B vitamins, including 0.36 mg of folic acid, in a nonplacebo intervention study; they found about a 70% reduction in recurrence of NTD in the women who took the supplement during the periconceptional period (before conception—about 1–3 mo, and during the early months of their pregnancies).

The definitive placebo-controlled, double-blind study of folic acid and prevention of recurrence of NTDs was published in 1991 by the Medical Research Council (MRC) and was led by Dr. Nicholas Wald (MRC Vitamin Study Research Group, 1991). In this study, recurrence of NTDs was reduced by 70% when a daily dose of 4-mg folic acid supplement was taken during the periconceptional period; additional supplementation with B vitamins did not confer further reduction in NTDs. Even though no other types of birth defects were reduced in the supplemented groups, this study clearly showed that a simple B vitamin, folic acid, could prevent the recurrence of NTDs.

NTDs occur during early pregnancy, often before a woman knows she is pregnant. The studies that found that folic acid prevented recurrence of NTDs cannot be underestimated, but the 1000-fold more prevalent event is the first occurrence of an NTD. In 1992 Czeizel and Dudas published the results of their impressive study that showed that a prenatal multivitamin supplement containing 0.8 mg of folic acid not only resulted in a greater than 90% reduction in the first occurrence of NTD, but also halved the rate of several major birth defects (Czeizel & Dudas, 1992). This study involved nearly 5000 pregnancies, and the results were greater than expected. Cardiovascular birth defects, which occur at a 5–10 times greater rate than NTD, were reduced by 60%, and there were fewer cleft lip/cleft palate defects, kidney defects, and limb reductions. The prenatal supplement or placebo was taken during the periconceptional period and throughout pregnancy. In addition to significant reductions in several classes of birth defects, the supplemented group experienced a 40% increase in multiple births (twins) and easier pregnancies with significantly less morning sickness. During the preconceptional period, the supplemented group's menstrual cycles became more regular, the time taken to become pregnant was shorter than in the placebo group, and there was a 7% increase in the rate of conception (Czeizel, 2001).

The supplement used in the Czeizel and Dudas trial is more comparable to the typical one-a-day type multivitamin/mineral supplement sold in the United States than the supplement used in the MRC trial. Thus, it is not surprising that survey data from the United States suggest that lowered cardiovascular birth defect risk is associated with periconceptional use of multivitamin/mineral supplements (Czeizel, 2001).

In 1992 the US Public Health Service (USPHS) recommended that all women capable of becoming pregnant consume 0.4 mg (400 μg) of folic acid daily. Three approaches to increasing folic acid consumption were suggested: improve dietary habits, fortify foods with folic acid, and use dietary supplements containing folic acid (Epidemiology Program Office, 1992). Mandatory fortification of cereal grain products went into effect in the United States in January 1998; during October 1998–December 1999, the reported prevalence of spina bifida declined 31% and the prevalence of anencephaly declined 16%. The CDC recently analyzed data from 23 population-based surveillance systems and reported that the number of NTD-affected pregnancies in the United States declined from 4000 in 1995–1996 to 3000 in 1999–2000. This decline in NTD-affected pregnancies highlights the partial success of the US folic acid fortification program as a public health strategy (Mersereau et al., 2004).

Unfortunately, few women (about 20%), even today, take a multivitamin daily during the periconceptional period before they have confirmed their pregnancy (Johnston & Staples, 1998). The majority of branded multivitamin supplements contain 0.4 mg of folic acid. Oakley, in an editorial in the *New England Journal of Medicine*, suggested that the right advice to American women is to eat the best diets possible and also take a multivitamin containing folic acid to assure that the birth-defect-preventive level of folic acid is consumed daily (Oakley, 1998). Further verification of the need for 0.4 mg of folic acid is seen in a recent study from China (Berry et al., 1999). There was a fourfold reduction in NTDs in the high-risk area and a 40% reduction in a lower-risk area when women anticipating pregnancy took supplemental folic acid during the periconceptional period.

The mechanism(s) by which folic acid prevents the incomplete closure of the neural tube have yet to be completely understood. One hypothesis suggests that there is an exceptional requirement of the embryo for folic acid during this period of cell duplication as the vitamin is required for the synthesis of nucleic acids and proteins; a second theory involves the presence of higher-than-normal levels of the amino acid homocysteine, which may preferentially destroy neural tube cells. There is an inverse relationship between the serum levels of folic acid and homocysteine (Czeizel, 2001).

2.4.2. Pregnancy Outcomes: Low Birthweight and Premature Birth Prevention

Low birthweight and preterm delivery often occur simultaneously. Preterm delivery is defined as birth following less than 37 wk of gestation; very preterm delivery is defined as less than 33 wk gestation. Low birthweight is defined as less than 2500 g and very low birthweight as less than 1500 g. Of all low-birthweight infants born, 60–70% are also preterm. In the United States, preterm delivery associated with low birthweight is the second leading cause of infant hospitalization and is also the second leading cause of infant mortality, following birth defects (Division of Reproductive Health, 1999). Low birthweight ranks second behind cardiovascular birth defects in annual hospitalization costs, exceeding $2.5 billion/yr (Bendich, Mallick, & Leader, 1997). Preterm births are more prevalent in teens, those with less than a high school education, and those with the lowest incomes.

Scholl et al. (1997) found in a prospective, case-control study that pregnant women in Camden, New Jersey, who took prenatal multivitamins during the first trimester had a fourfold reduction in very preterm births and a twofold reduction in preterm births. Even if supplementation began in the second trimester, there was a significant twofold reduction in very preterm as well as preterm births. The risk of very-low-birthweight outcomes (highly correlated with preterm delivery) was dramatically reduced by six- to sevenfold when prenatal multivitamins were taken during the first two trimesters. Low birthweight was also reduced significantly with supplementation. These results were found even though the women were at high risk for preterm/low-birthweight outcomes: they were poor, teens, and many had low weight gain during pregnancy. Prenatal supplements increased iron and folate status significantly, but did not alter serum zinc level. Previously, low iron and/or folate status had been associated with increased risk of preterm birth and low birthweight. Zinc-containing multivitamins have also been shown to reduce preterm births in an intervention study (Goldenberg et al., 1995).

Exposure to low nutrient intakes or substances that reduce dietary intakes in pregnant women may have effects that extend beyond the gestation period. Jones Riley, and Dwyer (1999) found that maternal smoking during pregnancy resulted in children having shorter stature linked to lower bone mass. Children of smoking mothers may be at greater risk for osteoporosis because their bones do not accumulate the mass needed to prevent this disease in later life. Importantly, infant bone mass has been shown to be increased if mothers are supplemented with calcium during pregnancy. Koo et al. (1999) showed that total bone mineral content was significantly greater in infant children born to mothers supplemented with 2000 mg/d of calcium during pregnancy compared to women in the placebo group, who consumed less than 600 mg/d of calcium. Recently, there have been links made between maternal diet during pregnancy, preterm birth, and cardiovascular disease in the offspring 50 or more years after birth (Barker, 1999; Klebanoff, Secher, Mednick, & Schulsinger, 1999). It may be that a program to provide folic-acid-containing multivitamins to all women of childbearing potential before as well as during the entire pregnancy may have far greater consequences than the immediate effects of reduction of either birth defects or preterm births. The full effects of reducing adverse birth outcomes may not be realized until the child reaches full maturity.

In developing countries, premature births are an even more serious problem; an additional problem is intrauterine growth retardation, which is often coincident with premature birth but may also occur with term delivery. de Onis, Villar, and Gulmezoglu (1998) reviewed the 12 nutritionally based intervention studies that examined the incidence of intrauterine growth retardation, preterm birth, and low birthweight. Only one of the interventions, balanced protein/energy supplementation during pregnancy, significantly reduced the risk of low birthweight. The authors also suggest that many of the micronutrients reviewed (vitamin D, folic acid, zinc, calcium, magnesium, and iron) were likely to prove beneficial. Ramakrishnan and Huffman (2001) extensively reviewed both observational and intervention studies from developing and developed countries that examined the role of micronutrients in optimizing pregnancy outcomes. In developing countries, one out of every five infants has low birthweight (20%) compared to a rate of 6% in developed countries. Moreover, in developing countries, the majority of low birthweight infants are carried to term. Intrauterine growth retardation is a significantly greater problem in developing countries and affects the physical and mental health of the child throughout life. Low maternal micronutrient intakes of zinc, calcium, magnesium, vitamin A, vitamin C, and possibly B vitamins, copper, and selenium are associated with premature birth and low birthweight. Deficiencies of iodine, folate, and/or iron are also linked to adverse pregnancy outcomes (Keen, Bendich, & Willhite, 1993).

Two large, well-controlled intervention studies in developing countries have found that micronutrient status can significantly enhance maternal health and pregnancy outcomes. West et al. (1999) examined, in a placebo-controlled trial, the effects of weekly supplementation with either the recommended dietary allowance of preformed vitamin A or β-carotene in more than 20,000 pregnant women in Nepal. They found a significant 40% reduction in maternal mortality in the supplemented group. The women were supplemented before conception and throughout the pregnancy. Interventions were a once-a-week supplement of either 20,000 IU of vitamin A as retinol or 42 mg of β-carotene or placebo. β-Carotene appeared to be more effective than retinol. Low β-carotene status has been reported in cases of pre-eclampsia in women from developing countries, and, as discussed below, the antioxidant potential of β-carotene (compared to the much lower antioxidant potential of retinol) may have been involved in reducing the incidence of maternal mortality seen in this study.

The second critical study involved more than 1000 HIV-infected pregnant women from Tanzania (Fawzi et al., 1998). In this placebo-controlled trial, the pregnant women received either placebo, β-carotene and retinol, a multivitamin containing vitamins B_1, B_2, B_6, B_{12}, niacin, folic acid, and vitamins C and E, or the multivitamin plus β-carotene and retinol from 12–27 wk gestation to birth. There was a 40% reduction in fetal death, 44% reduction in low birthweight, 39% reduction in very preterm birth, and a 43% reduction in small-for-gestational-age outcomes in the groups supplemented with the multivitamin independent of the vitamin A. Additionally, mothers taking the multivitamin had significantly heavier babies than those not taking the multivitamin ($p = 0.01$). Even though the supplement did not contain iron, the women in the multivitamin group had a significant increase in hemoglobin levels compared to those not taking the multivitamin. Because this study involved HIV-positive women, the investigators also measured the concentration of total T cells (CD3), T-helper cells (CD4) and T-suppressor cells (CD8). HIV-positive pregnant women who took the multivitamin supplement had significant increases in total T cells, mainly owing to increases in CD3 cells; CD8 cells also increased. Although vitamin A from either β-carotene or retinol did not show an effect in reducing transmission of HIV from mother to neonate, it may be that the HIV-infected women had low vitamin A status at the onset and the level provided may not have been sufficient and/or may not have been absorbed sufficiently to show an effect. It may also be that the vitamin A was administered too late in these pregnancies to see a reduction in HIV transmission. In the West et al. (1999) study, vitamin A supplementation, which is critical for early embryonic growth, was started before conception. An important finding in the Fawzi et al. (1998) study was that a multivitamin supplement containing modest doses of micronutrients significantly improved birth outcomes to levels similar to that seen when poor non-HIV-positive women in the United States used multivitamins during their pregnancies (Scholl, 2001).

3. MENOPAUSAL AND POSTMENOPAUSAL STRESSORS

Menopause is a stressful transition time for most women as it represents the loss of reproductive potential and the depletion of ovarian function culminating in the cessation of menses. The clinical definition of menopause and endocrine measures of menopause do not always correspond; therefore, in 2001 a menopause staging system was established (Soules et al., 2001). Stages of the menopause period span several years and include different symptoms. For example, in the perimenopausal period (newer definition of early and late menopause transition stages), menstruation has not completely ceased, yet there are symptoms associated with menopause, such as hot flashes. The progression of the menopause transition is associated with a loss in the feedback loop between the ovaries and the hypothalamic–pituitary axis, with significant reduction in the synthesis of pituitary gonadotropin follicle-stimulating hormone (FSH) and ovarian steroid hormones, including estrogen (Joffe, Soares, & Cohen, 2003). In addition to certain uncomfortable and stressful symptoms, the risk of age-related chronic diseases, such as autoimmune disease and osteoporosis, also increases.

3.1. Hot Fla(u)shes and Other Symptoms

Hot flashes, the most common menopausal complaint, affect about 75% of perimenopausal and postmenopausal women. Other symptoms, including sleep disruption and mood disturbances, are closely associated and may be partly induced by hot flashes. In the United States alone, more than 1 million women are expected to reach menopause every year. Medically induced menopause also often results in hot flashes. Despite its high prevalence and serious effects on quality of life, the physiology of hot flashes is not clearly understood (Joffe et al., 2003; Stearns, Beebe, Iyengar, & Dube, 2003). It is clear, however, that hot flashes are related to thermoregulation. Further, since hormones like estrogen, serotonin, and norepinephrine influence the thermoregulatory center, hormone therapy (mainly hormone-replacement therapy [HRT]) was the first and thus far the most successful avenue for treatment (Joffe et al., 2003). On the other hand, adverse effects associated with short-term (deep vein thrombosis) or long-term (cardiovascular and breast cancer) risks owing to the use of estrogen and progesterone have led to the development of other, nonhormonal therapies, which are now available (Rossouw et al., 2002). Nonhormonal prescription options including selective serotonin reuptake inhibitors (Stearns et al., 2003), psychoactive drugs, and an anticonvulsant have demonstrated some efficacy for treating hot flashes and are usually well tolerated (Joffe et al., 2003).

The strongest link between diet and menopausal symptoms involves soy products. Messina and Hughes (2003) reviewed the data from 19 clinical trials that examined the association of intake of soy foods or isolates from soy on the prevalence of hot flashes in perimenopausal women. The totality of the evidence supported a positive effect of soy on reducing the frequency of hot flashes, but because of the different types of products used as well as the intake levels, further studies are needed to clarify this relationship. This conclusion is supported by an independent review of 29 published studies in the literature on complementary and alternative medicine products used in the treatment of menopausal symptoms including hot flashes (Kronenberg & Fugh-Berman, 2002). Several other dietary supplements that have no nutritive value have been investigated for effects on menopausal symptoms. These are not reviewed in this chapter.

4. AUTOIMMUNE DISEASES

Autoimmune diseases are caused by an inappropriate response of the immune system to self antigens. Autoimmune diseases are noncontagious, although these may be triggered by an infectious agent and are often worsened by stressful life events. On the cellular level, the T cells no longer recognize self antigens and stimulate either the production of antibodies to the self antigens, autoantibodies, or there is destruction of self cells by the immune system. There is a strong genetic predisposition to autoimmune diseases, but the triggering event is considered to be environmental. Pathogens, pollutants, drugs, and even nutritional factors have been implicated as the initiating factors in autoimmune diseases. Certain autoimmune diseases are organ specific (thyroid, pancreas), and others are systemic, such as systemic lupus erythematosus (SLE) and rheumatoid arthritis (RA).

The autoimmune response is often used as an example of the differences between the sexes; women are affected to a much greater extent than men (Merrill, Dinu, & Lahita, 1996). Even though there are numerous (15) known diseases and many more (80) conditions that are aggravated by autoimmune disorders, the activation mechanisms are not known (Rose, 2002). Dramatic changes in the immune system are seen during pregnancy, menopause, and gonadectomy. The relationship stems partly from the fact that estrogen influences the expression of the immune system's regulatory proteins, which affect cell death (apoptosis) (Cruzan & Fagan, 2002; Mor et al., 2003). However, since the severity of some autoimmune diseases is similar in men and women, sex hormones may be only part of the explanation (Lockshin, 2002). Additionally, the balance between proliferative/apoptotic cycles that menstruating women are exposed to from puberty through menopause may affect the development of autoimmune diseases (Cruzan & Fagan, 2002). Finally, the female connection is further complicated in that different autoimmune diseases strike women of different ages with various hormone levels.

In the United States, immune-related conditions (e.g., diabetes, infections) are the third leading cause of death, surpassed only by heart disease and cancer (National Vital Statistics, 2002). A recent epidemiological study found that over 8 million adults—about 1 in 31 individuals or about 3% of the adult population—have an autoimmune disease (Jacobson, Gange, Rose, & Graham, 1997) and that women are at 2.7 times greater risk than men of suffering from an autoimmune disease.

4.1. Systemic Lupus Erythematosus

SLE is a chronic autoimmune inflammatory disease with an unknown etiology. It affects women predominantly, with a ratio of about 10:1 relative to men (Roitt & Delves, 2001). Worldwide, the incidence is 1 in 1000 in white women, and 1 in 250 in black women. In the United States, the disease affects about 1.4 million women. The differences between the prevalence of this disease between the sexes shows up mainly after puberty (after menarche) and lasts until menopause (McAlindon et al., 2001; Petri et al., 2002). Sex hormone metabolism seems to be different in SLE patients (Petri et al., 2002). Ex vivo experiments with SLE T cells showed that estradiol, working through estrogen receptors, could cause immune hyperstimulation and contribute to the pathogenesis of SLE (Rider et al., 2001).

There are few data associating nutritional status and risk of SLE. A prospective epidemiological study noted that low vitamin E status preceded diagnosis of both SLE and RA in a well-characterized population (Comstock et al., 1997). A limited number of studies suggest that certain food components and nutrients may affect the course of the disease. The data, however, are from small studies over relatively short periods of time. For example, indole-3-carbinol (I3C), a compound that is naturally present in cruciferous vegetables, has been suggested to reduce the severity of estrogen-dependent diseases through its increase in hydroxylation of estrone. Women with SLE appear to respond to I3C. It is hypothesized that I3C may attenuate the estrogen dependence of SLE disease activity (McAlindon et al., 2001). Corticosteroids are the most commonly used treatment to suppress end-organ inflammation and control and prevent disease flares in SLE; however, these drugs are not free of adverse effects. In addition to morbidity and even mortality owing to the toxicity associated with corticosteroids, adverse long-term effects include osteoporosis and cataract formation. These drugs also have negative consequences on nutritional status by increasing the excretion of vitamin B_6, magnesium, and potassium (Bendich & Zilberboim, 2004).

4.2. Rheumatoid Arthritis

RA is a chronic, progressive autoimmune disease of unknown origin that is associated with a genetic predisposition and an environmental trigger (Beers & Berkow, 1999a; Mongey & Hess, 1993; Newkirk, LePage, Niwa, & Rubin, 1998). It is the most common systemic autoimmune disease; about 1% of the US population suffers from adult-onset RA. More than 1.5 million US women (about 75% of all individuals affected) suffer from RA. Life expectancy for people with RA is reduced relative to the general population, perhaps as a result of increased cardiovascular disease (Meyer, 2001). This association is related to the involvement of inflammatory responses in the development of atherosclerosis (Solomon et al., 2003). RA causes a deterioration of articular joints, causing pain, stiffness, swelling, and deformity, which over time results in severe disability (Orstavik et al., 2004). The autoantibodies in RA are sometimes referred to as rheumatoid factor, and titers are used diagnostically. The autoantibodies are found in the joint fluids and are probably the initiators of the symmetrical inflammation seen in peripheral joints. Onset may occur in youth or young adulthood, resulting in juvenile oxidative damage to the joints and increased production of inflammatory cytokines, the hallmarks of RA. Patients with RA may also have symptoms of anemia unrelated to a lack of dietary intake of iron. Anemia of chronic disease (ACD) is associated with a reduction in red blood cell (RBC) iron. RA-associated ACD causes an increase in oxidative damage in the joints exposed to free iron (Beers et al., 1999a).

The progressive nature of RA necessitates successive use of more toxic drugs that have serious side effects on overall health and nutritional status (Balint & Gergely, Jr., 1996; Blanco, Martinez-Taboada, Rodriguez-Valverde, Sanchez-Andrade, & Gonzalez-Gay, 1997; Krensky, Storm, & Bluestone, 2001). The first medications given to reduce inflammation include aspirin and nonsteroidal anti-inflammatory drugs (NSAIDs), but their efficacy is often inadequate. Liver dysfunction and gastrointestinal (GI) tract discomfort are common with NSAIDs. A newer class of NSAID that targets only the type 2 cyclooxygenase (COX-2) enzyme may not cause as many GI tract problems as older drugs that targeted both COX-1 and COX-2.

As discussed above, corticosteroids are potent anti-inflammatory drugs that are used for many immune-related diseases to reduce inflammatory responses and/or immune response imbalances (Leong, Center, Henderson, & Eisman, 2001). The primary effect is to inhibit T-cell-mediated immune responses that result in both anti-inflammatory and antiadhesion responses by the immune cells. However, corticosteroids do not stop joint erosion, and their efficacy decreases with use (Axelrod, 2001; Cassidy & Hillman, 1997; Goldring, 2001).

Cytotoxic drugs are the next group of drugs given when RA continues to cause pain and joint erosion (Langford, Klippel, Balow, James, & Sneller, 1998), but despite pain reduction, disease progression continues. Most of the cytotoxic drugs are folate antagonists, and therefore these will decrease folate status and increase homocysteine levels. Increasing folate intake can overcome some of these effects, but there may be a concomitant decrease in drug efficacy (Morgan & Baggott, 1991). Liver dysfunction and GI tract discomforts are common with cytotoxic drugs and corticosteroids. In addition, drug-induced osteoporosis is significantly increased by both corticosteroids and cytotoxic drugs.

Several dietary components have been shown to reduce the formation of inflammatory prostaglandins that are the products of COX-2 enzyme activity (Cerhan, Saag, Merlino, Mikuls, & Criswell, 2003; de Sousa, 1993; Galperin, Fernandes, Oliveira, & Gershwin, 2000; Hanninen et al., 2000; Merlino et al., 2004). COX-2 inhibitors include vitamin E, vitamin C, and long-chain ω-3 and certain ω-6 fatty acids. Supplementation has resulted in pain reduction in some studies and reduction in pain medication use in others. In one study involving 49 RA patients, supplementation with γ-linolenic acid (ω-6) and eicosapentaenoic acid (ω-3) for 1 yr resulted in decreased pain and tapering of NSAID use in 80% of patients compared to 33% in the placebo group. A number of studies examining the effects of supplementation with ω-3 fatty acids have shown consistent reductions in tender joints and morning stiffness (Belluzzi, 2001).

4.3. Osteoporosis

Osteoporosis is defined as a progressive systemic skeletal disease characterized by low bone mass and deterioration of bone tissue architecture, with a consequent decrease in bone strength and increase in bone fragility and susceptibility to fracture (Beers & Berkow, 1999b). There can also be a concomitant loss of bone from the jaw resulting in dental complications including tooth loss (Krall, 2005). Results from NHANES III indicate that the majority of women aged 50–59 already have reduced BMD. The incidence increases with age such that 88% of women aged 70–79 have reduced BMD and osteoporosis is manifested in almost 30% of women above 65 yr (Welty, 2003). More than one-third of postmenopausal adult women will have one or more osteoporotic fractures in their lifetime. More than 6 million US adults, mainly women, have osteoporosis (Looker et al., 1997), which is defined as having bones two standard deviations below the peak BMD seen in young adults (Heaney, 2001; Looker et al., 1997). Osteoporosis is a known risk factor for hip fracture (Marshall, Johnell, & Wedel, 1996). There are nearly 300,000 annual hip fractures in the United States. Those with hip fractures experience increased risk of institutionalization and death (Kleerekoper, 1996). The lifetime risk for osteoporotic fractures in men is approximately one-half that in women. The decrease in BMD is the most important cause of fracture risk.

Postmenopausal osteoporosis is the primary cause of fractures and is linked to the loss of estrogen during menopause. Estrogen maintains the normal balance between bone formation and bone resorption that occurs throughout life. Estrogen also enhances the deposition of calcium in bone. The loss of estrogen is associated with an increased breakdown of bone tissue by osteoclasts that is not matched by an equivalent bone formation by the osteoblasts. Not only is there a loss of BMD, there can also be a loss of structural integrity and bone strength. Among other considerations, calcium and vitamin D deficiencies are important risk factors for a decrease in BMD and an increased risk of osteoporosis (Marcus, Feldman, & Kelsey, 2001a, 2001b). Calcium intake is considered to be inadequate in 90% of US adult women, and vitamin D intake is also considered to be low in the majority of adults over 65 yr (Heaney, 2001). Low calcium and vitamin D intakes are also common in Europe and Australia. When subjects with habitually low intakes were enrolled in clinical studies and provided supplemental calcium with or without vitamin D, there was a reduced risk of hip fractures (Chapuy et al., 1992; Dawson-Hughes, Harris, Krall, & Dallal, 1997; Reid, Ames, Evans, Gamble, & Sharpe, 1995).

Three placebo-controlled, double-blind studies have shown that calcium supplementation with or without vitamin D significantly reduced the risk of hip fracture in individuals over the age of 50 yr. The studies were mainly in women, although one of the studies included men. The studies were conducted in the United States, France, and Australia. There was an almost 50% reduction in hip fracture risk (Bendich, Leader, & Muhuri, 1999) when the studies were combined in a meta-analysis: the Mantel-Haenzel combined relative risk estimate was 0.53 (95% confidence interval [CI], 0.31–0.90) for hip fractures. The pooled relative risk for all nonvertebral fractures, including hip, was 0.61 (CI, 0.46–0.80). There was a 47% reduction in the risk of hip fracture in those individuals who took 500–1200 mg/d supplemental calcium for up to 3.4 yr. At the same time there was an additional benefit of a 39% reduction in all types of nonvertebral fractures (Bendich et al., 1999). LeBoff et al. (1999) measured the vitamin D and calcium status of postmenopausal women with hip fractures and found that 50% had deficient vitamin D levels and over 80% had low calcium levels. Since vitamin D is required for calcium absorption, the authors suggested that the low calcium status was linked to the low vitamin D status. These data suggest that individuals at risk for hip and other fractures should increase their calcium and vitamin D intakes.

In addition to calcium, antioxidant status has also been associated with hip fracture risk. Lifestyle factors, such as smoking, which decreases antioxidant status, also increase the risk of hip fracture. Melhus, Michaelsson, Holmberg, Wolk, and Ljunghall (1999) found a threefold increased risk of hip fracture in women who were current smokers and had the lowest intakes of either vitamin E or vitamin C compared to nonsmoking women with the highest antioxidant intakes. If the smokers had the lowest intakes of both vitamins, the odds ratio for hip fracture increased to 4.9. Smoking independent of antioxidant status has been shown to increase the risk of hip fracture, perhaps owing to its association with decreased calcium absorption (Krall & Dawson-Hughes, 1991).

Menopause in women and aging in both females and males are the major causes of osteoporosis (Orwoll, 1999). However, many osteoporotic fractures are the result of treatment of other diseases (secondary osteoporosis) as is seen with autoimmune diseases treated with corticosteroids (Andreassen, Rungby, Dahlerup, & Mosekilde, 1997; Bhattoa, Kiss, Bettembuk, & Balogh, 2001; Ebeling, 1999; Gennari, Martini, & Nuti, 1998; Heller & Sakhaee, 2001; Jamal, Browner, Bauer, & Cummings, 1998; Kaye, 2002; Lappe & Tinley, 1998; Orstavik et al., 2004; Valmadrid, Voorhees, Litt, & Schneyer, 2001).

Recent data suggest that fracture risks are actually greater in men when they are young compared to age-matched women, and that this risk changes as women age. Singer, McLauchlan, Robinson, and Christie (1998) documented the incidence of fractures in individuals 15–94 yr of age in Edinburgh, Scotland. They reported that between the ages of 15–49, men had 2.9 times the number of fractures as age-matched women; fractures of the wrist began to increase in women at 40 yr of age, before menopause, and that over the age of 60 women had 2.3-fold greater risk of fractures than men. Although this study did not examine nutritional factors, other studies have linked increased risk of fractures in young adults with low intakes of calcium and other micronutrients and low sun exposure (and, consequently, low vitamin D status), as found in Scotland.

4.3.1. Effect of Antiosteoporosis Drugs on Nutritional Status and Effects of Nutrients on Drugs Used to Treat Osteoporosis

Adequate calcium and vitamin D intakes are required for the efficacy of all drugs used to treat osteoporosis and reduce the risk of fracture (Becker, 2001; Sifton, 2001). Without adequate calcium and/or vitamin D, the efficacy of the drugs is diminished significantly (Eastell, 2005; Pereda & Eastell, 2001; Stock, 1996) For example, Nieves, Komar, Cosman, & Lindsay (1998) documented the importance of adequate calcium intake for the efficacy of both HRT and calcitonin in stopping bone loss.

HRT has been shown to reduce bone loss in women during menopause and afterwards (Cauley et al., 2003), but recent findings from the WHI suggest that HRT be used for relatively short periods of time (Rossouw et al., 2002). HRT has effects on many physiological functions, including dietary habits. HRT is associated with fluid retention and modest but consistent weight gain. HRT also enhances calcium absorption, thereby improving calcium balance.

Bisphosphonates, the most commonly used class of antiosteoporosis drugs, bind calcium and other minerals, and thus they should not be taken at the same time. Adequate calcium and vitamin D enhances the efficacy of bisphosphonates, and it is important that patients understand the dosing regimes for the drugs (Eastell, 2005). GI tract disturbances are common with bisphosphonates (Cummings et al., 1995; Meisler, 2003).

The National Institutes of Health (NIH) and the National Academy of Sciences recommend that postmenopausal women not taking HRT consume 1500 mg/d of calcium (NIH Consensus Development Panel on Optimal Calcium Intake, 1994; Standing Committee on the Scientific Evaluation of Dietary Reference Intakes Food and Nutrition Board Institute of Medicine, 1997). Since the benefit of antiosteoporosis drugs is predicated on the daily consumption of 1000 mg of calcium (Nieves et al., 1998), it is of interest to note that in a representative sample of US households, only half of the adults 60–94 yr of age drank one glass of milk (300 mg of calcium) every day; dairy products are the primary source of calcium in the US diet (Elbon, Johnson, & Fischer, 1998).

5. CONCLUSIONS

Women are exposed to many stressors, both physical and mental, during their adult lives. Compared to age-matched men, women have higher rates of depression, autoimmune diseases, and osteoporosis, and Alzheimer's disease is one of the 10 leading causes of death in women, but not in men. Cardiovascular disease and cancer are the number one and two killers of both men and women in the United States. Disease-prevention strategies differ between men and women, as seen in the greater usage of dietary supplements by women, especially female physicians.

Several stressful conditions that women suffer are associated with the menstrual cycle and can be affected by nutrient intakes. Dysmenorrheal pain may be lessened when diets contain foods rich in long-chain polyunsaturated fatty acids. PMS symptoms were significantly reduced in a well-controlled calcium supplementation clinical study. Amenorrhea is frequently seen when caloric intakes are severely restricted and can result in long-term negative effects, especially reduced BMD in growing girls. PCO, a metabolic syndrome that affects about 10% of menstruating women, includes risk factors such as obesity and diabetes. The infertility associated with PCO can be a major stressor for affected women. Weight loss as well as calcium supplementation have restored fertility in preliminary studies.

Pregnancy is a stressful time for the mother-to-be. The two leading causes of infant morbidity and mortality, birth defects and low birthweight, are directly linked to maternal nutrition. Folic acid, a B vitamin, has been definitively shown to reduce the risk of NTDs, and periconceptional multivitamin supplementation that includes folic acid and zinc can reduce the incidence of NTDs as well as several other serious birth defects. This same intervention can also reduce the risk of preterm delivery and low-birthweight outcomes in developed as well as developing countries. Even in HIV-infected pregnant women, multivitamin supplementation has improved birth outcomes as well as indices of maternal health.

Menopause can often involve stressful physical and mental symptoms. The time course of these changes can span several years, including a perimenopausal period in which menstruation has not completely ceased, and symptoms associated with menopause such as hot flashes may continue for many years after menses cessation. Soy and soy-containing products and/or extracts have been shown to reduce the frequency and severity of hot flashes. Other dietary supplements that do not provide nutritive value have also been examined for this indication, but are not reviewed.

Autoimmune diseases are significantly more prevalent in women and are often worsened by stressful life events. Women are at a 10-fold higher risk of suffering from SLE compared to men. Black women are at four times greater risk of having SLE compared to white women. Low antioxidant status appears to increase disease risk, and antioxidants may reduce disease symptoms. RA is the most common autoimmune disease seen in the United States and also affects women more frequently than men. Anti-inflammatory long-chain ω-3 fatty acids as well as antioxidant nutrients such as vitamins E and C reduce inflammation. Corticosteroids can cause secondary osteoporosis in patients with RA, and calcium and vitamin D supplementation is required to help slow this degenerative process.

In addition to secondary osteoporosis, postmenopausal loss of bone and the loss of bone associated with aging results in one of three women over 50 yr expected to have at least one fracture during her lifetime. Close to 90% of women over age 70 have significantly reduced BMD, a primary risk factor for osteoporotic fracture. Low intakes of calcium and vitamin D throughout the reproductive years predispose women to osteoporosis later in life. Low intakes of these essential nutrients during the postmenopausal years significantly increase the risk of fractures. For optimal efficacy, all of the currently approved antiosteoporosis drugs require adequate intakes of vitamin D and calcium. Antioxidants also appear to enhance bone mineral density and reduce fracture risk, especially if women have increased oxidative stress as a result of smoking.

REFERENCES

ACOG Committee Opinion. (1995). ACOG: Premenstrual syndrome. *International Journal of Gynecology and Obstetrics, 50*,, 80–84.

Ahluwalia, I. B., Holtzman, D., Mack, K. A., & Mokdad, A. (2003). Observations from the CDC. Health-related quality of life among women of reproductive age: Behavioral risk factor surveillance system (BRFSS), 1998–2001. *Journal of Women's Health, 12*, 5–9.

Andreassen, H., Rungby, J., Dahlerup, J. F., & Mosekilde, L. (1997). Inflammatory bowel disease and osteoporosis. *Scandinavian Journal of Gastroenterology, 32*, 1247–1255.

Axelrod, L. (2001). Corticosteroid therapy. In K. L. Becker (Ed.), *Principals and practice of endocrinology and metabolism* (3rd ed., pp. 751–772). Philadelphia: Lippincott Williams & Wilkins.

Balbi, C., Musone, R., Menditto, A., Di Prisco, L., Cassese, E., D'Ajello, M., Ambriosio, D., & Cardone, A. (2000). Influence of menstrual factors and dietary habits on menstrual pain in adolescence age. *European Journal of Obstetrics, Gynecology, and Reproductive Biology, 91*, 143–148.

Balint, G., & Gergely, P., Jr. (1996). Clinical immunotoxicity of antirheumatic drugs. *Inflammation Research, 45* (Suppl. 2), S91–S95.

Barker, D. J. (1999). Fetal origins of cardiovascular disease. *Annals of Medicine, 31* (Suppl. 1), 3–6.

Becker, K. L. (2001). *Principals and practice of endocrinology and metabolism.* (3rd ed.). Philadelphia: Lippincott Williams & Wilkins.

Beers, M. H., & Berklow, R. (1999a). Diffuse connective tissue disease. In M. H. Beers & R. Berkow (Eds.), *The merck manual of diagnosis and therapy* (17th ed., pp. 416–423). Whitehouse Station, NJ: Merck Research Laboratory.

Beers, M. H., & Berklow, R. (1999b). Osteoporosis. In M. H. Beers & R. Berkow (Eds.), *The Merck manual* (17th ed., pp. 469–473). Whitehouse Station, NJ: Merck Reserch Laboratories.

Belluzzi, A. (2001). Polyunsaturated fatty acids and autoimmune diseases. In A. Bendich & R. J. Deckelbaum (Eds.), *Primary and secondary preventive nutrition* (pp. 271–287). Totowa, NJ: Humana Press.

Bendich, A. (2000). The potential for dietary supplements to reduce premenstrual syndrome (PMS) symptoms. *Journal of the American College of Nutrition, 19*, 3–12.

Bendich, A., & Deckelbaum, R. J. (2001a). *Preventive nutrition: The comprehensive guide for health professionals* (2nd ed.). Totowa, NJ: Humana Press.

Bendich, A., & Deckelbaum, R. J. (2001b). *Primary and secondary preventive nutrition.* Totowa, NJ: Humana Press.

Bendich, A., Leader, S., & Muhuri, P. (1999). Supplemental calcium for the prevention of hip fracture: Potential health-economic benefits. *Clinical Therapeutics, 21*, 1058–1072.

Bendich, A., Mallick, R., & Leader, S. (1997). Potential health economic benefits of vitamin supplementation. *The Western Journal of Medicine, 166*, 306–312.

Bendich, A., & Zilberboim, R. (2004). Drug-nutrient interactions and immune function. In J. I. Boullata & V. T. Armenti (Eds.), *Handbook of drug–nutrient interactions* (pp. 441–478). Totowa, NJ: Humana Press.

Berman, M. K., Taylor, M. L., & Freeman, E. (1990). Vitamin B-6 in premenstrual syndrome. *Journal of the American Dietetic Association, 90*, 859–861.

Berry, R. J., Li, Z., Erickson, J. D., Li, S., Moore, C. A., Wang, H., et al. (1999). Prevention of neural-tube defects with folic acid in China. China-U.S. Collaborative Project for Neural Tube Defect Prevention. *The New England Journal of Medicine, 341*, 1485–1490.

Bhattoa, H. P., Kiss, E., Bettembuk, P., & Balogh, A. (2001). Bone mineral density, biochemical markers of bone turnover, and hormonal status in men with systemic lupus erythematosus. *Rheumatology International, 21*, 97–102.

Blanco, R., Martinez-Taboada, V. M., Rodriguez-Valverde, V., Sanchez-Andrade, A., & Gonzalez-Gay, M. A. (1997). Successful therapy with danazol in refractory autoimmune thrombocytopenia associated with rheumatic diseases. *British Journal of Rheumatology, 36*, 1095–1099.

Block, G., Cox, C., Madans, J., Schreiber, G. B., Licitra, L., & Melia, N. (1988). Vitamin supplement use, by demographic characteristics. *American Journal of Epidemiology, 127*, 297–309.

Cassidy, J. T., & Hillman, L. S. (1997). Abnormalities in skeletal growth in children with juvenile rheumatoid arthritis. *Rheumatic Diseases Clinics of North America, 23*, 499–522.

Cauley, J. A., Robbins, J., Chen, Z., Cummings, S. R., Jackson, R. D., LaCroix, A. Z., Le Boff, M., Lewis, C. E., McGowan, J., Neuner, J., Pettinger, M., Stefanick, M. L., Wactawski-Wende, J., & Watts, N. B. (2003). Effects of estrogen plus progestin on risk of fracture and bone mineral density: The Women's Health Initiative randomized trial. *The Journal of the American Medical Association, 290*, 1729–1738.

Cerhan, J. R., Saag, K. G., Merlino, L. A., Mikuls, T. R., & Criswell, L. A. (2003). Antioxidant micronutrients and risk of rheumatoid arthritis in a cohort of older women. *American Journal of Epidemiology, 157*, 345–354.

Chakmakjian, Z. H., Higgins, C. E., & Abraham, G. E. (1985). The effect of a nutritional supplement, Optivite® for women, on premenstrual tension syndromes: II. Effect on symptomatology, using a double blind cross-over design. *Journal of Applied Nutrition, 37*, 12–17.

Chapuy, M. C., Arlot, M. E., Duboeuf, F., Brun, J., Crouzet, B., Arnaud, S., Delmas, P. D., & Meunier, P. J. (1992). Vitamin D3 and calcium to prevent hip fractures in the elderly women. *The New England Journal of Medicine, 327*, 1637–1642.

Christian, R. C., Dumesic, D. A., Behrenbeck, T., Oberg, A. L., Sheedy, P. F., & Fitzpatrick, L. A. (2003). Prevalence and predictors of coronary artery calcification in women with polycystic ovary syndrome. *The Journal of Clinical Endocrinology and Metabolism, 88*, 2562–2568.

Chuong, C. J., Dawson, E. B., & Smith, E. R. (1990). Vitamin E levels in premenstrual syndrome. *American Journal of Obstetrics and Gynecology, 163*, 1591-1595.

Comstock, G. W., Burke, A. E., Hoffman, S. C., Helzlsouer, K. J., Bendich, A., Masi, A. T., Norkus, E. P., Malamet, R. I., & Gershwin, M. E. (1997). Serum concentrations of alpha tocopherol, beta carotene, and retinol preceding the diagnosis of rheumatoid arthritis and systemic lupus erythematosus. *Annals of the Rheumatic Diseases, 56*, 323–325.

Cruzan, C., & Fagan, T. (2002). *Proceedings from: Understanding the biology of sex differences: Sex differences in immunity and autoimmunity*. Washington, DC: Society for Women's Health Research.

Cummings, S. R., Nevitt, M. C., Browner, W. S., Stone, K., Fox, K. M., Ensrud, K. E., Cauley, J., Black, D., & Vogt, T. M. (1995). Risk factors for hip fracture in white women. Study of Osteoporotic Fractures Research Group. *The New England Journal of Medicine, 332*, 767–773.

Czeizel, A. E. (2001). Folic acid-containing multivitamins and primary prevention of birth defects. In A. Bendich & R. J. Deckelbaum (Eds.), *Preventive nutrition: The comprehensive guide for health professionals* (2nd ed., pp. 349–371). Totowa, NJ: Humana Press.

Czeizel, A. E., & Dudas, I. (1992). Prevention of the first occurrence of neural-tube defects by periconceptional vitamin supplementation. *The New England Journal of Medicine, 327*, 1832–1835.

Daugherty, J. E. (1998). Treatment strategies for premenstrual syndrome. *American Family Physician, 58*, 183–188.

Dawson-Hughes, B., Harris, S. S., Krall, E. A., & Dallal, G. E. (1997). Effect of calcium and vitamin D supplementation on bone density in men and women 65 years of age or older. *The New England Journal of Medicine, 337*, 670–676.

de Onis, M., Villar, J., & Gulmezoglu, M. (1998). Nutritional interventions to prevent intrauterine growth retardation: Evidence from randomized controlled trials. *European Journal of Clinical Nutrition, 52* (Suppl. 1), S83–S93.

de Sousa, M. (1993). Circulation and distribution of iron: A key to immune interaction. In S. Cunningham-Rundles (Ed.), *Nutrient modulation of the immune response*. New York: Marcel Dekker, Inc.

Diegoli, M. S., da Fonseca, A. M., Diegoli, C. A., & Pinotti, J. A. (1998). A double-blind trial of four medications to treat severe premenstrual syndrome. *International Journal of Gynecology and Obstetrics, 62*, 63–67.

Division of Reproductive Health. (1999). Preterm Singleton Births—United States, 1989–1996.

Douglas, S. (2002). Premenstrual syndrome. *Canadian Family Physician, 48*, 1789–1797.

Dunaif, A., & Lobo, R. A. (2002). Toward optimal health: The experts discuss polycystic ovary syndrome. *Journal of Women's Health & Gender-Based Medicine, 11*, 579–584.

Eastell, R. (2005). Calcium requirements during treatment of osteoporosis in women. In A. Bendich & R. J. Deckelbaum (Eds.), *Preventive nutrition: The comprehensive guide for health professionals* (3rd ed. pp. 425–432). Totowa, NJ: Humana Press.

Ebeling, P. R. (1999). Secondary causes of osteoporosis in men. In E. S. Orwoll (Ed.), *Osteoporosis in men: The effects of gender on skeletal health* (pp. 483–504). New York: Academic.

Elbon, S. M., Johnson, M. A., & Fischer, J. G. (1998). Milk consumption in older Americans. *American Journal of Public Health, 88*, 1221–1224.

Epidemiology Program Office. (1992). Recommendations for the use of folic acid to reduce the number of cases of spina bifida and other neural tube defects. http://www.cdc.gov/mmwr/preview/mmwrhtml/00019479.htm [on-line].

Facchinetti, F., Borella, P., Sances, G., Fioroni, L., Nappi, R. E., & Genazzani, A. R. (1991). Oral magnesium successfully relieves premenstrual mood changes. *Obstetrics and Gynecology, 78*, 177–181.

Facchinetti, F., Nappi, R. E., Sances, M. G., Neri, I., Grandinetti, G., & Genazzani, A. (1997). Effects of a yeast-based dietary supplementation on premenstrual syndrome. A double-blind placebo-controlled study. *Gynecologic and Obstetric Investigation, 43*, 120–124.

Facchinetti, F., Sances, G., Borella, P., Genazzani, A. R., & Nappi, G. (1991). Magnesium prophylaxis of menstrual migraine: Effects on intracellular magnesium. *Headache, 31*, 298–301.

Fairfield, K. M., & Fletcher, R. H. (2002). Vitamins for chronic disease prevention in adults: Scientific review. *The Journal of the American Medical Association, 287*, 3116–3126.

Fawzi, W. W., Msamanga, G. I., Spiegelman, D., Urassa, E. J., McGrath, N., Mwakagile, D., Antelman, G., Mbise, R., Herrera, G., Kapiga, S., Willett, W., & Hunter D. J. (1998). Randomised trial of effects of vitamin supplements on pregnancy outcomes and T cell counts in HIV-1-infected women in Tanzania. *Lancet, 351*, 1477–1482.

Frank, E., Bendich, A., & Denniston, M. (2000). Use of vitamin-mineral supplements by female physicians in the United States. *The American Journal of Clinical Nutrition, 72*, 969–975.

Freeman, E. W., Sammel, M. D., Rinaudo, P. J., & Sheng, L. (2004). Premenstrual syndrome as a predictor of menopausal symptoms. *Obstetrics and Gynecology, 103*, 960–966.

Galperin, C., Fernandes, G., Oliveira, R. M., & Gershwin, M. E. (2000). Nutritional modulation of autoimmune diseases. In M. E. Gershwin, J. B. German, & C. L. Keen (Eds.), *Nutrition and immunology principals and practice* (pp. 313–328). Totowa, NJ: Humana Press.

Gennari, C., Martini, G., & Nuti, R. (1998). Secondary osteoporosis. *Aging Clinical and Experimental Research, 10*, 214–224.

Goldenberg, R. L., Tamura, T., Neggers, Y., Copper, R. L., Johnston, K. E., DuBard, M. B., & Hauth, J. C. (1995). The effect of zinc supplementation on pregnancy outcome. *The Journal of the American Medical Association, 274*, 463–468.

Goldring, S. R. (2001). Osteoporosis associated with rheumatologic disorders. In R. Marcus, D. Feldman, & J. Kelsey (Eds.), Osteoporosis (2nd ed., Vol. 2, pp. 351–362). New York: Academic.

Gordon, C. M. (2003). Normal bone accretion and effects of nutritional disorders in childhood. *Journal of Women's Health, 12*, 137–143.

Hanninen, Kaartinen, K., Rauma, A. L., Nenonen, M., Torronen, R., Hakkinen, A. S., Adlercreutz, H., & Laakso, J. (2000). Antioxidants in vegan diet and rheumatic disorders. *Toxicology, 155*, 45–53.

Heaney, R. P. (2001). Osteoporosis: Mineral, vitamins, and other micronutrients. In A. Bendich & R. J. Deckelbaum (Eds.), *Preventive nutrition: The comprehensive guide for health professionals* (2nd ed., pp. 271–292). Totowa, NJ: Humana Press.

Heller, H. J., & Sakhaee, K. (2001). Anticonvulsant-induced bone disease: A plea for monitoring and treatment. *Archives of Neurology, 58*, 1352–1353.

Institute of Medicine. (1998). *Dietary reference intakes for thiamin, riboflavin, niacin, vitamin B6, folate, vitamin B12, pantothenic acid, biotin, and choline*. Washington, DC: National Academy Press.

Jacobson, D. L., Gange, S. J., Rose, N. R., & Graham, N. M. (1997). Epidemiology and estimated population burden of selected autoimmune diseases in the United States. *Clinical Immunology and Immunopathology, 84*, 223–243.

Jamal, S. A., Browner, W. S., Bauer, D. C., & Cummings, S. R. (1998). Warfarin use and risk for osteoporosis in elderly women. Study of Osteoporotic Fractures Research Group. *Annals of Internal Medicine, 128*, 829–832.

Joffe, H., Soares, C. N., & Cohen, L. S. (2003). Assessment and treatment of hot flushes and menopausal mood disturbance. *The Psychiatric Clinics of North America, 26*, 563–580.

Johnston, R. B., Jr., & Staples, D. A. (1998). Use of folic acid-containing supplements among women of childbearing age—United States, 1997. http://www.cdc.gov/mmwr/preview/mmwrhtml/00051435.htm [on-line].

Jones, G., Riley, M., & Dwyer, T. (1999). Maternal smoking during pregnancy, growth, and bone mass in prepubertal children. *Journal of Bone and Mineral Research, 14*, 146–151.

Kaye, P. S. (2002). Osteoporosis and fracture as a result of gastrointestinal and hepatic disorders. *Practical Gastroenterology*, 15–28.

Keen, C. L., Bendich, A., & Willhite, C. C. (1993). Maternal nutrition and pregnancy outcome. New York: The New York Academy of Science.

Kiddy, D. S., Hamilton-Fairley, D., Bush, A., Short, F., Anyaoku, V., Reed, M. J., & Franks, S. (1992). Improvement in endocrine and ovarian function during dietary treatment of obese women with polycystic ovary syndrome. *Clinical Endocrinology, 36*, 105–111.

Klebanoff, M. A., Secher, N. J., Mednick, B. R., & Schulsinger, C. (1999). Maternal size at birth and the development of hypertension during pregnancy: A test of the Barker hypothesis. *Archives of Internal Medicine, 159*, 1607–1612.

Kleerekoper, A. (1996). Evaluation and treatment of postmenopausal osteoporosis. In M. Fauvus (Ed.), *Primer on the metabolic bone disease and disorders of mineral metabolism* (pp. 264–271). Philadelphia: Lippincott-Raven.

Koo, W. W., Walters, J. C., Esterlitz, J., Levine, R. J., Bush, A. J., & Sibai, B. (1999). Maternal calcium supplementation and fetal bone mineralization. *Obstetrics and Gynecology, 94*, 577–582.

Koplan, J. P., Annest, J. L., Layde, P. M., & Rubin, G. L. (1986). Nutrient intake and supplementation in the United States (NHANES II). *American Journal of Public Health, 76*, 287–289.

Krall, E. A. (2005). Osteoporosis. In R. Touger-Decker, D. A. Sirois, & C. C. Mobley (Eds.), *Nutrition and oral medicine* (pp. 261–272). Totowa, NJ: Humana Press.

Krall, E. A., & Dawson-Hughes, B. (1991). Smoking and bone loss among postmenopausal women. *Journal of Bone and Mineral Research, 6*, 331–338.

Krensky, A. M., Storm, T. B., & Bluestone, J. A. (2001). Immunomodulators: Immunosuppressive agents, tolerogens, and immunomodulators. In J. G. Hardman, L. E. Limbird, & A. G. Gilman (Eds.), *The pharmacological basis of therapeutics* (10th ed., pp. 1463–1484). New York: McGraw-Hill.

Kronenberg, F., & Fugh-Berman, A. (2002). Complementary and alternative medicine for menopausal symptoms: A review of randomized, controlled trials. *Annals of Internal Medicine, 137*, 805–813.

Langford, C. A., Klippel, J. H., Balow, J. E., James, S. P., & Sneller, M. C. (1998). Use of cytotoxic agents and cyclosporine in the treatment of autoimmune disease. Part 2: Inflammatory bowel disease, systemic vasculitis, and therapeutic toxicity. *Annals of Internal Medicine, 129*, 49–58.

Lappe, J. M., & Tinley, S. T. (1998). Prevention of osteoporosis in women treated for hereditary breast and ovarian carcinoma: A need that is overlooked. *Cancer, 83*, 830–834.

LeBoff, M. S., Kohlmeier, L., Hurwitz, S., Franklin, J., Wright, J., & Glowacki, J. (1999). Occult vitamin D deficiency in postmenopausal US women with acute hip fracture. *The Journal of the American Medical Association, 281*, 1505–1511.

Lee, S. J., & Kanis, J. A. (1994). An association between osteoporosis and premenstrual symptoms and postmenopausal symptoms. *Bone and Mineral, 24*, 127–134.

Leong, G. M., Center, J. R., Henderson, N. K., & Eisman, J. A. (2001). Glucocorticoid-induced osteoporosis. In R. Marcus, D. Feldman, & J. Kelsey (Eds.), Osteoporosis (2nd ed., Vol. 2, pp. 169–193). New York: Academic Press.

Lockshin, M. D. (2002). Sex ratio and rheumatic disease: Excerpts from an Institute of Medicine report. *Lupus, 11*, 662–666.

London, R. S., Bradley, L., & Chiamori, N. Y. (1991). Effect of a nutritional supplement on premenstrual symptomatology in women with premenstrual syndrome: A double-blind longitudinal study. *Journal of the American College of Nutrition, 10*, 494–499.

London, R. S., Murphy, L., Kitlowski, K. E., & Reynolds, M. A. (1987). Efficacy of alpha-tocopherol in the treatment of the premenstrual syndrome. *Journal of Reproductive Medicine, 32*, 400–404.

Looker, A. C., Orwoll, E. S., Johnston, C. C., Jr., Lindsay, R. L., Wahner, H. W., Dunn, W. L., Calvo, M. S., Harris, T. B., & Heyse, S. P. (1997). Prevalence of low femoral bone density in older U.S. adults from NHANES III. *Journal of Bone and Mineral Research, 12*, 1761–1768.

Loucks, A. B. (2003). Energy availability, not body fatness, regulates reproductive function in women. *Exercise and Sport Sciences Reviews, 31*, 144–148.

Lyle, B. J., Mares-Perlman, J. A., Klein, B. E., Klein, R., Palta, M., Bowen, P. E., & Greger, J. L. (1999). Serum carotenoids and tocopherols and incidence of age-related nuclear cataract. *The American Journal of Clinical Nutrition, 69*, 272–277.

Mack, K. A. & Ahluwalia, I. B. (2003). Observations from the CDC: Monitoring women's health in the United States: Selected chronic disease indicators, 1991–2001 BRFSS. *Journal of Women's Health, 12*, 309–314.

Marcus, R., Feldman, D., & Kelsey, J. (2001a). Osteoporosis (2nd ed., Vol. 1). New York: Academic Press.

Marcus, R., Feldman, D., & Kelsey, J. (2001b). Osteoporosis (2nd ed., Vol. 2). New York: Academic Press.

Marjoribanks, J., Proctor, M., & Farquhar, C. (2003). Nonsteroidal anti-inflammatory drugs for primary dysmenorrhoea. *Cochrane Database of Systematic Reviews, 4*, CD001751.

Marshall, D., Johnell, O., & Wedel, H. (1996). Meta-analysis of how well measures of bone mineral density predict occurrence of osteoporotic fractures. *British Medical Journal, 312*, 1254–1259.

Mazure, C. M., Keita, G. P., & Blehar, M. C. (2002). Summit on women and depression proceedings and recommendations. http://www.apa.org/pi/wpo/women&depression.pdf [on-line].

McAlindon, T. E., Gulin, J., Chen, T., Klug, T., Lahita, R., & Nuite, M. (2001). Indole-3-carbinol in women with SLE: Effect on estrogen metabolism and disease activity. *Lupus, 10*, 779–783.

McLean, J. A., & Barr, S. I. (2003). Cognitive dietary restraint is associated with eating behaviors, lifestyle practices, personality characteristics and menstrual irregularity in college women. *Appetite, 40*, 185–192.

Meisler, J. G. (2003). Toward optimal health: The experts provide a current perspective on perimenopause. *Journal of Women's Health, 12*, 609–615.

Melhus, H., Michaelsson, K., Holmberg, L., Wolk, A., & Ljunghall, S. (1999). Smoking, antioxidant vitamins, and the risk of hip fracture. *Journal of Bone and Mineral Research, 14*, 129–135.

Merlino, L. A., Curtis, J., Mikuls, T. R., Cerhan, J. R., Criswell, L. A., & Saag, K. G. (2004). Vitamin D intake is inversely associated with rheumatoid arthritis: Results from the Iowa Women's Health Study. *Arthritis and Rheumatism, 50*, 72–77.

Merrill, J. T., Dinu, A. R., & Lahita, R. G. (1996). Autoimmunity: The female connection. *Medscape Women's Health, 1*, 5.

Mersereau, P., Kilker, M. N. K., Carter, H., Fassett, E., Williams, J., Flores, A., Prue, C., Williams, L., Mai, C., & Mulinare, J. (2004). Spina bifida and anencephaly before and after folic acid mandate—United States, 1995–1996 and 1999–2000. http://www.cdc.gov/mmwr/preview/mmwrhtml/mm5317a3.htm [on-line].

Messina, M., & Hughes, C. (2003). Efficacy of soyfoods and soybean isoflavone supplements for alleviating menopausal symptoms is positively related to initial hot flush frequency. *Journal of Medicinal Food, 6*, 1–11.

Meyer, O. (2001). Atherosclerosis and connective tissue diseases. *Joint Bone Spine, 68*, 564–575.

Michelmore, K. F., Balen, A. H., & Dunger, D. B. (2001). Polycystic ovaries and eating disorders: Are they related? *Human Reproduction, 16*, 765–769.

Miller, K. K. (2003). Mechanisms by which nutritional disorders cause reduced bone mass in adults. *Journal of Women's Health, 12*, 145–150.

Mira, M., Stewart, P. M., & Abraham, S. F. (1988). Vitamin and trace element status in premenstrual syndrome. *The American Journal of Clinical Nutrition, 47*, 636–641.

Mongey, A. B., & Hess, E. V. (1993). Drug and environmental effects on the induction of autoimmunity. *The Journal of Laboratory and Clinical Medicine, 122*, 652–657.

Mor, G., Sapi, E., Abrahams, V. M., Rutherford, T., Song, J., Hao, X. Y., et al. (2003). Interaction of the estrogen receptors with the Fas ligand promoter in human monocytes. *Journal of Immunology, 170*, 114–122.

Morgan, S. L., & Baggott, J. E. (1991). Role of dietary folate and oral folate supplements in the prevention of drug toxicity during anifolate therapy for nonneoplastic disease. In A. Bendich & C. E. Butterworth, Jr. (Eds.), *Micronutrients in health and in disease prevention* (pp. 333–358). New-York: Marcel Dekker, Inc.

Moss, A. J., Levy, A. S., Kim, I., & Park, Y. K. (1989). *Use of vitamin and mineral supplements in the United States; current users, types of products and nutrients* (Rep. No. Advanced Data no. 174). Hyattsville, MD: National Center for Health Statistics.

MRC Vitamin Study Research Group. (1991). Prevention of neural tube defects: Results of the Medical Research Council Vitamin Study. *Lancet, 338*, 131–137.

National Vital Statistics. (2002). Ten leading causes of death, by sex, race, and age. http://www.cdc.gov/nchs/fastats/pdf/nvsr50_16t1.pdf [on-line].

Newkirk, M. M., LePage, K., Niwa, T., & Rubin, L. (1998). Advanced glycation endproducts (AGE) on IgG, a target for circulating antibodies in North American Indians with rheumatoid arthritis (RA). *Cellular & Molecular Biology (Noisy-Le-Grand), 44*, 1129–1138.

Nieves, J. W., Komar, L., Cosman, F., & Lindsay, R. (1998). Calcium potentiates the effect of estrogen and calcitonin on bone mass: review and analysis. *The American Journal of Clinical Nutrition, 67*, 1824.

NIH Consensus Development Panel on Optimal Calcium Intake. (1994). NIH Consensus conference. Optimal calcium intake. *The Journal of the American Medical Association, 272*, 1942–1948.

Norman, R. J., Noakes, M., Wu, R., Davies, M. J., Moran, L., & Wang, J. X. (2004). Improving reproductive performance in overweight/obese women with effective weight management. *Human Reproduction Update, 10*, 267–280.

Norman, R. J., Wu, R., & Stankiewicz, M. T. (2004). 4: Polycystic ovary syndrome. *The Medical Journal of Australia, 180*, 132–137.

Oakley, G. P., Jr. (1998). Eat right and take a multivitamin. *The New England Journal of Medicine, 338*, 1060–1061.

Oakley, G. P., Jr., & Erickson, J. D. (1995). Vitamin A and birth defects. Continuing caution is needed. *The New England Journal of Medicine, 333*, 1414–1415.

Okey, R., Stewart, J. A., & Greenwood, M. L. (1930). Studies of the metabolism of women. IV. The calcium and inorganic phosphorus in the blood of normal women at the various stages of the monthly cycle. *The Journal of Biological Chemistry, 87*, 91–102.

Orstavik, R. E., Haugeberg, G., Mowinckel, P., Hoiseth, A., Uhlig, T., Falch, J. A., Halse, J. I., McCloskey, E., & Kvien, T. K. (2004). Vertebral deformities in rheumatoid arthritis: A comparison with population-based controls. *Archives of Internal Medicine, 164*, 420–425.

Orwoll, E. S. (1999). The prevention and therapy of osteoporsis in men. In E. S. Orwoll (Ed.), *Osteoporosis in men: The effects of gender on skeletal health* (pp. 553–569). New York: Academic.

Patterson, R. E., Kristal, A. R., & Neuhouser, M. L. (2001). Vitamin Supplements and Cancer Risk. In A. Bendich & R. J. Deckelbaum (Eds.), *Primary and secondary preventive nutrition* (pp. 21–43). Totowa, NJ: Humana Press.

Penland, J. G., & Johnson, P. E. (1993). Dietary calcium and manganese effects on menstrual cycle symptoms. *American Journal of Obstetrics and Gynecology, 168*, 1417–1423.

Pereda, C. A., & Eastell, R. (2001). Calcium requirements during treatment of osteoporosis in women. In A. Bendich & R. J. Deckelbaum (Eds.), *Primary and secondary preventive nutrition* (pp. 307–321). Totowa, NJ: Humana Press.

Petri, M. A., Lahita, R. G., Van Vollenhoven, R. F., Merrill, J. T., Schiff, M., Ginzler, E. M., Strand, V., Kunz, A., Gorelick, K. J., Schwartz, K. E, & GL601 Study Group. (2002). Effects of prasterone on corticosteroid requirements of women with systemic lupus erythematosus: A double-blind, randomized, placebo-controlled trial. *Arthritis and Rheumatism, 46*, 1820–1829.

Ramakrishnan, U., & Huffman, S. L. (2001). Multiple micronutrient malnutrition; What can be done? In R. D. Semba & M. W. Bloem (Eds.), *Nutrition and health in developing countries* (pp. 365–391). Totowa, NJ: Humana Press.

Reid, I. R., Ames, R. W., Evans, M. C., Gamble, G. D., & Sharpe, S. J. (1995). Long-term effects of calcium supplementation on bone loss and fractures in postmenopausal women: A randomized controlled trial. *The American Journal of Medicine, 98*, 331–335.

Rider, V., Jones, S., Evans, M., Bassiri, H., Afsar, Z., & Abdou, N. I. (2001). Estrogen increases CD40 ligand expression in T cells from women with systemic lupus erythematosus. *The Journal of Rheumatology, 28*, 2644–2649.

Roitt, I. M., & Delves, P. J. (2001). *Roitt's essential immunology* (10th ed.). Malden, MA: Blackwell Science, Inc.

Rose, N. R. (2002). Mechanisms of autoimmunity. *Seminars in Liver Disease, 22*, 387–394.

Rossouw, J. E., Anderson, G. L., Prentice, R. L., LaCroix, A. Z., Kooperberg, C., Stefanick, M. L., Jackson, R. D., Beresford, S. A., Howard, B. V., Johnson, K. C., Kotchen, J. M., Ockene, J., & The Writing Group for the Women's Health Initiative Investigators. (2002). Risks and benefits of estrogen plus progestin in healthy postmenopausal women: Principal results from the Women's Health Initiative randomized controlled trial. *The Journal of the American Medical Association, 288*, 321–333.

Satia-Abouta, J., Kristal, A. R., Patterson, R. E., Littman, A. J., Stratton, K. L., & White, E. (2003). Dietary supplement use and medical conditions: The VITAL study. *American Journal of Preventive Medicine, 24*, 43–51.

Scholl, T. O. (2001). Maternal nutrition and preterm delivery. In A. Bendich & R. J. Deckelbaum (Eds.), *Preventive nutrition: The comprehensive guide for health professionals* (2nd ed., pp. 387–413). Totowa, NJ: Humana Press.

Scholl, T. O., Hediger, M. L., Bendich, A., Schall, J. I., Smith, W. K., & Krueger, P. M. (1997). Use of multivitamin/mineral prenatal supplements: Influence on the outcome of pregnancy. *American Journal of Epidemiology, 146*, 134–141.

Schorah, C. J., & Smithells, R. W. (1991). A possible role for preconception multivitamin supplementation in the prevention or the recurrence of neural tube defects. In A. Bendich & C. E. Butterworth (Eds.), *Micronutrients in health and disease prevention* (pp. 263–285). New York: Marcel Decker.

Shikany, J. M., Patterson, R. E., Agurs-Collins, T., & Anderson, G. (2003). Antioxidant supplement use in Women's Health Initiative participants. *Journal of Women's Health, 36*, 379–387.

Sifton, D. W. (2001). *Physicians' desk reference*. (55th ed.) Montvale, NJ: Medical Economics Company, Inc.

Singer, B. R., McLauchlan, G. J., Robinson, C. M., & Christie, J. (1998). Epidemiology of fractures in 15,000 adults: The influence of age and gender. *The Journal of Bone and Joint Surgery. British Volume, 80*, 243–248.

Smithells, R. W., Sheppard, S., Schorah, C. J., Seller, M. J., Nevin, N. C., Harris, R., Read, A. P., & Fielding, D. W. (1980). Possible prevention of neural-tube defects by periconceptional vitamin supplementation. *Lancet, 1*, 339–340.

Solomon, D. H., Karlson, E. W., Rimm, E. B., Cannuscio, C. C., Mandl, L. A., Manson, J. E., Stampfer, M. J., & Curhan, G. C. (2003). Cardiovascular morbidity and mortality in women diagnosed with rheumatoid arthritis. *Circulation, 107*, 1303–1307.

Soules, M. R., Sherman, S., Parrott, E., Rebar, R., Santoro, N., Utian, W., & Woods, N. (2001). Executive summary: Stages of Reproductive Aging Workshop (STRAW). *Fertility and Sterility, 76*, 874–878.

Standing Committee on the Scientific Evaluation of Dietary Reference Intakes Food and Nutrition Board Institute of Medicine. (1997). *Dietary reference intake for calcium, phosphorous, magnesium, vitamin D, and fluoride* (S-9 ed.). Washington, DC: National Academy Press.

Stearns, V., Beebe, K. L., Iyengar, M., & Dube, E. (2003). Paroxetine controlled release in the treatment of menopausal hot flashes: a randomized controlled trial. *The Journal of the American Medical Association, 289*, 2827–2834.

Stock, J. L. (1996). Drug therapy. In C. J. Rosen (Ed.), *Osteoporosis: Diagnostic and therapeutic principles* (pp. 173–187). Totowa, NJ: Humana Press.

Subar, A. F., & Block, G. (1990). Use of vitamin and mineral supplements: Demographics and amounts of nutrients consumed. The 1987 Health Interview Survey. *American Journal of Epidemiology, 132*, 1091–1101.

Thomas, F., Renaud, F., Benefice, E., de Meeus, T., & Guegan, J. F. (2001). International variability of ages at menarche and menopause: Patterns and main determinants. *Human Biology; An International Record of Research, 73*, 271–290.

Thys-Jacobs, S., Alvir, J. M., & Fratarcangelo, P. (1995). Comparative analysis of three PMS assessment instruments—the identification of premenstrual syndrome with core symptoms. *Psychopharmacology Bulletin, 31*, 389–396.

Thys-Jacobs, S., Ceccarelli, S., Bierman, A., Weisman, H., Cohen, M. A., & Alvir, J. (1989). Calcium supplementation in premenstrual syndrome: A randomized crossover trial. *Journal of General Internal Medicine, 4*, 183–189.

Thys-Jacobs, S., Donovan, D., Papadopoulos, A., Sarrel, P., & Bilezikian, J. P. (1999). Vitamin D and calcium dysregulation in the polycystic ovarian syndrome. *Steroids, 64*, 430–435.

Thys-Jacobs, S., Starkey, P., Bernstein, D., & Tian, J. (1998). Calcium carbonate and the premenstrual syndrome: Effects on premenstrual and menstrual symptoms. Premenstrual Syndrome Study Group. *American Journal of Obstetrics and Gynecology, 179*, 444–452.

Valmadrid, C., Voorhees, C., Litt, B., & Schneyer, C. R. (2001). Practice patterns of neurologists regarding bone and mineral effects of antiepileptic drug therapy. *Archives of Neurology, 58*, 1369–1374.

Walker, A. F., De Souza, M. C., Vickers, M. F., Abeyasekera, S., Collins, M. L., & Trinca, L. A. (1998). Magnesium supplementation alleviates premenstrual symptoms of fluid retention. *Journal of Women's Health, 7*, 1157–1165.

Ward, M. W., & Holimon, T. D. (1999). Calcium treatment for premenstrual syndrome. *The Annals of Pharmacotherapy, 33*, 1356–1358.

Welty, F. K. (2003). Nutrition and Women's Health Symposium. Introduction. *Journal of Women's Health, 12*, 105–108.

West, K. P., Jr., Katz, J., Khatry, S. K., LeClerq, S. C., Pradhan, E. K., Shrestha, S. R., Connor, P. B., Dali, S. M., Christian, P., Pokhrel, R. P., & Sommer, A. (1999). Double blind, cluster randomised trial of low dose supplementation with vitamin A or beta carotene on mortality related to pregnancy in Nepal. The NNIPS-2 Study Group. *British Medical Journal, 318*, 570–575.

White, E., Patterson, R. E., Kristal, A. R., Thornquist, M., King, I., Shattuck, A. L., Evans, I., Satia-Abouta, J., Littman, A. J., & Potter, J. D. (2004). Vitamins and lifestyle cohort study: Study design and characteristics of supplement users. *American Journal of Epidemiology, 159*, 83–93.

Willett, W. C., Sampson, L., & Bain, C. (1981). Vitamin supplement use among registered nurses. *The American Journal of Clinical Nutrition, 34*, 1121–1125.

20 Long-Chain Polyunsaturated Fatty Acids and Metabolic Syndrome X

Undurti N. Das

KEY POINTS

- The incidence of metabolic syndrome X is increasing throughout the world and is characterized by insulin resistance.
- Adipose tissue of different regions is functionally different.
- Evidence suggests that abdominal obesity, one of the characteristic features of metabolic syndrome X, is a result of increased activity of 11β-hydroxysteroid dehydrogenase-1 in the abdominal adipose tissue.
- Low-grade systemic inflammation is a common feature of metabolic syndrome X.
- Insulin suppresses the production of tumor nucrosis factor-α, interleukin-6, and C-reactive protein and enhances the synthesis of endothelial nitric oxide, adiponectin, interleukin-4, and interleukin-10 and, thus, shows anti-inflammatory actions.
- Long-chain polyunsaturated fatty acids may function as endogenous statins, β-blockers, angiotensin-converting enzyme inhibitors, and anti-inflammatory and anti-hypertensive agents and are capable of enhancing adiponectin levels and reducing insulin resistance. Their deficiency increases the generation of tumor nucrosis factor-α and interleukin-6, which in turn induces insulin resistance, whereas increased concentrations of tumor nucrosis factor-α and interleukin-6 enhance the activity of 11β-hydroxysteroid dehydrogenase-1. This leads to the abdominal obesity seen in metabolic syndrome X. Prenatal exposure to tumor nucrosis factor-α produces obesity, and obese children and adults have high levels of tumor nucrosis factor-α and interleukin-6. It is possible that metabolic syndrome X starts in the perinatal period and is owing to perinatal deficiency of long-chain polyunsaturated fatty acids.

1. INTRODUCTION

Metabolic syndrome X is characterized by abdominal obesity, atherosclerosis, insulin resistance and hyperinsulinemia, hyperlipidemias, essential hypertension, type 2 diabetes mellitus, and coronary heart disease (CHD). Other minor features of metabolic syndrome X include hyperfibrinogenemia, increased plasminogen activator inhibitor-1 (PAI-1), low tissue plasminogen activator, nephropathy, microalbuminuria, and hyperuricemia (Das, 2002a). The incidence of metabolic syndrome X is increasing throughout

From: *Nutrients, Stress, and Medical Disorders*
Edited by: S. Yehuda and D. I. Mostofsky © Humana Press Inc., Totowa, NJ

the world. The cause(s) for this increasing incidence is not clear. Because genetics of various populations have not changed in the last 100 yr, it is likely that environmental factors play a major role in the increasing incidence of metabolic syndrome X.

Insulin resistance is common in metabolic syndrome X. Hyperinsulinemia may be a consequence of this. In the early stages of metabolic syndrome X, insulin resistance in muscle tissue is common whereas adipose tissue is not. This explains why exercise is beneficial in the prevention and treatment of insulin resistance.

2. BIOCHEMICAL AND FUNCTIONAL DIFFERENCES BETWEEN ADIPOSE TISSUES OF DIFFERENT REGIONS

Abdominal obesity or increased visceral fat is a marker of the presence of insulin resistance and hyperinsulinemia. Evidence suggests that distinct depot-specific differences exist. For instance, we observed that subcutaneous adipose tissue produces less interleukin (IL)-6 and corticosterone and more tumor necrosis factor (TNF)-α in comparison to mesenteric adipose tissue (Ramos et al., 2003). Peroxisome proliferator-activated receptor (PPAR)-γ is involved in adipocyte development and insulin sensitivity and exerts negative control on TNF-α synthesis. This suggests the existence of a complex network of events that regulate adipocyte accumulation, metabolism, and function. Furthermore, different depots of fat display distinct characteristics specific to each region of body (Das, 2003c).

3. WHAT CAUSES ABDOMINAL OBESITY?

Abdominal adipose tissue is different both biochemically and functionally from subcutaneous adipose tissue. Mice overexpressing 11β-hydroxysteroid dehydrogenase type 1 (11β-HSD-1) enzyme selectively in adipose tissue develop abdominal obesity and exhibit insulin resistance (Das, 2002c; Masuzaki et al., 2001). These features are similar to those seen in subjects with metabolic syndrome X. This led to the suggestion that abdominal obesity is like localized Cushing's syndrome, which is supported by the observation that 11β-HSD-1 activity is higher in abdominal adipose tissue than in subcutaneous adipose tissue (Bujalska, Kumar, & Stewart, 1997).

4. INFLAMMATORY NATURE OF METABOLIC SYNDROME X

Plasma levels of C-reactive protein (CRP), TNF-α, and IL-6, markers of inflammation, are elevated in subjects with obesity, insulin resistance, essential hypertension, type 2 diabetes, and CHD both before and after the onset of these diseases (Albert, Glynn, & Ridker, 2003; Das, 2001e; Das, 2002a, 2002c; Engstrom et al., 2003; Luc et al., 2003; Mosca, 2002; Ridker, Cushman, Stampfer, Tracy, & Hennekens, 1997; van der Meer et al., 2002). Weight reduction and moderate exercise decrease serum concentrations of TNF-α. A negative correlation has been described between plasma TNF-α and high-density lipoprotein (HDL) cholesterol, glycosylated hemoglobin, and serum insulin concentrations (Das, 2002d).

Subjects with elevated CRP levels were two times more likely to develop diabetes at 3–4 yr of follow-up. CRP levels greater than 3.0 mg/L were significantly associated with increased incidence of myocardial infarction, stroke, coronary revascularization, or cardiovascular death (reviewed in Das, 2002a).

An acute increase in plasma glucose levels in normal and impaired glucose tolerance (IGT) subjects resulted in increased plasma IL-6, TNF-α, and IL-18 levels. In IGT subjects, fasting IL-6 and TNF-α levels were higher than those of control subjects, and this increase lasted longer compared to controls (Esposito et al., 2002). Hyperglycemia induced the production of acute phase reactants from the adipose tissue (Lin et al., 2001). This suggests that low-grade systemic inflammation plays a significant role in the development of type 2 diabetes.

Elevated plasma IL-6 levels in women with hypertension and men with insulin resistance was reported (Fernandez-Real et al., 2001). A graded relationship between blood pressure and intercellular adhesion molecule-1 (ICAM-1) as well as IL-6 was noted in healthy men (Chae, Lee, Rifai, & Ridker, 2001). This suggests that low-grade systemic inflammation occurs in insulin resistance and hypertension. Systemic inflammation is a common feature in metabolic syndrome X and its associated conditions. On the other hand, concentrations of adiponectin, which is secreted by adipose tissue and has anti-inflammatory actions and enhances insulin action, are low in obesity, type 2 diabetes mellitus, hypertension, and metabolic syndrome X (Kern, Di Gregorio, Lu, Rassouli, & Ranganathan, 2003; Lindsay et al., 2002; Matsubara, Namioka, & Katayose, 2003; Spranger et al., 2003).

5. ANTI-INFLAMMATORY NATURE OF INSULIN

Insulin suppresses the production of TNF-α, IL-6, IL-1, IL-2, and macrophage migration inhibitory factor (MIF) and enhances the production of IL-4 and IL-10. Thus, insulin has anti-inflammatory effects. This suggests that one of the functions of hyperinsulinemia is to prevent or arrest the low-grade systemic inflammation that occurs in metabolic syndrome X. Leptin has pro-inflammatory actions (Das, 2001e). Hyperinsulinemia and hyperleptinemia are present in obese children (Kalhan, Puthawala, Agarwal, Amini, & Kalhan, 2001; Whincup et al., 2002), suggesting that low-grade systemic inflammation and metabolic syndrome X are initiated early in life.

Insulin and insulin-like growth factor (IGF)-I suppress, whereas TNF-α and IL-6 augment the activity of 11β-HSD-1 (Tomlinson et al., 2001). Elevated activity of 11β-HSD-1 in the visceral adipose tissue increases the accumulation of fat and causes abdominal obesity. Since IGF-I and insulin have a negative control on the activity of 11β-HSD-1, it is likely that insulin resistance and hyperinsulinemia could be protective against low-grade systemic inflammation. The activity of 11β-HSD-1 in adipose tissue depends on the balance between TNF-α and IL-6 and insulin and IGFs (Das, 2003b). In view of this, the presence of abdominal obesity can be considered a physical sign of elevated levels of TNF-α, IL-6, and CRP; hyperleptinemia; hypertriglyceridemia; increased expression and activity of 11β-HSD-1 in abdominal adipose tissue; low levels of HDL, endothelial nitric oxide (eNO), adiponectin, IL-4, and IL-10; insulin resistance; hyperinsulinemia; and glucose intolerance.

6. LONG-CHAIN POLYUNSATURATED FATTY ACIDS AND METABOLIC SYNDROME X

Metabolic syndrome X is believed to be 10 times more common in babies who are small with low birthweights compared to those whose birthweights were normal. However, this has been disputed, and postnatal nutrition and growth may also be important

(Lucas, Fewtrell, & Cole, 1999). If metabolic syndrome X has its origins in fetal life, it is reasonable to expect that improved obstetric care, a general increase in the standard of living, and better nutrition during pregnancy would decrease the incidence of metabolic syndrome X. Yet, the incidence of metabolic syndrome X is increasing (Mokdad et al., 2001). How can this paradox be explained?

The ω-3 and ω-6 fatty acids are essential for fetal growth and development (Das, 2002b). Dietary linoleic acid (LA) and α-linolenic acid (ALA), which are essential fatty acids (EFAs), are desaturated and elongated to form their respective long-chain metabolites. Newborn and preterm infants have a limited capacity to form eicosapentaenoic acid (EPA), docosahexaenoic acid (DHA), and arachidonic acid (AA). Dietary AA improves first-year growth of preterm infants (Carlson, Werkman, Peeples, Cooke, & Tolley, 1993), whereas EPA and DHA increase birthweight by prolonging gestation and/or by increasing the fetal growth rate (Baguma-Nibasheka, Brenna, & Nathaniesz, 1999; Olsen, Olsen, & Frische, 1990). EPA, DHA, and AA inhibit TNF-α and IL-6 production, enhance eNO generation (Das, 2002b), inhibit 3-hydroxy-3-methylglutaryl coenzyme A (HMG-CoA) reductase and angiotensin-converting enzyme (ACE) activities (Das, 2001c; Kumar & Das, 1997), function as endogenous ligands for PPARs, and suppress leptin gene expression (Reseland et al., 2001). Thus, long-chain polyunsaturated fatty acids (PUFAs) suppress inflammation, regulate cholesterol metabolism, enhance the production of adiponectin, and decrease insulin resistance. Long-chain PUFAs augment brain acetylcholine levels and, thus, enhance parasympathetic activity and increase heart rate variability (Das, 2001a). This suggests that long-chain PUFAs may function as endogenous statins (Das, 2001c), β-blockers, ACE inhibitors, and anti-inflammatory and antihypertensive molecules. Long-chain PUFAs bind to PPARs (similar to thiazolidinediones) and thus are capable of enhancing adiponectin levels and reducing insulin resistance. South Asian Indians, who are at high risk of developing metabolic syndrome X, have significantly lower concentrations of AA, EPA, and DHA compared to healthy Canadians and Americans (Das, Kumar, & Ramesh, 1994). Significant amounts of long-chain PUFAs in the cell membrane increase the number of insulin receptors on the cell membrane and their affinity to insulin by increasing membrane fluidity and thus decrease insulin resistance. On the other hand, saturated fatty acids have the opposite effect, namely they decrease the number of insulin receptors, decrease cell membrane fluidity, and cause insulin resistance (Das, 1994, 2002b, 2002e).

Maternal protein restriction or increased consumption of saturated and/or trans-fatty acids and energy-rich diets during pregnancy decrease the activity of the enzymes Δ^6 and Δ^5 desaturase, leading to both maternal and fetal deficiency of EPA, DHA, and AA. Perinatal protein depletion leads to almost complete absence of measurable activities of Δ^6 and Δ^5 desaturase in fetal liver and placenta (Mercuri, de Tomas, & Itarte, 1979). Thus, both protein deficiency and a high-energy diet decrease the activities of Δ^6 and Δ^5 desaturase.

EPA, DHA, and AA deficiency increases the generation of TNF-α and IL-6, which in turn induces insulin resistance. Increased concentrations of TNF-α and IL-6 enhance the activity of 11β-HSD-1, which in turn causes the abdominal obesity seen in metabolic syndrome X. Prenatal exposure to TNF-α produces obesity (Dhalgren et al., 2001), and obese children and adults have high levels of TNF-α and IL-6. Low plasma and tissue concentrations of EPA, DHA, and AA decrease the production of adiponectin, which also aggravates insulin resistance. Thus, metabolic syndrome X starts in the perinatal period and is owing to perinatal deficiency of EPA, DHA, and AA.

7. CONCLUSIONS

Based on the evidence presented above, the sequence of events that cause metabolic syndrome X could be as follows: even under normal conditions, food intake triggers the production of TNF-α and IL-6, increases plasma CRP levels, and decreases the levels of the anti-inflammatory cytokines IL-4 and IL-10 and adiponectin. This causes oxidative stress and activation of nuclear factor-κB (NF-κB), which induces insulin resistance and consequent hyperinsulinemia. Secretion of insulin in response to food intake not only normalizes plasma glucose concentrations, but also suppresses TNF-α and IL-6 and enhances IL-4 and IL-10 synthesis. Insulin stimulates activity of Δ^6 and Δ^5 desaturase (Das, 2001d, 2001e, 2002c) and restores the levels of long-chain PUFAs to normalcy, whereas long-chain PUFAs enhance insulin action (Das, 2001d, 2002e). This implies that Δ^6 and Δ^5 desaturases could be the elusive thrifty genes. TNF-α and IL-6 activate phospholipase A_2 (PLA2), inducing the release of long-chain PUFAs from the membrane lipid pool (Seeds, Jones, Chilton, & Bass, 1998). Long-chain PUFAs thus released, if adequate, suppress the synthesis of TNF-α and IL-6. This restores the balance between pro- and anti-inflammatory cytokines and oxidative stress to normal. In contrast, chronic consumption of an energy-rich diet and/or saturated and trans-fatty acids and/or suboptimal intake of long-chain PUFAs leads to a state of low-grade systemic inflammation and chronic oxidative stress. Dietary restriction, exercise, and weight loss suppress free radical generation and oxidative stress (Dandona et al., 2001; Yatagai et al., 2003), decrease production of TNF-α and IL-6, and enhance IL-4 and IL-10 and adiponectin synthesis. Saturated and trans-fats and hyperglycemia interfere with the synthesis of long-chain PUFAs, and hence, normal inhibitory control exerted by long-chain PUFAs on TNF-α and IL-6 will be defective or suboptimal. Adequate intake of EPA and DHA was inversely associated with plasma levels of soluble TNF receptors 1 and 2 and CRP, whereas ω-6 fatty acids did not inhibit the anti-inflammatory effects of ω-3 fatty acids (Pischon et al., 2003). It is interesting that a combination of ω-3 and ω-6 fatty acids is associated with the lowest levels of inflammation.

It is suggested that adequate intake or supplementation of long-chain PUFAs (especially EPA, DHA, and small amounts of γ-linolenic acid, dihomo-γ-linolenic acid, and AA) will prevent or postpone the development of metabolic syndrome X. It would be interesting to study whether maternal supplementation of long-chain PUFAs prevents or postpones the development of metabolic syndrome X in their offspring.

In experimental animals, DHA deficiency in the perinatal period raised blood pressure later in life, even when animals were subsequently replete with this fatty acid. DHA-deficient animals underdrank water and overingested sodium, suggesting an aberration in central osmo/sodium sensors or angiotensinergic mechanisms (Das, 2001b; Weisinger et al., 2001). This indicates that there is a critical window period during which adequate amounts of long-chain PUFAs are essential to the fetus and newborn to prevent diseases in later life (Das, 2001b, 2003a). It is likely that the availability of appropriate amounts of long-chain PUFAs during critical periods of growth programes the expression of various genes such that development of diseases such as hypertension, type 2 diabetes mellitus, CHD, and metabolic syndrome X are suppressed in adult life. This would explain why EPA, DHA, and AA supplementation after the onset of metabolic syndrome X is not highly beneficial.

REFERENCES

Albert, M. A., Glynn, R. J., & Ridker, P. M. (2003). Plasma concentration of C-reactive protein and the calculated Framingham coronary heart disease risk score. *Circulation, 108*, 161–165.

Baguma-Nibasheka, M., Brenna, J. T., & Nathaniesz, P. W. (1999). Delay of preterm delivery in sheep by omega-3 long-chain polyunsaturates. *Biology Reproduction, 60*, 698–701.

Bujalska, I. J., Kumar, S., & Stewart, P. M. (1997). Does central obesity reflect "Cushing's disease of the omentum"? *Lancet, 349*, 1210–1213.

Carlson, S. E., Werkman, S. H., Peeples, J. M., Cooke, R. J., & Tolley, E. A. (1993). Arachidonic acid status correlates with first year growth in preterm infants. *Proceedings of the National Academy of Sciences USA, 90*, 1073–1077.

Chae, C. U., Lee, R. T., Rifai, N., & Ridker, P. M. (2001). Blood pressure and inflammation in apparently healthy men. *Hypertension, 38*, 399–403.

Dandona, P., Mohanty, P., Ghanim, H., Aljada, A., Browne, R., Hamonda, W., Prabhala, A., Afzal, A., & Garg, R. (2001). The suppressive effect of dietary restriction and weight loss in the obese on the generation of reactive oxygen species by leukocytes, lipid peroxidation, and protein carbonylation. *Journal of Clinical Endocrinology and Metabolism, 86*, 355–362.

Das, U. N. (1994). Insulin resistance and hyperinsulinemia: Are they secondary to an alteration in the metabolism of essential fatty acids? *Medical Science Research, 22*, 243–245.

Das, U. N. (2001a). The brain-lipid connection. *Nutrition, 17*, 260–263.

Das, U. N. (2001b). Can perinatal supplementation of long-chain polyunsaturated fatty acids prevent hypertension in adult life? *Hypertension, 38*, e6–e8.

Das, U. N. (2001c). Essential fatty acids as possible mediators of the actions of statins. *Prostaglandins, Leukotrienes and Essential Fatty Acids, 65*, 37–40.

Das, U. N. (2001d). Is insulin an anti-inflammatory molecule? *Nutrition, 17*, 409–413.

Das, U. N. (2001e). Is obesity an inflammatory condition? *Nutrition, 17*, 953–966.

Das, U. N. (2002a). Is metabolic syndrome X an inflammatory condition? *Experimental Biology and Medicine, 227*, 989–997.

Das, U. N. (2002b). The lipids that matter from infant nutrition to insulin resistance. *Prostaglandins, Leukotrienes and Essential Fatty Acids, 67*, 1–12.

Das, U. N. (2002c). Metabolic syndrome X is common in South Asians, but why and how? *Nutrition, 18*, 774–776.

Das, U. N. (2002d). Obesity, metabolic syndrome X, and inflammation. *Nutrition, 18*, 430–432.

Das, U. N. (2002e). *A perinatal strategy for preventing adult diseases: The role of long-chain polyunsaturated fatty acids*. Boston: Kluwer Academic Publishers.

Das, U. N. (2003a) Can perinatal supplementation of long-chain polyunsaturated fatty acids prevent diabetes mellitus? *European Journal of Clinical Nutrition, 57*, 218–226.

Das, U. N. (2003b). Pathobiology of metabolic syndrome X in obese and non-obese South Asian Indians: Further discussion and some suggestions. *Nutrition, 19*, 560–562.

Das, U. N. (2003c). Sex differences in the number of adipose cells. *XX vs. XY, 1*, 132–133.

Das, U. N., Kumar, K. V., & Ramesh, G. (1994). Essential fatty acid metabolism in South Indians. *Prostaglandins, Leukotrienes and Essential Fatty Acids, 50*, 253–255.

Dhalgren, J., Nilsson, C., Jennische, E., Ho, H. P., Eriksson, E., Niklasson, A., Bjorntorp, P., Albertsson Wikland, K., & Holmang, A. (2001). Prenatal cytokine exposure results in obesity and gender-specific programming. *American Journal of Physiology, 281*, E326–E334.

Engstrom, G., Hedblad, B., Stavenow, L., Lind, P., Janzon, L., & Lindgarde, F. (2003). Inflammation-sensitive plasma proteins are associated with future weight gain. *Diabetes, 52*, 2097–2101.

Esposito, K., Nappo,F., Marfella,R., Giugliano, G., Giugliano, F., Ciotola, M., Quagliaro, L., Ceriello, A., & Gingliano, D. (2002). Inflammatory cytokine concentrations are acutely increased by hyperglycemia in humans. Role of oxidative stress. *Circulation, 106*, 2067–2072.

Fernandez-Real, J. M., Vayreda, M., Richart, C., Gutierrez, C., Broch, M., Vendrell, J., & Ricart, W. (2001). Circulating interleukins 6 levels, blood pressure, and insulin sensitivity in apparently healthy men and women. *Journal of Clinical Endocrinology and Metabolism, 86*, 1154–1159.

Kalhan, R., Puthawala, K., Agarwal, S., Amini, S. B., & Kalhan, S. C. (2001). Altered lipid profile, leptin, insulin, and anthropometry in offspring of South Asian immigrants in the United States. *Metabolism, 50*, 1197–1202.

Kern, P. A., Di Gregorio, G. B., Lu, T., Rassouli, N., & Ranganathan, G. (2003). Adiponectin expression from human adipose tissue. Relation to obesity, insulin resistance, and tumor necrosis factor-α expression. *Diabetes, 52*, 1779–1785.

Kumar, K. V., & Das, U. N. (1997). Effect of cis-unsaturated fatty acids, prostaglandins, and free radicals on angiotensin-converting enzyme activity in vitro. *Proceedings of the Society for Experimental Biology and Medicine, 214*, 374–379.

Lin, Y., Rajala, M. W., Berger, J. P., Moller, D. E., Barzilai, N., & Scherer, P. E. (2001). Hyperglycemia-induced production of acute phase reactants in adipose tissue. *Journal of Biological Chemistry, 276*, 42,077–42,083.

Lindsay, R. S., Funahashi, T., Hanson, R. L., Matsuzawa, Y., Tanaka, S., Tataranni, P. A., Knowler, W. C., & Krakoff, J. (2002). Adiponectin and development of type 2 diabetes in the Pima Indian population. *Lancet, 360*, 57–58.

Luc, G., Bard, J-M., Juhan-Vague, I., Ferrieres, J., Evans, A., Amonyel, P., Arveiler, D., Fruchart, J. C., Ducimetiere, P., & PRIME Study Group. (2003). C-reactive protein, interleukins-6, and fibrinogen as predictors of coronary heart disease. The PRIME study. *Arteriosclerosis, Thrombosis and Vascular Biology, 23*, 1255–1261.

Lucas, A., Fewtrell, M. S., & Cole, T. J. (1999). Fetal origins of adult disease—the hypothesis revisited. *British Medical Journal, 319*, 245–249.

Masuzaki, H., Paterson J., Shinyama, H., Morton, N. M., Mullins, J. J., Seckl, J. R., & Flier, J. S. (2001). A transgenic model of visceral obesity and the metabolic syndrome. *Science, 294*, 2166–2170.

Matsubara, M., Namioka, K., & Katayose, S. (2003). Decreased plasma adiponectin concentrations in women with low-grade C-reactive protein elevation. *European Journal of Endocrinology, 148*, 657–662.

Mercuri, O., de Tomas, E., & Itarte, H. (1979). Prenatal protein depletion and δ9, δ6, and δ5 desaturases in the rat. *Lipids, 14*, 822–825.

Mokdad, A. H., Bowman, B. A., Ford, E. S., Vinicor, F., Marks, J. S., & Koplan, J. P. (2001). The continuing epidemics of obesity and diabetes in the United States. *Journal of the American Medical Association, 286*, 1195–1200.

Mosca, L. (2002). C-reactive protein-to screen or not to screen. *The New England Journal of Medicine, 347*, 1615–1617.

Olsen, S. F., Olsen, J., & Frische, G. (1990). Does fish consumption during pregnancy increase fetal growth? A study of the size of the newborn, placental weight and gestational age in relation to fish consumption during pregnancy. *International Journal of Epidemiology, 19*, 971–977.

Pischon, T., Hankinson, S. E., Hotamisligil, G. S., Rifai, N., Willett, W. C., & Rimm, E. B. (2003). Habitual dietary intake of n-3 and n-6 fatty acids in relation to inflammatory markers among US men and women. *Circulation, 108*, 155–160.

Ramos, E. J. B., Xu, Y., Romanova, I., Middleton, F., Chen, C., Quinn, R., Inui, A., Das, U. N., & Meguid, M. M. (2003). Is obesity an inflammatory disease? *Surgery, 134*, 329–335.

Reseland, J. E., Haugen, F., Hollung, K., Solvoll, K., Halvorsen, B., Brude, I. R., Nenseter, M. S., Christiansen, E. N., & Drevon, C. A. (2001). Reduction of leptin gene expression by dietary polyunsaturated fatty acids. *Journal of Lipid Research, 42*, 743–750.

Ridker, P. M., Cushman, M., Stampfer, M. J., Tracy, R. P., & Hennekens, C. H. (1997). Inflammation, aspirin, and the risk of cardiovascular disease in apparently healthy men. *The New England Journal of Medicine, 336*, 973–979.

Seeds, M. C., Jones, D. F., Chilton, F. H., & Bass, D. A. (1998). Secretory and cytosolic phospholipase A2 are activated during TNF priming of human neutrophils. *Biochimica Biophysica Acta, 1389*, 273–284.

Spranger, J., Kroke, A., Mohlig, M., Bergmann, M. M., Ristow, M., Boeing, H., Pfeiffer, A. F. (2003). Adiponectin and protection against type 2 diabetes mellitus. *Lancet, 361*, 226–228.

Tomilinson, J. W., Moore, J., Cooper, M. S., Bujalska, I., Shahmanesh, M., Burt, C., Strain, A., Hewison, M., & Stewart, P. M. (2001). Regulation of expression of 11β-hydroxysteroid dehydrogenase type 1 in adipose tissue: Tissue-specific induction by cytokines. *Endocrinology, 142*, 1982–1989.

van der Meer, I. M., de Maat, M. P. M., Hak, A. E., Kiliaan, A. J., Del Sol, A. I., Van Dar Kuip, D. A., Nijhuis, R. L., Hofman, A., & Witteman, J. C. (2002). C-reactive protein predicts progression of atherosclerosis measured as various sites in the arterial tree. The Rotterdam study. *Stroke, 33*, 2750–2755.

Weisinger, H. S., Armitage, J. A., Sinclair, A. J., Vingrys, A. J., Burns, P. L., & Weisinger, R. S. (2001). Perinatal omega-3 deficiency affects blood pressure in later life. Nature *Medicine, 7*, 258–259.

Whincup, P. H., Gilg, J. A., Papacosta, O., Seymour, C., Miller, G. J., Alberti, K. G., & Cook, D. G. (2002). Early evidence of ethnic differences in cardiovascular risk: Cross sectional comparison of British South Asian and white children. *British Medical Journal, 324*, 1–6.

Yatagai, T., Nishida, Y., Nagasaka, S., Nakamura, T., Tokuyama, K., Shindo, M., Tanaka, H., & Ishibashi, S. (2003). Relationship between exercise training-induced increase in insulin sensitivity and adiponectinemia in healthy men. *Endocrinology Journal, 50*, 233–238.

21 Dietary Management of Stress Using Amino Acid Supplements

Miro Smriga and Kunio Torii

KEY POINTS

- Nine amino acids are essential nutrients, and their nutritional status is bidirectionally affected by the state of the organism.
- Prolonged stress that significantly threatens homeostasis of the organism produces situations in which the adaptive functional use of specific amino acids exceeds their dietary supply, resulting in a conditional deficiency.
- Insufficient intake of a nutritionally indispensable amino acid may decrease the ability of an organism to respond to stressful challenges.
- Amino acids promote health, enhance poststress recovery, and reduce the risk of stress-triggered chronic diseases.

1. INTRODUCTION

Amino acids, like carbohydrates and fatty acids, are basic nutrients. Twenty amino acids furnish the minimal requirements for growth, nitrogen equilibrium, maintenance of host defenses, neural (Fernstrom, 2000; Young, El-Khoury, Melchor, & Castillo, 1994) and muscular functions, as well as gene-expression regulation (Fafournoux, Bruhat, & Jousse, 2000). The catabolism of amino acids provides an energy source via the intermediate products of the glycolytic pathways and the citric acid cycle. The human body is incapable of storing large amounts of amino acids, and their homeostasis must be finely maintained by the integrated action of all tissues and organs. For this reason, the dietary requirement for amino acids has important health consequences (Millward, 1994; Rose, 1957; Young, 1998; Young & Borongha, 2000). Nine amino acids are considered indispensable in the diet, but the demarcation between dispensability and indispensability is blurred by discoveries that have revealed effects of age (Baertl, Placko, & Graham, 1974; Schober, Kurz, Musil, & Jarosch, 1989), nutritional status (Kurpad et al., 2003), and psycho-behavioral conditions, such as exposure to severe stress (Lacey & Wilmore, 1990; Obled, Papet, & Breuille, 2002; Smriga & Torii, 2002).

Over the centuries, consuming an amino-acid-balanced diet meant eating an adequate diet to avoid deficiency. Insufficient lysine (Lys) intake (FAO/Agrostat, 1991) still continues to plague developing regions, where low-income populations depend predomi-

From: *Nutrients, Stress, and Medical Disorders*
Edited by: S. Yehuda and D. I. Mostofsky © Humana Press Inc., Totowa, NJ

nantly on grains for their protein supply. Trials in rural areas of China and Pakistan showed that Lys supplementation of wheat flour improved growth in children along with a number of immunological indicators (Hussain, Abbas, Khan, & Serimshaw, 2004; Zhao et al., in press). A recent trial in Syria also showed that Lys deficiency detrimentally affects stress responses (Smriga et al., 2004). A deficiency in an indispensable amino acid may occur even if a person eats a well-balanced diet that contains enough protein because prolonged infection, stress, or drug abuse affects the pathways of amino acid utilization. In such conditions, amino acid supplementation promotes health and reduces the risk of chronic diseases often associated with psychosocial stress.

Like other special states, the stress system evolved because it offered net selective advantage. Arousal of the hypothalamic–pituitary–adrenal axis increased gluconeogenesis, and the entry of glucose into cells adjusted the metabolism for rapid expenditure (Johnson, Kamilaris, Chrousos, & Gold, 1992; Munck, Guyre, & Holbrook, 1984). But the stress response suffers from inherent trade-offs obvious in a modern industrialized society, characterized by a shift from physical to chronic psychosocial stress and a consequent increase in cardiovascular (hypertension), mental (anxiety, depression), and gastrointestinal (irritable bowel syndrome, gastric ulcers) disorders (Monnikes et al., 2001; Ressler & Nemeroff, 2000).

Figure 1 illustrates the principal hypothesis behind the use of dietary amino acids. The pool of amino acids meets the basal (structural) and adaptive (functional) needs of an organism. Behavioral patterns, such as excessive exercise, and exogenous influences, such as stress, have no effect on the use of amino acids as long as the homeostasis of the organism is not threatened. When psychosocial, nutritional, or physical stress endangers the homeostatic balance, adaptive needs for specific amino acids increase, requiring an increase in their intake. The increase in Lys, leucine, and methionine requirements during the stress of food deprivation and the greater need for glutamine during catabolic stress are examples of this phenomenon. The enhancement of adaptive needs shapes basic behaviors (i.e., diet selection) (Fig. 1) through a hypothetical feedback already studied in laboratory animals (Smriga & Torii, 2002). This feedback is masked in humans by social, cultural, and other exogenous influences; thus, the use of specific amino acids literally "supplements" the innate bodily function. Stress does not generally affect the structural use of amino acids, the exception being severe catabolic stress, such as trauma or sepsis, which depletes muscle protein. Because it is already clear that stress responses are specific, different types of stress require different nutritional approaches.

The notion that dietary amino acids can delay or even block stress pathologies is not new. Enteral diets containing glutamine (Gln) and arginine (Arg) have been tested for their potential in postinjury recovery (Obled et al., 2002). Tryptophan (Trp) and tyrosine (Tyr), two neurotransmitter precursors, have been studied with respect to their central nervous system actions, such as the reduction of stress-induced mood disturbances (Fernstrom, 2000). Yet the results, especially from the noncatabolic stress studies, are not straightforward. Much of the ambiguity lies in the complexity of behavioral and mental responses to stress and the perceptions regarding the effects of antistress supplements, which are characterized by a certain degree of subjectivity. This subjectivity stems from cumulating biological factors, such as genetics, nutrition, gender, age, and body composition, as well as from the sociocultural influences of tradition, education, and social status, creating a need for amino acid supplements that relief short-term stress but also ultimately enhance long-term well-being.

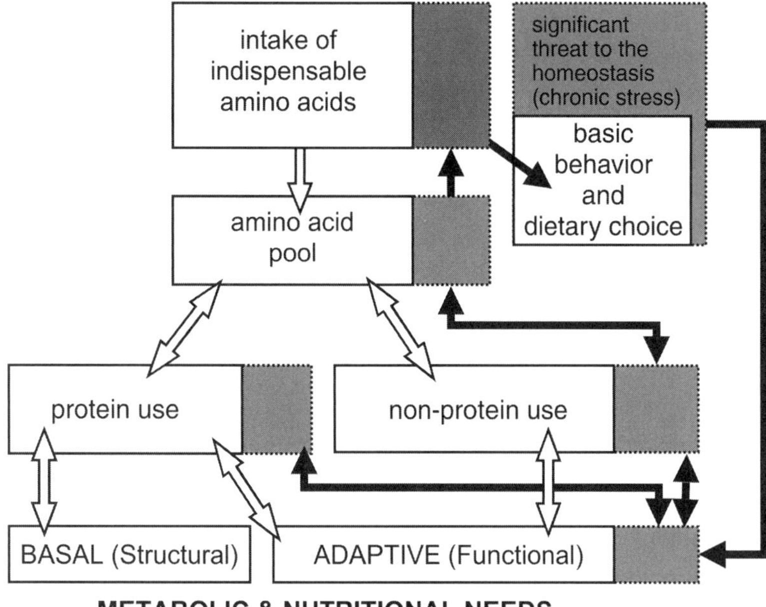

Fig. 1. Hypothesized relationship between the intake and the use/need for indispensable amino acids (white rectangles, white arrows). This relationship is not influenced by behavior, but a significant threat to homeostasis (e.g., stress) increases adaptive needs and nonprotein use of specific amino acids, via a set of feedbacks (black arrows), augments the requirement for a particular amino acid(s) and potentially alters behavioral patterns.

A range of amino acid supplements, either alone or in combination with minerals and vitamins, already exists on the market. Crystalline free-form amino acids, directly absorbable into the bloodstream, are extracted from a variety of grain products. Except for Gln, all amino acids may appear in both D- and L-forms, the latter being more compatible with human biochemistry because the proteins in human tissue consist of L-forms (the exception is D,L-phenylalanine). This chapter considers only the L-forms of amino acids and, therefore, omits the L- prefix. Furthermore, the analysis is simplified, by dividing stress exposure roughly into two categories: catabolic and noncatabolic, primarily psychosocial stress. The first part of the chapter examines the effectiveness of tryptophan, tyrosine, and Lys supplements in various models of mental stress, while the second part summarizes the value of glutamine, arginine, and the branched-chain amino acids (BCAAs) (leucine, isoleucine, valine) in catabolic stress caused by injury or exhaustive physical exercise.

2. TRYPTOPHAN, 5-HYDROXYTRYPTOPHAN, AND TYROSINE SUPPLEMENTS IN MENTAL STRESS

Although the relationship between stress and depression, on the one hand, and stress and anxiety, on the other, is still unclear, recent indications are that anxiety and depression have a common pathological mechanism. This mechanism includes the serotonin system (Ressler & Nemeroff, 2000; Riedel et al., 2002; Stahl, 1998), which is involved in the stress response as a result of its ability to keep behavioral reaction at its homeostatic

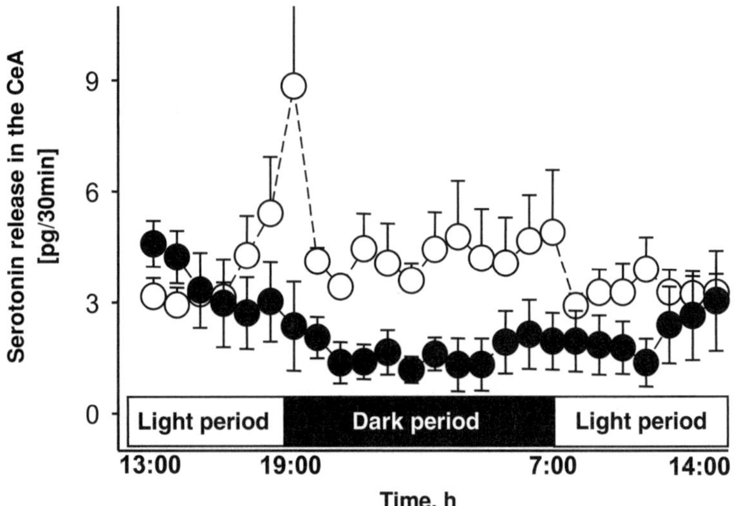

Fig. 2. Circadian pattern of serotonin release in the central nucleus of amygdala (CeA) of free-behaving male rats fed control (○) and Trp-deficient (●) diets. Wistar male rats (body weight, 250–280 g) were equipped with cannulae placed just above the left CeA. The experiment was conducted after a week-long recovery, when microdialysis probes were inserted into the cannulae at 8:00 h. (For technical details *see* Smriga et al., 2002a.) A Trp-deficient diet was given *ad libitum* for the first time at 8:00 h on the day of experiment (5 h before the start of recording). Control rats were fed a standard (control) diet; the amount equaled the average food intake measured in the Trp-deficient group. Dark period started at 19:00 h and finished at 7:00 h . The values measured in the Trp-deficient rats between 19:00 h and 7:00 h were significantly different from the values measured in controls ($p < 0.05$, one-way ANOVA followed by Duncan's multiple range test). Values are means ± SEM, $n = 4$.

setpoint. Consequently, the idea of using Trp to reduce mental stress is intuitive, because Trp influences the rate at which neuronal endings form serotonin. Brain Trp depends on the plasma supply of both Trp and carbohydrates (Fernstrom, 1991), and it is inversely affected by the circulating levels of other large neutral amino acids (LNAAs): Tyr, phenylalanine, leucine, isoleucine, and valine (Fernstrom, 1983). Chronic stress also adversely affects the brain's concentration of Trp (Young, Lopez, Murphy-Weinberg, Watson, & Akil, 2000). Thus, deficiency of Trp in the diet results in a rapid and severe decline in brain serotonin activity (Fig. 2). Trp deficiency worsens seasonal depression, anxiety, carbohydrate craving, premenstrual syndrome, and the ability to deal with daily stresses (Blokland, Lieben, & Deutz, 2002).

Numerous studies have demonstrated a positive correlation between Trp brain activity and the reduction of stress-induced mood disturbances in animals (e.g., Blokland et al., 2002; Gittos & Papp, 2001; Hussain & Mitra, 2000) and humans (Delgado, 2000). Recent human applications of the Trp deficiency model have suggested that the negative results of the deficiency originate not only from serotonin deficiency, but mainly from complex interactions between monoaminergic systems (Reilly, Delgado, 2000; McTavish, & Young, 1997; Van der Does, 2001). Indeed, a simultaneous depletion of Trp, Tyr, and phenylalanine (precursors of norepinephrine and dopamine) decreased mood more efficiently than Trp depletion alone (Hughes et al., 2003).

Controlled clinical studies indicate that Trp supplements alone or in combination with carbohydrates alleviate stress-induced mood (Maes et al., 1999; Markus et al., 1998) and cognitive deterioration (Markus, Olivier, & de Haan, 2002). However, in major mental dysfunctions, such as clinical depression, the effectiveness of Trp supplements significantly trailed that of selective serotonin reuptake inhibitors (SSRIs)—potent drugs that block serotonin reuptake on neuronal terminals. Nevertheless, Trp-containing supplements could still be utilized in milder forms of mood disturbances, for example, stress-induced sleep–wake problems. Combining Trp with an SSRI to reduce antidepressant dosages is another potential application (Walinder, Skott, Carlsson, Nagy, & Bjorn-Erik, 1976).

Human research on Trp supplements shrank suddenly 15 yr ago when nonprescription Trp preparations made by a single maker were linked to deadly outbreak of eosinophilia myalgia syndrome (EMS) and Trp was banned from the US market. Although pharmaceutically approved Trp has never been associated with symptoms of EMS, the ban is still imposed, hindering further research. One way to avoid this regulatory obstacle would be to use 5-hydroxytryptophan (5-HTP), a metabolic product of Trp and the direct precursor of serotonin. 5-HTP was effective in milder forms of stress exposure, especially those linked to jet lag and other chronopathologies, presumably because serotonin is involved in the control of arousal and sleepiness. Our data show that rats challenged with sudden light-reversal stress and fed a 5-HTP-enriched diet were able to adjust their diet intake significantly more efficiently than their normally fed counterparts (Fig. 3) (Smriga, Uneyama, & Torii, 2003).

The reason for Tyr being included in an antistress dietary supplement is qualitatively similar to that for Trp. Tyr is the precursor to the catecholamine neurotransmitters dopamine, epinephrine, and norepinephrine, which regulate mood responses to psychosocial stress (Ressler & Nemeroff, 2000). Unlike Trp, Tyr is not normally considered to be an indispensable amino acid, but some authors have suggested that under specific stress conditions the brain areas participating in stress-response regulation are not able to synthesize sufficient Tyr. Indeed, elevating Tyr concentration in actively firing but not in silent neurons (Wurtman, Hefti, & Melamed, 1980) stimulates norepinephrine production in the neuronal terminals. However, the relationship between blood and brain Tyr is not straightforward, since Tyr hydroxylase, which catalyzes the rate-limiting step in catecholamine synthesis, responds weakly to direct Tyr supply. For this reason, the use of dietary Tyr supplements to modulate brain catecholamines, and thus mood responses to stress, is questionable, as are the results of human trials. Tyr was tested in depressed patients without any significant effects on mood scores (Gelenberg, Wojcik, & Falk, 1990). However, when tested in healthy subjects under stressful conditions of combat or high altitude, Tyr significantly improved both performance and cognition (Banderet & Lieberman, 1989). Similar results were obtained in healthy subjects exposed to psychological stress (Deijin & Orlebeke, 1994). Tyr depletion impaired spatial working memory and recognition (Harmer, McTavish, Clark, Goodwin, & Cowen, 2001; Nathan et al., 2002) and in healthy women increased vulnerability to lowered mood, especially following exposure to stress (Leyton et al., 2000). The above results indicate that Tyr influences cognitive performance in mentally demanding stressful situations.

Animal studies yielded clearer results than clinical tests, but still required relatively high doses of Tyr to obtain positive effects. Rats pretreated with Tyr became more physically active following severe acute stress (Lehnert, Reinstein, Stowbridge, &

Normal light

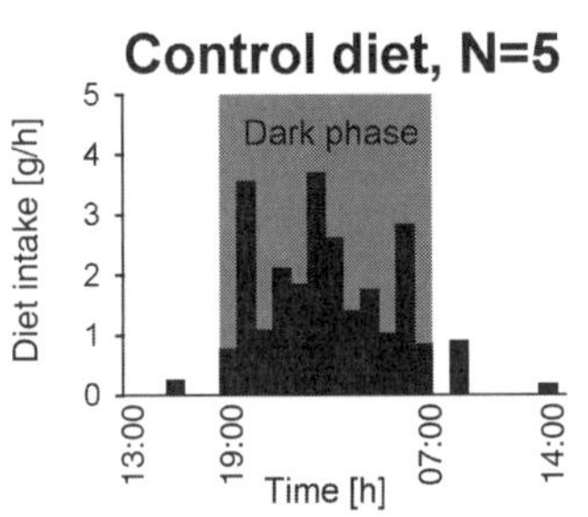

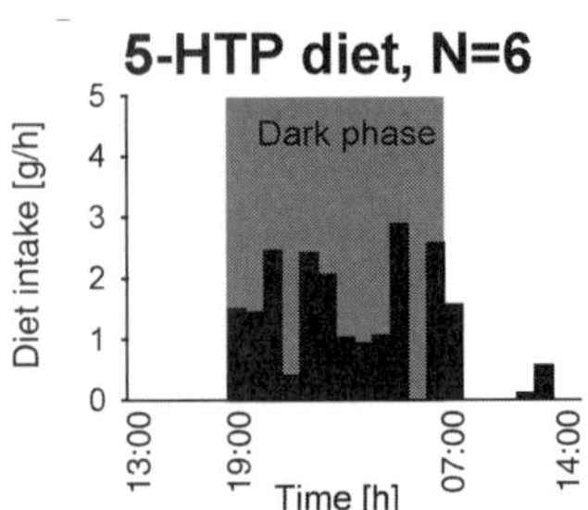

Light reversal

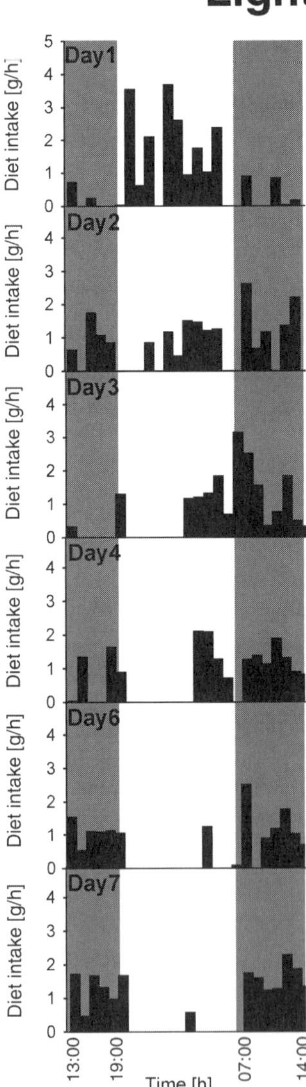

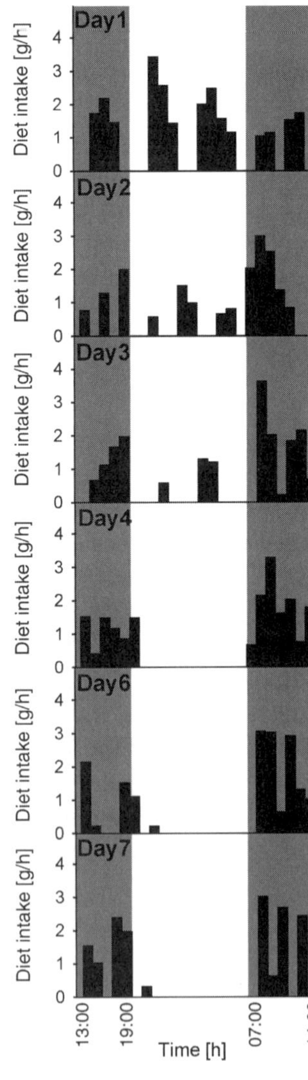

Wurtman, 1984), and their cognitive performance improved (Shurtleff, Thomas, Ahlers, & Schrot, 1993).

Trp and Tyr are precursors of neurotransmitters involved in stress regulation and thus provide logical targets for stress-modulating nutritional interventions. Several decades of clinical research, however, have not conclusively supported or refuted the effectiveness of Trp and Tyr supplements, and testing them in clinical depression or anxiety proved to be counterproductive. Specific groups, milder stress pathologies, such as sleep disturbances (Riemann et al., 2002), and long-term treatment with relatively high doses should maximize the potential of these amino acids to elevate performance and mood during mental stress. The simultaneous application of Trp and Tyr might be more effective than the use of either alone (Asnis, Wetzler, Sandrson, Kahn, & van Praag, 1992; Hughes et al., 2003).

3. LYSINE-BASED SUPPLEMENTS IN MENTAL STRESS

There are no indications that stress significantly reduces plasma or brain Lys, but recent studies documented that Lys deficiency increases the impact of stress exposure. Both rats and humans consuming a Lys-deficient diet exhibited increases in stress-induced anxiety and fecal excretion (Smriga, Kameishi, Uneyama, & Torii, 2002; Smriga et al., 2004). The anxiogenic effects in rats were traced to pathologies in circadian serotonin neurotransmission measured within the central nucleus of amygdala. Lys supplementation in normally fed rats reduced weight loss during protracted inescapable stress (Fig. 4), and treatment with Lys and arginine reduced stress-induced anxiety in rats (Smriga &Torii, 2003c) and pigs (Srinongkote, Smriga, Nakagawa, & Toride, 2003). The stress-relieving effect was attributed to Lys-induced blockade of both intestinal and central serotonin 4 receptors (Smriga & Torii, 2003a), although Lys itself did not directly affect serotonin metabolism or plasma concentration of stress hormones. Of the numerous serotonin receptors, the serotonin 4 receptor plays a "pro-stress" role in the gut and throughout the body by mobilizing energy and facilitating behavioral and gastrointestinal stress responses (Eglen, Wong, Dumuis, & Bockaert, 1995). Therefore, serotonin 4 receptor antagonists are promising targets for the treatment of diarrhea-predominant irritable bowel syndrome (Bharucha et al., 2000). Lys partly blocked serotonin 4 receptor in an in vitro assay system and mimicked anxiolytic and antidiarrhea effects of a serotonin 4 receptor antagonist in vivo, without directly affecting heart rate and cortisol release (Smriga & Torii, 2003a). In addition, Lys is a partial agonist on the central benzodiazepine receptors (Chang & Gao, 1995; Chang, Wing, Cauley, & Gao, 1993) and protects brain cells from stressful challenges by reducing the brain's metabolic rate (Guan & Ku,

---

Fig. 3. *(opposite page)* Hourly dietary intakes measured in Wistar male rats (body weight, 250–280 g) fed *ad libitum* a standard powdered diet (n = 5, left panel), or the same diet supplied with 5-hydroxytryptophan (5-HTP, 5.4 mg/1.0 g diet) (n = 6, right panel). Dark period started at 19:00 h and finished at 7:00 h. The light schedule of all rats was completely reversed on d 1 at 13:00 h (light reversal) and remained reversed for the following 7 d. Diet intake was measured each day, and the hourly values (means) calculated on d 1, 2, 3, 4, 6, and 7 are shown. Rats fed a 5-HTP-supplied diet synchronized their dietary intake significantly earlier than the controls (controls, 6.9 ± 0.6 d; 5-HTP rats, 4.5 ± 1.0 d) ($p < 0.05$, one-way ANOVA followed by Duncan's multiple range test; significance is not shown in the graph).

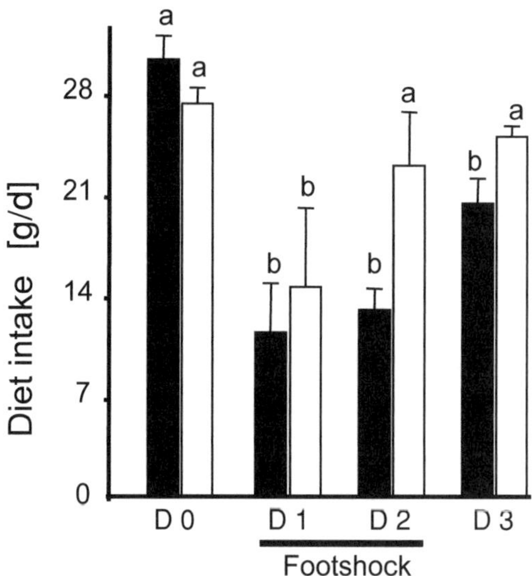

Fig. 4. Daily dietary intakes measured in Wistar male rats (body weight, 380–450 g) fed *ad libitum* a standard powdered diet (□) or the same diet supplied with Lys (3.14 mg/1.0 g diet) (■). Pairs of rats were housed in sound-attenuated, ventilated operant boxes. Footshocks were applied randomly (at least once per 2 h) to the floor of the boxes during d 1 and 2 of the experiment, and the summarized daily intakes were measured. Footshock resulted in a significant decrease in diet intake in both groups during the first day of stress exposure. Rats fed a Lys-supplied diet normalized their dietary intake significantly more efficiently on d 2 of the footshock exposure, as well as on the day immediately following the footshock exposure (d 3). The bars with different superscript letters differ significantly at $p < 0.05$ (two-way ANOVA).

1999). Consequently, the mechanism of a Lys-triggered anxiolytic effect is probably mediated via a concurrent blockage of the brain serotonin 4 receptors and stimulation of the benzodiazepine receptors (Smriga & Torii, 2003a, 2003c; Srinongkote et al., 2003). Yet research on the mechanism of the effects of Lys is in an early period, and the gastrointestinal results are especially obscure. Because secretory glycoprotein synthesis, rather than catabolism (Van der Schoor et al., 2002), appears to be a major metabolic role of Lys in the gut, it is possible that its antistress effects were mediated partly via an increased rate of glycoprotein synthesis.

Any dietary amino acid supplement causes transient imbalances in other amino acids triggered by complex metabolic and biochemical interrelationships. Although Lys has been documented as safe and well tolerated (Flodin, 1997), it worsened stress-induced decrease in plasma arginine (Smriga & Torii, 2003b). The effect was observable only when stress and oral Lys were co-administered, suggesting that the principal trigger of arginine deficiency was the high metabolic cost of stress defense.

Lys is not a direct precursor of brain neurotransmitters and does not intervene in the metabolism of stress hormones. Therefore, the possibility of treatment-related adverse effects is lower when compared to Trp or Tyr supplements. To the extent that it is possible to extrapolate from animal results to humans, Lys-based antistress supplements may offer a completely new approach to managing intestinal and other problems related to severe mental stress.

4. GLUTAMINE AND ARGININE SUPPLEMENTS IN CATABOLIC STRESS AND EXERCISE

Dysfunctional metabolism, a compromised immune system (Newsholme et al., 1987), reduced plasma levels of some amino acids (Castell, 2002; Coghlin-Dickson et al., 2000; Parry-Billings, Leighton, Dimitriadis, de Vasconcelos, & Neursholme, 1989; Roth, Funovics, Muhlbacher, & Schemper, 1982; Yu, Ryan, & Burke, 1995), and a strong endocrine stress response (Boelens, Nijveld, Houdijk, Meijir, & van Leeuwen, 2001) characterize catabolic stress (i.e., accidental injury or major surgery). Both protein and amino acid supplements have been tested in catabolic stress. Protein supplements did not block the impact of catabolic stress, mainly because of the discrepancy between the variation of amino acids needed for the synthesis of stress defense compounds and the variation provided by muscle proteolysis (Obled et al., 2002). Among the free amino acids supplements tested so far, Gln and Arg, regarded as dispensable under normal conditions, have received the greatest attention because of the inability of mammals to synthesize them sufficiently during periods of catabolic stress (Lacey & Wilmore, 1990; Smriga & Torii, 2003b; Yu et al., 1995). Both amino acids are especially important for the rapidly multiplying gut cells, as both mucosal cells and lymphoid tissue use Gln and Arg as fuel to maintain the integrity of the intestinal flora (Brzozowski et al., 1997; Okabe et al., 1976; Takagi & Okabe, 1967). Gln and Arg are closely related biochemically; Arg is synthesized in mammals from Gln via pyrroline-5-carboxylate synthetase and proline oxidase in a multistep metabolic conversion (Wu, Davis, & Flynn, 1997). Supplemental Gln and Arg are easily absorbed (Preiser, Berre, & Van Gossum, 2001), with half of Arg being readily converted to ornithine.

It is noteworthy that the positive effects of Gln differ, depending on the route of administration. Although intravenous administration of Gln improves the nitrogen balance in catabolic patients without producing clear clinical benefits (Sacks, 1999), oral or enteral Gln positively influences clinical outcomes of catabolic stress at the gut level, while not significantly altering nitrogen balance (Reeds & Jahoor, 2001).

Because catabolic stress enhances urea production and thus increases Arg degradation (Yu et al., 1995), and because Arg serves several important nonmetabolic functions, including nitric oxide synthesis, Arg supplementation positively contributes to the recovery from catabolic stress. Arg orally given in catabolic stress protected myocardium (Britten, Zeiher, & Schachinger, 1999; Kronon et al., 1999; Taddei et al., 2000), sheltered stomach mucosal cells (Brzozowski et al., 1997), prevented platelet coagulation, and reduced potentially toxic accumulation of blood ammonia (Colombani et al., 1999).

Comparabe to direct injury, the stress of exhaustive exercise suppresses immune and gut functions (Bassit, Sawada, Bacurau, Navarro, & Costa Rosa, 2000; Castell & Newsholme, 1997) and decreases plasma Gln (Castell, 2000). In fact, there is high prevalence of incidence illness in professional endurance athletes, supposedly linked to an exercise-triggered decrease of plasma Gln, increase in stress hormones, and impairment of neutrophil and T-lymphocyte function. Fukatsu (1996) reported that neutrophil bactericidal activity decreased after a 50-mile walking race, mainly owing to high cortisol levels. In marathon runners, plasma levels of Gln, the branched-chain amino acids (leucine, isoleucine, valine), and T lymphocytes all declined following a run. Although Gln supplementation did not directly affect T lymphocytes, it decreased the number of postexercise infections (Castell & Newsholme, 1997). The precise mechanism for this effect of Gln has not yet been established, but evidence suggests that the beneficial effects of Gln are dependent on neutrophil function (for review, *see* Castell, 2002).

In conclusion, Gln and Arg have been extensively studied for their effects in injury, postoperative recovery, and exhaustive exercise. The results of clinical studies are encouraging, although the mode of action is questionable, as the recovery of plasma Gln and Arg levels does not always lead to clear clinical benefits. Recent studies of the exhaustive exercise model of physical stress also indicate the usefulness of Gln and Arg, especially in the stress-protection of gut and immune cells. Gln and Arg supplements mainly support the poststress recovery responses of the gut and immune system, with the exception of the promising pre-stress Gln effects in the the immune systems of athletes. Finally, a combination of Gln and Arg, or even a broader amino acid mixture with the Gln precursors (BCAAs), rather than a separate treatment, may increase their efficacy (Ohtani, Maruyama, Sugita, & Kobayashi, 2001).

5. BRANCHED-CHAIN AMINO ACID SUPPLEMENTS IN EXHAUSTIVE EXERCISE

Exhaustive exercise increasingly oxidizes muscle BCAAs (Fitts, 1994), eventually contributing to fatigue, which is explainable not only by peripheral (Fitts, 1994) but also by central (brain) mechanisms. The "central fatigue" hypothesis is based on exercise-triggered oxidation of the peripheral BCAAs and freeing of Trp from albumin (Davis et al., 1992). These effects result in decreased BCAA:free Trp ratio in plasma during and after exercise (Blomstrand, 2001). Because BCAAs and Trp compete at the blood–brain barrier and the rate-limiting step in the synthesis of the brain serotonin is Trp transport across the barrier, sustained exercise increases brain serotonin activity (Kirby, Allen, & Lucki, 1995; Smriga, Kameishi, Tanaka, Kondoh, & Torii, 2002). Serotonin controls arousal, sleepiness, and mood, and it is assumed that the activation of the serotonin system in specific brain areas causes the feelings of fatigue (Newsholme, 1987). Central fatigue is a particularly important factor in chronic fatigue syndrome and postoperative recovery. Chronic fatigue syndrome patients reportedly cannot adjust the BCAA:Trp ratio during or after exercise (Cleare et al., 1995). Postoperative elderly patients are characterized by increased plasma free Trp (Yamamoto et al., 1997).

Studies have been conducted on the effects of BCAA supplements and avoidance of calming, Trp-containing products during exercise. Supporting data showed increases in time to fatigue induced by BCAA supplements in both humans (Castell, Yamamoto, Phoenix, & Newsholme, 1999; Newsholme et al., 1987; Yamamoto & Newsholme, 2000) and rats (Calders, Motthys, Derave, & Pannier, 1999; Smriga, Kameishi, Tanaka, et al., 2002). However, several studies failed to observe a significant effect (Gastman & Lehmann, 1998; Van Hall et al., 1995). Proponents of central fatigue argue that the discrepancies are caused by the differences in stressful aspects of exercise and that the ergogenic effects of BCAAs are observable during exercise in the heat or in a competitive race, when the mental stress component of fatigue is stronger (Blomstrand, 2001).

Time to fatigue has been used as the main measure of the effectiveness of an ergogenic treatment. Recently our group tested the effects of BCAA in conventional laboratory rats (Smriga, Kameishi, Tanaka, et al., 2002) using a different paradigm. We concentrated on the solution preference pattern (water vs BCAA solution) in exercising rats, hypothesizing that rats with free access to water and a BCAA solution would adjust fluid intake in such a way that the BCAA solution would be preferably ingested over water during times of increased physical activity. Indeed, BCAA solution intake (volume and timing) positively correlated with running pattern (Smriga, Kumeishi, Tanaka, et al., 2002). In addition, we evaluated serotonin release in several brain regions in exercising rats, postulating that some of the discrepancies in the central effects of BCAAs are owing to an inability to measure the brain serotonin release in human, and differences in recording sites in rats. We speculated that serotonin release during exercise would be specifically increased only in those brain areas involved in the recognition of peripheral amino acids and emotional responses to physical stress. Rats were trained for 10 d on a specially constructed treadmill. Thereafter, plasma amino acids, corticosterone, and brain serotonin were measured during a 1-h run. No effect of BCAA pretreatment on corticosterone was found, whereas the BCAA solution increased the plasma BCAA:Trp ratio at the end of the exercise (Smriga, Kameishi, Tanaka, et al., 2002). In control rats, lateral hypothalamus serotonin activity was significantly elevated at the end of the 1-h run and thereafter. This increase was blunted in BCAA-pretreated rats, with the main effects being observed 60–80 min after the offset of exercise. Similar but less pronounced effects were observed in the amygdala, while other brain regions were unaffected. These results from controlled laboratory tests indicate that BCAAs have a positive effect on physical performance and that a part of this effect might be mediated specifically via serotonin-dependent processes of brain areas involved in emotional reactions to exercise—the lateral hypothalamus and the amygdala. It is, however, improbable that these specific shifts in serotonin responses to exercise are responsible for the whole ergogenic effect of BCAAs. Rather, the final outcome is probably created by a combination of peripheral and central effects. In parallel, DePalo et al. (1993) reported positive effects of BCAA supplements on the physical capacity of athletes, but argued that the effect was mediated predominantly via an increase in fatty acid metabolism, rather than suppression of central fatigue.

BCAA effects during exhaustive exercise and postoperative fatigue were successfully tested in clinical trials, and the pharmacological basis of the effects is relatively established. Because at least part of the BCAA ergogenic effect is centrally mediated, it is likely that the effect of BCAA supplements is significantly greater during serotonin system sensitization, for example, during exercise in stressful situations.

6. CONCLUSIONS

A high-quality protein diet together with balanced lifestyle makes the use of amino acid supplements unnecessary. However, prolonged stress that significantly threatens the homeostasis of the organism produces situations in which the adaptive functional use of specific amino acids exceeds their dietary supply, resulting in a conditional deficiency. Specific amino acids would appear to promote health, enhance poststress recovery, and reduce the risk of stress-triggered chronic diseases.

REFERENCES

Asnis, G. M., Wetzler, S., Sanderson, W. C., Kahn, R. S., & van Praag, H. M. (1992). Functional interrelationship of serotonin and norepinephrine: Cortisol response to MCPP and DMI in patients with panic disorder, patients with depression, and normal control subjects. *Psychiatry Research, 43*, 65–76.

Baertl, J. M., Placko, R. P., & Graham, G. G. (1974). Serum proteins and plasma free amino acids in severe malnutrition. *American Journal of Clinical Nutrition, 27*, 733–742.

Banderet, L. E., & Lieberman, H. R. (1989). Treatment with tyrosine, a neurotransmitter precursor, reduces environmental stress in humans. *Brain Research Bulletin, 22*, 759–762.

Bassit, R. A., Sawada, L. A., Bacurau, R. F. P., Navarro, F., & Costa Rosa, L. F. B. P. (2000). The effect of BCAA supplementation upon the immune response of triathletes. *Medicine and Science in Sports and Exercise, 32*, 1214–1219.

Bharucha, A. E., Camilleri, M., Haydock, S., Ferber, I., Burton, D., Cooper, S., Tompson, D., Fitzpatrick, K., Higgins, R., & Zinsmeister, A. R. (2000). Effects of a serotonin 5-HT(4) receptor antagonist SB-207266 on gastrointestinal motor and sensory function in humans. *Gut, 47*, 667–674.

Blokland, A., Lieben, C., & Deutz, N. E. (2002). Anxiogenic and depressive-like effects, but no cognitive deficits, after repeated moderate tryptophan depletion in the rat. *Journal of Psychopharmacology, 16*, 39–49.

Blomstrand, E. (2001). Amino acids and central fatigue. *Amino Acids, 20*, 25–34.

Boelens, P. G., Nijveldt, R. J., Houdijk, A. P. J., Meijir, S., & van Leeuwen P. A. M. (2001). Glutamine alimentation in catabolic state. *Journal of Nutrition, 131*, 2569S–2577S.

Britten, M. B., Zeiher, A. M., & Schachinger, V. (1999). Clinical importance of coronary endothelial vasodilator dysfunction and therapeutic options. *Journal of Internal Medicine, 245*, 315–327.

Brzozowski, T., Konturek, S. J., Sliwowski, Z., Drozdowicz, D., Zaczek, M., & Kedra, D. (1997). Role of L-arginine, a substrate for nitric oxide-synthase, in gastroprotection and ulcer healing. *Journal of Gastroenterology, 32*, 442–452.

Calders, P., Matthys, D., Derave, W., & Pannier, J. L. (1999). Effects of BCAA, glucose, and glucose plus BCAA on endurance performance in rats. *Medicine and Science in Sports and Exercise, 31*, 583–587.

Castell, L. M. (2002). Can glutamine modify the apparent immunodepression observed after prolonged, exhaustive exercise? *Nutrition, 18*, 371–375.

Castell, L. M., & Newsholme, E. A. (1997). The effects of oral glutamine supplementation on athletes after prolonged, exhaustive exercise. *Nutrition, 13*, 738–742.

Castell, L. M., Yamamoto, T., Phoenix, J., & Newsholme, E. A. (1999). The role of tryptophane in fatigue in different conditions of stress. *Advances in Experimental Medicine and Biology, 467*, 697–704.

Chang, Y. F., & Gao, X. M. (1995). L-Lysine is a barbiturate-like anticonvulsant and modulator of the benzodiazepine receptor. *Neurochemical Research, 20*, 931–937.

Chang, Y. F., Wing, Y., Cauley, R. K. & Gao, X. M. (1993). Chronic L-lysine develops anti-pentylenetetrazol tolerance and reduces synaptic GABAergic sensitivity. *European Journal of Pharmacology, 233*, 209–217.

Cleare, A. J., Bearne, J., Allain, T., McGregor, A., Wessely, S., Murray, K. M., & O'Keanne, V. (1995). Contrasting neuroendocrine responses in depression and chronic fatigue syndrome. *Journal of Affective Disorders, 35*, 283–289.

Coghlin-Dickson, D. T., Wong, R. M., Offrin, R. S., Shizuru, J. A., Johnston, L. H. J., Hu, W. W., Blume, K. G., & Stockerl-Goldstein, K. E. (2000). Effect of oral glutamine supplementation during bone marrow transplantation. *Journal of Parenteral and Enteral Nutrition, 24*, 61–66.

Colombani, P. C., Bitzi, R., Frey-Rindova, P., Frey, W., Arnold, M., Langhans, W., & Wenk, C. (1999). Chronic arginine-aspartate supplementation in runners reduces total plasma amino acid level at rest and during a marathon run. *European Journal of Nutrition, 38*, 263–270.

Davis, J. M., Bailey, S. P., Woods, J. A., Galiano, F. J., Hamilton, M. T., & Bartoli, W. P. (1992). Effects of carbohydrate feedings on plasma free tryptophan and branched-chain amino acids during prolonged cycling. *European Journal of Applied Physiology, 65*, 513–519.

Deijin, J. B., & Orlebeke, J. F. (1994). Effect of tyrosine on cognitive function and blood pressure under stress. *Brain Research Bulletin, 33*, 319–323.

Delgado, P. L. (2000). Depression: The case for a monoamine deficiency. *Journal of Clinical Psychiatry, 61*, 7–11.

DePalo, E. F., Metus, P., Gatti, R., Previti, O., Bigon, L., & dePalo, C. B. (1993). BCAA chronic treatment and muscular exercise performance in athletes: A study through plasma acetyl-carnitine levels. *Amino Acids, 14*, 255–266.

Eglen, R. M., Wong, E. H. F., Dumuis, A., & Bockaert, J. (1995). Central 5-HT4 receptors. *Trends Pharmaceutical Science, 16*, 391–398.

Fafournoux, P., Bruhat, A., & Jousse C. (2000). Amino acid regulation of gene expression. *Biochemical Journal, 351*, 1–12.
FAO/Agrostat. (1991). Food balance sheet 1961–89. Computerized information series n1.
Fernstrom, J. D. (1983). Role of precursos availability in control of monoamine biosynthesis in brain. *Physiological Reviews, 63*, 484–486.
Fernstrom, J. D. (1991). Effects of the diet and other metabolic phenomena on brain tryptophan uptake and serotonin synthesis. *Advances in Experimental Medicine and Biology, 294*, 369–376.
Fernstrom, J. D. (2000). Can nutrient supplements modify brain function? *American Journal of Clinical Nutrition, 71*, 1669S–1673S.
Fitts, R. H. (1994). Cellular mechanisms of muscle fatigue. *Physiological Reviews, 74*, 49–94.
Flodin, N. W. (1997). The metabolic roles, pharmacology and toxicology of lysine. *Journal of American College of Nutrition, 16*, 7–21.
Fukatsu, A., Sato, N., & Shimizu, H. (1996). 50-Mile walking race suppresses neutrophil bactericidal function by inducing increases in cortisol and ketone bodies. *Life Science, 58*, 2337–2341.
Gastman, U. A., & Lehmann, M. J. (1998). Overtraining and BCAA hypothesis. *Medicine and Science in Sports and Exercise, 30*, 1173–1178.
Gelenberg, A. J., Wojcik, J. D., & Falk, W. E. (1990). Tyrosine for depression: A double blind trial. *Journal of Affective Disorders, 19*, 125–132.
Gittos, M. W., & Papp, M. (2001). Antidepressant-like action of AGN 2979, a tryptophan hydroxylase activation inhibitor, in a chronic mild stress model of depression in rats. *European Journal of Neuropsychopharmacology, 11*, 351–357.
Guan, H. P., & Ku, B. S. (1999). Neuroprotective effect of L-lysine HCl on acute iterative anoxia in rats with quantitative analysis of electrocorticogram. *Life Science, 65*, PL19–PL25.
Harmer, C. J., McTavish, S. F., Clark, L., Goodwin, G. M., & Cowen, P. J. (2001). Tyrosine depletion attenuates dopamine function in healthy volunteers. *Psychopharmacology, 154*, 105–111.
Hughes, J., Matrenza, C., Kemp, A., Harrison, B. J., Liley, D., & Nathan, P. J. (2004). The selective effects of monoamine depletion on mood and emotional regulation. *International Journal of Neuropsychopharmacology, 7*, 9–17.
Hussain, A. M., & Mitra, A. K. (2000). Effect of aging on tryptophan hydroxylase in rat brain: Implications on serotonin level. *Drug Metabolism and Disposal, 28*, 1038–1042.
Hussain, T., Abbas, S., Khan, M. A., & Scrimshaw, N. S. (2004). Effect of lysine fortification of wheat flour on predominantly cereal-eating families in Pakistan. *Food and Nutritional Bulletin, 25*, 114–122.
Johnson, E., Kamilaris, T., Chrousos, G., & Gold, P. (1992). Mechanisms of stress—a dynamic overview of hormonal and behavioral homeostasis. *Neuroscience and Biobehavioral Reviews, 16*, 115–130.
Kirby, L. G., Allen, A. R., & Lucki, I. (1995). Regional differences in the effects of forced swimming on extracellular levels of levels of 5-HT and 5-HIAA. *Brain Research, 682*, 189–196.
Kronon, M. T., Allen, B. S., Halldorsson, A., Rahman, S., Wang, T., & Ilbawi, M. (1999). L-Arginine, prostaglandin, and white cell filtration equally improve myocardial protection in stressed neonatal hearts. *Journal of Thoracic Cardiovascular Surgery, 118*, 665–772.
Kurpad, A. V., Regan, M. M., Raj, T., Vasudevan, J., Kuriyan, R., Gnanou, J., & Young, V. R. (2003). Lysine requirements of chronically undernourished adult Indian men, measured by a 24-h indicator amino acid oxidation and balance technique. *American Journal of Clinical Nutrition, 77*, 101–108.
Lacey, J. M., & Wilmore, D. W. (1990). Is glutamine a conditionally dependable amino acid? *Nutritional Reviews, 48*, 297–309.
Lehnert, H. R., Reinstein, D. K., Strowbridge, B. W., & Wurtman, R. J. (1984). Neurochemical and behavioral consequences of acute, uncontrollable stress: Effects of dietary tyrosine. *Brain Research, 303*, 215–223.
Leyton, M., Young, S. N., Pihl, R. O., Etezadi, S., Lauze, C., Blier, P., Baker, G. B., & Benkelfat, C. (2000). Effecst on mood of acute phenylalanine/tyrosine depletion in healthy women. *Neuropsychopharmacology, 22*, 52–63.
Maes, M., Lin, A. H., Verkerk, R., Delmeire, L., Van Gastel, A., Van der Planken, M., & Scharpe, S. (1999). Serotonergic and noradrenergic markers of post-traumatic stress disorder with and without major depression. *Neuropsychopharmacology, 20*, 188–197.
Markus, C. R., Olivier, B., & de Haan, E. H. F. (2002). Whey protein rich in α–lactalbumin increases the ration of plasma tryptophan to the sum of the other large neutral amino acids and improves cognitive performance in stress-vulnerable subjects. *American Journal of Clinical Nutrition, 75*, 1051–1056.

Markus, C. R., Panhuysen, G., Tuiten, A., Koppeschaar, H., Fekkes, D., & Peters, M. L. (1998). Does carbohydrate-rich, protein-poor food prevent a deterioration of mood and cognitive performance of stress-prone subjects when subjected to a stressful task? *Appetite, 31*, 49–65.

Millward, J. (1994). Can we define indispensable amino acid requirements and assess protein quality in adults? *Journal of Nutrition, 124*, 1509S–1516S.

Monnikes, H., Tebbe, J. J., Hildebrandt, M., Arck, P., Osmanoglou, E., Rose, M., Klapp, B., Wiedenmann, B., & Hyemann-Monnikes, I. (2001). Role of stress in functional gastrointestinal disorders. *Digestive Disorders, 19*, 201–211.

Munck, A., Guyre, P. M., & Holbrook, N. J. (1984). Physiological functions of glucocorticoids in stress and their relation to pharmacological actions. *Endocrinological Reviews, 5*, 25–44.

Nathan, P. J., Harrison, B. J., Olver, J. S., Norman, T. R., & Burrows, G. D. (2002). Depletion of serotonin versus dopamine produces double dissociation on tests of mnemonic function in healthy volunteers. *International Journal of Neuropsychopharmacology, 5*, S191.

Newsholme, E. A., Acworth, I. N., & Blomstrand, E. (1987). Amino acids, neurotransmitters and a functional link between muscle and brain that is important in sustained exercise. In *Advances in myochemistry* (127–138.). London: John Libbey Eurotext.

Obled, C., Papet, I., & Breuille, D. (2002). Metabolic bases of amino acid requirements in acute diseases. *Current Opinions in Clinical Nutrition and Metabolic Care, 5*, 189–197.

Ohtani, M., Maruyama, K., Sugita, M., & Kobayashi, K. (2001). Amino acid supplementation affects hematological and biochemical parameters in elite rugby players. *Bioscience, Biotechnology and Biochemistry, 65*, 1970–1976.

Parry-Billings, M., Leighton, B., Dimitriadis, G., de Vasconcelos, P. R., & Newsholme, E. A. (1989). Skeletal muscle glutamine metabolism during sepsis in the rat. *International Journal of Biochemistry, 21*, 419–423.

Preiser, J. C., Berre, P. J., & Van Gossum, A. 2001. Metabolic effects of arginine addition to the enteral feeding of critically ill patients. *Journal of Parenteral and Enteral Nutrition, 25*, 182–187.

Reeds, P. J., & Jahoor, F. (2001). The amino acid requirements of disease. *Clinical Nutrition, S1*, 15–22.

Reilly, J. G., McTavish, S. F., & Young, A. H. (1997). Rapid depletion of plasma tryptophan: A review of studies and experimental methodology. *Journal of Psychopharmacology, 11*, 381–392.

Ressler, K. J. & Nemeroff, C. B. (2000). Role of serotonergic and noradrenergic systems in the pathophysiology of depression and anxiety disorders. *Depression and Anxiety, 12*, 2–19.

Riedel, W. J., Klaasen, T., Griez, E., Honig, A., Menheere, P. P. C. A., & van Praag, H. M. (2002). Dissociable hormonal cognitive and mood responses to neuroendocrine challenge: Evidence for receptor-specific serotonergic dysregulation in depressed mood. *Neuropsychopharmacology, 26*, 358–367.

Riemann, D., Feige, B., Hornyak, M., Koch, S., Hohagen, F., & Voderholzer, U. (2002). The tryptophan depletion test: Impact on sleep in primary insomnia—a pilot study. *Psychiatry Research, 15*, 129–135.

Rose, W. C. (1957). The amino acid requirement of adult man. *Nutritional Abstracts and Reviews, 27*, 489–497.

Roth, E., Funovics, J., Muhlbacher, F., & Schemper, M. (1982). Metabolic disorders in sever abdominal sepsis: Glutamine deficiency in skeletal muscle. *Clinical Nutrition, 1*, 25–41.

Sacks, G. S. (1999). Glutamine supplementation in catabolic patients. *Annals of Pharmacotherapy, 33*, 348–354.

Schober, P. H., Kurz, R., Musil, H. E., & Jarosch, E. (1989). Stress adapted parenteral amino acid substitution in operated premature and newborn infants. *Infusionstherapie, 16*, 68–74.

Shurtleff, D., Thomas, D. J., Ahlers, S. T., & Schrot, J. (1993). Tyrosine ameliorates a cold-induced delayed matching-to-sample performance decrement in rats. *Psychopharmacology, 112*, 228–232.

Smriga, M., Ghosh, S., Mouneimne, Y., Toride, Y., Pellett, P., & Scrimshaw, N. (2004). Lysine fortification reduces anxiety and lessens stress in family members in economically weak Middle East communities. *Proceedings of the National Academy of Sciences USA, 101*, 8285–8288.

Smriga, M., Kameishi, M., Tanaka, T., Kondoh, T., & Torii, K. (2002). Preference for a solution of branched-chain amino acids plus glutamine and arginine correlates with free running activity in rats: Involvement of serotonergic-dependent processes of lateral hypothalamus. *Nutritional Neuroscience, 5*, 189–199.

Smriga, M., Kameishi, M., Uneyama, H., & Torii, K. (2002). Deficiency of dietary L-lysine increases stress-induced anxiety and fecal excretion in rats. *Journal of Nutrition, 132*, 3744–3746.

Smriga, M., Mori, M., & Torii, K. (2000). Circadian release of hypothalamic norepinephrine in rats in vivo is depressed during early L-lysine deficiency. *Journal of Nutrition, 130*, 1641–1644.

Smriga, M., & Torii, K. (2002). Behaviorally dependent intake of nutritionally essential amino acids. *Recent Research Developments in Nutrition, 5*, 1–14.

Smriga, M., & Torii, K. (2003a). L-Lysine acts like a partial serotonin receptor 4 antagonist and inhibits serotonin-mediated intestinal pathologies and anxiety in rats. *Proceedings of National Academy of Sciences USA, 100*, 15,370–15,375.

Smriga, M., & Torii, K. (2003b). Metabolic interactions between restraint stress and L-lysine: The effect on urea cycle components. *Amino Acids, 24*, 435–437.

Smriga, M., & Torii, K. (2003c). Prolonged treatment with L-lysine and L-arginine reduces stress-induced anxiety in an elevated plus maze. *Nutritional Neuroscience, 6*, 125–128.

Smriga, M., Uneyama, H., & Torii, K. (2003). An adjuster of circadian rhythms. Japanese patent, disclosure number 2003-081829.

Srinongkote, S., Smriga, M., Nakagawa, K., & Toride, Y. (2003). A diet fortified with L-lysine and L-arginine normalizes growth of broilers during stressful conditions of high stock density. *Nutritional Neuroscience, 6*, 283–287.

Stahl, S. M. (1998). Mechanism of action of serotonin selective reuptake inhibitors. Serotonin receptors and pathways mediate therapeutic effects and side effects. *Journal of Affective Disorders, 51*, 215–235.

Taddei, S., Galetta, F., Virdis, A., Ghiadoni, L., Salvetti, G., Franzoni, F., Giusti, C., & Salvetti, A. (2000). Physical activity prevents age-related impairment in nitric oxide availability in elderly athletes. *Circulation, 101*, 2896–2901.

Takagi, T., & Okabe, S. (1967). The effects of drugs on the production and recovery processes of the stress ulcer. *Japanese Journal of Pharmacology, 18*, 9–18.

Van der Does, A. J. (2001). The effect of tryptophan depletion on mood and psychiatric symptoms. *Journal of Affective Disorders, 64*, 107–119.

Van der Schoor, S. R. D., Reeds, P. J., Stoll, B., Henry, J. F., Rosenberger, J. R., Burrin, D. G., & Van Goudoever, J. B. (2002). The high metabolic cost of a functional gut. *Gastroenterology, 123*, 1931–1940.

Van Hall, G., Raaymakers, J. S. H., Saris, W. H. M., & Wagenmakers, A. J. M. (1995). Ingestion of branched-chain amino acids and tryptophan during sustained exercise in man: failure to affect performance. *Journal of Physiology, 486*, 789–794.

Walinder, J., Skott, A., Carlsson, A., Nagy, A., & Bjorn-Erik, R. (1976). Potentiation of the antidepressant action of clomipramine by tryptophan. *Archives of General Psychiatry, 33*, 1384–1389.

Wu, G., Davis, P. K., & Flynn, N. E. (1997). Endogenous synthesis of arginine plays an important role in maintaining arginine homeostasis in postweaning growing pigs. *Journal of Nutrition, 127*, 2342–2349.

Wurtman, R. J., Hefti, F., & Melamed, E. (1980). Precursor control of neurotransmitter synthesis. *Pharmacological Revue, 32*, 315–335.

Yamamoto, T., Castell, L. M., Botella, J., Powell, H., Hall, G. M., Young, A., & Newsholme, E. A. (1997). Changes in the albumine binding of Trp during post-operative recovery: A possible link with central fatigue. *Brain Research Bulletin, 43*, 43–46.

Yamamoto, T., & Newsholme, E. A. (2000). Diminished central fatigue by inhibition of L-system transporter for the uptake of tryptophan. *Brain Research Bulletin, 52*, 35–38.

Young, E. A., Lopez, J. F., Murphy-Weinberg, V., Watson, S. J., & Akil, H. (2000). Hormonal evidence for altered responsiveness to social stress in major depression. *Neuropsychopharmacology, 23*, 411–418.

Young, V. R. (1998). Human amino acid requirements: Counterpoint to Millward and the importance of tentative revised estimates. *Journal of Nutrition, 128*, 1570–1573.

Young, V. R., & Borgonha, S. (2000). Nitrogen and amino acid requirements: The Massachusetts Institute of Technology amino acid requirement pattern. *Journal of Nutrition, 130*, 1841S–1849S.

Young, V. R., El-Khoury, A. E., Melchor, S., & Castillo, L. (1994). The biochemistry and physiology of protein and amino acid metabolism, with reference to protein nutrition. In Protein metabolism during infancy (pp. 1–28). New York: Vevey/Raven.

Yu, Y. M., Ryan, C. M., & Burke, J. F. (1995). Relations among arginine, citrulline, ornithine, and leucine kinetics in adult burn patients. *American Journal of Clinical Nutrition, 62*, 960–966.

Yu, Y. M., Young, V. R., Castillo, L., Chapman, T. E., Tompkins, R. G., Ryan, C. M., & Burke, J. F. (1995). Plasma arginine and leucine kinetics and urea production rates in burn patients. *Metabolism, 44*, 659–666.

Zhao, W., Zhai, F., Zhang, D., An, Y., Liu, Y., He, Y., Ge K., & Scrimshaw, N. S. (2004). The impact of lysine fortified wheat flour on the nutritional and immunological status of wheat eating families in China. *Food and Nutritional Bulletin, 25*, 123–129.

22 Conditioned Nutritional Requirements of the Failing Heart

Michael J. Sole

KEY POINTS

- Disease, genetic predisposition, or certain drug therapies may alter the nutritional requirements (conditioned nutritional requirements) of specific organs.
- The failing myocardium exhibits deficiencies in carnitine, taurine, coenzyme Q10, and thiamine.
- Supplementation of both animal models and humans with heart failure with these nutrients restores myocardial levels and improves myocardial function and structure.
- Restoration of adequate myocyte nutrition is an important component of the therapy of heart failure.

1. INTRODUCTION

Congestive heart failure has emerged as a major health problem during the past four decades (Bourassa et al., 1993). In spite of our advances, the underlying heart disease is relentlessly progressive in almost all patients who develop symptoms of overt failure, and mortality continues to be unacceptably high—approx 40% in 5 yr (Bourassa et al., 1993). Heart transplantation appears to be the only prospect to improve long-term survival for many patients.

The modern pharmacological therapy of heart failure has focused on the amelioration of fluid overload, hemodynamic abnormalities, and inappropriate neurohormonal stimulation. Attention is now being turned to the evaluation and management of etiological factors that lead to progressive, long-term myocardial damage, particularly factors that result in myocyte loss or dysfunction (Sole, 1995). Several metabolic abnormalities are important contributors to the pathogenesis of this deterioration. In particular, there is a progressive accumulation of calcium in myocytes, which in turn results in increased calcium in the mitochondria. The progressive increase in mitochondrial calcium decreases myocyte energy production and increases oxidative stress resulting in free radical damage, myocyte dysfunction, and death (Katz, 1989; Vogt & Kubler, 1998). In addition, these processes may influence skeletal muscle and contribute to fatigue and disability (Clark, Sparrow, & Coats, 1995).

From: *Nutrients, Stress, and Medical Disorders*
Edited by: S. Yehuda and D. I. Mostofsky

The presence of protein–energy malnutrition in congestive heart failure has been recognized by surveys of hospitalized patients using anthropometric, biochemical, and immunological measures of nutritional status. These surveys have indicated that 50–68% of patients with congestive heart failure were significantly malnourished (Carr, Stevenson, Walden, & Heber, 1989; Freeman & Roubenoff, 1994). Cardiac failure results in a cascade of metabolic effects such as tissue hypoxia, hypermetabolism, weakness, dyspnea, and hypomotility of the gastrointestinal tract, all leading to poor nutrient intake. Anorexia and early satiety have been reported in congestive heart failure patients and may be aggravated by unpalatable dietary restrictions or a variety of cardiac drugs. These factors may lead to compromised food and nutrient intake and subsequently contribute to the poor nutritional status of these patients. In addition, patients with heart failure have been shown to have increased resting metabolic rates, possibly owing to the increased work of breathing or elevated sympathetic nervous system outflow (Anker et al., 1997). There appears to be a significant correlation between the loss of lean body mass in heart failure patients and increases in circulating catabolic neuroendocrine factors and cytokines; the neuroendocrine anabolic response reported in these patients is inadequate (Anker et al., 1997).

Simple protein–calorie feeding does not resolve the issue. For example, a randomized controlled trial with a protein supplement of 30 g and a daily energy supplement of 750 kcal did not show clinical benefit in either heart or skeletal muscle in spite of a marked positive energy balance (Broqvist et al., 1994). There is increasing evidence that patients with cardiac failure are deficient in specific micronutrients important in the effective metabolism of protein–energy foods, maintenance of intracellular calcium homeostasis, and control of oxidative stress rather than merely protein–calorie malnutrition (Sole & Jeejeebhoy, 2002; Witte, Clark, & Cleland, 2001). Indeed, the failing myocardium may exhibit specific nutritional requirements long before they become clinically evident (Sole & Jeejeebhoy, 2002). This chapter is not meant to comprehensively review all of the micronutrients one may consider in heart failure, but rather discusses some nutritional principles important in the pathogenesis of myocardial disease and specific nutrients particularly relevant to the treatment of heart failure.

2. CONDITIONED NUTRITIONAL REQUIREMENTS AND THE NEED FOR SUPPLEMENTS

The need for increased folic acid and iron in pregnancy or calcium and vitamin D supplements in aging are well recognized. Less well understood is the concept that the advent of disease, genetic predisposition, or certain drug therapies may significantly alter the recommended daily intake for specific nutrients published by government agencies and established in healthy people (Zeisel, 2000). The nutritional demands of a given physiological state or pathological process such as myocardial failure may result in "conditioned nutrient requirements or deficiencies" for the affected organ—in this case the myocardium and perhaps skeletal muscle (Sole & Jeejeebhoy, 2002). The need for a given nutrient may not be readily detected, as its level in the blood may not reflect a deficiency or increased requirements in the diseased organ. Even normal levels may be insufficient to maintain full functional status in the face of pathological metabolic demands.

The use of a supplement for a given disorder, such as heart failure, can be justified through decision analysis:

1. Are there data supporting an important role for the nutrient in cellular or organ function?
2. Is the level of the nutrient reduced in tissues (organ) affected by the disorder?
3. Are there data suggesting impairment of biological pathways that require the nutrient?
4. Is there evidence that tissue levels respond to the intake of the nutrient?
5. Is there evidence for biological benefit from restoration of normal nutrient levels?
6. Can simple dietary modification achieve the nutrient intake required to restore tissue levels, or is a supplement needed?

3. MAINTAINING MYOCARDIAL ENERGETICS

Myocardial energy production from nutrients requires the assistance of a number of cofactors. Reduction in the level of these, namely, carnitine (critical for the transport of long-chain fatty acid substrate and maintenance of adequate glucose oxidation), coenzyme Q10 (a key transducer for mitochondrial oxidative phosphorylation and an important endogenous antioxidant), creatine (important as a storage reservoir and shuttle of high-energy phosphate) and thiamine (important for carbohydrate metabolism), has been described in heart failure.

3.1. L-Carnitine

L-Carnitine, an amino acid derivative (3-hydroxy-4-*N*-trimethylaminobutyric acid), is essential for the transport of long-chain fatty acids from the cytoplasm into the sites of β-oxidation within the mitochondrial matrix (Arsenian, 1997). In addition to promoting the entry of fat into the mitochondria, carnitine binds acyl groups and releases free coenzyme A (CoA). This benefits the myocyte by removing toxic short-chain acyl groups to form acylcarnitines, which can freely diffuse out of the cell and be eliminated through the urine. Furthermore, the reduced acetyl CoA:CoA ratio promotes the activation of pyruvate dehydrogenase and hence glucose oxidation; this in turn improves the coupling between glycolysis and glucose oxidation, reducing the lactate and H^+ burden on the cells (Arsenian, 1997; Schonekess, Allard, & Lopaschuk, 1995).

Body stores of L-carnitine are supplied both by diet and via endogenous biosynthesis from trimethyllysine. The concentration of carnitine in normal adult cardiac and skeletal muscle is approx 8–15 nmol/mg noncollagen protein; plasma levels are approx 35–50 μmol/L. Thus, plasma levels are not a good measure of tissue concentrations. A 20–50:1 intracellular:extracellular carnitine gradient is maintained by a sodium-dependent plasma membrane transport system.

Carnitine deficiency occurs in several genetically determined metabolic abnormalities, where it is associated with the development of cardiomyopathy and skeletal muscle dysfunction (Engel, 1986). L-Carnitine administration to these patients ameliorates the cardiac and skeletal muscle dysfunction.

Evaluation of carnitine metabolism in several cardiac pathologies has led to the realization that carnitine deficiency may also be acquired and organ selective. Failing myocardium generally exhibits a marked depletion (up to 50%) of both free and total carnitine (Arsenian, 1997; Pepine, 1991).

The administration of L-carnitine (3–5 g in divided doses) or one of its analogs (e.g., proprionyl-carnitine) has been reported to result in significant hemodynamic improvement and an overall benefit in the functional capacity of animals and patients with myocardial dysfunction (Arsenian, 1997; Pepine 1991). A recent multicenter, placebo-controlled, double-blind, randomized clinical trial showed a significant beneficial effect, including a reduction in adverse cardiac remodeling, when L-carnitine was taken for 6 mo following myocardial infarction (Illiceto et al., 1995).

3.2. Ubiquinone or Coenzyme Q10

Coenzyme Q10 or ubiquinone (2,3-dimethoxy-5-methyl-6-decaprenyl benzoquinone), sited within the inner mitochondrial membrane, is a vital rate-limiting carrier for the flow of electrons through complexes I, II, and III of the mitochondrial respiratory chain (Littaru, 1995). It is associated with the membranes of other intracellular organelles as a major endogenous lipophilic antioxidant (Villalba et al., 1995) and is an important component of circulating low-density lipoprotein (LDL) particles, protecting LDL from oxidation (Littaru, 1995).

Ubiquinone is actively biosynthesized with the cells. The quinone ring is synthesized from the amino acid tyrosine, and the polyisoprenoid side chain is formed through the acetyl CoA–mevalonate pathway (Littaru, 1995). The latter pathway is under the control of the enzyme hydroxymethylglutaryl coenzyme A (HMG-CoA) reductase, which is also used for cholesterol synthesis. Inhibition of this pathway using HMG-CoA reductase inhibitors—drugs that decrease plasma cholesterol—also results in a parallel decrease in plasma ubiquinone and may also reduce tissue ubiquinone levels (Folkers et al., 1990). The significance of this in heart disease is unknown.

Ubiquinone is widespread throughout all food groups, and thus body stores may also be partially supplied by diet. The concentration of ubiquinone in normal cardiac muscle is approximately 0.4–0.5 μg/mg dry weight, slightly less in skeletal muscle, and 0.6–1.3 μg/mL in plasma. Oral absorption is slow, and there is a large hepatic first-pass effect, so that only 2–5% of an oral dose is taken up by the myocardium.

The failing heart exhibits both impaired energy production and increased oxidative stress, suggesting a particular dependence on ubiquinone. However, the role of ubiquinone in cardiac disease is unclear. Reductions of myocardial ubiquinone of up to 50% are well documented in heart failure in both animal models and humans (Folkers, Vadhanavikit, & Mortensen, 1985; Jeejeebhoy et al., 2002). The relevance of this degree of reduction to myocyte membrane structure and function through impairment of mitochondrial oxidation or increased oxidative stress is uncertain.

Oral ubiquinone therapy has been shown to beneficially affect the course of heart disease in a wide variety of animal paradigms (Guarnieri et al., 1987; Momomura, Serizawa, Ohtani, Izuka, & Sugimoto, 1991). The results of trials in patients with heart failure are mixed, but these studies were small or had methodological problems or utilized doses of ubiquinone of 100 mg/d or less (Hofman-Bang, Rehnqvist, Swedberg, Wiklund, & Astrom, 1995; Langsjoen, Vadhanavikit, & Folkers, 1985; Soja & Mortenson, 1997). It has been suggested that at least 150–200 mg/d of a highly bioavailable formulation are required.

3.3. Creatine

Creatine phosphate (PCr) is the primary high-energy phosphate reservoir of the heart and skeletal muscle and a critical carrier of high-energy phosphate from the mitochondria to sites of utilization in the cytoplasm. High-energy phosphate is transferred from PCr to adenosine diphosphate (ADP) to form adenosine triphosphate (ATP) through catalysis by creatine kinase:

$$PCr + ADP + H^+ \leftrightarrow ATP + Cr$$

Muscle creatine stores are maintained through myocardial uptake of creatine biosynthesized from the endogenous precursors arginine, glycine, and methionine in the liver, pancreas, and kidneys and through the ingestion of meat and fish (Wyss & Walliman, 1994). The concentration of total creatine in normal adult human myocardium or skeletal muscle is approx 140 μmol/g protein (Nascimben et al., 1996).

Experimental creatine depletion in animals results in structural, metabolic and functional abnormalities in muscle (Wyss & Walliman, 1994). Myocardial creatine content is reduced up to 50% with the expected concomitant reduction in creatine phosphate in a wide variety of animal paradigms and humans with heart failure (Nasciben et al., 1996; Neubauer, et al., 1997). The myocardial PCr:ATP ratio has been reported to be a better predictor of patient mortality in dilated cardiomyopathy than left ventricular ejection fraction or the patient's functional class (Neubauer et al., 1997).

The role of creatine supplementation may not be observed in cardiac muscle under normal levels of performance, because creatine has only been shown to improve short-term intense exercise in skeletal muscle, where it reduces lactate accumulation. The administration of a creatine supplement (5 g four times daily) for 10 d to nine patients with heart failure did not increase cardiac ejection fraction but did increase skeletal muscle creatine phosphate and muscle strength and endurance relative to placebo-treated control patients (Gordon, Hultman, & Kaijser, 1995)

3.4. Thiamine

Thiamine is a water-soluble vitamin that functions as a coenzyme in metabolic pathways related to carbohydrate energy metabolism. It is stored in very small quantities (approx 30 mg) with any daily excess excreted. Thus, thiamine requirements must be met daily; patients with poor intakes may be at increased risk for deficiency during acute illness. Necropsy studies indicate that thiamine deficiency is underdiagnosed in life (Harper, Giles, & Finlay-Jones, 1986). The classical deficiency signs of beriberi are often absent, or they are not recognized.

Patients with heart failure may be at risk for thiamine deficiency as a result of poor dietary intake as well as increased thiamine requirements owing to alterations in metabolic rate. Thiamine intake in patients with heart disease has been reported in only one study using a semi-quantitative food frequency questionnaire focusing on foods high in thiamine (Brady, Rock, & Horneffer, 1995). Nutrient analysis indicated a low overall intake of thiamine of 0.966 mg/d, with 33% of patients not meeting the Recommended Dietary Allowance (RDA) of 0.8 mg/d for thiamine.

It is reported that the use of diuretics causes increased urinary losses of thiamine (Seligmann et al., 1991). Studies in patients with heart failure report the incidence of thiamine deficiency to be between 13 and 91%, depending on the population studied (Pfitzenmeyer, Guilland, d'Athis, Petit-Marnier, & Gaudet, 1994; Seligmann et al., 1991). We examined thiamine status (erythrocyte thiamine pyrophosphate concentrations) in 100 hospitalized heart failure patients and 50 age- and sex-matched controls. The prevalence of thiamine deficiency was 33% in patients with heart failure compared to 12% in controls. There was no association between thiamine deficiency and age, gender, hospitalization, diabetes, left ventricular dysfunction, or urine volume; preadmission spironolactone use exhibited a weak correlation (Douglas et al., 2003).

Thiamine supplementation was reported to be of benefit in patients with heart failure in a randomized double-blind trial of 30 patients with heart failure and on long-term furosemide (Shimon et al., 1995). No other trial addressing the possible benefits of thiamine in patients suffering from congestive heart failure could be found.

4. REGULATING INTRACELLULAR CALCIUM

The failing myocardium exhibits an increase in calcium content and impaired movement of intracellular calcium. Impaired uptake of calcium adversely affects diastolic relaxation, whereas the kinetics of transsarcolemmal calcium flux and calcium release by the sarcoplasmic reticulum is a principal determinant of systolic function. Chronic intracellular calcium overload ultimately leads to cell death.

Taurine (2-aminoethanesulfonic acid) is a unique amino acid that lacks a carboxyl group and as such it does not enter into protein synthesis. It is an important amino acid for the modulation of cellular calcium levels, exhibiting a remarkable biphasic action by increasing or decreasing calcium levels appropriate to the maintenance of intracellular calcium homeostasis by affecting several myocardial membrane systems particularly calcium channels and ion exchangers in the sarcoplasmic reticulum and sarcolemma (Azuma, Sawamura, & Awata, 1992). Taurine is also an antioxidant, reacting with a variety of potentially toxic intracellular aldehydes including acetaldehyde and malonyldialdehyde (Ogasawara, Nakamura, Koyama, Nemoto, & Yoshida, 1994). Taurine comprises approx 60% of the free amino acid pool of the cardiomyocytes of small animals and 25–30% in humans (Huxtable, Chubb, & Azari, 1980).

Taurine is not an essential amino acid in mature, healthy humans, because it can be synthesized in the liver and pancreas from cysteine or methionine, but most taurine in humans is obtained directly through dietary sources. Biosynthetic capacity is almost absent in the human fetus and newborn but progressively increases until adulthood (Sturman, 1993). Active taurine transport into cells is regulated by the activation of two calcium sensitive enzymes: protein kinase C, which inhibits the transporter, and calmodulin, which stimulates transport (Ganapathy & Leibach, 1994). This reciprocal regulation of intracellular taurine levels by these two enzymes is consistent with a physiological role for taurine in the maintenance of intracellular calcium homeostasis.

Cats have very little taurine biosynthetic capacity and may exhibit a taurine-deficient cardiomyopathy (Pion, Kittleson, Rogers, & Morris, 1987). In humans, cardiac taurine concentrations are altered in heart disease (Azuma et al., 1992; Huxtable et al., 1980). In myocardial ischemia, concentrations are reduced, whereas in nonischemic forms of heart failure, levels may be normal but inadequate relative to the intracellular calcium burden. Cytokine activity, particularly that of tumor necrosis factor (TNF)-α and interleukin (IL)-6 is increased in heart failure. The infusion of TNF-α into experimental animals has been shown to reduce the transsulfuration of dietary methionine to cysteine and in consequence decrease the levels of taurine and glutathione unless the animals are supplemented with cysteine (Grimble et al., 1992). These findings suggest that the increased cytokine activity in heart failure may increase the need for cysteine and taurine.

Taurine depletion has been shown to render the heart more susceptible to doxorubicin toxicity or to ischemic damage (Schaffer, Allo, Harada, & Mozaffari, 1987). Prolonged depletion of the myocardium has also been shown to decrease contractile force through reduction of myofibrils (Lake, 1994). This finding is of interest because increased calcium levels in the myocyte can activate calcium-dependent proteinases, which in turn may breakdown myofibrils. In animal models, orally administered taurine has been shown to significantly reduce myocardial damage induced by the calcium paradox, doxorubicin, isoproterenol, or in hamster cardiomyopathy (Azari, Brumbaugh, Barbeau, & Huxtable, 1980; Azuma et al., 1992). It also has been reported to increase the survival of rabbits with aortic regurgitation (Takihara, Azuma, & Awata, 1986). We reported a remarkable beneficial cardiac protective effect of taurine in a murine model of iron overload cardiomyopathy (Oudit et al., 2004). Studies of taurine administration in humans with congestive heart failure have been very limited and uncontrolled. However, taurine given in an oral dose of 1 g three times daily, has been reported to be extremely well tolerated and to improve both hemodynamic state and functional capacity. Toxicity has not been noted with large doses in either animal or human studies (Azuma et al., 1992).

5. REDUCING OXIDATIVE STRESS

Cells are constantly subjected to interplay between free radical injury and protective mechanisms to prevent or minimize free radical injury. Oxidative stress has been defined as a disturbance in the equilibrium between pro- and antioxidative systems. A number of different challenges in heart failure increase oxidative stress, resulting in damage to membranes, proteins, and DNA in the myocardium.

Oxidative stress may be an important contributor to the deterioration of the hypertrophied or failing myocardium. This finding is not surprising because a number of factors associated with heart failure, such as activation of the sympathetic and the renin–angiotensin system, microvascular reperfusion injury, cytokine stimulation, activated inflammatory cells, and mitochondrial DNA mutations (particularly related to respiratory complex I), are known stimuli for free radical production and oxidative stress (Ball & Sole, 1998). Coenzyme Q10 and taurine, discussed above, are both important endogenous antioxidants.

Oxidative stress or peroxidative damage has been demonstrated in the hearts of dogs and rats with heart failure owing to pressure or volume overload or following myocardial infarction (Ball & Sole, 1998; Singh, Dhalla, & Singal, 1995). We have observed decreases in the levels of glutathione peroxidase and α-tocopherol and a concomitant increase in protein oxidation in the myocardium of cardiomyopathic hamsters during the late stages of cardiomyopathy (Li, Sole, Mickle, Schimmer, & Goldstein, 1997); an elevation of myocardial free radicals and lipid peroxides has also been demonstrated in this model. The administration of vitamin E appears to completely normalize these findings (Li et al., 1997).

We have demonstrated a significant increase in the plasma lipid peroxide and malonyldialdehyde levels, markers of oxidative stress, in patients suffering from congestive heart failure (Geranmaygan et al., 1998). The increase in oxidative stress was related to the clinical severity of heart failure, with the highest levels of lipid peroxidation and malonyldialdehydes being observed in class 3 and 4 patients. These observations and similar data from other laboratories (Diaz-Velez, Garcia-Castineiras, Mendoza-Ramos, & Hernandez-Lopez, 1996) suggest that antioxidant supplements may be important additions to the therapy of heart failure. However, we have completed a double-blind randomized, placebo-controlled study of 50 patients with class II–IV heart failure (Keith et al., 2001). Vitamin E (1000 IU) or placebo was taken for 3 mo. There was a twofold increase in plasma vitamin E in the active group, but plasma catecholamines, atrial ratriuretic peptide, TNF-α, and malonyldialdehyde were not affected. These negative findings mirror the disappointing results seen in numerous studies of antioxidants, such as vitamins E and C, for the prevention of atherosclerotic vascular disease and the endpoints of heart attack and stroke.

6. NUTRITIONAL SUPPLEMENTATION

In each of the deficiencies discussed here, restoration of a single nutrient by dietary supplementation of affected animals or humans suffering from myocardial failure has yielded mixed results. Replacement of one nutritional constituent in the traditional pharmacological paradigm is unlikely to correct the cascade of interconnected abnormalities found in the failing myocardium. Furthermore, the need for a given nutrient may not be readily apparent, as tissue levels differ significantly from those in the blood.

Therefore, we randomized a placebo diet against one including a supplement containing taurine, coenzyme Q10, carnitine, thiamine, creatine, vitamin E, vitamin C, and selenium to cardiomyopathic Syrian hamsters during the late stages of their disease (Keith et al., 2001). We observed a depletion of myocardial vitamin E, creatine, carnitine, taurine, and coenzyme Q10 in the diseased animals. Supplementation for 3 mo markedly improved myocyte sarcomeric ultrastructure, developed pressure, +dp/dt, -dp/dt, measured in a Langendorff apparatus. A supplement containing these nutrients was given for 30 d in a double-blind, randomized, placebo-controlled trial to 41 patients with ischemic cardiomyopathy awaiting bypass surgery (Jeejeebhoy et al., 2002). Myocardial biopsies taken from patients on the placebo exhibited significant reductions in carnitine, coenzyme Q10, and taurine. Supplemented patients exhibited restored myocardial levels of taurine, coenzyme Q10, and carnitine and a significant decrease in left ventricular end diastolic volume.

7. NUTRITIONAL SUPPLEMENTATION AS A NEW THERAPEUTIC STRATEGY FOR HEART FAILURE

The recommended daily intake of vitamins and related micronutrients established by federal nutrition authorities in Canada, the United States, and western Europe are often relied upon by healthcare professionals to determine the nutritional requirements of their patients. However, these recommendations are commonly determined through the analysis of deficiency data from otherwise healthy humans and animals. We believe that these data cannot be relied upon for determining the nutritional requirements of patients suffering from cardiac or other diseases.

Investigators, with an interest in nutritional deficiencies, have used single specific nutrients to treat heart failure and other diseases. This is the traditional pharmacological paradigm—one molecule for a specific function or receptor. However, the replacement of only one nutritional constituent would not correct the cascade of interconnected abnormalities, such as we have described for the failing myocardium.

Finally, it should be noted that the population of myocytes within the failing heart is heterogeneous with respect to composition and structure. The failing heart deteriorates over a span of several years; thus, only a small minority of cells at any given time can be irreversibly injured; that is, the vast majority of myocytes in the failing heart must be capable of recovery under the appropriate conditions. The contemporary treatment of heart failure has focused on normalizing myocyte environment through correcting hemodynamic and neurohormonal stressors. We contend that addressing cellular nutritional needs, i.e., conditioned nutritional requirements, is also important and worthy of intensive study.

8. CONCLUSIONS

The failing myocardium exhibits conditioned nutritional requirements, resulting in significant nutritional deficiencies even with normal dietary intake. These deficiencies impair myocardial protein synthesis, energy metabolism, and calcium balance and increase oxidative stress. It is probable that skeletal muscle nutrition in heart failure is similarly impaired. Nutritional deficiency appears to be an integral contributor to myocyte dysfunction and loss and possibly the fatigue and exercise intolerance seen in heart failure. Thus, restoring adequate myocyte nutrition would seem to be essential to any therapeutic strategy designed to benefit patients suffering from this disease. Both basic and clinical research in this area is sorely needed.

REFERENCES

Anker, S. D., Chua, T. P., Ponikowski, P., Harrington, D., Swan, J. W., Kox, W. J., Poole-Wilson, P. A., & Coats, J. S. (1997). Hormonal changes and catabolic/anabolic imbalance in chronic heart failure and their importance for cardiac cachexia. *Circulation, 96*, 526–534.

Arsenian, M. A. (1997). Carnitine and its derivatives in cardiovascular disease. *Progress in Cardiovascular Disease, 40*, 265–286.

Azari, J., Brumbaugh, P., Barbeau, A., & Huxtable, R. (1980). Taurine decreases lesion severity in the hearts of cardiomyopathic Syrian hamsters. *Canadian Journal of Neurological Sciences, 7*, 435–440.

Azuma, J., Sawamura, A., & Awata, N. (1992). Usefulness of taurine in chronic congestive heart failure and its prospective application. *Japanese Circulation Journal, 56*, 95–99.

Ball, A. M. M. M., & Sole, M.J. (1998). Oxidative stress and the pathogenesis of heart failure. *Cardiology Clinics, 16*, 665–675.

Bourassa, M. G., Gurne, O., Bangdiwala, S. I., Ghali, J. K., Young, J. B., Rousseau, M., Johnstone, D. E., & Yusuf, S., for the Studies of Left Ventricular Dysfunction (SOLVD) Investigators. (1993). Natural history and patterns of current practice in heart failure. *Journal of the American College of Cardiology, 22* (Suppl. A), 14A–19A.

Brady, J. A., Rock, C. L., & Horneffer, M. R. (1995). Thiamine status, diuretic medications and the management of congestive heart failure. *Journal of the American Dietetic Association, 95*, 541–544.

Broqvist, M., Arnqvist, H., Dahlstrom, U., Larsson, J., Nylander, E., & Permet, J. (1994). Nutritional assessment and muscle energy metabolism in severe chronic congestive heart failure: Effects of long-term dietary supplementation. *European Heart Journal, 15*, 1641–1650.

Carr, J. G., Stevenson, L. W., Walden, J. A., & Heber, D. (1989). Prevalence and hemodynamic correlates of malnutrition in severe congestive heart failure secondary to ischemic or idiopathic dilated cardiomyopathy. *American Journal of Cardiology, 63*, 709–713.

Clark, A. L., Sparrow, J. L., & Coates, A. J. S. (1995). Muscle fatigue and dyspnea in chronic heart failure: Two sides of the same coin? *European Heart Journal, 16*, 49–52.

Diaz-Velez, C. R., Garcia-Castineiras, S., Mendoza-Ramos, E., & Hernandez Lopez, E. (1996). Increased malondialdehyde in peripheral blood of patients with congestive heart failure. *American Heart Journal, 131*, 146–152.

Douglas, S., Darling, P.B., Barr, A., Kurian, R., Sole, M., & Keith, M. (2003). Prevalence of thiamin deficiency in hospitalized patients with congestive heart failure. *Canadian Journal of Cardiology, 19* (Suppl. A), 193A.

Engel, A. G. (1986). Carnitine deficiency syndromes and lipid storage myopathies. In A. G. Engel & B. Q. Banker (Eds.) *Myology, basic and clinical.* (pp. 1663–1696). Toronto: McGraw-Hill.

Folkers, K., Langsjoen, P., Willis, R., Richardson, P., Xia, L. J., Ye, C. Q., & Tamagama, H. (1990). Lovastatin decreases coenzyme Q levels in humans. *Proceedings of the National Academy of Sciences USA, 87*, 8931–8934.

Folkers, K., Vadhanavikit, S., & Mortensen, S. A. (1985). Biochemical rationale and myocardial tissue data on the effective therapy of cardiomyopathy with coenzyme Q10. *Proceedings of the National Academy of Sciences USA, 82*, 4240–4244.

Freeman, L., & Roubenoff, R. (1994). The nutrition implications of cardiac cachexia. *Nutrition Reviews, 52*, 340–347.

Ganapathy, V., & Leibach, F. H. (1994). Expression and regulation of the taurine transporter in cultured cell lines of human origin. In R. Huxtable & D.V. Michalk (Eds.), *Taurine in health and disease. Advances in experimental medical biology* (Vol. 359, pp. 51–57). New York: Plenum.

Geranmaygan, A., Keith, M., Sole, M. J., Kurian, R., Robinson, A., Omran, A. S., & Jeejeebhoy, K. N. (1998). Increased oxidative stress in patients with congestive heart failure. *Journal of the American College of Cardiology, 31*, 1352–1356.

Gordon, A., Hultman, E., & Kaijser, L. (1995). Creatine supplementation in chronic heart failure increases skeletal muscle creatine phosphate and muscle performance. *Cardiovascular Research, 30*, 413–418.

Grimble, R. F., Jackson, A. A., Persaud, C., Wride, M. J., Delers, F., & Engler, R. (1992). Cysteine and glycine supplementation modulate the metabolic response to tumor necrosis factor alpha in rats fed a low protein diet. *Journal of Nutrition, 122*, 2066–2073.

Guarnieri, C., Muscari, C., Manfroni, S., Caldarera, I., Stefanelli, C., & Pretolani, E. (1987). The effect of treatment with coenzyme Q10 on the mitochondrial function and superoxide radical formation in cardiac muscle hypertrophied by mild aortic stenosis. *Journal of Molecular and Cellular Cardiology, 19*, 63–71.

Harper, C. G., Giles, M., & Finlay-Jones, R. (1986). Clinical signs in the Wernicke-Korsakoff complex: A retrospective analysis of 131 cases diagnosed at necropsy. *Journal of Neurological Neurosurgical Psychiatry, 49*, 341–345.

Hofman-Bang, C., Rehnqvist, N., Swedberg, K., Wiklund, I., & Astrom, H., for the Q10 Study Group. (1995). Coenzyme Q10 as an adjunctive in the treatment of chronic congestive heart failure. *Journal of Cardiac Failure, 1*, 101–107.

Huxtable, R.J., Chubb, J., & Azari J. (1980). Physiological and experimental regulation of taurine content in the heart. *Federation Proceedings, 39*, 2685–2690.

Iliceto, S., Scrutinio, D., Bruzzi, P., D'Ambrosio, G., Boni, L., Di Biase, M., Biasco, G., Hugenholtz, P. G., & Rizzon, P. J. (1995). Effects of L-carnitine administration on left ventricular remodeling after acute anterior myocardial infarction: The L-Carnitine Ecocardiografia Digitalizzata Infarto Miocardico (CEDIM) Trial. *Journal of the American College of Cardiology, 26*, 380–387.

Jeejeebhoy, F., Keith, M., Freeman, M., Barr, A., McCall, M., Kurian, R., Mazer, D., & Errett, L. (2002). Nutritional supplementation with MyoVive repletes essential cardiac myocyte nutrients and reduces left ventricular size in patients with left ventricular dysfunction. *American Heart Journal, 143*, 1092–1100.

Katz, A. M. (1989). The myocardium in congestive heart failure. *American Journal of Cardiology, 63*, 12A–16A.

Keith, M. E., Ball, A., Jeejeebhoy, K. N., Kurian, R., Butany, J., Dawood, F., Wen, W. H., Madapallimattam, A., & Sole, M. J. (2001) Conditioned nutritional deficiencies in the cardiomyopathic hamster heart. *Canadian Journal of Cardiology, 17*, 449–458.

Keith, M. E., Jeejeebhoy, K. N., Langer, A., Kurian, R., Barr, A., O'Kelly, B., & Sole, M. J. (2001). A controlled clinical trial of vitamin E supplementation in patients with congestive heart failure. *American Journal of Clinical Nutrition, 73*, 219–224.

Lake, N. (1994). Alterations of ventricular contractility and myofibrillar loss in taurine deficient hearts In R. Huxtable & D.V. Michalk (Eds.), *Taurine in health and disease. Advances in experimental medical biology* (Vol. 359, pp. 335–342). New York: Plenum.

Langsjoen, P. H., Vadhanavikit, S., & Folkers, K. (1985). Response of patients in classes III and IV of cardiomyopathy to therapy in a blind and crossover trial with coenzyme Q10. *Proceedings of the National Academy of Sciences USA, 82*, 4240–4244.

Li, R. K., Sole, M. J., Mickle, D. A. G., Schimmer, J., & Goldstein, D. (1997). Vitamin E and oxidative stress in the heart of the cardiomyopathic Syrian hamster. *Free Radicals in Biology and Medicine, 24*, 252–258.

Littaru, G. P. (1995). *Energy and defence: Facts and perspectives on coenzyme Q10 in biology and medicine.* Rome: Casa Editrice Scientifica Internazionale.

Momomura, S., Serizawa, T., Ohtani, Y., Izuka, M., & Sugimoto, T. (1991). Coenzyme Q10 attenuates the progression of cardiomyopathy in hamsters. *Japanese Heart Journal, 32*, 101–110.

Nascimben, L., Ingwall, J. S., Pauletto, P., Freidrich, J., Gwathmey, J. K., Saks, V., Pessina, A. C., & Allen, P. D. (1996). Creatine kinase system in failing and nonfailing human myocardium. *Circulation, 94*, 1894–1901.

Neubauer, S., Horn, M., Cramer, M., Harre, K., Newell, J. B., Peters, W., Pabst, T., Ertl, G., Hahn, D., Ingwall, J. S., & Kochsiek, K. (1997). In patients with cardomyopathy the myocardial phosphocreatine/ ATP ratio predicts mortality better than ejection fraction or NYHA class. *Circulation, 96*, 2190–2196.

Ogasawara, M., Nakamura, T., Koyama, I., Nemoto, M., & Yoshida, T. (1994). Reactivity of taurine with aldehydes and its physiological role. In R. Huxtable & D.V. Michalk (Eds.), *Taurine in health and disease. Advances in experimental medical biology.* (Vol. 359, pp. 71–78). New York: Plenum.

Oudit, G. Y., Trivieri, M. G., Khaper, N., Husain, T., Wilson, G. J., Liu, P., Sole, M. J., & Backx, P. H. (2004). Taurine supplementation reduces oxidative stress and improves cardiovascular function in an iron-overload murine model. *Circulation, 109*, 1877–1885.

Pepine, C. J. (1991). The therapeutic potential of carnitine in cardiovascular disorders. *Clinical Therapeutics, 13*, 2–18.

Pfitzenmeyer, P., Guilland, J. C., d'Athis, Ph., Petit-Marnier, C., & Gaudet, M. (1994). Thiamine status of elderly patients with cardiac failure including the effects of supplementation. *International Journal of Vitamin and Nutrition Research, 64*, 113–118.

Pion, P. D., Kittleson, M. D,, Rogers, Q.R., & Morris, J. G. (1987). Myocardial failure in cats associated with low plasma taurine: A reversible cardiomyopathy. *Science, 237*, 764–768.

Schaffer, S. W., Allo, S., Harada, H., Mozaffari, M. (1987). Potentation of myocardial ischemic injury by drug-induced taurine depletion. In R. J. Huxtable, F. Franconi, & A. Giotti (Eds.), *The biology of taurine* (pp. 15–158). New York: Plenum.

Schonekess, B. O., Allard, M. F., & Lopaschuk, G. D. (1995). Proprionyl L-carnitine improvement of hypertrophied heart function is accompanied by an increase in carbohydrate oxidation. *Circulation Research, 77*, 726–734.

Seligmann, H., Halkin, H., Rauchfleisch, S., Kaufman, N., Motro, M., Vered, Z., & Ezra, D. (1991). Thiamine deficiency in patients with congestive failure receiving long-term furosemide therapy: A pilot study. *American Journal of Medicine, 91*, 151–155.

Shimon, I., Almong, S., Vered, Z., Seligmann, H., Shefi, M., Peleg, E., Rosenthal, T., Motro, M., Halkin, H., & Ezra, D. (1995). Improved left ventricular function after thiamine supplementation in patients with congestive heart failure receiving long-term furosemide therapy. *American Journal of Medicine, 98*, 485–490.

Singh, N., Dhalla, A.K., & Singal, P.K.(1995). Oxidative stress and heart failure. *Molecular and Cellular Biochemistry,147*, 77–81.

Soja, A. M., & Mortenson, S. A. (1997). Treatment of congestive heart failure with coenzyme Q10 illuminated by meta-analysis of clinical trials. *Molecular Aspects of Medicine, 18* (Suppl.), S159–168.

Sole, M. J. (1995). Shifting the paradigm for the treatment of dilated cardiomyopathy. *European Heart Journal, 16* (Suppl. O), 176-179.

Sole, M. J., & Jeejeebhoy, K. N. (2002). Conditioned nutritional requirements: Therapeutic relevance to heart failure. *Herz, 27*, 174–179.

Sturman, J. A. (1993). Taurine in development. *Physiological Reviews, 73*, 119–147.

Takihara, K., Azuma, J., & Awata, N. (1986). Beneficial effect of taurine in rabbits with chronic congestive heart failure. *American Heart Journal, 112*, 1278–1284.

Villalba, J. M., Navarro, F., Cordoba, F., Serrano, A., Arroyo, A., Crane, F. L., & Navas, P. (1995). Coenzyme Q reductase from liver plasma membrane: Purification and role in trans-plasma-membrane electron transport. *Proceedings of the National Academy of Sciences U S A, 92*, 4887–4891.

Vogt, A. M., & Kubler, W. (1998). Heart failure: Is there an energy deficit contributing to contractile dysfunction? *Basic Research in Cardiology, 93*, 1-10.

Witte, K. K. A,, Clark, A. L., & Cleland, J. G. F. (2001). Chronic heart failure and micronutrients. *Journal of the American College of Cardiology, 37*, 1765–1774.

Wyss, M., & Walliman, T. (1994). 1-4 Creatine metabolism and the consequences of creatine depletion in muscle. *Molecular and Cellular Biochemistry, 133/134*, 51–66.

Zeisel, S.H. (2000). Is there a metabolic basis for dietary supplementation? *American Journal of Clinical Nutrition, 72* (Suppl.), 507s–511s.

23 Polyunsaturated Fatty Acids and Neuro-Inflammation

Sophie Layé and Robert Dantzer

KEY POINTS

- Pro-inflammatory cytokines are expressed in the brain during peripheral inflammatory events and the aging process by microglial cells
- The functional consequences of brain cytokine action (neuro-inflammation) are alterations in cognition, affect, and behavior or neurotoxicity. Therefore, pro-inflammatory cytokines play a key role in depression and neurodegenerative diseases linked to aging.
- Prostaglandins mediate the actions of pro-inflammatory cytokines in the brain as well as pro-inflammatory cytokine production.
- Polyunsaturated fatty acids from the diet regulate both prostaglandin and pro-inflammatory cytokine production in the immune system. *n*-3 fatty acids are highly anti-inflammatory, while *n*-6 fatty acids are precursors of prostaglandins.
- Inappropriate amounts of dietary *n*-6 and *n*-3 fatty acids could lead to neuro-inflammation because of their abundance in the brain. Depending on which polyunsaturated fatty acids are present in the diet, neuro-inflammation will be kept at a minimum or exacerbated. This could explain the protective role of *n*-3 fatty acids in neurodegenerative diseases linked to aging.

1. INTRODUCTION

Inflammation is an active defense reaction against diverse insults that aims at neutralizing noxious agents. Although inflammation serves a protective function in controlling infection and promoting tissue repair, it can also cause tissue damage. Inflammatory mediators include complement, adhesion molecules, products of cyclooxygenase (COX) enzymes, eicosanoids, and cytokines. Cytokines are polypeptides that are generally associated with inflammation, immune activation, and cell differentiation or death. They include interleukins (ILs), interferons (IFNs), tumor necrosis factors (TNFs), chemokines, and growth factors. Although most have little or no function in healthy tissues, they are rapidly induced locally in response to tissue injury, infection, or inflammation.

Inflammatory mediators including cytokines are expressed not only at the site of injury but also in distant organs, including the brain, where they coordinate the central component of the acute-phase reaction. This brain-mediated response involves profound meta-

From: *Nutrients, Stress, and Medical Disorders*
Edited by: S. Yehuda and D. I. Mostofsky © Humana Press Inc., Totowa, NJ

bolic alterations in the form of an increased setpoint for thermoregulation resulting in fever and drastic behavioral changes commonly labeled as sickness behavior (anorexia, decreased locomotor activity, withdrawal from social contacts, etc.). Brain expression of cytokines also plays a key role in the pathophysiology of immune (e.g., multiple sclerosis) and nonimmune (e.g., brain injury, stroke, Alzheimer's disease) neurological disorders. The expression and action of pro-inflammatory cytokines in the brain is a rapidly growing area of experimental and clinical research. Because of the number of cytokines and the diversity of their actions, this chapter will focus primarily on the cytokine that has been studied most extensively in the brain—IL-1.

In the brain, inflammatory mediators are mainly produced by endothelial cells and glial cells, including astrocytes and microglia. The expression of pro-inflammatory cytokines in the brain is increased in response to various conditions, such as infection, lesions, trauma, and oxidative stress. Neuro-inflammation, the inflammatory response in the brain, has many cellular and biochemical features that make it different from the peripheral inflammatory response (Combrinck, Perry, & Cunningham, 2002; Neuhaus, Archelos, & Hartung, 2003; Perry, Bell, Brown, & Matyszak, 1995; Rothwell & Luheshi, 2000).

Functional consequences of neuro-inflammation include alterations in cognition, affect, and behavior, and they usually take place in the absence of neurotoxicity (Dantzer, 2001; Konsman, Parnet, & Dantzer, 2002). The behavioral repertoire of humans and animals is well known to change dramatically during the course of an infection. Ill individuals have little motivation to eat, are listless, complain of fatigue and malaise, lose interest in social activities, and have significant changes in sleep patterns (Dantzer, 2001; Kent, Bluthe, Kelley, & Dantzer, 1992). They feel sick and in pain, display an inability to experience pleasure, and experience difficulties in attention, concentration, and memory (Reichenberg et al., 2001). These functional alterations can be reproduced in naïve individuals by peripheral or central injection of pro-inflammatory cytokines (Kent, Bluthe, & Dantzer, 1992). When neuro-inflammation is exacerbated or prolonged, it can lead to neuronal cell death and neurodegeneration as a consequence of the deprivation of neurons from their growth factors (Rothwell & Luheshi, 2000; Venters, Dantzer, & Kelley, 2000) or the overproduction of reactive oxygen species (Mattson, 1994). As far as neurodegeneration is concerned, it is unclear if this condition is propagated through inflammation or whether, in contrast, the inflammatory response reflects an attempt to protect against further cellular injury.

There are multiple aspects of neuro-inflammation, all occurring simultaneously. Following exposure to noxious stimuli, components of neuro-inflammation include activation of microglia release of cytokines and induction of tissue repair enzymes, all of which limit cellular damage and promote repair. At the behavioral level, cytokine-induced sickness behavior is nothing more than the outward manifestation of a central motivational state that helps the body to fight infection and promote recovery (Dantzer, 2001). The extent of neuro-inflammation is normally regulated by a variety of opposing processes involving anti-inflammatory cytokines such as IL-10, growth factors such as insulin-like growth factor (IGF)-1, hormones such as glucocorticoids, and neuropeptides such as vasopressin and α-melanotropin (Allan, 2000; Lipton, Zhao, Ichiyama, Barsh, & Catania, 1999; Strle et al., 2001).

Micronutriments in the diet in the form of antioxidants and polyunsaturated fatty acids (PUFAs) are also able to regulate neuro-inflammation. PUFAs are incorporated into cell membranes. The composition of cell membranes determines the type of inflammatory mediators that will be produced during the inflammatory response. It is generally admitted that humans evolved on a diet with a *n*-6:*n*-3 PUFA ratio of approx 1, whereas today this ratio is closer to 10–20, indicating that Western diets are usually deficient in *n*-3 fatty acids (Raper, Cronin, & Exler, 1992; Simopoulos, 2001, 2003). The relative excess of *n*-6 fatty acids stimulates the formation of arachidonic acid (ARA), the fatty acid precursor of prostaglandins (PGs) and other eicosanoids involved in inflammation, which accounts for their importance in chronic inflammatory disease (Okuyama, Kobayashi, & Watanabe, 1996). Eicosanoids derived from eicosapentaenoic acid (EPA) are less physiologically potent than mediators synthesized from ARA (Calder, 2003). Moreover, *n*-3 fatty acids such as docosahexaenoic acid (DHA) display anti-inflammatory effects and inhibit the production of pro-inflammatory cytokines independent of the production of eicosanoids (Calder & Grimble, 2002). Since feeding animals or human subjects with regimens enriched with DHA and EPA results in a decrease in ARA in glial cell membranes, less substrate will be available for the synthesis of eicosanoids from ARA (Anderson & Connor, 1994; Champeil-Potokar et al., 2004; Rosenberger et al., 2004). Because *n*-3 fatty acids are highly anti-inflammatory and are preferentially incorporated in the brain, inappropriate amounts of dietary *n*-6 and *n*-3 fatty acids could lead to neuro-inflammation. Depending on which PUFAs are present in the diet, neuro-inflammation will therefore be kept at a minimum or exacerbated. This chapter will review the mechanisms of neuro-inflammation, its functional consequences, and its modulation by PUFAs.

2. NEURO-INFLAMMATION

For a long time the brain was considered to be a privileged organ from an immunological point of view because of its inability to mount an immune response and process antigens (Rivest, 2001). Although this is partly true, the central nervous system (CNS) shows a well-organized innate immune reaction in response to systemic bacterial infection and cerebral injury. The hallmark of brain inflammation is the activation of glia, particularly microglia (Nguyen, 2002). Microglial cells are sensor cells in the CNS that respond to injury and brain disease (Guillemin & Brew, 2004; Kreutzberg, 1996). These cells are able to scavenge invading microorganisms and dead cells and to act as immune or immunoeffector cells (Kloss, Bohatschek, Kreutzberg, & Raivich, 2001). In physiological conditions, the brain contains resting microglia, perivascular macrophages, and pericytes, as well as a few patrolling lymphocytes. The origin of pericytes, perivascular macrophages, and microglia found in the adult brain is probably systemic monocytes that infiltrate the CNS during embryogenesis (Guillemin & Brew, 2004; Theele & Streit, 1993). In pathological conditions, all these cells become activated and are strongly involved in the local inflammatory response. In particular, resting microglia become activated and change phenotype to amoeboid microglia capable of phagocytosis. This is accompanied by the production of pro-inflammatory cytokines, in particular IL-1, nitric oxide, superoxide anions, and eicosanoids (Kloss et al., 2001; Nakamura, 2002; Streit, Walter, & Pennell, 1999).

Cell wall components of Gram-negative or Gram-positive bacteria (lipopolysaccharide [LPS] and peptidoglycan, respectively) function as pathogen-associated molecular patterns (PAMPs) that are recognized by specific membrane receptors on innate immune cells (Akira, Takeda, & Kaisho, 2001). LPS and peptidoglycan bind to Toll-like receptors

(TLRs) (Akira et al., 2001; O'Neill, Fitzgerald, & Bowie, 2003). Although TLR2 recognizes PAMPs produced by Gram-positive bacterial cell wall components, TLR4 is critical for the recognition of LPS (Muzio & Mantovani, 2000; Poltorak et al., 1998; Schwandner, Dziarski, Wesche, Rothe, & Kirschning, 1999). Flagellin, the principal element of bacterial flagella, is recognized by TLR5, and TLR9 is required for the inflammatory response triggered by bacterial DNA (Hayashi et al., 2001; Hemmi et al., 2000). TLR3 induces an innate immune response to double-stranded RNA (dsRNA) viruses (Alexopoulou, Holt, Medzhitov, & Flavell, 2001). Microglia are the main cellular component of the innate immune system in the brain (Akira et al., 2001; Nguyen et al., 2002). The peripheral administration of LPS activates systemic innate immune cells, which results in the production and extracellular release of pro-inflammatory cytokines (Konsman, Kelley, & Dantzer, 1999; Laflamme & Rivest, 2001; Quan, Zhang, Emery, Bonsall, & Weiss, 1994). Once present in the bloodstream, these cytokines are believed to mediate most of the effects of systemically injected LPS, although circulating levels of cytokines are not necessarily detectable prior to the occurrence of the early physiological responses induced by the endotoxin (Kluger, 1991). The best example is fever that takes place within minutes in response to a systemic injection of LPS, even though cytokines are not yet detectable in the bloodstream (Kluger, 1991). Because of this temporal constraint, LPS has been proposed to be a direct ligand in the brain (Laflamme and Rivest, 2001). In accordance with this hypothesis, cytokine gene expression in response to a peripheral LPS challenge is first detected in the circumventricular organs (CVOs) that are devoid of a blood–brain barrier (BBB), leptomeninges, and choroid plexus (ChP) (Konsman et al., 1999; Laflamme & Rivest, 2001; Quan et al., 1994). The demonstration that CD14 and TLR4 receptors are constitutively expressed in the CVOs reinforces this idea (Laflamme & Rivest, 1999, 2001; Nguyen et al., 2002). Circulating LPS also causes a rapid increase in CD14 in these brain regions, and a delayed response takes place in cells located at the boundaries of the CVOs and in microglia across the brain parenchyma (Laflamme, Echchannaoui, Landmann, & Rivest, 2003). A similar expression pattern was recently found for the gene that encodes TLR2 in the brains of mice after a single systemic injection of LPS (Laflamme, Soucy, & Rivest, 2001). The signal was first detected in regions devoid of BBB, and a second wave was detected in parenchymal microglial cells (Laflamme et al., 2003).

Interestingly, TLRs and IL-1 receptors share a cytoplasmic motif, the Toll/IL-1 receptor (TIR) domain, which is required for initiating intracellular signaling (O'Neill, 2002). The TIR family of receptors uses very similar signaling mechanisms to activate downstream effector mechanisms (Fig. 1). Although some components of the downstream signaling machinery such as the adapter TNF-receptor-associated factor 6 (TRAF6) are shared by other receptors of pro-inflammatory cytokines, one signaling module is exclusively employed by the TIR family. This consists of MyD88, IL-1 receptor (IL-1R) associated kinase (IRAK) family members, and Tollip (Wesche, Henzel, Shillinglaw, Li, & Cao, 1997; Xu et al., 2000). TRAF6 directly facilitates full activation of the nuclear factor-κB (NF-κB) pathway and the mitogen-activated protein kinase (MAPK) signaling cascades (Chang & Karin, 2001; Wang et al., 2001). In unstimulated cells, NF-κB family proteins exist as heterodimers or homodimers that are sequestered in the cytoplasm by virtue of their association with a member of the inhibitor-κB (I-κB) family of inhibitory proteins (Karin & Ben-Neriah, 2000) (Fig. 1). These interactions mask the nuclear local-

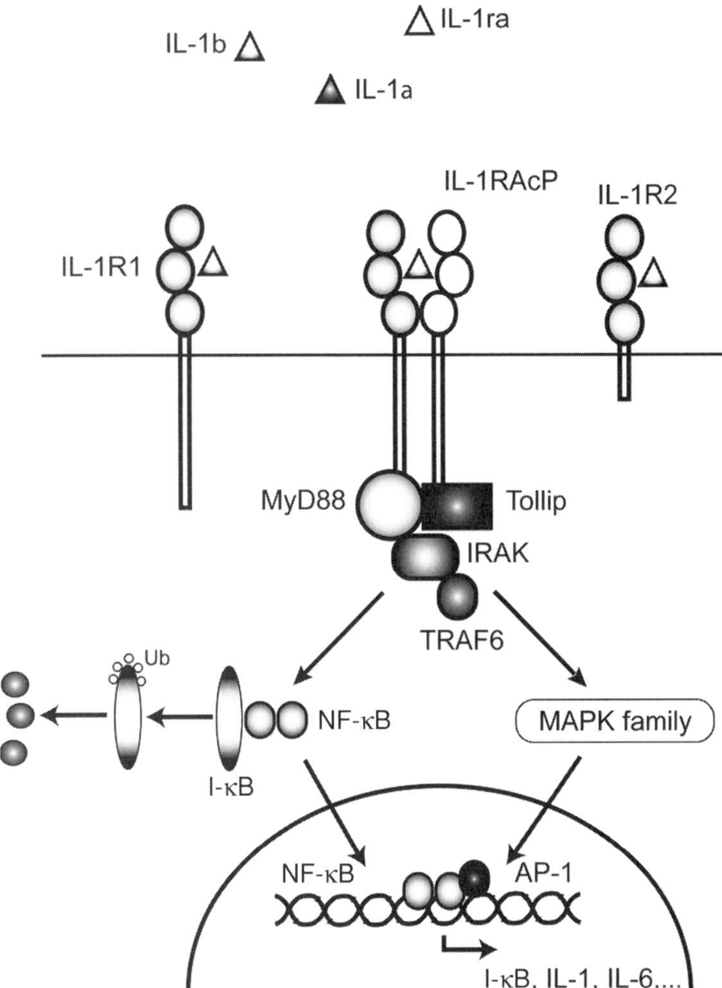

Fig. 1. Signaling pathways activated by the IL-1 family and receptor complex. The IL-1 family is composed of two agonists, IL-1α and IL-1β, and a natural antagonist, IL-1ra. IL-1 agonists bind to the type 1 IL-1 receptor (IL-1R1) and then interact with IL-1 receptor accessory protein (IL-1RAcP). They form a functional heterodimeric complex that activates dowstream signaling pathways involving NF-κB and the MAPK family. This activation requires the formation of a complex between IRAK (IL-1-receptor associated kinase), MyD88, and Tollip. This complex activates TNF-receptor-associated factor 6 (TRAF6), leading to the phosphorylation and degradation of the NF-kB inhibitor, I-κB, and the activation of the MAPK family.

ization sequence of NF-κB and interfere with sequences important for DNA binding (Huang, Huxford, Chen, & Ghosh, 1997). The destruction of I-κB unmasks the nuclear localization signal of NF-κB, leading to its nuclear translocation and binding to the promoters of target genes (Karin & Ben-Neriah, 2000). The detection of I-κB induction reveals the extent and cellular location of brain-derived immune molecules in response to peripheral immune challenges. I-κBα mRNA is induced in brain after peripheral LPS injection, beginning in cells lining the blood side of the BBB and progressing to cells inside the brain parenchyma (Laflamme & Rivest, 1999; Quan, Whiteside, Kim, & Herkenham, 1997). The same results were obtained after a peripheral injection of IL-1 and TNF-α, but not IL-6 (Laflamme & Rivest, 1999). This spatiotemporal pattern indicates that under the effect of LPS, cells of the BBB synthesize immune signal molecules to activate cells inside the CNS. The cerebrospinal fluid appears to be a conduit for these signal molecules. Because LPS induces the expression of bioactive IL-1 in microglial cells, it is not clear whether the induction of I-κB expression in the brain is due to a direct LPS effect on brain cells or to LPS-induced IL-1 produced in the brain (Eriksson, Nobel, Winblad, & Schultzberg, 2000; Quan, Zhang, Emery, Bonsall, & Weiss, 1996). A recent study analyzed NF-κB translocation and I-κB expression in the brain of rats treated with IL-1 (Nadjar et al., 2003). In this study the expression of I-κB mRNA did not strictly parallel NF-κB nuclear translocation. This important finding indicates that peripheral IL-1 can reach the brain across the CVOs that lack a BBB and endothelial cells all over the brain and interact with its receptors to induce NF-κB translocation (Nadjar et al., 2003).

IL-1 is bioactive in the brain because there are IL-1Rs in the brain. Ligands of the IL-1Rs (two agonists, IL-1α and IL-1β, and the natural antagonist, IL-1ra) bind to a transmembrane receptor and to soluble forms of the receptor, which are characterized by extracellular immunoglobulin (Ig)-like domains. The prototypes of this family are the IL-1R type 1 (IL-1R1) (Sims et al., 1988) and an accessory protein that functions as a coreceptor molecule, the IL-1RAcP (Greenfeder et al., 1995). The receptor chains contain the ligand-binding site, whereas the coreceptor IL-1RAcP is unable to bind the cytokine alone (Greenfeder et al., 1995). Indeed, deletion of IL-1R1 or IL-1RAcP, administration of antibodies to IL-1R1 or inhibition of specific MAPKs or NF-κB abolishes most actions of IL-1 in vivo and in vitro (O'Neill, 2002). The type 2 IL-1R (IL-1R2) is a negative regulator of the IL-1 system and functions as a decoy receptor (Colotta, Dower, Sims, & Mantovani, 1994; McMahan et al., 1991). In the brain, IL-1R1 mRNA is diffusely spread across the rodent brain, with the highest level of binding in the granular layer of the dentate gyrus, the granule cell layer of the cerebellum, the hypothalamus, and the pyramidal cell layer of the hippocampus (Cunningham et al., 1991; Ericsson, Liu, Hart, & Sawchenko, 1995; Wong & Licinio, 1994). IL-1R1 is expressed in cells of the choroid plexus and endothelial cells of brain capillaries (Konsman, Vigues, Mackerlova, Bristow, & Blomqvist, 2004; Nadjar et al., 2003). Neuronal expression appears mostly in the hippocampus (French et al., 1999). IL-1RacP mRNA is highly expressed throughout the rat brain (Ilyin, Gayle, Flynn, & Plata-Salaman, 1998; Liu, Chalmers, Maki, & De Souza, 1996). However, the presence of IL-1RAcP in brain areas that lack type 1 IL-1 receptors indicates additional functions for this protein that are still obscure. Interestingly, no NF-κB activation is observed in the brain of IL-1R1 and IL-1RAcP knockout (KO) mice treated with IL-1 (Nadjar et al., 2003). The same effect is observed in mixed glial cells in vitro, indicating that IL-1R1 is essential for IL-1β signaling in the brain (Pinteaux, 2002). The MAPK p38, c-Jun N-terminal kinase (JNK), and the extracellular signal-regulated protein kinase (ERK1/2) are also activated in glial cells from wild-type mice but not from IL-1R1 KO mice (Pinteaux et al., 2002). Selective inhibition of p38 or ERK1/2 MAPKs significantly reduced IL-1β-induced IL-6 release. Whether this pathway is involved in IL-1 signaling in the brain is still unknown. This is very important since brain-produced IL-1 is a key regulator of the synthesis of other pro-inflammatory cytokines such as IL-6 and TNF-α (Laye et al., 2000; Luheshi et al., 1996).

Prostanoids represent another key component of neuro-inflammation. Particularly, PG E_2 (PGE2) is highly synthesized in the brain during inflammation (Konsman et al., 2004; Quan, Whiteside, Herkenham, Bakhle, & Botting, 1998; Vane, 1998). COX is involved in the first two steps of the synthesis of PGE2 from its substrate ARA, an *n*-6 PUFA. There are two known COX isoenzymes (Vane et al., 1998): COX-1 is expressed constitutively in various tissues, whereas COX-2 has a low expression level in human tissues under normal conditions but can be induced by cytokines at sites of inflammation (Vane et al., 1998). Under peripheral treatment by LPS or IL-1, COX-2 expression is induced in endothelial cells of the brain vasculature and perivascular microglial cells (Cao, Matsumura, Yamagata, & Watanabe, 1996; Ericsson, Arias, & Sawchenko, 1997; Konsman et al., 2004; Lacroix & Rivest, 1998; Schiltz & Sawchenko, 2002). PGE2 mediates many central actions of IL-1, including fever. However, PGE2 can also act as an inhibitor of IL-1 and TNF-α production (Caggiano & Kraig, 1999; Petrova, Akama, & Van Eldik, 1999; Zhang & Rivest, 2001).

3. CONSEQUENCES OF NEURO-INFLAMMATION: FROM "SICKNESS BEHAVIOR" TO DEPRESSION

Pro-inflammatory cytokines act in the brain to induce nonspecific symptoms of infection, including fever and profound psychological and behavioral changes, termed "sickness behavior" (Kent, Bluthe, Kelley, et al., 1992). Sick individuals experience weakness, malaise, cognitive alterations and listlessness, hypersomnia, depressed activity, and loss of interest in social activities (Dantzer, 2001; Hart, 1988). Although these symptoms are usually regarded as the result of the debilitation process that occurs during infection, they are actually part of a natural homeostatic reaction that the body uses to fight infection (Hart, 1988). These changes in behavior have been shown to be the expression of a motivational state that resets the organism's priorities to promote resistance to pathogens and recovery from infection. By preventing the occurrence of activities that are metabolically expensive (e.g., foraging) and favoring expression of those that decrease heat loss (e.g., rest) and increase heat production (e.g., shivering), sickness behavior positively contributes to recovery following infection (Dantzer, 2001; Konsman et al., 2002). Sickness behavior is initiated by cytokines that are induced by infectious agents in the periphery and relayed by centrally produced cytokines (Laye et al., 2000). This role of centrally produced cytokines in sickness behavior was first discovered by comparison of dose-response curves in vivo. In general, centrally injected cytokines induce dramatic behavioral effects at doses that are 100–1000 times less than those needed when they are injected peripherally (Kent, Bluthe, Dantzer, et al., 1992). Moreover, the behavioral effects of peripherally injected IL-1 were strongly attenuated by central administration of the specific antagonist of IL-1Rs, IL-1ra, at a dose that was able to inhibit the effects of centrally injected IL-1 (Kent, Bluthe, Dantzer, et al., 1992). The use of neutralizing antibodies directed against specific IL-1R subtypes strengthen these data. A monoclonal neutralizing antibody specific to IL-1R1 injected into the lateral ventricle of the brain fully abrogated the behavioral effects of centrally and peripherally injected IL-1 (Cremona, Goujon, Kelley, Dantzer, & Parnet, 1998). The blockade of brain IL-1R1 using antisense strategies was found to abrogate the anorexic, but not the adipsic effects of centrally injected IL-1 (Sonti, Flynn, Plata-Salaman, 1997). In contrast, the blockade of brain IL-1R2 potentiated IL-1 effects on food intake but not on body temperature, indicating that some IL-1 actions in the brain are specifically regulated by this receptor (Cremona, Laye, Dantzer, & Parnet, 1998). The use of KO mice for IL-1R1 and IL-1RAcP reinforces the idea of a specific role for these receptors in mediating IL-1 effects on sickness behavior (Bluthe et al., 2000; Laye, Liege, Li, Moze, & Neveu, 2001; Liege, Laye, Li, Moze, & Neveu, 2000). However, while the cytotoxic effect of IL-1 in traumatic brain injury was blocked by centrally injected IL-1ra, no blockade was observed in IL-1R1 KO mice (Touzani et al., 2002). Furthermore, central injection of IL-1 exacerbated ischemic brain damage but had no effect on food intake in IL-1R1 KO mice (Touzani et al., 2002). These intriguing data indicate that IL-1 effects in the ischemic brain are independent of IL-1R1. In other words, IL-1R1 mediates the behavioral but not the cytotoxic effects of IL-1.

LPS-induced sickness behavior has been assessed in a strain of mice (C3H/HeJ) that is hyporesponsive to LPS. These mice have a mutation in TLR4, and it is this deficiency that leads to endotoxin hyporesponsiveness (Poltorak et al., 1998). The hyporesponsive C3H/HeJ mice are completely resistant to the sickness-inducing effects of LPS when injected intracerebroventricularly, but they remain fully responsive to central injections of IL-1 (Johnson, Gheusi, Segreti, Dantzer, & Kelley, 1997; Segreti, Gheusi, Dantzer, Kelley, & Johnson, 1997). These experiments show that CNS cells derived from C3H/HeJ endotoxin hyporesponders, such as microglia, share with peripheral macrophages the inability to respond to LPS and to synthesize pro-inflammatory cytokines, therefore impeding development of sickness behavior. From a practical perspective, these data show that the C3H/HeJ mouse strain is an excellent model that can be used to avoid any potential confounding effects of endotoxin contamination in preparations of recombinant cytokines injected in the CNS.

Like at the periphery, the lack of a cytokine in the brain cytokine network can result in compensation by other cytokines that are still present in the network. For instance, peripheral or central administration of LPS still induced sickness behavior in IL-1R1 KO and IL-1RacP KO mice (Bluthe et al., 2000; Laye et al., 2000, 2001; Liege et al., 2000) that did not respond any longer to IL-1. The sensitivity of IL-1R1 KO mice to LPS was a result of TNF-α replacing IL-1 since central administration of an antagonist of TNF-α blocked LPS action in IL-1R1 KO mice but not in wild-type mice (Bluthe et al., 2000).

The pyrogenic actions of LPS and pro-inflammatory cytokines are mediated by PGE2. PGE2 released in the preoptic area acts on preoptic neurons bearing E prostanoid (EP) receptors, alter their intrinsic firing rate, and evoke an elevation in the thermoregulatory setpoint (Kluger, Kozak, Leon, Soszynski, & Conn, 1995). There are four known cellular receptors for PGE2: EP1 through EP4 (Ushikubi et al., 1998). The particular receptor subtype involved in the induction of fever is unknown. Although mice lacking neuronal EP3 demonstrate an impaired febrile response to both exogenous (endotoxin) and endogenous pyrogens, studies in rats appear to implicate the EP4 receptor (Oka et al., 2000; Ushikubi et al., 1998). PGs are also involved in inflammation-induced anorexia. COX-2 inhibition during LPS-induced inflammation resulted in preserved food intake and maintenance of body weight, whereas COX-1 inhibition resulted in augmented and prolonged weight loss (Johnson, Vogt, Burney, & Muglia, 2002; Lugarini, Hrupka, Schwartz, Plata-Salaman, & Langhans, 2002). This effect could be mediated by PGE2 (Lugarini et al., 2002).

Evidence in favour of a role of cytokines in mediating mood disorders and cognitive disturbances that develop in patients receiving cytokine immunotherapy is growing fast

(Capuron and Dantzer, 2003). The same mechanisms appear to be at work for the wide variety of nonspecific sickness symptoms that develop in patients suffering from somatic diseases with an inflammatory component, inluding coronary heart disease, rheumatoid arthritis, asthma, cancer, stroke, and various neuropathologies (Cleeland et al., 2003; Eikelenboom et al., 2002; Gidron, Gilutz, Berger, & Huleihel, 2002; Kiecolt-Glaser & Glaser, 2002). Many patients complain of pain, fatigue, anorexia, sleep disturbances, and cognitive and mood disorders. These nonspecific neurovegetative and psychiatric symptoms are not necessarily the result of a chain of events linked to each other with a more or less direct cause (e.g., pain induces sleep disorders that impact on cognition and induce fatigue and lassitude, culminating in anorexia) (Cleeland et al., 2003). They could actually just represent another facet of the inflammatory process. These nonspecific symptoms are a major source of suffering for the patient, often more so than the diseased organ itself. Physicians, whatever their skills, are not always well equipped to deal with these important nonspecific symptoms that drastically affect the quality of life of sick patients. The challenge is not only to bring these symptoms to the forefront of the clinician's attention, but also to be able to treat them adequately (e.g., by molecules that target cytokine production and action in the CNS).

4. NEURO-INFLAMMATION IN THE AGING BRAIN

Microglial cell activation contributes to the onset and exacerbation of inflammation and neuronal degeneration in many brain diseases (Liu & Hong, 2003; Merrill & Benveniste, 1996). Nonetheless, microglial cells also act in a neuroprotective manner by eliminating excess excitotoxins in the extracellular space (Liu & Hong, 2003; Merrill & Benveniste, 1996). Moreover, there is accumulating evidence that microglia produce neurotrophic and/or neuroprotective molecules; in particular, it has been proposed that they promote neuronal survival in cases of brain injury. CNS inflammation occurs in myelin degenerative disorders such as multiple sclerosis (MS) (Martino et al., 2002) and in neurodegenerative disorders such as Alzheimer's disease (McGeer & Rogers, 1992), human immunodeficiency virus (HIV) encephalopathy (Gendelman et al., 1998), ischemia (Chopp et al., 1994), and traumatic brain injury (Dusart & Schwab, 1994). A general consequence of brain inflammation is reactive gliosis, typified by astrocyte hypertrophy and proliferation of astrocytes and microglia (Aschner, 1998; Kreutzberg, 1996). Changes in gap junction intercellular communication as reflected by alterations in dye coupling and connexin expression have been associated with numerous CNS inflammatory diseases, which may have dramatic implications in the survival of neuronal and glial populations in the context of neuro-inflammation (Kielian & Esen, 2004; Nakase et al., 2003).

IL-1 exerts a number of diverse actions in the brain, and it is currently well accepted that it contributes to experimentally induced neurodegeneration. In response to local brain injury or insult, like acute head trauma, IL-1 is overexpressed by microglia (Allan & Rothwell, 2001; Griffin et al., 1994; Hetier et al., 1988). Such acute overexpression of IL-1 has been implicated in the pathogenesis of some forms of acute brain injury (Allan and Rothwell, 2001). Moreover, patients with MS have elevated levels of IL-1 in the cerebrospinal fluid when their disease is active (Hauser, Doolittle, Lincoln, Brown, & Dinarello, 1990). Brain microglia may chronically overexpress IL-1 under repeated or persistent injurious stimuli or chronic neurological conditions (Down syndrome, HIV, epilepsy). Chronic overexpression of IL-1 is also observed in normal aging brain and in

Alzheimer's disease (Griffin et al., 1985; Katafuchi, Takaki, Take, Kondo, & Yoshimura, 2003). Recent microarray studies assessing gene expression of Alzheimer-related cytokines show selective overexpression of IL-1 in Alzheimer's disease (Loring, Wen, Lee, Seilhamer, & Somogyi, 2001). This increase is coupled with an increase in the expression of IL-1R1 and increased activity of IL-1R-associated MAPK (Hacham, Argov, White, Segal, & Apte, 2002; Lynch, 1998). There are genetic associations between IL-1 gene polymorphisms and Alzheimer's disease, chronic epilepsy, and Parkinson's disease (Kanemoto, Kawasaki, Miyamoto, Obayashi, & Nishimura, 2000; Mrak and Griffin, 2000; Nishimura et al., 2000).

IL-1 overexpression has been implicated in both the initiation and progression of neuropathological changes (Griffin et al., 1985). Brain from Tg2576 mice (a model for Alzheimer's disease) showed significant increases in IL-1 expression compared to controls. Moreover, aged Tg2576 mounted an exacerbated cytokine response to LPS that could have amplified the degenerative processes (Sly et al., 2001). IL-1 administration depressed food intake more in aged mice than in adults (Nelson, Marks, Heyen, & Johnsone, 1999). Attenuation of the fever response in old age could be owing to the lack of entry of peripheral IL-1 into the brain and not to a lack of brain IL-1R functionality (McLay, Kastin, & Zadina, 2000; Plata-Salaman et al., 1998). Age-induced IL-1 overproduction in the brain, and more particularly in the hippocampus, is associated with a decrease in synaptic plasticity, measured by long-term potentiation (LTP) in the dentate gyrus, which could explain cognitive impairment observed in the elderly (Lynch, 1998; Murray and Lynch, 1998). Receptors for IL-1 are distributed with a high density in the hippocampus, where IL-1 exerts inhibitory effects on release of calcium (Campbell, Segurado, & Lynch, 1998). There is also evidence for a role of endogenous brain IL-1 in the normal physiological regulation of hippocampal plasticity and learning processes (Coogan, O'Neill, & O'Connor, 1999; Schneider et al., 1998; Wolf et al., 2003; Yirmiya, Winocur, & Goshen, 2002). Low levels of IL-1 are essential for memory and plasticity, whereas higher levels of IL-1, such as those achieved during aging and neurodegeneration, can be detrimental.

Overexpression of IL-1 in Alzheimer brains is linked to an increase in microglia activity frequently associated with amyloid plaques (Griffin et al., 1989; Sheng, Griffin, Royston, & Mrak, 1998). This specific distribution suggests a role for IL-1 in the initiation and progression of neuritic and neuronal injury in Alzheimer's disease because of its appearance in early plaque formation and its absence in plaques that are devoid of injured neuritic elements (Griffin, Sheng, Roberts, & Mrak, 1995). No microglia have been observed in amyloid deposits in nondemented elderly (Griffin et al., 1998; Sheng, Mrak, & Griffin, 1998). IL-1 overexpression can also result in cholinergic neurotransmission impairment (Rada et al., 1991). The soluble form of amyloid protein (sAPP) released from neurons activates microglia and induces excessive microglial expression of IL-1 (Barger and Harmon, 1997). IL-1 increases the production and activity of the acetylcholine-degrading enzyme acetylcholinesterase, which results in a decrease in brain acetylcholine levels (Li et al., 2000). The increased levels of IL-1 in Alzheimer's disease could be due to increased production and activity of the IL-1β-converting enzyme (ICE), which converts pro-IL-1β to mature IL-1β and is specifically produced by microglia (Chauvet et al., 2001). ICE activity and expression are increased in Alzheimer's disease, and this increase is related to neuronal DNA damage as well as to compromised neuronal function (Zhu et al., 1999).

All these data point to a pathophysiolgical role of IL-1 overexpression in the aging brain. Epidemiological studies show that subjects who take anti-inflammatory agents or suffer from arthritis in general or rheumatoid arthritis in particular have a lower risk of developing Alzheimer's disease (Broe et al., 2000; McGeer and Rogers, 1992; Stewart, Kawas, Corrada, & Metter, 1997; Zandi et al., 2002). A role for neuro-inflammation in Alzheimer pathogenesis has received further support from epidemiological studies showing a protective effect of anti-inflammatory medications on the occurrence of Alzheimer's disease (Andersen et al., 1995; Breitner et al., 1994, 1995) and from the recent finding that oral administration of ibuprofen suppresses plaque pathology and IL-1 expression in a transgenic mouse model of Alzheimer's disease (Lim et al., 2000). However, anti-inflammatory agents are effective if used at an early stage of the disease (Van Gool, Aisen, & Eikelenboom, 2003). In addition, in order to make anti-inflammatory drugs effective, it is very important that they act on the right molecular targets. This is very well illustrated by the failures in clinical trials of prednisone, the COX-2 inhibitors celecoxib and nimesulide, and hydroxychloroquine (Aisen, 2000; Aisen, Schmeider, & Pasinetti, 2002). The fact that COX-2 inhibitors, known to be effective in treating arthritis, are poorly useful in neuro-inflammation linked to Alzheimer's disease could be owing to the overproduction of pro-inflammatory cytokines by activated microglia. Although PGE2 has frequently been considered as a possible inducer of brain damage and degeneration, it may exert beneficial effects in the CNS (Candelario-Jalil et al., 2003; Sasaki et al., 2004). Indeed, in spite of its classic role as a pro-inflammatory molecule, recent in vitro and in vivo observations indicate that PGE2 can inhibit microglial activation and release of pro-inflammatory cytokines (Caggiano and Kraig, 1999; Petrova et al., 1999; Zhang and Rivest, 2001). It has been shown that exogenous PGE2, through the activation of EP2 receptor, protects the brain against excitotoxic and anoxic injury (McCullough et al., 2004). Therefore, the exact role of PGE2 in brain damage needs to be clarified.

5. PUFAS AND NEURO-INFLAMMATION

The PUFA linoleic acid and its *n*-6 derivative ARA, and α-linolenic acid and its *n*-3 derivatives, EPA and DHA, play a key role in both energy production and cell structure and are indispensable for brain development (Neuringer, Anderson, & Connor, 1988). ARA and DHA are found in large concentrations in brain lipids. Nearly 6% of the dry weight of brain consists of *n*-3 PUFAs (Bourre et al., 1991). They are incorporated as phospholipids and are key components of brain cell membranes. They provide fluidity and the proper environment for active integral protein functions (Bourre et al., 1992; Spector, 1999; Yehuda, Rabinovitz, Carasso, & Mostofsky, 2002; Zerouga, Jenski, & Stillwell, 1995). Moreover, phospholipids have a role in cellular function because they are a reservoir of signaling messengers for neurotransmitters or growth factors. There are some data on PUFA contents of neurons and astrocytes, but nothing is known concerning microglial cells (Bourre et al., 1992; Champeil-Potokar et al., 2004). In culture, astrocytes elongate and desaturate precursors of the long-chain PUFAs, whereas neurons are unable to do so (Moore, 2001; Moore, Yoder, Murphy, Dutton, & Spector, 1991). Indeed, neurons cocultured with astrocytes accumulate DHA synthesized by glial cells in their membrane.

DHA and ARA have beneficial effects when available in moderation. As already mentioned, human beings originally consumed a diet rich in *n*-3 PUFAs and low in saturated fatty acids because wild and free-range food animals have much higher *n*-3 fatty acid levels than do present-day commercial livestock. An excess of *n*-6 precursors stimulates the formation of ARA. Although some ARA is essential, the current high ratio of *n*-6 to *n*-3 fatty acids may be responsible for the increase in chronic inflammatory diseases (Horrocks and Yeo, 1999a, 1999b). A high intake of *n*-3 PUFAs such as DHA or EPA may have anti-inflammatory effects in patients with neuro-inflammation. Conversely, high dietary intake of *n*-6 PUFAs, which lowers intake of *n*-3 PUFAs, may contribute to the development of neuro-inflammation. For example, ARA is the principal substrate for COX (O'Banion, 1999). Additional substrates include cannabinoids and lipoamino acids, which can also be oxidized to produce PG precursors, the pathophysiological of which role is not known (Chang, Lee, & Lin, 2001; Kozak, Prusakiewicz, Rowlinson, Schneider, & Marnett, 2001). PGs have the ability to play either a protective or an injurious role, depending on the context and quantity produced. Therefore, the membrane levels of their precursor, ARA, are important. Moreover, EPA contained in membrane phospholipids competes with ARA as a substrate for COX and lipooxygenase (LOX) (Calder, 2003). The consequences of such a competition are a decrease in the production of inflammatory metabolites such as PGE2, leukotriene A4 (LTA4), and thromboxane A2 (TXA2) and an increase in the synthesis of less inflammatory eicosanoids or even anti-inflammatory ones (Calder & Grimble, 2002; Zaloga and Marik, 2001). This has been demonstrated in many cells throughout the body, including glial cells (Petroni, Salami, Blasevich, Papini, & Galli, 1994). A 6-d LPS infusion in the brain increased phospholipase A_2 activities and brain concentrations of linoleic acid and ARA and of PGE2 and PGD2 (Rosenberger et al., 2004). Alteration in *n*-6 metabolism in the brain in response to LPS emphasizes again the link between *n*-3/*n*-6 brain composition and neuro-inflammation.

Numerous studies have revealed that *n*-3 PUFAs inhibit the in vitro production of pro-inflammatory cytokines by macrophages and their in vivo synthesis in healthy adults and those with autoimmune diseases (Calder, 1997, 2001; Meydani et al., 1991). However, little is known concerning microglial cell that produce pro-inflammatory cytokines in the brain. It has been shown that in the brain and in microglia, DHA is converted to potent anti-inflammatory products called 17-resolvins by aspirin-induced acetylated COX-2 (Serhan et al., 2000). Resolvins block production of cytokines by microglial cells (Serhan et al., 2000). Moreover, they protect from ischemia by blocking NF-κB activation and pro-inflammatory cytokine production (Marcheselli et al., 2003).

A short time *n*-3 supplemention attenuated the fever responses induced in rats by both ip and icv IL-1 without altering the thermogenic capacity of the organism (Cooper and Rothwell, 1993; Pomposelli, Mascioli, Bistrian, Lopes, & Blackburn, 1989). However, the group of Kluger reported that fever, lethargy, and anorexia were differentially regulated by a fish oil diet depending on the inflammatory stimulus used (Kozak, 1997). Turpentine is a model of local inflammation that induces a robust acute-phase response consisting of fever, anorexia, cachexia, and acute-phase protein production. Fish oil diet exacerbated LPS-induced lethargia and decreased temperature, whereas it blocked turpentine-induced fever, lethargia, and anorexia (Kozak et al., 1997). These changes were associated with a decrease in circulating LPS-induced PGE2 and an increase in LPS-induced TNF-α. Because TNF-α production is partially regulated by PGE2, fish oil could upregulate TNF-α production by decreasing PGE2 production (Kunkel et al., 1988). In mice, the early hypothermic phase of fever to a high dose of LPS was exacerbated by TNF-α treatment, whereas administration of the soluble TNF receptor, a blocker of TNF-α activity, attenuated hypothermia (Klir et al., 1995; Kozak, Conn, Klir, Wong, & Kluger, 1995). It is questionable, therefore, whether ingesting high amounts of n-3 PUFA during inflammatory events is beneficial. Further studies on the role of PUFA in neuro-inflammation are clearly needed.

Elderly people who eat fish or seafood rich in *n*-3 PUFAs at least once a week are at lower risk of developing dementia, including Alzheimer's disease (Barberger-Gateau et al., 2002; Kalmijn et al., 1997, 2004). Because aging is associated with a decrease in membrane PUFAs, including ARA, and an increase in brain IL-1 production, Lynch proposed that the increase in IL-1 seen in aging is linked to aging decreased membrane ARA (Lynch, 1998; Murray & Lynch, 1998). Therefore IL-1, by affecting membrane composition, would contribute to age-related impairments in neuronal function (Lynch, 1998; Murray, Clements, & Lynch, 1999; Murray & Lynch, 1998). IL-1 increased lipid peroxidation in hippocampal tissue from young but not old rats, and this effect was associated with decreased long-term potentiation (LTP) (Lynch, 1998; Murray et al., 1999; Murray and Lynch, 1998). A short-time supplementation of ARA in combination with another long-chain *n*-6 PUFA, γ-linolenic acid (GLA), reversed the age-related impairment in LTP (McGahon, Murray, Clements, & Lynch, 1998). EPA had a similar effect, and in this last case there was evidence that this effect was a consequence of its ability to block the effects of IL-1 (Martin et al., 2002), providing support for the hypothesis that EPA acts as an anti-inflammatory agent (Babcock, Helton, & Espat, 2000; Babcock, Helton, Hong, & Espat, 2002; McCarthy & Kenny, 1992). The anti-inflammatory effect of EPA could be owing to the blockade by EPA of the IL-1 signaling pathway MAPK, and more particularly p38, in the brain (Martin et al., 2002). The blockade of p38 activation by EPA or DHA has been reported in other cell types (Denys, Hichami, & Khan, 2001). Interestingly, LPS-induced p38 activation in the hippocampus is accompanied by an increased activation of NF-κB (Kelly et al., 2003), the pharmacological inhibition of which partially suppresses the inhibitory effects of LPS and IL-1 on LTP (Kelly et al., 2003; Nadjar et al., 2003). It has been reported in a human monocytic cell line that TNF-α expression was reduced by EPA through its inhibitory effect on NF-κB activation by preventing the phosphorylation of I-κBα (Zhao, Joshi-Barve, Barve, & Chen, 2004). In addition, *n*-3 PUFAs might protect the brain from the deleterious effects of IL-1. Irradiation induced increases in IL-1, IL-1R1, and IL-1RAcP concentrations in the hippocampus (Lynch et al., 2003). These changes were coupled with an increased activation of JNK and apoptotic cell death. Rats that had been fed a diet rich in EPA did not display any of these events (Lynch et al., 2003). The anti-inflammatory cytokine IL-10 could explain EPA anti-inflammatory and neuroprotective effects in the brain, because EPA increased IL-10 levels and IL-10 blocked the IL-1 effect (Bluthe et al., 1999; Lynch et al., 2003; Pousset, Cremona, Dantzer, Kelley, & Parnet, 1999). EPA-supplemented diet, but not ARA, significantly attenuated centrally injected IL-1-induced anxiety behavior (Song & Horrobin, 2004; Song, Li, Leonard, & Horrobin, 2003). This was accompanied by a decrease in IL-1-induced PGE2 and an increase in IL-10 (Song & Horrobin, 2004; Song et al., 2003).

6. CONCLUSION

There is growing evidence that the expression and action of pro-inflammatory cytokines in the brain are responsible not only for the development and maintenance of sickness behavior during the host response to infection, but also for the occurrence of nonspecific symptoms of sickness during chronic inflammatory disorders. In addition, neuroinflammation can have detrimental consequences on neuronal viability, especially when maintained over long periods of time and transiently amplified by peripheral infectious episodes (Holmes et al., 2003; Perry, Cunningham, & Boche, 2002; Perry, Newman, & Cunningham, 2003). All of this points to the interest in finding new ways of controlling inflammation in the brain. Because of their abundance in the brain and their modulatory role in inflammation and cell functions, PUFAs certainly have a role to play. However, this role needs to be better characterized by way of multidisciplinary studies aimed at assessing the effects of these molecules at different levels of functioning, from the molecular to the organism level.

REFERENCES

Aisen, P. S. (2000). Anti-inflammatory therapy for Alzheimer's disease: Implications of the prednisone trial. *Acta Neuropathologica Scandinavian (Suppl.), 176*, 85–89.

Aisen, P. S., Schmeidler, J., & Pasinetti, G. M. (2002). Randomized pilot study of nimesulide treatment in Alzheimer's disease. *Neurology, 58*(7), 1050–1054.

Akira, S., Takeda, K., & Kaisho, T. (2001). Toll-like receptors: Critical proteins linking innate and acquired immunity. *Nature Immunology, 2*(8), 675–680.

Alexopoulou, L., Holt, A. C., Medzhitov, R., & Flavell, R. A. (2001). Recognition of double-stranded RNA and activation of NF-kappaB by Toll-like receptor 3. *Nature, 413*(6857), 732–738.

Allan, S. M. (2000). The role of pro- and antiinflammatory cytokines in neurodegeneration. *Annual New York Academical Sciences, 917*, 84–93.

Allan, S. M., & Rothwell, N. J. (2001). Cytokines and acute neurodegeneration. *Nature Review Neurosciences, 2*(10), 734–744.

Andersen, K., Launer, L. J., Ott, A., Hoes, A. W., Breteler, M. M., & Hofman, A. (1995). Do nonsteroidal anti-inflammatory drugs decrease the risk for Alzheimer's disease? The Rotterdam Study. *Neurology, 45*(8), 1441–1445.

Anderson, G. J., & Connor, W. E. (1994). Accretion of n-3 fatty acids in the brain and retina of chicks fed a low-linolenic acid diet supplemented with docosahexaenoic acid. *American Journal of Clinical Nutrition, 59*(6), 1338–1346.

Aschner, M. (1998). Astrocytes as mediators of immune and inflammatory responses in the CNS. *Neurotoxicology, 19*(2), 269–281.

Babcock, T., Helton, W. S., & Espat, N. J. (2000). Eicosapentaenoic acid (EPA): An antiinflammatory omega-3 fat with potential clinical applications. *Nutrition, 16*(11–12), 1116–1118.

Babcock, T. A., Helton, W. S., Hong, D., & Espat, N. J. (2002). Omega-3 fatty acid lipid emulsion reduces LPS-stimulated macrophage TNF-alpha production. *Surgical Infection, 3*(2), 145–149.

Barberger-Gateau, P., Letenneur, L., Deschamps, V., Peres, K., Dartigues, J. F., & Renaud, S. (2002). Fish, meat, and risk of dementia: Cohort study. *British Medical Journal 325*(7370), 932–933.

Barger, S. W., & Harmon, A. D. (1997). Microglial activation by Alzheimer amyloid precursor protein and modulation by apolipoprotein E. *Nature 388*(6645), 878–881.

Bluthe, R. M., Castanon, N., Pousset, F., Bristow, A., Ball, C., Lestage, J., Michaud, B., Kelley, K. W., & Dantzer, R. (1999). Central injection of IL-10 antagonizes the behavioral effects of lipopolysaccharide in rats. *Psychoneuroendocrinology, 24*(3), 301–311.

Bluthe, R. M., Laye, S., Michaud, B., Combe, C., Dantzer, R., & Parnet, P. (2000). Role of interleukin-1beta and tumour necrosis factor-alpha in lipopolysaccharide-induced sickness behavior: A study with interleukin-1 type I receptor-deficient mice. *European Journal of Neurosciences, 12*(12), 4447–4456.

Bourre, J. M., Bonneil, M., Chaudiere, J., Clement, M., Dumont, O., Durand, G., Lafont, H., Nalbone, G., Pascal, G., & Piciotti, M. (1992). Structural and functional importance of dietary polyunsaturated fatty acids in the nervous system. *Advanced Experimental Medical Biology, 318*, 211–229.

Bourre, J. M., Dumont, O., Piciotti, M., Clement, M., Chaudiere, J., Bonneil, M., Nalbone, G., Lafont, H., Pascal, G., & Durand, G. (1991). Essentiality of omega 3 fatty acids for brain structure and function. *World Review in Nutritional Diet, 66*, 103–117.

Breitner, J. C., Gau, B. A., Welsh, K. A., Plassman, B. L., McDonald, W. M., Helms, M. J., & Anthony, J. C. (1994). Inverse association of anti-inflammatory treatments and Alzheimer's disease: Initial results of a co-twin control study. *Neurology, 44*(2), 227–232.

Breitner, J. C., Welsh, K. A., Helms, M. J., Gaskell, P. C., Gau, B. A., Roses, A. D., Pericak-Vance, M. A., & Saunders, A. M. (1995). Delayed onset of Alzheimer's disease with nonsteroidal anti-inflammatory and histamine H2 blocking drugs. *Neurobiology of Aging, 16*(4), 523–530.

Broe, G. A., Grayson, D. A., Creasey, H. M., Waite, L. M., Casey, B. J., Bennett, H. P., Brooks, W. S., & Halliday, G. M. (2000). Anti-inflammatory drugs protect against Alzheimer disease at low doses. *Archive of Neurology, 57*(11), 1586–1591.

Caggiano, A. O., & Kraig, R. P. (1999). Prostaglandin E receptor subtypes in cultured rat microglia and their role in reducing lipopolysaccharide-induced interleukin-1beta production. *Journal of Neurochemistry, 72*(2), 565–575.

Calder, P. C. (1997). n-3 polyunsaturated fatty acids and cytokine production in health and disease. *Annals of Nutritional Metabolism, 41*(4), 203–234.

Calder, P. C. (2001). Polyunsaturated fatty acids, inflammation, and immunity. *Lipids, 36*(9), 1007–1024.

Calder, P. C. (2003). N-3 polyunsaturated fatty acids and inflammation: From molecular biology to the clinic. *Lipids, 38*(4), 343–352.

Calder, P. C., & Grimble, R. F. (2002). Polyunsaturated fatty acids, inflammation and immunity. *European Journal of Clinican Nutrition, 56* (Suppl. 3), S14–19.

Campbell, V. A., Segurado, R., & Lynch, M. A. (1998). Regulation of intracellular Ca2[1] concentration by interleukin-1beta in rat cortical synaptosomes: An age-related study. *Neurobiology of Aging, 19*(6), 575–579.

Candelario-Jalil, E., Gonzalez-Falcon, A., Garcia-Cabrera, M., Alvarez, D., Al-Dalain, S., Martinez, G., Leon, O. S., & Springer, J. E. (2003). Assessment of the relative contribution of COX-1 and COX-2 isoforms to ischemia-induced oxidative damage and neurodegeneration following transient global cerebral ischemia. *Journal of Neurochemistry, 86*(3), 545–555.

Cao, C., Matsumura, K., Yamagata, K., & Watanabe, Y. (1996). Endothelial cells of the rat brain vasculature express cyclooxygenase-2 mRNA in response to systemic interleukin-1 beta: A possible site of prostaglandin synthesis responsible for fever. *Brain Research, 733*(2), 263–272.

Capuron, L., & Dantzer, R. (2003). Cytokines and depression: The need for a new paradigm. *Brain Behavior and Immunity, 17* (Suppl. 1), S119–124.

Champeil-Potokar, G., Denis, I., Goustard-Langelier, B., Alessandri, J. M., Guesnet, P., & Lavialle, M. (2004). Astrocytes in culture require docosahexaenoic acid to restore the n-3/n-6 polyunsaturated fatty acid balance in their membrane phospholipids. *Journal of Neuroscience Research, 75*(1), 96–106.

Chang, L., & Karin, M. (2001). Mammalian MAP kinase signaling cascades. *Nature 410*(6824), 37–40.

Chang, Y. H., Lee, S. T., & Lin, W. W. (2001). Effects of cannabinoids on LPS-stimulated inflammatory mediator release from macrophages: involvement of eicosanoids. *Journal of Cellular Biochemistry, 81*(4), 715–723.

Chauvet, N., Palin, K., Verrier, D., Poole, S., Dantzer, R., & Lestage, J. (2001). Rat microglial cells secrete predominantly the precursor of interleukin-1beta in response to lipopolysaccharide. *European Journal of Neurosciences, 14*(4), 609–617.

Chopp, M., Zhang, R. L., Chen, H., Li, Y., Jiang, N., & Rusche, J. R. (1994). Postischemic administration of an anti-Mac-1 antibody reduces ischemic cell damage after transient middle cerebral artery occlusion in rats. *Stroke, 25*(4), 869–875.

Cleeland, C. S., Bennett, G. J., Dantzer, R., Dougherty, P. M., Dunn, A. J., Meyers, C. A., Miller, A. H., Payne, R., Reuben, J. M., Wang, X. S., & Lee, B. N. (2003). Are the symptoms of cancer and cancer treatment due to a shared biologic mechanism? A cytokine-immunologic model of cancer symptoms. *Cancer, 97*(11), 2919–2925.

Colotta, F., Dower, S. K., Sims, J. E., & Mantovani, A. (1994). The type II 'decoy' receptor: A novel regulatory pathway for interleukin 1. *Immunology Today, 15*(12), 562–566.

Combrinck, M. I., Perry, V. H., & Cunningham, C. (2002). Peripheral infection evokes exaggerated sickness behavior in pre-clinical murine prion disease. *Neuroscience, 112*(1), 7–11.

Coogan, A. N., O'Neill, L. A., & O'Connor, J. J. (1999). The P38 mitogen-activated protein kinase inhibitor SB203580 antagonizes the inhibitory effects of interleukin-1beta on long-term potentiation in the rat dentate gyrus in vitro. *Neuroscience, 93*(1), 57–69.

Cooper, A. L., & Rothwell, N. J. (1993). Inhibition of the thermogenic and pyrogenic responses to interleukin-1 beta in the rat by dietary N-3 fatty acid supplementation. *Prostaglandins, Leukotrienes, and Essential Fatty Acids, 49*(2), 615–626.

Cremona, S., Goujon, E., Kelley, K. W., Dantzer, R., & Parnet, P. (1998). Brain type I but not type II IL-1 receptors mediate the effects of IL-1 beta on behavior in mice. *American Journal of Physiology, 274*(3 Pt. 2), R735-740.

Cremona, S., Laye, S., Dantzer, R., & Parnet, P. (1998). Blockade of brain type II interleukin-1 receptors potentiates IL1beta-induced anorexia in mice. *Neuroscience Letters, 246*(2), 101–104.

Cunningham, E. T., Jr., Wada, E., Carter, D. B., Tracey, D. E., Battey, J. F., & De Souza, E. B. (1991). Localization of interleukin-1 receptor messenger RNA in murine hippocampus. *Endocrinology, 128*(5), 2666–2668.

Dantzer, R. (2001). Cytokine-induced sickness behavior: Mechanisms and implications. *Annual New York Academical Sciences, 933*, 222–234.

Denys, A., Hichami, A., & Khan, N. A. (2001). Eicosapentaenoic acid and docosahexaenoic acid modulate MAP kinase (ERK1/ERK2) signaling in human T cells. *Journal of Lipid Research, 42*(12), 2015–2020.

Dusart, I., & Schwab, M. E. (1994). Secondary cell death and the inflammatory reaction after dorsal hemisection of the rat spinal cord. *European Journal of Neurosciences, 6*(5), 712–724.

Eikelenboom, P., Bate, C., Van Gool, W. A., Hoozemans, J. J., Rozemuller, J. M., Veerhuis, R., & Williams, A. (2002). Neuroinflammation in Alzheimer's disease and prion disease. *Glia, 40*(2), 232–239.

Ericsson, A., Arias, C., & Sawchenko, P. E. (1997). Evidence for an intramedullary prostaglandin-dependent mechanism in the activation of stress-related neuroendocrine circuitry by intravenous interleukin-1. *Journal of Neurosciences, 17*(18), 7166–7179.

Ericsson, A., Liu, C., Hart, R. P., & Sawchenko, P. E. (1995). Type 1 interleukin-1 receptor in the rat brain: Distribution, regulation, and relationship to sites of IL-1-induced cellular activation. *Journal of Comparative Neurology, 361*(4), 681–698.

Eriksson, C., Nobel, S., Winblad, B., & Schultzberg, M. (2000). Expression of interleukin 1 alpha and beta, and interleukin 1 receptor antagonist mRNA in the rat central nervous system after peripheral administration of lipopolysaccharides. *Cytokine, 12*(5), 423–431.

French, R. A., VanHoy, R. W., Chizzonite, R., Zachary, J. F., Dantzer, R., Parnet, P., Bluthe, R. M., & Kelley, K. W. (1999). Expression and localization of p80 and p68 interleukin-1 receptor proteins in the brain of adult mice. *Journal of Neuroimmunology, 93*(1–2), 194–202.

Gendelman, H. E., Zheng, J., Coulter, C. L., Ghorpade, A., Che, M., Thylin, M., Rubocki, R., Persidsky, Y., Hahn, F., Reinhard, J., Jr., & Swindells, S. (1998). Suppression of inflammatory neurotoxins by highly active antiretroviral therapy in human immunodeficiency virus-associated dementia. *Journal of Infectious Disease, 178*(4), 1000–1007.

Gidron, Y., Gilutz, H., Berger, R., & Huleihel, M. (2002). Molecular and cellular interface between behavior and acute coronary syndromes. *Cardiovascular Research, 56*(1), 15–21.

Greenfeder, S. A., Nunes, P., Kwee, L., Labow, M., Chizzonite, R. A., & Ju, G. (1995). Molecular cloning and characterization of a second subunit of the interleukin 1 receptor complex. *Journal of Biological Chemistry, 270*(23), 13,757–13,765.

Griffin, D. E., Moser, H. W., Mendoza, Q., Moench, T. R., O'Toole, S., & Moser, A. B. (1985). Identification of the inflammatory cells in the central nervous system of patients with adrenoleukodystrophy. *Annals of Neurology, 18*(6), 660–664.

Griffin, W. S., Sheng, J. G., Gentleman, S. M., Graham, D. I., Mrak, R. E., & Roberts, G. W. (1994). Microglial interleukin-1 alpha expression in human head injury: Correlations with neuronal and neuritic beta-amyloid precursor protein expression. *Neuroscience Letters, 176*(2), 133–136.

Griffin, W. S., Sheng, J. G., Roberts, G. W., & Mrak, R. E. (1995). Interleukin-1 expression in different plaque types in Alzheimer's disease: Significance in plaque evolution. *Journal of Neuropathology and Experimental Neurology, 54*(2), 276–281.

Griffin, W. S., Sheng, J. G., Royston, M. C., Gentleman, S. M., McKenzie, J. E., Graham, D. I., Roberts, G. W., & Mrak, R. E. (1998). Glial-neuronal interactions in Alzheimer's disease: The potential role of a 'cytokine cycle' in disease progression. *Brain Pathology, 8*(1), 65–72.

Griffin, W. S., Stanley, L. C., Ling, C., White, L., MacLeod, V., Perrot, L. J., White, C. L., 3rd, & Araoz, C. (1989). Brain interleukin 1 and S-100 immunoreactivity are elevated in Down syndrome and Alzheimer disease. *Proceedings of the National Academy of Sciences, 86*(19), 7611–7615.

Guillemin, G. J., & Brew, B. J. (2004). Microglia, macrophages, perivascular macrophages, and pericytes: A review of function and identification. *Journal of Leukocyte Biology, 75*(3), 388–397.

Hacham, M., Argov, S., White, R. M., Segal, S., & Apte, R. N. (2002). Different patterns of interleukin-1alpha and interleukin-1beta expression in organs of normal young and old mice. *European Cytokine Network, 13*(1), 55–65.

Hart, B. L. (1988). Biological basis of the behavior of sick animals. *Neuroscience and Biobehavioral Reviews, 12*(2), 123–137.

Hauser, S. L., Doolittle, T. H., Lincoln, R., Brown, R. H., & Dinarello, C. A. (1990). Cytokine accumulations in CSF of multiple sclerosis patients: Frequent detection of interleukin-1 and tumor necrosis factor but not interleukin-6. *Neurology, 40*(11), 1735–1739.

Hayashi, F., Smith, K. D., Ozinsky, A., Hawn, T. R., Yi, E. C., Goodlett, D. R., Eng, J. K., Akira, S., Underhill, D. M., & Aderem, A. (2001). The innate immune response to bacterial flagellin is mediated by Toll-like receptor 5. *Nature, 410*(6832), 1099–1103.

Hemmi, H., Takeuchi, O., Kawai, T., Kaisho, T., Sato, S., Sanjo, H., Matsumoto, M., Hoshino, K., Wagner, H., Takeda, K., & Akira, S. (2000). A Toll-like receptor recognizes bacterial DNA. *Nature, 408*(6813), 740–745.

Hetier, E., Ayala, J., Denefle, P., Bousseau, A., Rouget, P., Mallat, M., & Prochiantz, A. (1988). Brain macrophages synthesize interleukin-1 and interleukin-1 mRNAs in vitro. *Journal of Neuroscience Research, 21*(2–4), 391–397.

Holmes, C., El-Okl, M., Williams, A. L., Cunningham, C., Wilcockson, D., & Perry, V. H. (2003). Systemic infection, interleukin 1beta, and cognitive decline in Alzheimer's disease. *Journal of Neurology and Neurosurgical Psychiatry, 74*(6), 788–789.

Horrocks, L. A., & Yeo, Y. K. (1999a). Docosahexaenoic acid-enriched foods: Production and effects on blood lipids. *Lipids, 34* (Suppl.), S313.

Horrocks, L. A., & Yeo, Y. K. (1999b). Health benefits of docosahexaenoic acid (DHA). *Pharmacological Research, 40*(3), 211–225.

Huang, D. B., Huxford, T., Chen, Y. Q., & Ghosh, G. (1997). The role of DNA in the mechanism of NFkappaB dimer formation: Crystal structures of the dimerization domains of the p50 and p65 subunits. *Structure, 5*(11), 1427–1436.

Ilyin, S. E., Gayle, D., Flynn, M. C., & Plata-Salaman, C. R. (1998). Interleukin-1beta system (ligand, receptor type I, receptor accessory protein and receptor antagonist), TNF-alpha, TGF-beta1 and neuropeptide Y mRNAs in specific brain regions during bacterial LPS-induced anorexia. *Brain Research Bulletin, 45*(5), 507–515.

Johnson, P. M., Vogt, S. K., Burney, M. W., & Muglia, L. J. (2002). COX-2 inhibition attenuates anorexia during systemic inflammation without impairing cytokine production. *American Journal of Physiology, 282*(3), E650–656.

Johnson, R. W., Gheusi, G., Segreti, S., Dantzer, R., & Kelley, K. W. (1997). C3H/HeJ mice are refractory to lipopolysaccharide in the brain. *Brain Research, 752*(1–2), 219–226.

Kalmijn, S., Launer, L. J., Ott, A., Witteman, J. C., Hofman, A., & Breteler, M. M. (1997). Dietary fat intake and the risk of incident dementia in the Rotterdam Study. *Annals of Neurology, 42*(5), 776–782.

Kalmijn, S., van Boxtel, M. P., Ocke, M., Verschuren, W. M., Kromhout, D., & Launer, L. J. (2004). Dietary intake of fatty acids and fish in relation to cognitive performance at middle age. *Neurology, 62*(2), 275–280.

Kanemoto, K., Kawasaki, J., Miyamoto, T., Obayashi, H., & Nishimura, M. (2000). Interleukin (IL)1beta, IL-1alpha, and IL-1 receptor antagonist gene polymorphisms in patients with temporal lobe epilepsy. *Annals of Neurology, 47*(5), 571–574.

Karin, M., & Ben-Neriah, Y. (2000). Phosphorylation meets ubiquitination: The control of NF-[kappa]B activity. *Annual Review of Immunology, 18*, 621–663.

Katafuchi, T., Takaki, A., Take, S., Kondo, T., & Yoshimura, M. (2003). Endotoxin inhibitor blocks heat exposure-induced expression of brain cytokine mRNA in aged rats. *Molecular Brain Research, 118*(1–2), 24–32.

Kelly, A., Vereker, E., Nolan, Y., Brady, M., Barry, C., Loscher, C. E., Mills, K. H., & Lynch, M. A. (2003). Activation of p38 plays a pivotal role in the inhibitory effect of lipopolysaccharide and interleukin-1 beta on long term potentiation in rat dentate gyrus. *Journal of Biological Chemistry, 278*(21), 19,453–19,462.

Kent, S., Bluthe, R. M., Dantzer, R., Hardwick, A. J., Kelley, K. W., Rothwell, N. J., & Vannice, J. L. (1992). Different receptor mechanisms mediate the pyrogenic and behavioral effects of interleukin 1. *Proceedings of the National Academy of Sciences, 89*(19), 9117–9120.

Kent, S., Bluthe, R. M., Kelley, K. W., & Dantzer, R. (1992). Sickness behavior as a new target for drug development. *Trends in Pharmacological Sciences, 13*(1), 24–28.

Kiecolt-Glaser, J. K., & Glaser, R. (2002). Depression and immune function: Central pathways to morbidity and mortality. *Journal of Psychosomatic Research, 53*(4), 873–876.

Kielian, T., & Esen, N. (2004). Effects of neuroinflammation on glia-glia gap junctional intercellular communication: A perspective. *Neurochemistry International, 45*(2–3), 429–436.

Klir, J. J., McClellan, J. L., Kozak, W., Szelenyi, Z., Wong, G. H., & Kluger, M. J. (1995). Systemic but not central administration of tumor necrosis factor-alpha attenuates LPS-induced fever in rats. *American Journal of Physiology, 268*(2 Pt. 2), R480–486.

Kloss, C. U., Bohatschek, M., Kreutzberg, G. W., & Raivich, G. (2001). Effect of lipopolysaccharide on the morphology and integrin immunoreactivity of ramified microglia in the mouse brain and in cell culture. *Experimental Neurology, 168*(1), 32–46.

Kluger, M. J. (1991). Fever: Role of pyrogens and cryogens. *Physiological Reviews, 71*(1), 93–127.

Kluger, M. J., Kozak, W., Leon, L. R., Soszynski, D., & Conn, C. A. (1995). Cytokines and fever. *Neuroimmunomodulation, 2*(4), 216–223.

Konsman, J. P., Kelley, K., & Dantzer, R. (1999). Temporal and spatial relationships between lipopolysaccharide-induced expression of Fos, interleukin-1beta and inducible nitric oxide synthase in rat brain. *Neuroscience, 89*(2), 535–548.

Konsman, J. P., Parnet, P., & Dantzer, R. (2002). Cytokine-induced sickness behavior: Mechanisms and implications. *Trends in Neurosciences, 25*(3), 154–159.

Konsman, J. P., Vigues, S., Mackerlova, L., Bristow, A., & Blomqvist, A. (2004). Rat brain vascular distribution of interleukin-1 type-1 receptor immunoreactivity: Relationship to patterns of inducible cyclooxygenase expression by peripheral inflammatory stimuli. *Journal of Comparative Neurology, 472*(1), 113–129.

Kozak, K. R., Prusakiewicz, J. J., Rowlinson, S. W., Schneider, C., & Marnett, L. J. (2001). Amino acid determinants in cyclooxygenase-2 oxygenation of the endocannabinoid 2-arachidonylglycerol. *Journal of Biological Chemistry, 276*(32), 30,072–30,077.

Kozak, W., Conn, C. A., Klir, J. J., Wong, G. H., & Kluger, M. J. (1995). TNF soluble receptor and antiserum against TNF enhance lipopolysaccharide fever in mice. *American Journal of Physiology, 269*(1 Pt. 2), R23–29.

Kozak, W., Soszynski, D., Rudolph, K., Conn, C. A., & Kluger, M. J. (1997). Dietary n-3 fatty acids differentially affect sickness behavior in mice during local and systemic inflammation. *American Journal of Physiology, 272*(4 Pt. 2), R1298–1307.

Kreutzberg, G. W. (1996). Microglia: A sensor for pathological events in the CNS. *Trends in Neurosciences, 19*(8), 312–318.

Kunkel, S. L., Spengler, M., May, M. A., Spengler, R., Larrick, J., & Remick, D. (1988). Prostaglandin E2 regulates macrophage-derived tumor necrosis factor gene expression. *Journal of Biological Chemistry, 263*(11), 5380–5384.

Lacroix, S., & Rivest, S. (1998). Effect of acute systemic inflammatory response and cytokines on the transcription of the genes encoding cyclooxygenase enzymes (COX-1 and COX-2) in the rat brain. *Journal of Neurochemistry, 70*(2), 452–466.

Laflamme, N., Echchannaoui, H., Landmann, R., & Rivest, S. (2003). Cooperation between toll-like receptor 2 and 4 in the brain of mice challenged with cell wall components derived from gram-negative and gram-positive bacteria. *European Journal of Immunology, 33*(4), 1127–1138.

Laflamme, N., & Rivest, S. (1999). Effects of systemic immunogenic insults and circulating proinflammatory cytokines on the transcription of the inhibitory factor kappaB alpha within specific cellular populations of the rat brain. *Journal of Neurochemistry, 73*(1), 309–321.

Laflamme, N., & Rivest, S. (2001). Toll-like receptor 4: The missing link of the cerebral innate immune response triggered by circulating gram-negative bacterial cell wall components. *FASEB Journal, 15*(1), 155–163.

Laflamme, N., Soucy, G., & Rivest, S. (2001). Circulating cell wall components derived from gram-negative, not gram-positive, bacteria cause a profound induction of the gene-encoding Toll-like receptor 2 in the CNS. *Journal of Neurochemistry, 79*(3), 648–657.

Laye, S., Gheusi, G., Cremona, S., Combe, C., Kelley, K., Dantzer, R., & Parnet, P. (2000). Endogenous brain IL-1 mediates LPS-induced anorexia and hypothalamic cytokine expression. *American Journal of Physiology, 279*(1), R93–98.

Laye, S., Liege, S., Li, K. S., Moze, E., & Neveu, P. J. (2001). Physiological significance of the interleukin 1 receptor accessory protein. *Neuroimmunomodulation, 9*(4), 225–230.

Li, Y., Liu, L., Kang, J., Sheng, J. G., Barger, S. W., Mrak, R. E., & Griffin, W. S. (2000). Neuronal-glial interactions mediated by interleukin-1 enhance neuronal acetylcholinesterase activity and mRNA expression. *Journal of Neurosciences, 20*(1), 149–155.

Liege, S., Laye, S., Li, K. S., Moze, E., & Neveu, P. J. (2000). Interleukin 1 receptor accessory protein (IL-1RAcP) is necessary for centrally mediated neuroendocrine and immune responses to IL-1beta. *Journal of Neuroimmunology, 110*(1–2), 134–139.

Lim, G. P., Yang, F., Chu, T., Chen, P., Beech, W., Teter, B., Tran, T., Ubeda, O., Ashe, K. H., Frautschy, S. A., & Cole, G. M. (2000). Ibuprofen suppresses plaque pathology and inflammation in a mouse model for Alzheimer's disease. *Journal of Neurosciences, 20*(15), 5709–5714.

Lipton, J. M., Zhao, H., Ichiyama, T., Barsh, G. S., & Catania, A. (1999). Mechanisms of antiinflammatory action of alpha-MSH peptides. In vivo and in vitro evidence. *Annual New York Academical Sciences, 885,* 173–182.

Liu, B., & Hong, J. S. (2003). Role of microglia in inflammation-mediated neurodegenerative diseases: Mechanisms and strategies for therapeutic intervention. *Journal of Pharmacology and Experimental Therapy, 304*(1), 1–7.

Liu, C., Chalmers, D., Maki, R., & De Souza, E. B. (1996). Rat homolog of mouse interleukin-1 receptor accessory protein: Cloning, localization and modulation studies. *Journal of Neuroimmunology, 66*(1–2), 41–48.

Loring, J. F., Wen, X., Lee, J. M., Seilhamer, J., & Somogyi, R. (2001). A gene expression profile of Alzheimer's disease. *DNA and Cellular Biology, 20*(11), 683–695.

Lugarini, F., Hrupka, B. J., Schwartz, G. J., Plata-Salaman, C. R., & Langhans, W. (2002). A role for cyclooxygenase-2 in lipopolysaccharide-induced anorexia in rats. *American Journal of Physiology, 283*(4), R862–868.

Luheshi, G., Miller, A. J., Brouwer, S., Dascombe, M. J., Rothwell, N. J., & Hopkins, S. J. (1996). Interleukin-1 receptor antagonist inhibits endotoxin fever and systemic interleukin-6 induction in the rat. *American Journal of Physiology, 270*(1 Pt. 1), E91–95.

Lynch, A. M., Moore, M., Craig, S., Lonergan, P. E., Martin, D. S., & Lynch, M. A. (2003). Analysis of interleukin-1 beta-induced cell signaling activation in rat hippocampus following exposure to gamma irradiation. Protective effect of eicosapentaenoic acid. *Journal of Biological Chemistry, 278*(51), 51,075–51,084.

Lynch, M. A. (1998). Age-related impairment in long-term potentiation in hippocampus: A role for the cytokine, interleukin-1 beta? *Progress in Neurobiology, 56*(5), 571–589.

Marcheselli, V. L., Hong, S., Lukiw, W. J., Tian, X. H., Gronert, K., Musto, A., Hardy, M., Gimenez, J. M., Chiang, N., Serhan, C. N., & Bazan, N. G. (2003). Novel docosanoids inhibit brain ischemia-reperfusion-mediated leukocyte infiltration and pro-inflammatory gene expression. *Journal of Biological Chemistry, 278*(44), 43,807–43,817.

Martin, D. S., Lonergan, P. E., Boland, B., Fogarty, M. P., Brady, M., Horrobin, D. F., Campbell, V. A., & Lynch, M. A. (2002). Apoptotic changes in the aged brain are triggered by interleukin-1beta-induced activation of p38 and reversed by treatment with eicosapentaenoic acid. *Journal of Biological Chemistry, 277*(37), 34,239–34,246.

Martino, G., Adorini, L., Rieckmann, P., Hillert, J., Kallmann, B., Comi, G., & Filippi, M. (2002). Inflammation in multiple sclerosis: The good, the bad, and the complex. *Lancet Neurology, 1*(8), 499–509.

Mattson, M. P. (1994). Mechanism of neuronal degeneration and preventative approaches: Quickening the pace of AD research. *Neurobiology of Aging, 15* (Suppl. 2), S121–125.

McCarthy, G. M., & Kenny, D. (1992). Dietary fish oil and rheumatic diseases. *Seminar in Arthritis Rheumatoid, 21*(6), 368–375.

McCullough, L., Wu, L., Haughey, N., Liang, X., Hand, T., Wang, Q., Breyer, R. M., & Andreasson, K. (2004). Neuroprotective function of the PGE2 EP2 receptor in cerebral ischemia. *Journal of Neurosciences, 24*(1), 257–268.

McGahon, B., Murray, C. A., Clements, M. P., & Lynch, M. A. (1998). Analysis of the effect of membrane arachidonic acid concentration on modulation of glutamate release by interleukin-1: An age-related study. *Experimental Gerontology, 33*(4), 343–354.

McGeer, P. L., & Rogers, J. (1992). Anti-inflammatory agents as a therapeutic approach to Alzheimer's disease. *Neurology, 42*(2), 447–449.

McLay, R. N., Kastin, A. J., & Zadina, J. E. (2000). Passage of interleukin-1-beta across the blood-brain barrier is reduced in aged mice: A possible mechanism for diminished fever in aging. *Neuroimmunomodulation, 8*(3), 148–153.

McMahan, C. J., Slack, J. L., Mosley, B., Cosman, D., Lupton, S. D., Brunton, L. L., Grubin, C. E., Wignall, J. M., Jenkins, N. A., & Brannan, C. I. (1991). A novel IL-1 receptor, cloned from B cells by mammalian expression, is expressed in many cell types. *EMBO Journal, 10*(10), 2821–2832.

Merrill, J. E., & Benveniste, E. N. (1996). Cytokines in inflammatory brain lesions: Helpful and harmful. *Trends in Neurosciences, 19*(8), 331–338.

Meydani, S. N., Endres, S., Woods, M. M., Goldin, B. R., Soo, C., Morrill-Labrode, A., Dinarello, C. A., & Gorbach, S. L. (1991). Oral (n-3) fatty acid supplementation suppresses cytokine production and lymphocyte proliferation: Comparison between young and older women. *Journal of Nutrition, 121*(4), 547–555.

Moore, S. A. (2001). Polyunsaturated fatty acid synthesis and release by brain-derived cells in vitro. *Journal of Molecular Neurosciences, 16*(2–3), 195–221.

Moore, S. A., Yoder, E., Murphy, S., Dutton, G. R., & Spector, A. A. (1991). Astrocytes, not neurons, produce docosahexaenoic acid (22:6 omega-3) and arachidonic acid (20:4 omega-6). *Journal of Neurochemistry, 56*(2), 518–524.

Mrak, R. E., & Griffin, W. S. (2000). Interleukin-1 and the immunogenetics of Alzheimer disease. *Journal of Neuropathology and Experimental Neurology, 59*(6), 471–476.

Murray, C. A., Clements, M. P., & Lynch, M. A. (1999). Interleukin-1 induces lipid peroxidation and membrane changes in rat hippocampus: An age-related study. *Gerontology, 45*(3), 136–142.

Murray, C. A., & Lynch, M. A. (1998). Evidence that increased hippocampal expression of the cytokine interleukin-1 beta is a common trigger for age- and stress-induced impairments in long-term potentiation. *Journal of Neurosciences, 18*(8), 2974–2981.

Muzio, M., & Mantovani, A. (2000). Toll-like receptors. *Microbes and Infection, 2*(3), 251–255.

Nadjar, A., Combe, C., Laye, S., Tridon, V., Dantzer, R., Amedee, T., & Parnet, P. (2003). Nuclear factor kappaB nuclear translocation as a crucial marker of brain response to interleukin-1. A study in rat and interleukin-1 type I deficient mouse. *Journal of Neurochemistry, 87*(4), 1024–1036.

Nakamura, Y. (2002). Regulating factors for microglial activation. *Biological and Pharmacological Bulletin, 25*(8), 945–953.

Nakase, T., Fushiki, S., Sohl, G., Theis, M., Willecke, K., & Naus, C. C. (2003). Neuroprotective role of astrocytic gap junctions in ischemic stroke. *Cell Communication and Adhesion, 10*(4–6), 413–417.

Nelson, K. P., Marks, N. L., Heyen, J. R., & Johnson, R. W. (1999). Behavior of adult and aged mice before and after central injection of interleukin-1beta. *Physiology of Behavior, 66*(4), 673–679.

Neuhaus, O., Archelos, J. J., & Hartung, H. P. (2003). Immunomodulation in multiple sclerosis: from immunosuppression to neuroprotection. *Trends in Pharmacological Sciences, 24*(3), 131–138.

Neuringer, M., Anderson, G. J., & Connor, W. E. (1988). The essentiality of n-3 fatty acids for the development and function of the retina and brain. *Annual Review of Nutrition, 8*, 517–541.

Nguyen, M. D., Julien, J. P., & Rivest, S. (2002). Innate immunity: The missing link in neuroprotection and neurodegeneration? *Nature Reviews Neuroscience, 3*(3), 216–227.

Nishimura, M., Mizuta, I., Mizuta, E., Yamasaki, S., Ohta, M., & Kuno, S. (2000). Influence of interleukin-1beta gene polymorphisms on age-at-onset of sporadic Parkinson's disease. *Neuroscience Letters, 284*(1–2), 73–76.

O'Banion, M. K. (1999). Cyclooxygenase-2: Molecular biology, pharmacology, and neurobiology. *Critical Review in Neurobiology, 13*(1), 45–82.

Oka, T., Oka, K., Scammell, T. E., Lee, C., Kelly, J. F., Nantel, F., Elmquist, J. K., & Saper, C. B. (2000). Relationship of EP(1-4) prostaglandin receptors with rat hypothalamic cell groups involved in lipopolysaccharide fever responses. *Journal of Comparative Neurology, 428*(1), 20–32.

Okuyama, H., Kobayashi, T., & Watanabe, S. (1996). Dietary fatty acids—the *n*-6/*n*-3 balance and chronic elderly diseases. Excess linoleic acid and relative *n*-3 deficiency syndrome seen in Japan. *Progress in Lipid Research, 35*(4), 409–457.

O'Neill, L. A. (2002). Signal transduction pathways activated by the IL-1 receptor/toll-like receptor superfamily. *Current Topics in Microbiology and Immunology, 270*, 47–61.

O'Neill, L. A., Fitzgerald, K. A., & Bowie, A. G. (2003). The Toll-IL-1 receptor adaptor family grows to five members. *Trends in Immunology, 24*(6), 286–290.

Perry, V. H., Bell, M. D., Brown, H. C., & Matyszak, M. K. (1995). Inflammation in the nervous system. *Current Opinion in Neurobiology, 5*(5), 636–641.

Perry, V. H., Cunningham, C., & Boche, D. (2002). Atypical inflammation in the central nervous system in prion disease. *Current Opinion in Neurology, 15*(3), 349–354.

Perry, V. H., Newman, T. A., & Cunningham, C. (2003). The impact of systemic infection on the progression of neurodegenerative disease. *Nature Reviews Neuroscience, 4*(2), 103–112.

Petroni, A., Salami, M., Blasevich, M., Papini, N., & Galli, C. (1994). Inhibition by n-3 fatty acids of arachidonic acid metabolism in a primary culture of astroglial cells. *Neurochemistry Research, 19*(9), 1187–1193.

Petrova, T. V., Akama, K. T., & Van Eldik, L. J. (1999). Selective modulation of BV-2 microglial activation by prostaglandin E(2). Differential effects on endotoxin-stimulated cytokine induction. *Journal of Biological Chemistry, 274*(40), 28,823–28,827.

Pinteaux, E., Parker, L. C., Rothwell, N. J., & Luheshi, G. N. (2002). Expression of interleukin-1 receptors and their role in interleukin-1 actions in murine microglial cells. *Journal of Neurochemistry, 83*(4), 754–763.

Plata-Salaman, C. R., Peloso, E., & Satinoff, E. (1998). Interleukin-1beta-induced fever in young and old Long-Evans rats. *American Journal of Physiology, 275*(5 Pt. 2), R1633–1638.

Poltorak, A., He, X., Smirnova, I., Liu, M. Y., Van Huffel, C., Du, X., Birdwell, D., Alejos, E., Silva, M., Galanos, C., Freudenberg, M., Ricciardi-Castagnoli, P., Layton, B., & Beutler, B. (1998). Defective LPS signaling in C3H/HeJ and C57BL/10ScCr mice: mutations in Tlr4 gene. *Science, 282*(5396), 2085–2088.

Pomposelli, J. J., Mascioli, E. A., Bistrian, B. R., Lopes, S. M., & Blackburn, G. L. (1989). Attenuation of the febrile response in guinea pigs by fish oil enriched diets. *Journal of Parenteral and Enteral Nutrition, 13*(2), 136–140.

Pousset, F., Cremona, S., Dantzer, R., Kelley, K., & Parnet, P. (1999). Interleukin-4 and interleukin-10 regulate IL1-beta induced mouse primary astrocyte activation: A comparative study. *Glia, 26*(1), 12–21.

Quan, N., Sundar, S. K., & Weiss, J. M. (1994). Induction of interleukin-1 in various brain regions after peripheral and central injections of lipopolysaccharide. *Journal of Neuroimmunology, 49*(1–2), 125–134.

Quan, N., Whiteside, M., & Herkenham, M. (1998). Cyclooxygenase 2 mRNA expression in rat brain after peripheral injection of lipopolysaccharide. *Brain Research, 802*(1–2), 189–197.

Quan, N., Whiteside, M., Kim, L., & Herkenham, M. (1997). Induction of inhibitory factor kappaBalpha mRNA in the central nervous system after peripheral lipopolysaccharide administration: An in situ hybridization histochemistry study in the rat. *Proceedings of the National Academy of Sciences, 94*(20), 10,985–10,990.

Quan, N., Zhang, Z., Emery, M., Bonsall, R., & Weiss, J. M. (1996). Detection of interleukin-1 bioactivity in various brain regions of normal healthy rats. *Neuroimmunomodulation, 3*(1), 47–55.

Rada, P., Mark, G. P., Vitek, M. P., Mangano, R. M., Blume, A. J., Beer, B., & Hoebel, B. G. (1991). Interleukin-1 beta decreases acetylcholine measured by microdialysis in the hippocampus of freely moving rats. *Brain Research, 550*(2), 287–290.

Raper, N. R., Cronin, F. J., & Exler, J. (1992). Omega-3 fatty acid content of the US food supply. *Journal of American College of Nutrition, 11*(3), 304–308.

Reichenberg, A., Yirmiya, R., Schuld, A., Kraus, T., Haack, M., Morag, A., & Pollmacher, T. (2001). Cytokine-associated emotional and cognitive disturbances in humans. *Archive of General Psychiatry, 58*(5), 445–452.

Rivest, S. (2001). How circulating cytokines trigger the neural circuits that control the hypothalamic-pituitary-adrenal axis. *Psychoneuroendocrinology, 26*(8), 761–788.

Rosenberger, T. A., Villacreses, N. E., Hovda, J. T., Bosetti, F., Weerasinghe, G., Wine, R. N., Harry, G. J., & Rapoport, S. I. (2004). Rat brain arachidonic acid metabolism is increased by a 6-day intracerebral ventricular infusion of bacterial lipopolysaccharide. *Journal of Neurochemistry, 88*(5), 1168–1178.

Rothwell, N. J., & Luheshi, G. N. (2000). Interleukin 1 in the brain: Biology, pathology and therapeutic target. *Trends in Neurosciences, 23*(12), 618–625.

Sasaki, T., Kitagawa, K., Yamagata, K., Takemiya, T., Tanaka, S., Omura-Matsuoka, E., Sugiura, S., Matsumoto, M., & Hori, M. (2004). Amelioration of hippocampal neuronal damage after transient forebrain ischemia in cyclooxygenase-2-deficient mice. *Journal of Cerebral Blood Flow Metabolism, 24*(1), 107–113.

Schiltz, J. C., & Sawchenko, P. E. (2002). Distinct brain vascular cell types manifest inducible cyclooxygenase expression as a function of the strength and nature of immune insults. *Journal of Neurosciences, 22*(13), 5606–5618.

Schneider, H., Pitossi, F., Balschun, D., Wagner, A., del Rey, A., & Besedovsky, H. O. (1998). A neuromodulatory role of interleukin-1beta in the hippocampus. *Proceedings of the National Academy of Sciences, 95*(13), 7778–7783.

Schwandner, R., Dziarski, R., Wesche, H., Rothe, M., & Kirschning, C. J. (1999). Peptidoglycan- and lipoteichoic acid-induced cell activation is mediated by toll-like receptor 2. *Journal of Biological Chemistry, 274*(25), 17,406–17,409.

Segreti, J., Gheusi, G., Dantzer, R., Kelley, K. W., & Johnson, R. W. (1997). Defect in interleukin-1beta secretion prevents sickness behavior in C3H/HeJ mice. *Physiology of Behavior, 61*(6), 873–878.

Serhan, C. N., Clish, C. B., Brannon, J., Colgan, S. P., Gronert, K., & Chiang, N. (2000). Anti-microinflammatory lipid signals generated from dietary N-3 fatty acids via cyclooxygenase-2 and transcellular processing: a novel mechanism for NSAID and N-3 PUFA therapeutic actions. *Journal of Physiology and Pharmacology, 51*(4 Pt. 1), 643–654.

Sheng, J. G., Griffin, W. S., Royston, M. C., & Mrak, R. E. (1998). Distribution of interleukin-1-immunoreactive microglia in cerebral cortical layers: Implications for neuritic plaque formation in Alzheimer's disease. *Neuropathology and Applied Neurobiology, 24*(4), 278–283.

Sheng, J. G., Mrak, R. E., & Griffin, W. S. (1998). Enlarged and phagocytic, but not primed, interleukin-1 alpha-immunoreactive microglia increase with age in normal human brain. *Acta Neuropathologica, 95*(3), 229–234.

Simopoulos, A. P. (2001). n-3 Fatty acids and human health: defining strategies for public policy. *Lipids, 36* (Suppl.), S83–89.

Simopoulos, A. P. (2003). Importance of the ratio of omega-6/omega-3 essential fatty acids: evolutionary aspects. *World Review in Nutritional Diet, 92,* 1–22.

Sims, J. E., March, C. J., Cosman, D., Widmer, M. B., MacDonald, H. R., McMahan, C. J., Grubin, C. E., Wignall, J. M., Jackson, J. L., Call, S. M., et al. (1988). cDNA expression cloning of the IL-1 receptor, a member of the immunoglobulin superfamily. *Science, 241*(4865), 585–589.

Sly, L. M., Krzesicki, R. F., Brashler, J. R., Buhl, A. E., McKinley, D. D., Carter, D. B., & Chin, J. E. (2001). Endogenous brain cytokine mRNA and inflammatory responses to lipopolysaccharide are elevated in the Tg2576 transgenic mouse model of Alzheimer's disease. *Brain Research Bulletin, 56*(6), 581–588.

Song, C., & Horrobin, D. (2004). Omega-3 fatty acid ethyl-eicosapentaenoate, but not soybean oil, attenuates memory impairment induced by central IL-1beta administration. *Journal of Lipid Research, 45*(6), 1112–1121.

Song, C., Li, X., Leonard, B. E., & Horrobin, D. F. (2003). Effects of dietary n-3 or n-6 fatty acids on interleukin-1beta-induced anxiety, stress, and inflammatory responses in rats. *Journal of Lipid Research, 44*(10), 1984–1991.

Sonti, G., Flynn, M. C., & Plata-Salaman, C. R. (1997). Interleukin-1 (IL-1) receptor type I mediates anorexia but not adipsia induced by centrally administered IL-1beta. *Physiology of Behavior, 62*(5), 1179–1183.

Spector, A. A. (1999). Essentiality of fatty acids. *Lipids, 34* (Suppl.), S1–3.

Stewart, W. F., Kawas, C., Corrada, M., & Metter, E. J. (1997). Risk of Alzheimer's disease and duration of NSAID use. *Neurology, 48*(3), 626–632.

Streit, W. J., Walter, S. A., & Pennell, N. A. (1999). Reactive microgliosis. *Progress in Neurobiology, 57*(6), 563–581.

Strle, K., Zhou, J. H., Shen, W. H., Broussard, S. R., Johnson, R. W., Freund, G. G., Dantzer, R., & Kelley, K. W. (2001). Interleukin-10 in the brain. *Critical Review in Immunology, 21*(5), 427–449.

Theele, D. P., & Streit, W. J. (1993). A chronicle of microglial ontogeny. *Glia, 7*(1), 5–8.

Touzani, O., Boutin, H., LeFeuvre, R., Parker, L., Miller, A., Luheshi, G., & Rothwell, N. (2002). Interleukin-1 influences ischemic brain damage in the mouse independently of the interleukin-1 type I receptor. *Journal of Neurosciences, 22*(1), 38–43.

Ushikubi, F., Segi, E., Sugimoto, Y., Murata, T., Matsuoka, T., Kobayashi, T., Hizaki, H., Tuboi, K., Katsuyama, M., Ichikawa, A., Tanaka, T., Yoshida, N., & Narumiya, S. (1998). Impaired febrile response in mice lacking the prostaglandin E receptor subtype EP3. *Nature 395*(6699), 281–284.

Vane, J. R., Bakhle, Y. S., & Botting, R. M. (1998). Cyclooxygenases 1 and 2. *Annual Review of Pharmacology and Toxicology, 38,* 97–120.

van Gool, W. A., Aisen, P. S., & Eikelenboom, P. (2003). Anti-inflammatory therapy in Alzheimer's disease: Is hope still alive? *Journal of Neurology, 250*(7), 788–792.

Venters, H. D., Dantzer, R., & Kelley, K. W. (2000). A new concept in neurodegeneration: TNFalpha is a silencer of survival signals. *Trends in Neurosciences, 23*(4), 175–180.

Wang, C., Deng, L., Hong, M., Akkaraju, G. R., Inoue, J., & Chen, Z. J. (2001). TAK1 is a ubiquitin-dependent kinase of MKK and IKK. *Nature, 412*(6844), 346–351.

Wesche, H., Henzel, W. J., Shillinglaw, W., Li, S., & Cao, Z. (1997). MyD88: An adapter that recruits IRAK to the IL-1 receptor complex. *Immunity, 7*(6), 837–847.

Wolf, G., Yirmiya, R., Goshen, I., Iverfeldt, K., Holmlund, L., Takeda, K., & Shavit, Y. (2003). Impairment of interleukin-1 (IL-1) signaling reduces basal pain sensitivity in mice: Genetic, pharmacological and developmental aspects. *Pain, 104*(3), 471–480.

Wong, M. L., & Licinio, J. (1994). Localization of interleukin 1 type I receptor mRNA in rat brain. *Neuroimmunomodulation, 1*(2), 110–115.

Xu, Y., Tao, X., Shen, B., Horng, T., Medzhitov, R., Manley, J. L., & Tong, L. (2000). Structural basis for signal transduction by the Toll/interleukin-1 receptor domains. *Nature, 408*(6808), 111–115.

Yehuda, S., Rabinovitz, S., Carasso, R. L., & Mostofsky, D. I. (2002). The role of polyunsaturated fatty acids in restoring the aging neuronal membrane. *Neurobiology of Aging, 23*(5), 843–853.

Yirmiya, R., Winocur, G., & Goshen, I. (2002). Brain interleukin-1 is involved in spatial memory and passive avoidance conditioning. *Neurobiology of Learning Memory, 78*(2), 379–389.

Zaloga, G. P., & Marik, P. (2001). Lipid modulation and systemic inflammation. *Critical Care Clinical, 17*(1), 201–217.

Zandi, P. P., Anthony, J. C., Hayden, K. M., Mehta, K., Mayer, L., & Breitner, J. C. (2002). Reduced incidence of AD with NSAID but not H2 receptor antagonists: The Cache County Study. *Neurology, 59*(6), 880–886.

Zerouga, M., Jenski, L. J., & Stillwell, W. (1995). Comparison of phosphatidylcholines containing one or two docosahexaenoic acyl chains on properties of phospholipid monolayers and bilayers. *Biochemistry and Biophysical Acta, 1236*(2), 266–272.

Zhang, J., & Rivest, S. (2001). Anti-inflammatory effects of prostaglandin E2 in the central nervous system in response to brain injury and circulating lipopolysaccharide. *Journal of Neurochemistry, 76*(3), 855–864.

Zhao, Y., Joshi-Barve, S., Barve, S., & Chen, L. H. (2004). Eicosapentaenoic acid prevents LPS-induced TNF-alpha expression by preventing NF-kappaB activation. *Journal of American College of Nutrition, 23*(1), 71–78.

Zhu, S. G., Sheng, J. G., Jones, R. A., Brewer, M. M., Zhou, X. Q., Mrak, R. E., & Griffin, W. S. (1999). Increased interleukin-1beta converting enzyme expression and activity in Alzheimer disease. *Journal of Neuropathology and Experimental Neurology, 58*(6), 582–587.

24 Pathophysiological Effects of Inflammatory Mediators and Stress on Distinct Memory Systems

Lisa A. Teather

KEY POINTS

- Memory is processed in multiple brain systems, including the hippocampal- and the dorsal striatal-based systems.
- Consolidation processes in the hippocampus and in the dorsal striatal memory systems share several common neurochemical mediators, such as glutamate and extracellular platelet-activating factor.
- Hippocampal, but not dorsal striatal, consolidation requires inflammatory mediators such as intracellular platelet-activating factor and prostaglandins derived from cyclooxygenase-2 activity.
- Dependency on inflammatory signals in physiological memory processing may predispose the hippocampus to age-related neuropathology and cognitive deficits.
- Stress may contribute to age-related neurodegeneration of the hippocampal system by interactions with central inflammatory mediators.

1. THE EXISTENCE OF MULTIPLE MEMORY SYSTEMS

Findings of studies examining the organization of memory provide compelling evidence that memory is processed in multiple brain systems that differ in terms of the type of memory they mediate (Packard & Teather, 1997a). Dissociations between the roles of the hippocampal system (e.g., Cohen & Squire, 1980; Hirsh, 1974; Packard & Teather, 1998) and the dorsal striatum (i.e., caudate nucleus) (e.g., Packard, Hirsh & White, 1989; Packard & Teather, 1998; Packard & White, 1990) in the acquisition of various learning tasks have been observed following damage to these structures. These and other results suggest that the hippocampus and dorsal striatum may be part of distinct memory systems. For example, lesions of the hippocampal system selectively impair acquisition of tasks that require "cognitive" or "reference" forms of memory (McDonald & White, 1993; Packard et al., 1989; Packard & Teather, 1998). In contrast, lesions of the dorsal striatum selectively impair acquisition of tasks requiring "stimulus-response" (S-R) or "habit" forms of memory (McDonald & White, 1993; Packard et al., 1989; Packard & Teather, 1998).

From: *Nutrients, Stress, and Medical Disorders*
Edited by: S. Yehuda and D. I. Mostofsky © Humana Press Inc., Totowa, NJ

Although lesion studies have provided evidence for differential roles of the hippocampus and dorsal striatum in memory, recent evidence is also mounting in regard to the nature of the neurochemical bases of memory storage in these systems. Although glutamate (Packard & Teather, 1999), NMDA receptor activation (Packard & Teather, 1997a, 1997b), dopamine (Packard & White, 1991), and acetylcholine (Power, Vazdarjanova, & McGaugh, 2003) are required for both hippocampal and dorsal striatal memory processing, how these neural systems differ in their actions to consolidate memory with respect to other neurochemical signals are now becoming clear. In particular, mediators previously shown to be involved in immune/inflammatory events appear to be critical for hippocampal-dependent, but not for dorsal striatal-dependent, memory processing. Furthermore, stress can have opposing effects on hippocampal and dorsal striatal memory; the distinct effects of stress may be related to the use of inflammatory mediators by the hippocampus in physiological memory processing. As various neurodegenerative brain disorders can selectively affect the striatum and hippocampus, such neurochemical dissociations may impact our understanding of the basic principles of the molecular events underlying learning and memory, as well as our understanding of the neurobiology of various neurodegenerative disorders.

2. THE HIPPOCAMPUS AND DORSAL STRIATUM SHARE SEVERAL NEUROBIOLOGICAL MECHANISMS DURING EARLY MEMORY CONSOLIDATION

The dorsal striatum receives dense glutamatergic projections from the cortex via the corticostriatal pathway and contains a moderate density of NMDA receptors (Ottersen, Hjelle, Osen, & Laake, 1995). It has been hypothesized that corticostriatal glutamatergic input provides the dorsal striatum with sensory information critical for the participation of this structure in S-R memory (White, 1989). In support of this hypothesis, administration of glutamate directly into the dorsal striatum of rats was found to enhance consolidation of S-R memory (Packard & Teather, 1999). Moreover, intrastriatal administration of a selective NMDA receptor antagonist (i.e., 2-amino-5-phosphopentaenoic acid [AP-5]) impairs S-R memory in rats (Packard & Teather, 1997a), suggesting that glutamate is required, at least in part, to activate NMDA receptors in the striatum during early S-R memory consolidation.

The hippocampus receives glutamatergic innervation from the entorhinal cortex via the perforant pathway and contains a high density of NMDA receptors (Otterson & Storm-Mathisen, 1989). Glutamate is also the principal neurotransmitter in the trisynaptic pathways through the hippocampal formation (for review, *see* Otterson & Storm-Mathisen, 1989). Glutamate administration directly into the hippocampus of rats enhances consolidation of cognitive forms of memory (Packard & Teather, 1999). Intrahippocampal administration of various NMDA receptor antagonists impairs consolidation of cognitive memory (Izquierdo et al., 1992; Packard & Teather, 1997a), suggesting that glutamate is required, at least in part, to activate NMDA receptors in the hippocampus during early cognitive memory consolidation. These findings not only demonstrate a double dissociation of the mnemonic functions of the hippocampus and dorsal striatum, but also suggest glutamate and NMDA receptor function to be integral during early consolidation mechanisms in both structures.

Platelet-activating factor (PAF) (1-*O*-alkyl-2-acetyl-*sn*-glycero-3-phosphocholine) is a potent phospholipid mediator that participates in normal cell function as well as in pathological conditions (Bazan, 1995). Interaction of PAF with plasma membrane (i.e., cell surface) PAF receptors activates heterotrimeric GTP-binding proteins, which triggers the activation of various protein kinases, including protein kinase C (PKC), protein kinase A (PKA), and mitogen-activated protein kinase (MAPK). Activation of these protein kinases occurs in various forms of synaptic plasticity. Thus, it is not surprising that PAF modulates synaptic plasticity. For instance, PAF applied to CA1 neurons of the hippocampus elicits glutamate release from presynaptic collateral terminals, suggesting that PAF is a retrograde messenger in long-term potentiation (LTP) (Kato, Clark, Bazan, & Zorumski, 1994), a putative cellular model of memory formation (Bliss & Collingridge, 1993). PAF-induced glutamate release is attenuated by preadministration of a selective cell surface PAF receptor antagonist (i.e., BN 52021) (Kato et al., 1994). These results suggest that postsynaptically synthesized PAF enhances glutamate release by diffusing across the synaptic cleft, where it activates presynaptic PAF receptors. Postsynaptic PAF may be generated via activation of cytosolic phospholipase A_2 (cPLA_2), following NMDA receptor-activation-induced enhancement of intracellular calcium levels, suggesting the potential for a positive-feedback loop.

A similar mechanism of PAF action (i.e., at the cell surface) may occur in both hippocampal- and dorsal-striatal-dependent memory processing. Posttraining administration of the nonhydrolyzable analog of PAF, methylcarbamyl-PAF (mc-PAF), into the hippocampus (Izquierdo et al., 1995; Teather, Packard, & Bazan, 1998) or dorsal striatum (Teather at al., 1998) enhances the consolidation of cognitive and S-R forms of memory, respectively. Moreover, posttraining administration of BN 52021 into the dorsal striatum (Teather et al., 1998) or hippocampus (Teather et al., 1998) impairs consolidation of S-R and cognitive forms of memory, respectively. These findings suggest that PAF, acting at cell surface PAF receptors, is an endogenous mediator in early dorsal-striatal-dependent and hippocampal-dependent memory processing.

It is feasible that PAF enhances cognitive and S-R forms of memory by increasing the release of glutamate, which ultimately increases activation of NMDA receptors within the dorsal striatum and hippocampus. In a study designed to assess this possibility, the first evidence of a dissociation of the neurochemical bases of hippocampal and dorsal striatal memory consolidation was demonstrated (Teather, Packard, & Bazan, 2001). Specifically, the S-R memory-enhancing effect of intrastriatal injections of mc-PAF was completely attenuated by prior systemic administration of the NMDA receptor antagonist MK-801. In contrast, peripheral administration of MK-801, which impairs cognitive memory when administered alone, did not prevent the cognitive memory-enhancing effect of intrahippocampal mc-PAF. Thus, it appears that PAF may be acting in a distinct fashion in the mechanisms underlying hippocampal and dorsal striatal memory consolidation. In both structures PAF can influence memory storage by eliciting glutamate release, thereby increasing NMDA receptor activation. However, in the hippocampus, part of the memory-enhancing effect of PAF appears to be downstream of NMDA receptor activation, possibly at intracellular binding sites within the hippocampus (Teather et al., 2001).

3. CONSOLIDATION OF HIPPOCAMPAL-DEPENDENT MEMORY REQUIRES INFLAMMATION/IMMUNE SIGNALS

Many biological responses induced by PAF result from its interaction with cell-surface PAF receptors; other effects of PAF have been attributed to the lipid interacting with intracellular binding sites. Activation of the intracellular PAF binding sites in neurons and glial cells increases the expression and/or activation of genes and proteins associated with immune/inflammatory reactions (Bazan, 1994), suggesting that these sites mediate the inflammatory responses to PAF in central nervous system (CNS) tissue (Teather & Wurtman, 2003). In fact, the intracellular sites are involved in inflammatory pain processing (Teather, Magnusson, & Wurtman, 2002).

Rapid inactivation of PAF is carried out by various species of PAF acetylhydrolase (PAF-AH). The primary intracellular isoform of PAF-AH in brain, PAF-AH 1b, is a heterotrimer comprised of three subunits (Hattori, Adachi, Tsujimoto, Arai, & Inoue, 1994). The β-subunit of PAF-AH 1b is a regulatory (i.e., noncatalytic) subunit that harnesses the two catalytic subunits: α_2, and the more catalytically active, α_1. Transgenic rats that express high brain levels of the α_1 subunit display hippocampal-dependent memory impairment; dorsal-striatal-dependent memory remains intact (Teather, 1998). These results suggest that increased brain expression of the most catalytically active intracellular PAF-AH 1b subunit (i.e., α_1), which would theoretically deplete cells of intracellular PAF, causes selective deficits in hippocampal-dependent memory.

Furthermore, posttraining intrahippocampal administration of BN 50730, a selective antagonist for the intracellular PAF binding sites, was found to impair cognitive memory formation; administration of BN 50730 into the dorsal striatum had no affect on S-R memory formation (Teather et al., 2001). Taken together, these findings support a role for intracellular PAF in hippocampal-dependent, but not dorsal striatal-dependent, memory processing. While the mechanism of action of intracellular PAF in hippocampal-dependent memory processing is not known, recent findings suggest that cytosolic PAF may participate in mnemonic functions via activation of an inflammatory enzyme.

Cyclooxygenase (COX) enzymes synthesize prostaglandins (PGs) from arachidonic acid. Two isoforms of COX have thus far been characterized; the housekeeping isoform COX-1, and the inducible inflammatory-immune isoform, COX-2 (Vane, Bakhl, & Botting, 1998). We recently demonstrated that activation of intracellular PAF binding sites with physiologically relevant concentrations of PAF rapidly elicits prostaglandin E_2 (PGE_2) release from primary rat astrocytes (Teather, Lee, & Wurtman, 2002). PAF-induced PGE_2 mobilization is dependent on COX-2 activity (Teather & Wurtman, 2003). Interestingly, PAF does not elicit PGE_2 release from primary rat cortical or hippocampal neurons or from human neuroblastoma cell lines.

Although COX-2 is undetectable in most tissues under basal conditions, marked constitutive expression has been observed in the CNS, particularly in hippocampus and cortex (Breder, Dewitt, & Kraig, 1995; Yamagata, Andreasson, Kaufmann, Barnes, & Worley, 1993), suggesting a role for this inflammatory isoform in physiological signaling within the CNS. Indeed, we (Teather, Packard, & Bazan, 2002), and others (Rall, Mach, & Dash., 2003) have shown that inhibition of COX-2 impairs hippocampal-dependent memory processing. In contrast, COX-2 inhibitors have no influence on striatal-dependent forms of memory (Teather, Packard, & Bazan, 2002). A dissociation of COX-2 mnemonic function in the striatum and hippocampus may stem from the fact that the striatum expresses low or even undetectable basal levels of COX-2 protein, while the hippocampus expresses very high constitutive levels of COX-2 (Teather, 1998). Thus, it appears that during early consolidation processes in the hippocampus, intracellular PAF induces the release of COX-2-derived mediators from astrocytes.

4. INFLAMMATORY SIGNALS IN PHYSIOLOGICAL MEMORY PROCESSING AND AGE-RELATED NEURODEGENERATION

Several mediators associated with inflammatory/immune events appear to be involved in hippocampal-based memory; these agents do not play an integral role in striatal-based memory. It is tempting to speculate that the use of inflammatory signals, such as intracellular PAF and COX-2-derived lipid mediators, for physiological memory formation in the hippocampus may predispose this neural system to age-related degenerative pathology. In fact, several lines of evidence suggest that this may indeed be the case.

Aging and Alzheimer's disease (AD) are characterized by progressive hippocampal-dependent cognitive decline combined with deterioration of the hippocampus, among other areas. Inflammatory mechanisms contribute to the neurodegeneration that accompanies AD and normal aging. In fact, a number of epidemiological and clinical studies indicate that long-term administration of non-steroidal anti-inflammatory drugs (NSAIDs) reduces the risk of developing AD (McGeer & McGeer, 1995). Recent findings suggest that chronic NSAID use also protects against age-associated cognitive deficits (Casolini, 2002). Interestingly, inhibition of COX-2 accounts largely for the therapeutic actions of many of these agents.

It would appear that an age-related shift in the brain status of COX-2 in the hippocampus occurs; inhibition of COX-2 in young brains impairs hippocampal-dependent memory formation, whereas COX-2 inhibition in pathological states alleviates cognitive deterioration. Thus, in physiological situations, with moderate levels of COX-2 expression and activation, this isoform is beneficial for hippocampal memory formation. However, overexpression of COX-2, such as that which occurs in aging and AD (Lukiw & Bazan, 1998), may be a result of overproduction related to chronic inflammatory events.

A loss of cholinergic neurons in basal forebrain nuclei is a prominent neuropathological hallmark of AD (Bartus, Dean, Beer, & Lippa, 1982) and aging (McGeer & McGeer 1995). An important role of brain inflammatory reaction in cholinergic degeneration has recently been demonstrated in rats (Scali et al., 2003). Specifically, quisqualic acid injection into the nucleus basalis induced reactive astrogliosis, increased the expression of several pro-inflammatory mediators, and induced a marked loss of cholinergic cells; COX-2 inhibitors prevented these effects. These findings support the contention that COX-2-derived PGs, possibly from activated astrocytes, could be a key element in the etiopathologies underlying AD and aging.

Following an immune/inflammatory challenge, astrocytes undergo a phenotypic alteration—a response known as activation. Activated astrocytes then release cytokines and other pro-inflammatory signals, including COX-2-derived PGs (Teather & Wurtman, 2003). In fact, astrocytes are a major source of PGs in the CNS; in culture these cells synthesize up to 20 times more PGs than do neurons. PGs and several enzymes involved in PG production are increased in AD (Lukiw & Bazan, 1998; Stephenson, Lemere,

Selkoe, & Clemens, 1996) and aging (Casolini et al., 2002). A role for astrocyte-derived PGs in neuronal cell death has been demonstrated. For example, PGE_2 stimulates astrocytic glutamate release and prevents astrocytes from taking up glutamate (Bezzi et al., 1998), the consequent increase in extracellular glutamate is neurotoxic (Drachman & Rothstein, 2000).

PAF concentrations in plasma show significant age-related increases (Zhang et al., 2003). Although PAF levels in AD have not yet been assessed, several interesting findings suggest that this lipid mediator may be involved in age-related hippocampal pathogenesis. First, mice inoculated with LP-BM5 murine leukemia viruses (resulting in murine acquired immunodeficiency syndrome) display hippocampal-dependent cognitive deficits, hippocampal pathology similar to AD, and increased brain PAF levels (Nishida et al., 1996). Moreover, in HIV-infected patients brain PAF levels were found to correlate with hippocampal-dependent cognitive deficits (Gelbard et al., 1994). Finally, it has been suggested that the reduction in PAF platelet binding observed in AD patients is a result of an increase in PAF levels, which can cause a decrease in PAF receptors via negative-feedback mechanisms (Hershkowitz & Adunsky, 1996). Thus, increased brain levels of PAF could be involved in the age-related shift in COX-2 function in the hippocampus (i.e., from beneficial in young brains to damaging in aged brains).

5. STRESS AND INFLAMMATORY MEDIATORS IN HIPPOCAMPAL-BASED MEMORY PROCESSING AND NEURODEGENERATION

The hypothalamic–pituitary–adrenocortical (HPA) axis is activated in response to stress and inflammation, resulting in the enhanced release of adrenal glucocorticoids, such as corticosterone (CORT), the principal glucocorticoid synthesized by rodents (cortisol being the equivalent compound in humans). Numerous studies have shown that stress can impair cognitive processes (for review, *see* de Kloet, Vereugdenhil, Oitzl, & Joels, 1998), although others suggest a facilitative role for stress in memory storage (for review, *see* Roozendaal, 2000). The reason for the contrasting results could be owing to the nature and/or memory systems responsible for the processing of the various tasks. Acute stress impairs hippocampal-dependent memory, while enhancing striatal-dependent memory, suggesting that stress can bias the brain toward the use of a specific memory system (Kim, Lee, Han, & Packard, 2001). Perhaps the increase in CORT that occurs during the stress response affects hippocampal learning and memory processes via actions on mnemonic inflammatory-related mediators.

It is well known that CORT has anti-inflammatory and immunosuppressive properties. Thus, it is possible that CORT impairs hippocampal memory processing by suppressing the required inflammatory-related signals necessary for consolidation. As the hippocampal and dorsal striatal memory systems appear to be dynamically interactive rather than independent modules, it is not surprising that dysfunction of the hippocampal system often has beneficial effects on the striatal system owing to the competitive interaction between the systems.

Inflammatory stimuli elicit HPA axis activation, and it is well established that the inflammatory/immune and HPA systems are mutually regulatory and that their interactions partly determine stress effects on immune function. It is tempting to speculate that the interaction between the HPA axis and inflammatory mediators also determine the effects on cognitive function and potentially the development of hippocampal-based age-related neurodegeneration. Interestingly, the hippocampus plays a prominent role in modulating the negative feedback effect of glucocorticoids on HPA axis activity (Jacobsen & Sapolosky, 1991). In fact, the hippocampus may have evolved as an immune structure to monitor the internal state of the organism; thus, the hippocampus has the mechanisms for inflammatory/immune signaling. Perhaps as memory processing became a hippocampal function (during the evolution of multiple memory systems), this structure used the available inflammatory mediators for mnemonic purposes. In fact, early hippocampal consolidation appears to be similar to acute inflammatory reactions with respect to signal transduction cascades (Teather et al., 2001). It is reasonable to assume that the reliance on such signals may predispose the hippocampal system to age-related degeneration.

Aging and AD are associated with HPA axis dysfunction, and elevations in CORT are correlated with the decline in hippocampal function (Lupien et al., 1998). It has been suggested that the mechanism underlying brain aging involves chronically elevated levels of glucocorticoids, which damage and/or kill hippocampal cells, ultimately leading to the progressive inability of limbic-driven mechanisms to mediate the HPA axis to control or shut off the neuroendocrine response to stress (Sapolsky, Krey, & McEwen, 1986). In fact, prolonged stress or exposure to CORT accelerates the age-related loss and/or dysfunction of neurons in the hippocampus of rats and increases reactive glia at this site (Sapolsky et al., 1986), suggesting an interaction between stress and inflammatory components in the hippocampus.

It has been suggested that the increased CORT levels associated with brain degenerative processes may be an adaptive response to the progression of the inflammatory components (Casolini et al., 2002). During aging, the hippocampal content of various inflammatory markers and the plasma corticosterone levels increase significantly in rats (Casolini et al., 2002). However, although CORT has previously been shown to inhibit the production of inflammatory mediators in brain (Chrousos, 1995; Lee et al., 1988), recent evidence suggests that higher concentrations may actually have pro-inflammatory effects (Dinkel, MacPherson, & Sapolsky, 2003).

6. CONCLUSIONS

The mammalian brain is comprised of distinct memory systems, including the dorsal striatal and hippocampal systems. While these neural structures use several common mediators during early memory consolidation, an important distinction has been revealed. The hippocampus, possibly owing to its role as an immune structure, requires the use of acute inflammatory response mediators for physiological consolidation. As several neurodegenerative disorders are associated with chronic central inflammation processes, it is feasible that the reliance of the hippocampal system on inflammatory mediators predisposes this system to age-related cognitive dysfunction and cell death.

While excitoxicity via the glutamatergic/NMDA receptor cascade has often been implicated in neurodegenerative disorders affecting both the striatum (e.g., Parkinson's disease) and hippocampus (e.g., AD and aging), it is possible that the hippocampus is selectively affected by age-related degenerative processes due the use of intracellular PAF and COX-2. A myriad of cell types, including the immune/inflammatory resident cell astrocytes, produce and/or respond to PAF and COX-2-derived lipids, suggesting the possibility that a shift in production and/or response may occur as a function of aging.

Although systemic CORT has immunosuppressive and anti-inflammatory effects, recent evidence suggests that high levels of CORT induce pro-inflammatory effects in the CNS and exacerbate excitotoxin-induced hippocampal cell death (Dinkel, MacPherson, & Sapolsky, 2003). Perhaps part of the mnemonic effects of stress can be attributed to interaction between the HPA axis-derived CORT and inflammatory agents in the hippocampus. Much work remains to be done to assess the interactions between HPA axis-derived stress and inflammatory mediators, both in physiological memory processing and pathological degeneration.

REFERENCES

Bartus, R. T., Dean, R. L., Beer, B., & Lippa, A. S. (1982). The cholinergic hypothesis of geriatric memory dysfunction. *Science, 217*, 408–417.

Bazan, N. G. (1994). Platelet-activating factor is a synapse messenger and an intracellular modulator of gene expression. *Journal of Lipid Mediators and Cell Signaling, 10*, 83–86.

Bazan, N. G. (1995). Inflammation: A signal terminator. *Nature, 374*, 501–502.

Bezzi, P., Carmignoto, G., Pasti, L., Vesce, S., Rossi, D., Rizzini, B. L., Pozzan, T., & Volterra, A. (1998). Prostaglandins stimulate calcium-dependent glutamate release in astrocytes. *Nature, 391*, 281–285.

Bliss, T. V. P., & Collingridge, G. L. (1993). A synaptic model of memory: Long-term potentiation in the hippocampus. *Nature, 361*, 31–39.

Breder, C. D., Dewitt, D., & Kraig, R. P. (1995). Characterization of inducible cyclooxygenase in rat brain. *Journal of Comparative Neurology, 355*, 296–315.

Casolini, P., Catalani, A., Zuena, A. R., & Angelucci, L. (2002). Inhibition of COX-2 reduces the age-dependent increase of hippocampal inflammatory markers, corticosterone secretion, and behavioral impairments in the rat. *Journal of Neuroscience Research, 68*, 337–343.

Chrousos, G. P. (1995). The hypothalamic-pituitary-adrenal axis and immune-mediated inflammation. *New England Journal of Medicine, 332*, 1351–1362.

Cohen, N. J., & Squire, L. R. (1980). Preserved learning of pattern analyzing skill in amnesia: dissociation of knowing how and knowing that. *Science, 210*, 207–210.

de Kloet, E. R., Vereugdenhil, E., Oitzl, M. S., & Joels, M. (1998). Brain corticoidsteroid receptor balance in health and disease. *Endocrinological Review, 19*, 269–301.

Drachman, D. B., & Rothstein, J. D. (2000). Inhibition of cyclooxygenase-2 protects motor neurons in an organotypic model of amyotrophic lateral sclerosis. *Annals of Neurology, 48*, 792–795.

Gelbard, H. A., Nottet, H. S. L. M., Swindells, S., Jett, M., Dzenko, K. A., Genis, P., White, R., Wang, L., Choi, Y. -B., Zhang, D., Lipton, S. A., Tourtellotte, W. W., Epstein, L. G., & Gendelman, H. (1994). Platelet-activating factor: A candidate human immunodeficiency virus type 1-induced neurotoxin. *Journal of Virology, 68*, 4628–4635.

Hattori, M., Adachi, H., Tsujimoto, M., Arai, H., & Inoue, K. (1994). Miller-Dieker lissencephaly gene encodes a subunit of brain platelet-activating factor. *Nature, 370*, 216–218.

Hershkowitz, M., & Adunsky, A. (1996). Binding of platelet-activating factor to platelets of Alzheimer's disease and multipinfarct dementia patients. *Neurobiology of Aging, 17*, 865–868.

Hirsh, R. (1974). The hippocampus and contextual retrieval of information from memory: A theory. *Behavioral Biology, 12*, 421–442.

Izquierdo, I., da Chuna, C., Rosat, R., Jerusalinsky, D., Ferreiara, M. B. C., & Medina, H. (1992). Neurotransmitter receptors involved in post-training memory processing by the amygdala, medial septum, and hippocampus of the rat. *Behavioral and Neural Biology, 58*, 16–26.

Izquierdo, I., Fin, C., Schmitz, P. K., Da Silva, R., Jerusalinsky, D., Quillfeldt, J. A., Ferreiara, M. B. C., Medina, J. H., & Bazan, N. G. (1995). Memory enhancement by intrahippocampal, intraamygdala, or intraentorhinal infusion of platelet-activating factor measured in an inhibitory avoidance task. *Proceedings of the National Academy of Science, 92*, 5047–5051.

Jacobson, L., & Sapolsky, R. M. (1991). The role of the hippocampus in feedback regulation of the hypothalamic-pituitary-adrenocortical axis. *Endocrinological Review, 12*, 118–134.

Kadoyama, K., Takahashi, Y., Higashida, H., Tanabe, T., & Yoshimoto, T. (2001). COX-2 stimulates production of amyloid beta-peptide in neuroblastoma X glioma hybrid NG108-15 cells. *Biochemica Biophysica Research Communications, 281*, 483–488.

Kato, K., Clark, G. D., Bazan, N. G., & Zorumski, C. F. (1994). Platelet-activating factor as a potential retrograde messenger in CA1 hippocampal long-term potentiation. *Nature, 367*, 175–179.

Kim, J. J., Lee, H. J., Han, J. -S., Packard, M. G. (2001). Amygdala is critical for stress-induced modulation of hippocampal long-term potentiation and learning. *Journal of Neuroscience, 21*, 5222–5228.

Lukiw, W. J., & Bazan, N. G. (1998). Strong nuclear factor-kb-DNA binding parallels cyclooxygenase-2 gene transcription in aging and in sproradic Alzheimer's disease superior temporal lobe cortex. *Journal of Neuroscience Research, 53*, 583–592.

Lupien, S. J., de Leon, M., de Santi, S., Convit, A., Tarhish, C., Nair, N. P., Thakur, M., McEwen, B. S., Hauger, R. L., & Meaney, M. J. (1998). Corisol levels during human aging predict hippocampal atrophy and memory deficits. *Nature Neuroscience, 1*, 69–73.

McDonald, R. J., & White, N. M. (1993). A triple dissociation of memory systems: Hippocampus, amygdala, and dorsal striatum. *Behavioral Neuroscience, 107*, 3–22.

McGeer, P. L., & McGeer, E. G. (1995). The inflammatory response system of brain: Implications for therapy of Alzheimer and other neurodegenerative diseases. *Brain Research Reviews, 21*, 195–218.

Nishida, K., Markey, S. P., Kustova, Y., Morse, H. C., III, Skolnick, P., Basile, A. S., & Sei, Y. (1996). Increased brain levels of platelet-activating factor in a murine aquired immune deficiency syndrome are NMDA receptor-mediated. *Journal of Neurochemistry, 66*, 433–435.

Ottersen, O. P., Hjelle, O. P., Osen, K. K., & Laake, J. H. (1995). Amino acid transmitters. In G. Paxinos (Ed.), *The rat nervous system* (pp. 1017–1040). New York: Academic.

Ottersen, O. P., & Storm-Mathisen, J. (1989). Excitatory and inhibitor amino acids in the hippocampus. In V. Chan-Palay & C. Kohler (Eds.), *The hippocampus: New vistas* (pp. 97–117). New York: Liss.

Packard, M. G., Hirsh, R., & White, N. M. (1989). Differential effects of fornix and caudate nucleus lesions on two radial maze tasks: Evidence for multiple memory systems. *Journal of Neuroscience, 9*, 1465–1472.

Packard, M. G., & Teather, L. A. (1997a). Double dissociation of hippocampal and dorsal-striatal memory systems by posttraining injections of 2-amino-5-phosphopentanoic acid. *Behavioral Neuroscience, 111*, 543–551.

Packard, M. G., & Teather, L. A. (1997b). Posttraining injections of MK-801 produce a time-dependent impairment of memory in two water maze tasks. *Neurobiology of Learning and Memory, 68*, 42–50.

Packard, M. G., & Teather, L. A. (1998). Amygdala modulation of multiple memory systems: Hippocampus and caudate-putamen. *Neurobiology of Learning and Memory, 69*, 163–203.

Packard, M. G., & Teather, L. A. (1999). Dissociation of multiple memory systems by posttraining intracerebral injections of glutamate. *Psychobiology, 27*, 40–50.

Packard, M. G., & White, N. M. (1990). Lesions of the caudate nucleus selectively impair acquisition of "reference memory" in the radial maze. *Behavioral and Neural Biology, 53*, 39–50.

Packard, M. G., & White, N. M. (1991). Dissociation of hippocampus and caudate nucleus memory systems by posttraining intracerebral injection of dopamine agonists. *Behavioral Neuroscience, 105*, 295–306.

Power, A. E., Vazdarjanova, A., & McGaugh, J. L. (2003). Muscarinic cholinergic influences in memory consolidation. *Neurobiology of Learning and Memory, 80*, 178–193.

Rall, J. M., Mach, S. A., & Dash, P. K. (2003). Intrahippocampal infusion of a cyclooxygenase-2 inhibitor attenuates memory acquisition in rats. *Brain Research, 968*, 273–276.

Roozendaal, B. (2000). Glucocorticoids and the regulation of memory consolidation. *Psychoneuroendocrinology, 25*, 213–238.

Sapolsky, R. M., Krey, L. C., & McEwen, B. S. (1986). The neuroendocrinology of stress and aging: the glucocorticoid cascade hypothesis. *Endocrinological Review, 7*, 284–301.

Scali, C., Giovannini, M. G., Prosperi, C., Bellucci, A., Pepeu, G., & Casamenti, F. (2003). The selective cyclooxygenase-2 inhibitor rofecoxib suppresses brain inflammation and protects neurons from excitotoxic degeneration in vivo. *Neuroscience, 117*, 909–919.

Stephenson, D. T., Lemere, C. A., Selkoe, D. J., & Clemens, J. A. (1996). Cytosolic phospholipase A_2 ($cPLA_2$) immunoreactivity is elevated in Alzheimer's disease brain. *Neurobiology of Disease, 3*, 51–63.

Teather, L. A. (1998). Neurobiological mechanisms of anatomically and functionally distinct mammalian memory systems. In *Neuroscience* (p. 334). New Orleans: Louisiana State University Medical Center.

Teather, L. A., Lee, R. K. K., & Wurtman, R. J. (2002). Platelet-activating factor increases prostaglandin E2 release from astrocyte-enriched cortical cell cultures. *Brain Research, 946,* 87–95.

Teather, L. A., Magnusson, J. E., & Wurtman, R. J. (2002). Platelet-activating factor antagonists decrease the inflammatory nociceptive response in rats. *Psychopharmacology, 163,* 430–433.

Teather, L. A., Packard, M. G., & Bazan, N. G. (1998). Effects of post-training intra-hippocampal injections of platelet-activating factor and PAF antagonists on memory. *Neurobiology of Learning and Memory, 70,* 349–363.

Teather, L. A., Packard, M. G., & Bazan, N. G. (2001). Differential interaction of platelet-activating factor and NMDA receptor function in hippocampal and dorsal striatal memory processes. *Neurobiology of Learning and Memory, 75,* 310–324.

Teather, L. A., Packard, M. G., & Bazan, N. G. (2002). Post-training cyclooxygenase-2 (COX-2) inhibition impairs memory consolidation. *Learning and Memory, 9,* 41–47.

Teather, L. A., & Wurtman, R. J. (2003). Cyclooxygenase-2 mediates platlet-activating factor-induced prostaglandin E2 release from primary astrocytes. *Neuroscience Letters, 340,* 177–180.

White, N. M. (1989). A functional hypothesis concerning the striatal matrix and patches: Mediation of S-R memory and reward. *Life Sciences, 45,* 1943–1957.

Vane, J. R., Bakhl, Y. S., & Botting, R. M. (1998). Cyclooxygenases 1 and 2. *Annual Review of Pharmacology and Toxicology, 38,* 97–120.

Yamagata, K., Andreasson, K. I., Kaufmann, W. E., Barnes, C. A., & Worley, P. F. (1993). Expression of a mitogen-inducible cyclooxygenase in brain neurons: Regulation by synaptic activity and glucocorticoids. *Neuron, 11,* 371–386.

25 The Interaction Between Nutrition and Inflammatory Stress Throughout the Life Cycle

Robert F. Grimble

KEY POINTS

- Inflammation not only is an essential process for recovery from infection and injury, but plays an adverse role in chronic inflammatory diseases, heart disease, and diabetes mellitus.
- Inflammation is controlled by cytokines.
- Polymorphisms in cytokine genes influence the inherent level of cytokine production in individuals and have been linked with an increased propensity for the adverse effects of inflammation.
- Polymorphisms in cytokine genes influence longevity.
- Obesity and aging increase the level of inflammatory stress in the body.
- Dietary supplementation with antioxidants and *n*-3 polyunsaturated fatty acids suppress adverse aspects of cytokine biology.

1. INTRODUCTION: THE IMMUNE RESPONSE AS A PURPOSEFUL ACTIVITY

The human race inhabits a world in which it is surrounded by a myriad of different microorganisms—yeasts, bacteria, protozoa, and viruses. Most of these are benign, and some, such as the normal gut flora, play an important part in promoting health via the synthesis of vitamins and stimulation of normal function of gut epithelia. Approximately 0.1% of microbes in our environment have catastrophic effects if they penetrate the epithelial surfaces of the body (Bryson, 2003). History reveals many instances in which armies have been defeated and civilizations have collapsed because of encounters between humans and such microorganisms (Diamond, 1999).

Humans, like all mammals, have evolved with a complex immune system, which is present as specialized organs (spleen, thymus) or cell types (lymphocytes, macrophages, and mast cells) throughout the body. The system can detect and destroy any cell or particle that is not "self," i.e., a normal component of the body. A complex series of events follows from contact between components of the immune system and microbes invading the body

From: *Nutrients, Stress, and Medical Disorders*
Edited by: S. Yehuda and D. I. Mostofsky © Humana Press Inc., Totowa, NJ

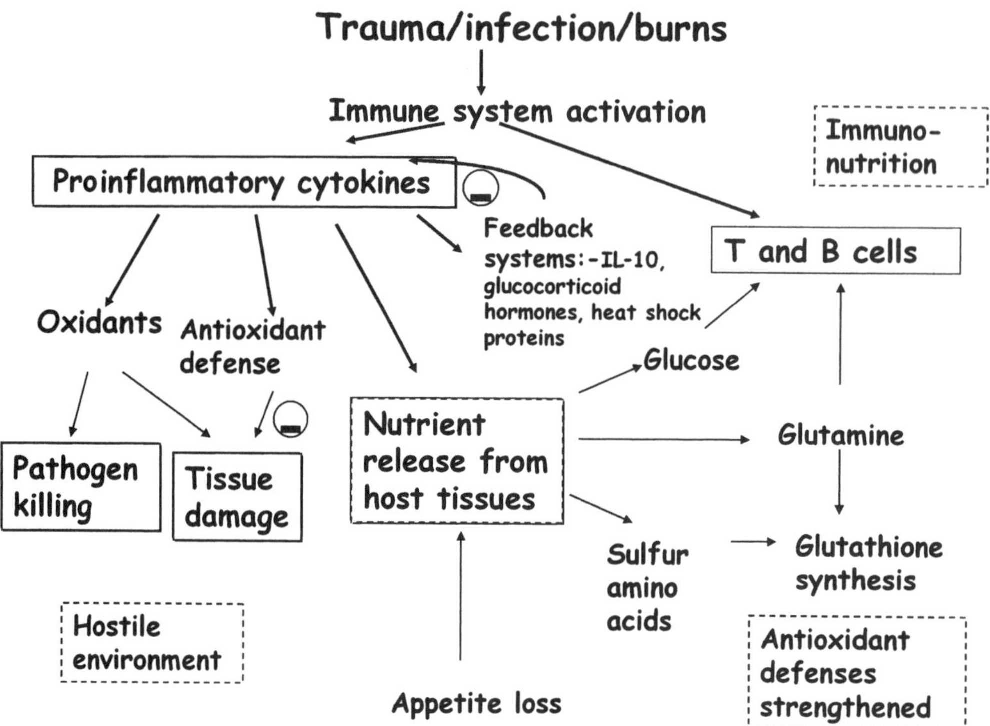

Fig. 1. Overview of the metabolic and immunological response to injury and infection. Proinflammatory cytokine production orchestrates the nonspecific inflammatory response; T and B cells carry out the specific immune response.

(Fig. 1). The response can be divided into two main categories. The first is the acquired immune response, in which the immune system recognizes specific chemical motifs on the invader and "remembers" the encounter so that a more rapid, specific, and intense response can be produced at any future meeting. The second category is the nonspecific response in which the response to each encounter is similar for all invaders of the body. The process of inflammation is a central part of the second category of response. The immune response is also activated by a wide range of adverse events, such as surgery, burns, and trauma.

The primary purposes of the response are to kill pathogens and initiate the curative processes that will restore body function to normal. The first purpose is achieved by creating a hostile tissue environment through production of oxidant molecules and activation of T and B lymphocytes. Part of the response ensures a supply of substrate, from endogenous sources, for supporting the activity of T and B lymphocytes and enhancement of antioxidant defenses. The latter event is important for protecting healthy tissue from the oxidants produced as part of the inflammatory response (Grimble, 2001a). The response exerts considerable biological demands and stress on the body. A central part of substrate provision is the release of amino acids into the blood from the breakdown of proteins in skeletal muscle, skin, and bone matrix, and fatty acids released from triglycerides stored in adipose tissue. Enhanced gluconeogenesis, catabolic hormone production, and decreased insulin sensitivity occurs to facilitate this redistribution of tissue

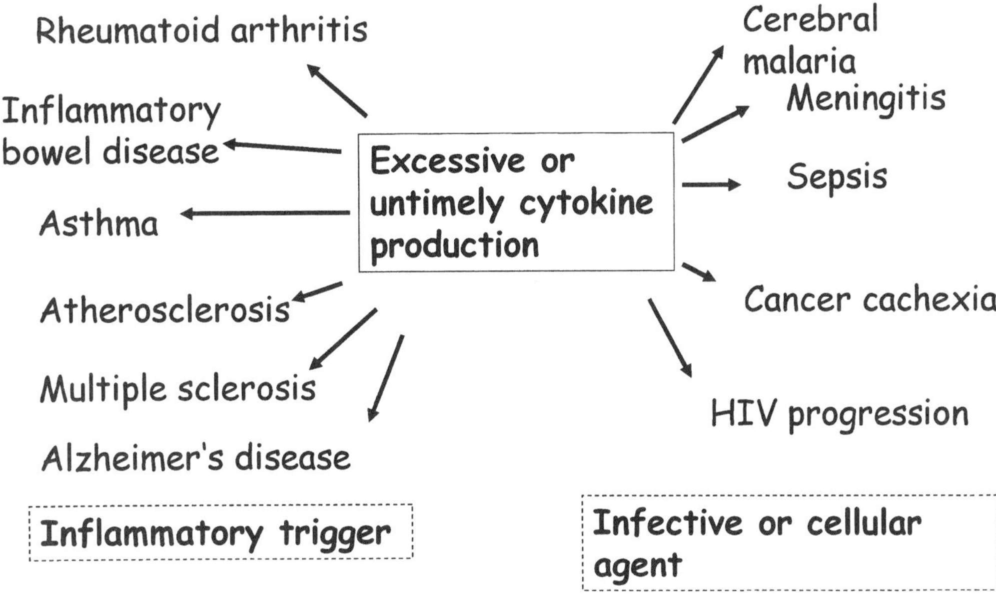

Fig. 2. Diseases and conditions in which inappropriate or excessive amounts of pro-inflammatory cytokines exert adverse or lethal effects on the host.

components (Fig. 1). The animal loses the desire to carry out many day-to-day activities. Physical weakness ensues, exploratory activity declines, appetite is decreased, and apathy and sleep may occur. The response thus exerts physiological and mental stress upon the body.

Inflammation comes under the control of signaling proteins (cytokines) that possess hormone-like actions. The pro-inflammatory cytokines interleukin (IL)-1β, IL-6, and tumor necrosis factor (TNF)-α, are major activators and modulators of the events described above. To modulate the degree of stress imposed on the body, in achieving the essential functions of inflammation, the response comes under the control of powerful anti-inflammatory mechanisms. These will impose their biological effects with increasing vigor as the original stimulus for the inflammatory response (infection, injury) declines in intensity. Heat-shock proteins, endorphins, glucocorticoid hormones, and cytokine receptor antagonists are important components of this anti-inflammatory system.This system is essential for closing down the inflammatory response once it has achieved its primary purposes because of the high biological cost it imposes on the body (Grimble, 2001a).

1.1. Pathological Effects of the Inflammatory Response

Although cytokines play an important role in the response to infection and injury, they can exert damaging and lethal effects on the host. Many studies have shown that excessive or prolonged production of cytokines is associated with increased morbidity and mortality in a wide range of acute and chronic inflammatory conditions (Fig. 2). These include sepsis, adult respiratory distress syndrome, malaria, meningitis, cancer, cystic fibrosis, systemic lupus erythematosus, inflammatory bowel disease, rheumatoid arthritis, and asthma.

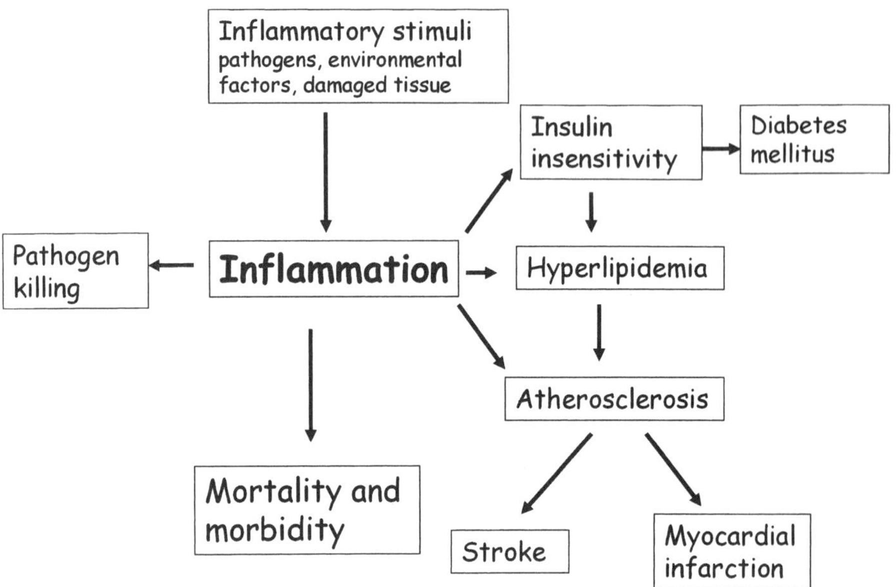

Fig. 3. Overview of the interrelationships between the inflammatory response to pathogens and diseases and pathology with a covert inflammatory basis.

Events similar to those seen in the inflammatory response to injury and infection can be observed during the course of overt inflammatory diseases such as rheumatoid arthritis and Crohn's disease and in diseases that have a covert inflammatory basis, for example, atherosclerosis and diabetes mellitus (Fig. 3). Clearly the inflammatory response in these situations does not have a purposeful nature and contribute to the disease process. Recent studies indicate that low-intensity inflammation occurs in elderly and obese individuals (Grimble 2002, 2003). Thus, the inflammatory response, which has evolved to allow humankind to survive infection and injury, is indiscriminate in both its triggers and targets. As a result, the process is a two-edged sword capable of both defending and damaging its bearer.

During the remainder of this chapter we will be exploring the biological and nutritional factors that determine the intensity of, and outcome from, the inflammatory process.

2. MAJOR FACTORS INFLUENCING THE STRENGTH AND OUTCOME OF THE INFLAMMATORY RESPONSE

2.1. Interactions Between Components of the Inflammatory Response

Various components of the inflammatory response interact to modulate its intensity. Predominant among these interactions are the relative amounts of pro- and anti-inflammatory cytokines produced during the response to microbes and injury and the effect of oxidant molecules on cytokine production.

2.1.1. The Balance Between Pro- and Anti-Inflammatory Cytokine Production

Early work on cytokines and the response to infection linked excessive pro-inflammatory cytokine production with increased morbidity and mortality in a wide range of conditions, such as malaria, meningitis, and sepsis. However, research in the last 5 yr has shown that the balance in production between pro- and anti-inflammatory cytokines has a more direct bearing on the outcome of infection and injury. For example, in sepsis, plasma IL-6 concentrations were higher and IL-10 concentrations were lower in patients who died than in those who survived (Arnalich et al., 2000;Taniguchi et al., 1999). A survey of over 400 patients admitted to hospital in the Netherlands with fever showed that, independently of how the patients were clinically classified (positive blood cultures, presence of endotoxin), those who subsequently died had a higher plasma IL-10:TNF-α ratio than patients who survived (Van Dissell, van Langervelde, Westendorp, Kwappenberg, & Frolich, 1998).

2.1.2. Interaction Between Oxidant Stress and Inflammation

Powerful oxidant molecules (e.g., superoxide, hydrogen peroxide, hypochlorous acid) are produced as part of the inflammatory response. Their biological purpose is to destroy invading microbes. However, these molecules also have the capacity to damage host tissues and to increase the intensity of the inflammatory response. Clearly both of these biological events can have adverse effects upon the host.

The oxidant molecules activate at least two important families of proteins in the host that are sensitive to changes in cellular redox state. The families are nuclear transcription factor κ B (NF-κB) and activator protein 1 (AP1). These transcription factors act as "control switches" for biological processes, not all of which are of advantage to the individual. NF-κB is present in the cytosol in an inactive form, by virtue of being bound to an inhibitory unit I-κB. Phosphorylation and dissociation of I-κB renders the remaining NF-κB dimer active. The dissociated I-κB is degraded, and the active NF-κB is translocated to the nucleus, where it binds to response elements in the promoter regions of genes. A similar translocation of AP1, a transcription factor composed of the protooncogenes *c-fos* and *c-jun*, from cytosol to nucleus, also occurs in the presence of oxidant stress. Binding of the transcription factors is implicated in activation of a wide range of genes associated with inflammation and the immune response, including those encoding cytokines, cytokine receptors, cell adhesion molecules, acute-phase proteins, and growth factors (Schreck, Rieber, & Baeurerle, 1991) (Fig. 4). Activation of NF-κB can be brought about by a wide range of stimuli including pro-inflammatory cytokines, hydrogen peroxide, mitogens, bacteria and viruses and their related products, and ultraviolet (UV) and ionizing radiations. The extent of activation of NF-κB will depend in part upon the strength and efficiency of the antioxidant defenses of the body. These comprise endogenous components such as glutathione (GSH) and enzymatic components of antioxidant defenses, such as catalase, superoxide dismutase (SOD), and GSH peroxidase, and dietary components that have antioxidant properties (e.g., vitamins C and E and polyphenolic compounds). The influence of modulation of inflammation by these dietary factors are dealt with later.

An unfortunate side effect of activation of NF-κB arises from the ability of the transcription factor to activate transcription of the genes of some viruses, such as human immunodeficiency virus (HIV) (Fig. 4). This sequence of events, in the case of HIV, accounts for the ability of minor infections to speed the progression of individuals who are infected with HIV towards acquired immunodeficiency syndrome (AIDS). Thus, if antioxidant defenses are poor, each encounter with general infections results in cytokine and oxidant production, NF-κB activation, and an increase in HIV replication. It is thus

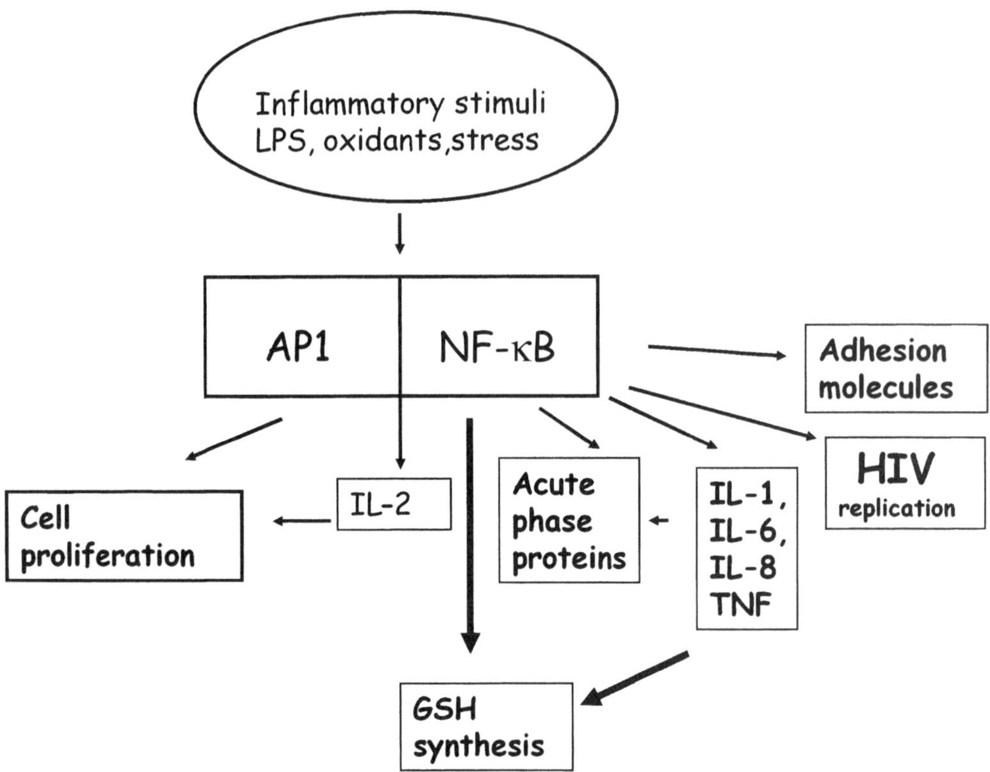

Fig. 4. Gene products whose synthesis is enhanced following activation of transcription factors by oxidant stress. NF-κB, nuclear factor κB; AP1, activator protein 1; IL-2, interleukin-2; HIV, human immunodeficiency virus.

unfortunate that reduced cellular concentrations of GSH are a common feature of infections, including that from the HIV (Staal, Ela, & Roederer, 1992).

Oxidant damage to cells will indirectly create a pro-inflammatory effect by the production of lipid peroxides. This situation may also lead to upregulation of NF-κB activity.

As will be seen in later sections, genetic and dietary factors change the intensity of the inflammatory response. Thus, although the inflammatory response has evolved to ensure the survival of the human species, individuals may die as a result primarily of the response to invasion rather than from the invasive agent itself.

2.2. Genetic Influences on the Intensity of the Inflammatory Process

2.2.1. Genomic Effects on Cytokine Production

It has recently become apparent that single base changes (single-nucleotide polymorphisms [SNPs]), usually in the promoter region of genes responsible for producing the molecules involved in the inflammatory process, exert a modulatory effect on the intensity of inflammation. In vitro production of TNF-α by peripheral blood mononuclear cells (PBMCs) from healthy and diseased subjects stimulated with inflammatory agents shows remarkable individual constancy in males and postmenopausal females (Jacob et al., 1990). This constancy suggests that genetic factors exert a strong influence. A number of studies have shown that SNPs in the promoter regions for the TNF-α and lymphotoxin

Table 1
Single Nucleotide Polymorphisms (SNPs) in Cytokine Genes Associated With Altered Levels of Cytokine Production[a]

Gene and location of polymorphism in promoter region	*Genotype associated with raised cytokine production and/or altered clinical outcome to inflammation[b]*
Pro-inflammatory cytokines	
TNF-α – 308	TNF-α – 308 A allele (TNF2)
LT-α + 252	LT-α + 252 AA (TNFB2:2)
IL-1β – 511	CT or TT
IL-6 – 174	G allelle
Anti-inflammatory cytokines	
IL-10 – 1082[c]	GG
TGF-1β+915 (arg-25-pro)[c]	GG

TNF, tumor necrosis factor; LT, lymphotoxin; IL, interleukin; TGF, transforming growth factor; C, cytosine; G, guanosine; T, thymidine, A, adenine.

[a]The location of the polymorphism is indicated by the nucleotide position in the promotor region.

[b]Poor clinical outcome for pro-inflammatory cytokines.

[c]Improved clinical outcome for anti-inflammatory cytokines.

(LT)-α genes are associated with differential TNF-α production (Allen, 1999; Messer et al., 1991; Wilson et al., 1993). The TNF2 (A) and TNFB2 (A) alleles (at -308 and +252 for the TNF-α and LT-α genes, respectively) are linked to high TNF production, particularly in homozygous individuals. The SNP in the LT-α gene (+252) is found in linkage disequilibrium with major histocompatibility molecules HLA-A1, B8, DR3 (Messer et al., 1991; Wilson et al., 1993). This genotype has also been reported to define a TNF "high expresser" haplotype (Warzocha et al., 1998), in addition to modifying expression of LT-α itself (Messer et al., 1991). A large body of research has indicated that SNPs occur in the upstream regulatory (promoter) regions of many cytokine genes (Bidwell et al., 2001). Many of these genetic variations influence the level of expression of genes and the outcome from the inflammatory response. Both pro- and anti-inflammatory cytokines are influenced by the differences in genotype (Allen 1999; Turner, Williams, & Sankeran, 1997). A number of SNPs that have been implicated in the outcome of inflammatory stress are shown in Table 1.

2.2.2. Genomic Effects on Induction of Oxidant Molecules

NF-κB is activated by oxidants and switches on many of the genes involved in the inflammatory response (cytokines, adhesion molecules, and acute-phase proteins). Enhancement of antioxidant defenses is important in protecting healthy tissues and in preventing excessive activation of NF-κB by the oxidative cellular environment during inflammation (Schreck et al., 1991). NF-κB upregulates cytokine and adhesion molecule expression, increasing the risk of host damage (Jersmann, Hii, Ferrante, & Ferrante, 2001).

Genetic factors also influence the propensity of individuals to produce oxidant molecules and thereby influence NF-κB activation. Natural resistance-associated macrophage protein 1 (NRAMP1) has effects on macrophage functions, including TNF-α production and activation of inducible nitric oxide synthase (iNOS), which occurs by cooperation between the NRAMP1, TNF-α, and LT-α genes (Ables et al., 2001). There are four variations in the NRAMP1 gene, resulting in different basal levels of activity and differential sensitivity to stimulation by inflammatory agents. Alleles 1, 2, and 4 are poor promoters, whereas allele 3 causes high gene expression. Hyperactivity of macrophages, associated with allele 3, is linked to autoimmune disease susceptibility and high resistance to infection, whereas allele 2 increases susceptibility to infection and protects against autoimmune disease (Searle & Blackwell, 1999).

As indicated earlier, a number of molecules suppress production of pro-inflammatory cytokines and exert an anti-inflammatory influence. These include antioxidant defenses and IL-10 (Chernoff et al., 1995; Espevik et al., 1987). Production is modulated by genetic factors. There are at least three polymorphic sites (-1082, -819, -592) in the IL-10 promoter that influence production (Perrey, Pravice, Sinnott, & Hutchinson, 1998). SNPs also occur in genes encoding enzymatic components of antioxidant defenses, such as catalase, SOD, and GSH peroxidase, which influence levels of activity (Chorazy, Schumacher, & Edlind, 1992; Forsberg, Lyrenas, de Faire, & Morgenstern, 2001; Mitrunen et al., 2001).

There is circumstantial evidence, that at an individual level, an inflammatory genotype exists that can adversely effect the host. In a study of inflammatory lung disease caused by exposure to coal dust, the TNF2 (LT-α+252 A) allele was almost twice as common in miners with the disease than in those who were healthy (Zhai, Jetten, Schins, Franssen, & Borm, 1998). Development of farmer's lung from exposure to hay dust was 80% greater in individuals with the TNF2 allele than in those without the allele (Schaaf, Seitzer, Pravica, Aries, & Zabel, 2001). The TNF2 allele was also twice as common in smokers who developed chronic obstructive pulmonary disease than in those who remained disease-free (Sakao et al., 2001). In addition to disease progression, genetic factors have important effects on mortality and morbidity in infectious and inflammatory disease. During malaria, children who were homozygous for TNF2 had a sevenfold greater risk of death or serious pathology than children who were homozygous for the TNF1 allele (McGuire, Hill, Allsopp, Greenwood, & Kwiatkowski, 1994). In intensive-care patients the occurrence of 1082*G high-producing allele for IL-10 was present in those who developed multiorgan failure with a frequency of one-fifth of that of the normal population (Reid, Hutchinson, Campbell, & Little, 1999). In sepsis, patients possessing the TNF2 allele had a 3.7-fold greater risk of death than those without the allele, and patients who were homozygous for the LT-α+252 A allele had twice the mortality rate and higher peak plasma TNF-α concentrations than heterozygotic individuals (Mira et al., 1999; Stuber, Peterson, Bokelmann, & Schade, 1996). The TNF2 allele also been found in increased frequencies in systemic lupus erythromatosus, dermatitis hepetiformis, and insulin-dependent diabetes mellitus and noninsulin-dependent diabetes mellitus (NIDDM) (Jacob et al., 1990, Wilson, Clay, & Crane, 1995; Wilson, Gordon, & di Giovine, 1994).

Thus, it now appears that each individual possesses combinations of SNPs in their genes associated with inflammation corresponding to inflammatory drives of differing intensities when microbes or tissue injury are encountered. At an individual level this may express itself as differing degrees of morbidity and mortality (Fig. 5). The strength of the genomic influence on the inflammatory process may affect the chances of an individual developing inflammatory disease, particularly if their antioxidant defenses are poor. In addition to disease progression, genetic factors have important effects on mortality and morbidity in infectious and inflammatory disease and following injury (Paolini-Giacobino, Grimble, & Pichard, 2003).

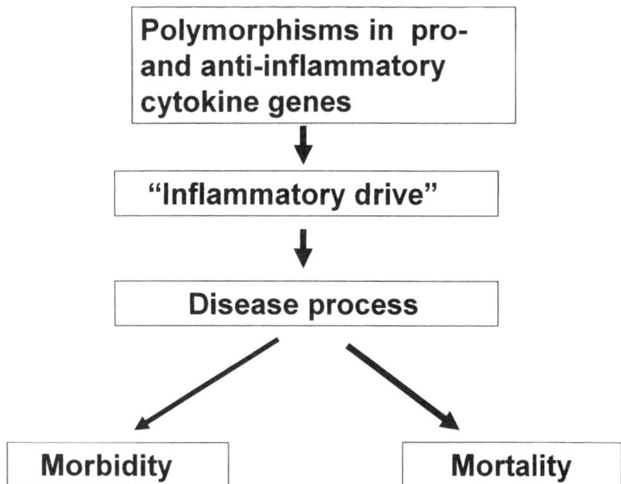

Fig. 5. Combined influences of single nucleotide polymorphisms in pro- and anti-inflammatory cytokine genes in modulating the inherent strength of the inflammatory response to injury and infection: the "inflammatory drive."

There are sex-linked differences in the influence of genotype on the inflammatory processes. In general, males are more sensitive to the genomic influences on the strength of the inflammatory process than females. In a study on LT-α genotype and mortality from sepsis, it was found that men possessing a TNFB22 (LT-α+252 AA) genotype had a mortality of 72% compared with men who were TNFB11 (LT-α+252 GG), who had a 42% mortality rate. In female patients the mortalities for the two genotypes were 53% and 33%, respectively (Schroder, Kahlke, Book, & Stuber, 2000). In a study on patients undergoing surgery for gastrointestinal cancer, it was found that postoperative C-reactive protein (CRP) and IL-6 concentrations were higher in men than in women. Multivariate analysis showed that males possessing the TNF2 (TNF-α-308 A) allele had greater responses than men without it. The genomic influence was not seen in females (Table 2) (Grimble, Thorell, et al., 2003). Furthermore, possession of the IL-1-511 T allele was associated with a 48% greater length of stay in hospital in old men admitted for geriatric care (Table 3) (Grimble, Anderson, et al., 2003). Women were unaffected by these genetic influences.

Paradoxically, with improvements in hygiene and vaccination programs against infectious diseases, two major changes in public health and population characteristics have led to a general increase in inflammatory stress in populations of industrialized countries in the last half century. These are, respectively, an increase in the number of overweight and obese subjects and an increase in longevity. We will now examine the mechanisms underlying this phenomenon.

3. EVIDENCE FOR A LINK BETWEEN INFLAMMATION, OBESITY, INSULIN INSENSITIVITY, AND ATHEROSCLEROSIS FROM POPULATION STUDIES

It has been recognized for many years that there is a strong link between the "diseases of affluence"—obesity, insulin sensitivity, and atherosclerosis. However, it is only quite recently that the realization came that inflammation provided a link between the three

Table 2
Influence of TNF-α – 308 Polymorphism and Gender on the Inflammatory Response to Surgery in Gastrointestinal Cancer Patients

	Males (n = 65)	*Females (n = 56)*
Duration of operation (min)	214 ± 125 (65)	172 ± 76 (56)
Blood loss (mL)	473 ± 521 (65)	258 ± 348 (54)
Peak CRP concentration (mg/mL)[a]	150 ± 81 (45)	126 ± 48 (38)
TNF-α−308		
without A allele	132 ± 46 (33)	128 ± 57 (25)
with A allele	193 ± 116 (12)*	121 ± 37 (13)
Peak IL-6 concentration (pg/mL)[b]	467 ± 411 (31)	342 ± 310 (20)
TNF-α–308		
without A allele	439 ± 402 (24)	362 ± 376 (15)
with A allele	676 ± 544 (7)*	315 ± 147 (5)

TNF, tumor necrosis factor; IL, interleukin; CRP, C-reactive protein.
[a]2 d postoperatively.
[b]1 d postoperatively.
*Significantly different from females with same genotype by multivariate analysis allowing for longer operation time and greater blood loss; $p = 0.013$ and $p = 0.027$ for CRP and IL-6, respectively.
Means ± SD, values in parentheses are the number of patients.

Table 3
Influence of Genotype and Gender on Hospital Length of Stay and Survival in Geriatric Care Patients (Mean Age 83 ± 7 yr[a])

	Males (n = 50)	*Females (n = 39)*
Hospital length of stay (days)		
Patients with IL-1β– 511 CC genotype	9 ± 11 (9)	15 ± 7 (26)
Patients with IL-1β – 511 CT or TT genotype	14 ± 6 (13)*	14 ± 12 (28)
Survival posthospitalization (months)		
Patients with TNFB11 or 12 genotype	21 ± 12 (11)	21 ± 15 (19)
Patients with TNFB22 genotype	10 ± 12 (10)*	22 ± 15 (28)
Patients with IL-1β– 511 CC genotype	27 ± 13 (9)	19 ± 15 (26)
Patients with IL-1β – 511 CT or TT genotype	14 ± 13 (16)*	25 ± 14 (28)

TNF, tumor necrosis factor; IL, interleukin; C, cytosine; T, thymidine; A, adenine; G, guanine.
[a]The location of the polymorphism is indicated by the nucleotide position in the IL-1β and LT-α genes, TNFB11 (GG), TNFB12(AG), TNFB22(AA) .
*Significantly different from value for same sex possessing the other genotype; $p < 0.05$ using Mann-Whitney Test.
Means ± SD, values in parentheses are the number of patients.

biological phenomena (Fig. 3). Many studies have shown a clear link between obesity, oxidant stress, and inflammation (Grimble 2002). The link may lie in the ability of adipose tissue to produce pro-inflammatory cytokines, particularly TNF-α. There is a positive relationship between adiposity and TNF production. A positive correlation

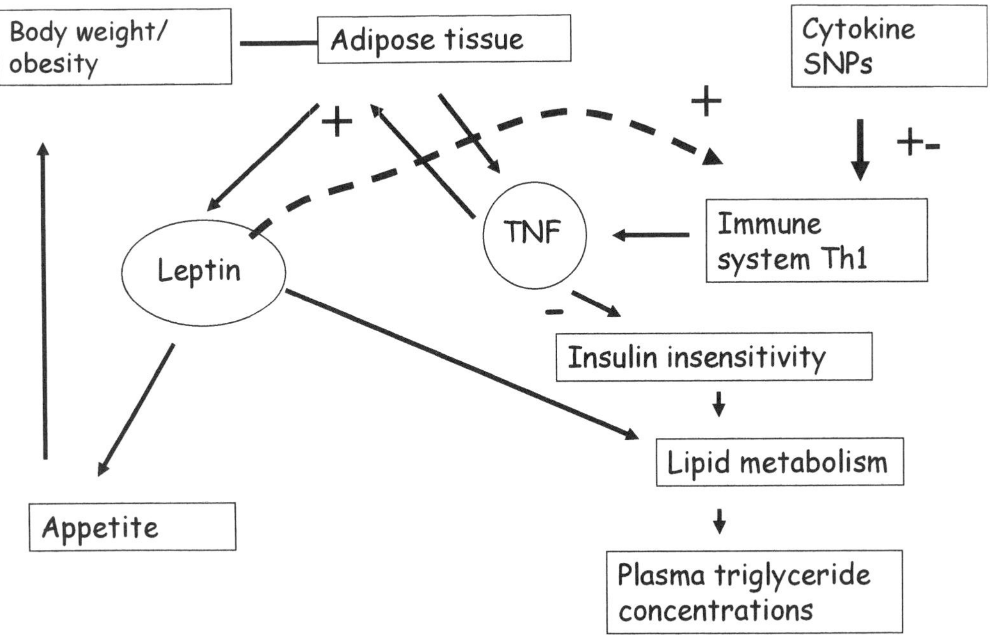

Fig. 6. Interaction between leptin and tumor necrosis factor (TNF) with adipose tissue mass, lipid metabolism, and inflammation. TNF and leptin stimulate the immune system and adipose tissue, respectively. Both also act on lipid metabolism and plasma triglyceride concentrations.

between serum TNF-α production and body mass index (BMI) has been noted in NIDDM patients and healthy women (Nilsson, Jovinge, Niemann, Reneland, & Lithell, 1998; Yaqoob, Newsholme, & Calder, 1999). Leptin has been shown to influence pro-inflammatory cytokine production (Fig. 6). Thus, plasma triglycerides, body fat mass, and inflammation may be loosely associated because of these endocrine relationships.

A number of population studies have been conducted to explore the extent and nature of the relationship of inflammation to these diseases of affluence. The studies have examined populations in which there is a high incidence of insulin insensitivity, such as Pima Indians and individuals with a South Asian background.

TNF-α is overexpressed in adipose and muscle tissues of obese subjects compared with tissues from lean individuals (Hotamisligl & Spiegelman. 1994). In a study of a group of nondiabetic Pima Indians, employing the hyperinsulinemic euglycemic clamp to assess insulin action, strong evidence of the links between inflammation, insulin insensitivity, and obesity emerged. Plasma IL-6 was found to be related positively to adiposity and negatively to insulin sensitivity. The investigators concluded that the relationship between IL-6 and insulin action appeared to be mediated through adiposity (Vozarova, Weyer, & Hanson, 2001).

A number of studies have looked at the extent of the interaction between insulin insensitivity and inflammation by studying the extreme form of diabetes, type 1 diabetes mellitus. A study assessed endothelial cell perturbation by measurement of von Willebrand factor and tissue-plasminogen activator (t-PA), in type 1 diabetics who had had the disease for <1 or >1 yr. Compared with normal subjects, children with diabetes for <1year had the highest concentrations of von Willebrand factor, indicating that endothelial perturbation represents an early event in type 1 diabetes (Romano, Pomilio, & Vigneri, 2001).

Studies that have attempted either to remove the cause of inflammation, to lower plasma lipids, or improve insulin sensitivity have supported the hypothesis that inflammation, insulin sensitivity, and atherosclerosis are intimately interlinked. When a study of the potential anti-inflammatory effect of weight loss was conducted in obese women, it was found that a 1 yr weight-reduction program resulted in lowering of plasma IL-6, TNF-α, and adhesion molecule concentrations (Ziccardi, Nappo, & Giugliano, 2002).

3.1. Inflammation and Atherosclerosis

Since the 1990s large population studies have indicated that inflammation plays a key role in cardiovascular disease (CVD) (Grimble, 1990; Ross, 1993). Periodontal disease and other low-grade infections, such as *Chlamydia pneumoniae* infection, have been linked closely with atherosclerosis. Development of atherosclerotic plaques to which macrophages have already been recruited occurs by cytokines inducing hypertriglyceridemia and hypercholesterolemia (Kol, Sukhova, Lichtman, & Libby, 1998; Saldeen & Rand 1998). Chlamydial infection induces production of TNF-α. The cytokine inhibits the action of lipoprotein lipase, leading to changed lipid metabolism, elevation of serum triglycerides, and a decrease in serum high-density lipoprotein (HDL) cholesterol, thereby exerting an atherogenic influence (Armitage, 2000). In the Bruneck study, raised plasma bacterial lipopolysaccharide (LPS) was associated with an increased rate of thickening of the coronary artery intima. Smoking, a further inflammatory stress, exacerbated this effect (Williet & Kiechl, 2000). LPS binds in human serum to both low-density lipoprotein (LDL) and HDL cholesterol and makes LDL cholesterol immunogenic or toxic to endothelial cells. Thus, the link between specific infections and atherosclerosis may be a nonspecific effect of chronic inflammation on the atherosclerotic process.

It is well recognized that alterations in plasma protein concentrations invariably occur among the many metabolic changes that occur during inflammation. Proteins that increase during inflammation (positive acute-phase proteins, e.g., CRP and fibrinogen) and those that decrease (negative acute-phase proteins, e.g., serum albumin and retinol-binding protein) are used to diagnose inflammation in population nutritional surveys. The early indications that inflammation was involved in atherosclerosis came from the findings that there were links between concentrations of positive and negative acute-phase proteins in blood and CVD (Grimble, 1990). In the Bruneck study of a group of 826 40- to 79-yr-old Italians, it was found that impaired glucose tolerance and, to a greater extent, type 2 diabetes were strong independent predictors of advanced atherosclerosis (measured by high-resolution ultrasound of the carotid artery) (Bonora, Kiechl, & Oberhollenzer, 2000). A cross-sectional study of obesity, plasma CRP, fibrinogen, and carotid artery intima media thickness (an index of atherosclerosis) in more than 1500 multiethnic subjects showed a positive relationship between plasma CRP and body fat. Intima media thickness was related to CRP and fibrinogen in men. The relationship was attenuated by adjustment for BMI (Festa, D'Agostino, & Williams, 2001). A cross-sectional study of more than 1800 men and women examined the link between elevated plasma CRP concentrations and prevalent CVD, ankle/brachial blood pressure, and carotid artery intima media thickness. After adjustment for age and family type, there was a weak association between CRP and intima media thickness in both sexes and with prevalent heart disease in women (Folsom, Pankow, & Tracy, 2001). A study on a Turkish population of 1046 individuals with low cholesterol concentration but a high prevalence of other risk factors for coronary heart disease investigated whether CRP acted as a predictor of coronary heart disease . Among the risk factors, only CRP and systolic blood pressure were independent risk factors for CVD (Onat, Sansoy, & Yildirim, 2001). In a study in which CRP concentrations and conventional risk factors for CVD in 500 healthy Indian Asians were compared with values in a similar number of healthy European white subjects, CRP and CVD risk factors were higher in the former group. However, differences were eliminated when adjustment was made for central obesity and insulin resistance score (Chambers, Eda, & Bassett, 2001). A study on a Brazilian population found that markers of inflammation correlated with components of the metabolic syndrome—cardiovascular and diabetes risk factors, insulin resistance, and central obesity (Duncan & Schmidt, 2001). In a study of 574 healthy elderly subjects in the Netherlands, acute-phase proteins, soluble adhesion molecules, IL-6, and insulin were measured and associated with cholesterol and obesity. The association between insulin, obesity, and cholesterol was as strong as between insulin, acute-phase proteins, and adhesion molecules (Hak, Pols, & Stehouwer, 2001).

3.2. Inflammation and Insulin Insensitivity

Insulin insensitivity occurs as part of the normal inflammatory response to pathogens. During inflammation the secretion of catabolic hormones, which enhances muscle protein breakdown and glutamine release, will oppose insulin action. Paradoxically, however, although insulin insensitivity may initially exert a beneficial effect during the response to infection and injury, it has an adverse influence in chronic disease processes.

Glucose and glutamine act as major fuels for immune cells during the normal response to infection. Large increases in glucose and glutamine utilization by immune cells occur during the response to infection and injury (Spitzer, Bagby, Meszaros, & Lang, 1988, 1989). Studies in rats given LPS and observations in patients with sepsis show that the flow of amino acids into the circulation increases and gluconeogenesis is enhanced under the influence of pro-inflammatory cytokines. An insulin-insensitive state will reduce glucose uptake by tissues in which the process is insulin dependent (muscle), thereby increasing availability to tissues in which the process is not insulin dependent (immune tissue).

A study in the United States investigated whether elevated plasma IL-6 and CRP was associated with the development of type 2 diabetes mellitus in more than 27,000 healthy women. In the 4-yr follow-up period, 188 women developed type 2 diabetes. For these women, baseline IL-6 and CRP were higher than in controls. The relative risk of future type 2 diabetes in women between the highest and lowest quartiles of these inflammatory markers was 7.5 for IL-6 and 15.7 for CRP (Pradhan, Manson, & Rifai, 2001) These data suggest a possible role for inflammation in diabetogenesis. Furthermore, data collected from the Third National Health and Nutrition Examination Survey (NHANES III) in the United States provide further evidence for a possible role of inflammation in insulin resistance and glucose intolerance. More than 2500 men and women were studied for associations between plasma CRP, fasting insulin, glucose, and glycosylated hemoglobin (HbA1c). Elevated CRP was associated with higher insulin and HbA1c in both sexes and with raised glucose in women (Wu, Dorn, & Donahue, 2002). A study on the link between CRP, central adiposity, and fasting glucose and insulin in more than 200 healthy

Italian women showed an independent relationship of adiposity to insulin resistance and CRP concentrations (Pannacciulli, Cantatore, & Minenna, 2001).

In a review, Nishimura and Murayama (2001) discussed the possibility that treatment of periodontal infection may improve insulin sensitivity. Their conclusions about the efficacious effect of an anti-infective approach are supported by a study in which 13 type 2 diabetic patients with periodontal disease were given antimicrobial treatment with minocycline. Blood TNF-α concentrations and glycosylated hemoglobin decreased (Iwamoto, Nishimura, & Nakagawa, 2001). Conversely, improvement in insulin sensitivity exerted an anti-inflammatory effect. A group of 18 hyperlipidemic patients and 20 normolipidemic controls who were insulin resistant and hypertriglyceridemic with low HDL cholesterol concentrations and raised TNF-α production and plasma IL-6 and fibrinogen concentrations were studied. All subjects were treated with the lipid-lowering drug bezafibrate. The drug normalized all parameters.The drug thus exerts an anti-inflammatory effect associated with its ability to normalize lipid metabolism and insulin sensitivity (Jonkers, Mohrschladt, & Westendorp, 2002). In an in vitro study on a lung epithelial cell line, the oral hypoglycemic agent thiazolidinedione exerted an anti-inflammatory influence by suppressing production of monocyte chemoattractant protein (MCP-1) (Momoi, Murao, & Imachi, 2001).

3.3. Mechanisms for the Link Between Inflammation and Insulin Insensitivity

It can be concluded from the studies reported in the above sections that inflammation is closely linked to obesity, CVD, insulin insensitivity, and diabetes mellitus. Although this interaction is a relatively novel concept, it has been known for many years that these diseases are interlinked and that insulin insensitivity is a common factor in their pathology. A number of recent studies have examined the mechanisms underlying the link between inflammation and the conditions and diseases in which insulin insensitivity plays a part (Fig. 3).

A difficult question to address is whether chronic inflammation leads to a condition of insulin insensitivity and associated diseases, or whether insulin insensitivity, which is associated with obesity, diabetes, and atherosclerosis, brings about a condition of chronic inflammatory stress. Many studies suggest that the former is more likely to be the case. Reviews have highlighted the risk of inflammation and infection of atherosclerotic plaques associated with poor diabetic control and the importance of elevated nonesterified fatty acid concentrations, glucocorticoids, and low-grade inflammation as causative agents in atherosclerosis and insulin insensitivity (Bell, 2000; Corry & Tuck, 2001). A study on type 2 diabetes mellitus patients determined the extent to which PBMCs contributed to oxidative stress and inflammation. A linear correlation between HbA1c and superoxide release was found. The authors concluded that type 2 diabetes mellitus is accompanied by priming of PBMCs and increased self-necrosis. The necrosis may start a chain of events that results ultimately in oxidant stress and endothelial dysfunction (Shurtz-Swirski, Sela, & Herskovitis, 2001). In a study on Pima Indians, who are characterized by high incidence of obesity and insulin resistance but not atherosclerotic disease, CRP, ICAM-1, and secretory phospholipase A_2 are correlated with body fat but not E-selectin and von Willebrand factor. In addition to showing that markers of inflammation increase with adiposity, the study showed that markers of endothelial dysfunction increase in proportion to insulin resistance and inflammation (Weyer, Yudkin, & Stehouwer, 2002). A further study on Pima Indians examined whether a raised white blood cell count predicted a worsening of insulin action, insulin secretory function, and the development of type 2 diabetes. A high white blood cell count predicted the development of diabetes with a relative risk of 2.7 when adjusted for age and sex (Vozarova, Weyer, & Lindsay, 2002).

TNF-α has been shown to play a key role in mediating insulin resistance as a result of obesity in patients and in numerous rodent models of obesity—diabetes syndromes (Hotamiligil & Spiegelman, 1994). Multiple mechanisms have been suggested to account for these metabolic effects of TNF-α. These include the downregulation of genes that are required for normal insulin action, direct effects on insulin signaling, induction of elevated plasma free fatty acids via stimulation of lipolysis, and negative regulation of PPAR-γ, an important insulin-sensitizing nuclear receptor (Moller, 2000). The induction of insulin resistance is mediated through its ability to produce serine phosphorylation of insulin receptor substrate (IRS)-1, decreasing the tyrosine kinase activity of the insulin receptor (Hotamisligil, Budavari, Murray, & Spiegelman, 1994). Neutralization of TNF-α in obese fa/fa rats by intravenous administration of a soluble TNF receptor immunoglobulin G chimeric protein substantially improved insulin sensitivity and restored the tyrosine kinase activity in fat and muscle (Hotamisligil et al., 1996). In an in vitro study using 3T3-L1 adipocytes, TNF-α was shown to induce sustained suppressor of cytokine signaling protein 3 (SOCS-3) production. SOCS-3 has been shown to decrease insulin-induced IRS1 tyrosine phosphorylation and its association with the p85 regulatory subunit of phosphatidylinositol-3 kinase (Emanuelli, Peraldi, & Filloux, 2001). These observations therefore suggest that SOCS-3 may be a key mediator in the development of insulin sensitivity during inflammation.

Obesity is associated with insulin resistance, particularly when body fat has a central distribution. While elevated plasma leptin concentrations are associated with obesity, some studies have suggested that insulin sensitivity is an additional determinant of circulating leptin concentrations. Leptin is produced by adipose tissue in proportion to adipose tissue mass and is a pleiotropic molecule. In addition to playing a role in appetite and adipose tissue regulation, leptin influences immune functions. Leptin concentrations increase acutely during inflammation and regulate T-cell responses, polarizing T-helper (Th) cells toward a Th1 phenotype. Thus, increased leptin production during obesity, may exert a pro-inflammatory influence (Faggioni, Feingold, & Grunfeld, 2001). Further complexity is added to the concept of a link between insulin sensitivity, inflammation, and obesity by the results of a study of 268 individuals selected from the Health Professionals follow-up study in the United States (Chu, Spiegelman, & Hotamisligil, 2001). In the study plasma insulin, leptin, and soluble TNF receptor (sTNF-R, an index of TNF-α production) concentrations were measured and correlated with BMI and the CVD risk factors insulin, triglyceride, t-PA antigen levels, and apolipoprotein (Apo)-A1. In a multivariate regression model controlling for age, smoking, alcohol intake, physical activity, and diet, BMI was inversely associated with HDL cholesterol and Apo-A1 and positively associated with trigyceride, Apo-B, and t-PA antigen levels. The associations between BMI and these CVD risk factors were only slightly changed after adjusting for leptin and/or sTNF-R, but were substantially attenuated after controlling for insulin levels. These data suggest that the association between obesity and biological predictors of CVD may be mediated through changes in plasma insulin, rather than leptin or sTNF-R levels, and that insulin may be exerting an anti-inflammatory effect. (Cnop, Landchild, & Vidal, 2002).

3.4. Genomic Influences on Interrelationships Between Inflammation, Insulin Sensitivity, and Obesity

Genetic factors may play a part in the interaction between inflammation, insulin insensitivity, and obesity. NF-κB is an important mediator of inflammation by increasing transcription of a range of genes central to the inflammatory process (cytokines, adhesion molecules, acute-phase proteins). SNPs in the NF-κB gene were investigated in a group of 217 type 1 diabetic patients and compared with gene frequencies in 111 normal controls. It was found that there was a higher frequency of allele 138 bp (A10) (high bioactivity) and a lower frequency of allele 146 bp (A14) (less bioactive) in diabetics than in controls. Genotype may thus contribute to inflammatory stress in diabetes mellitus (Hegazy, O'Reilly, & Yang, 2001). NF-κB may also provide an important focus for PPAR-γ action, because it has been shown in a number of studies that PPAR-γ in combination with retinoid X receptor is able to inhibit NF-κB activation (Wada, Nakajima, & Blumberg, 2001; Fruchart, Staels, & Duriez, 2001; Debril, Renaud, Fajas, & Auwerx, 2001). It is interesting to note that the *n*-3 polyunsaturated fatty acids (PUFAs), found in abundance in fish oil, are PPAR-γ agonists, raising the possibility that the oil may exert its anti-inflammatory effects partly via this mechanism.

In an investigation of cytokine production in 139 healthy males, the author found that in the study population as a whole there were no statistically significant relationships between BMI, plasma fasting triglycerides, and the ability of PBMCs to produce TNF-α. However, individuals with the LT-α+252 AA genotype (associated with raised TNF production) showed significant relationships between TNF production and BMI and fasting triglycerides (Fig. 7). Thus, despite the study population being comprised of healthy subjects, within that population were individuals with a genotype that resulted in an "aged" phenotype as far as plasma lipids, BMI, and inflammation were concerned (Paolini-Giacobino et al., 2003).

4. AGE-RELATED INCREASE IN OXIDATIVE AND INFLAMMATORY STRESS

4.1. Inflammation and Immune Function in the Elderly

It is well known that the incidence of diseases of affluence and recognizable inflammatory diseases, such as rheumatoid arthritis, increase with aging. Are these phenomena an unfortunate side effect of maturity, or is there a common mechanism that determines the appearance of these diseases patterns in the elderly?

Paradoxically, aging is associated with a decline in T-lymphocyte function and an increase in inflammatory stress. A number of elements of the chronic inflammatory response are apparent in otherwise healthy elderly subjects. The elements of the response include muscle protein loss, a rise in plasma acute-phase protein concentrations, and a decrease in plasma zinc. An age-related increase in IL-6 concentration has been found in serum, plasma, and supernatants of mononuclear blood cell cultures from apparently healthy elderly people and centenarians (Fagiolo et al., 1993; Baggio, Donnazzan, Monti, & Mari, 1998; Ershler & Kerller, 2000). Because IL-6 is a pleiotropic cytokine capable of regulating proliferation, differentiation, and activity of a variety of cell types (Ershler & Kerller, 2000) and plays a pivotal role in neuroendocrine and immune system homeostasis, it is not surprising that the rise in production of pro-inflammatory cytokines might have long-term pathological effects (Bethin, Vogt, & Muglia, 2000). Increases in serum

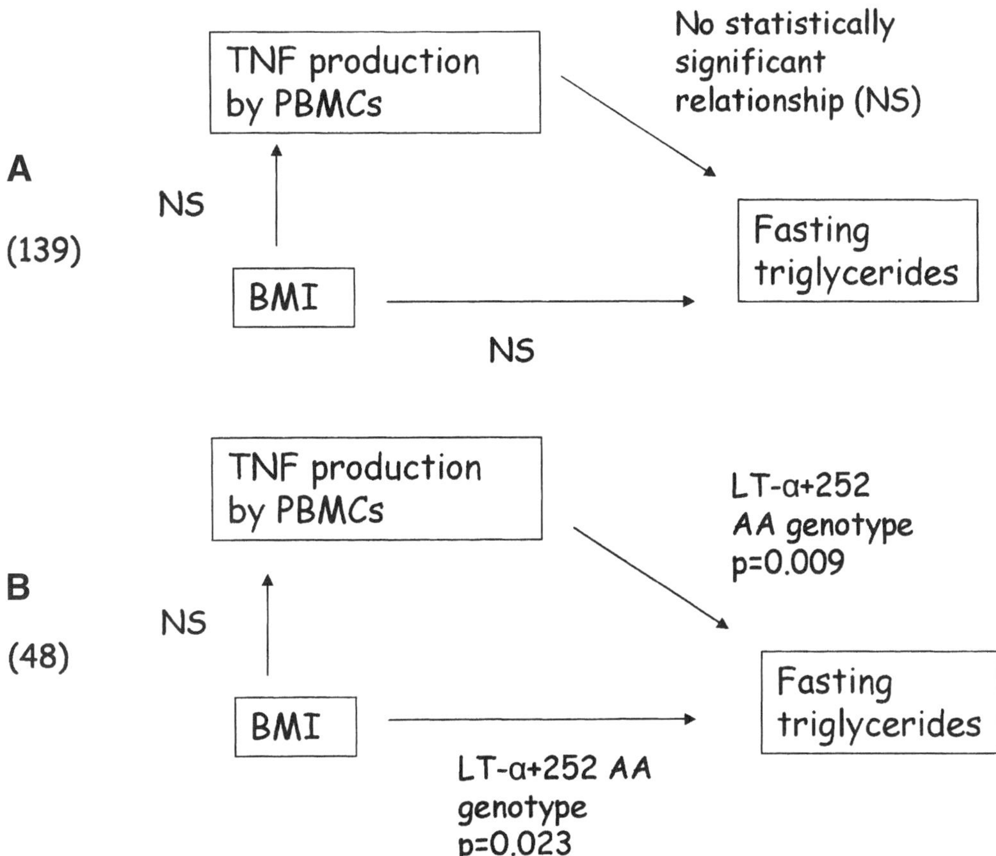

Fig. 7. Relationships between TNF production, BMI and fasting triglycerides, and the ability of PBMCs to produce TNF-α in the study populations: (**A**) all subjects irrespective of genotype, (**B**) individuals with the LT-α+252 AA genotype, associated with raised TNF production. NS, non-significant relationship; BMI, body mass index; PBMCs, peripheral blood mononuclear cells. The number of subjects is shown in parentheses; the correlations were examined by Spearman's rank correlation.

levels of this cytokine have also been found as early as at 30–40 yr of age (Mysliwska, Bryl, Foerster, & Mysliwski, 1998), particularly in men (Young, Skibinski, Mason, & James, 1999). Population studies have shown that the magnitude of increase in the concentration of IL-6 is a reliable marker for functional disability and a predictor of mortality in the elderly (Ferrucci, Harris, Guralnik, & Tracy, 1999; Harris, Ferrucci, Tracy, & Corti, 1999). Antioxidant status may decline with age (Nuttall, Dunne, Kendall, & Martin, 1999) and may thus be linked to increased TNF-α production (Kudoh, Katagai, Takazawa, & Matsuki, 2001; Rink, Cakman, & Kirchner, 1998).

An enhanced capacity for the release of pro-inflammatory cytokines by white blood cells may contribute to the pathogenesis of ischemic stroke. Grau et al. (2001) investigated the LPS-induced release of IL-1β, IL-6, IL-8, and TNF-α in whole blood from patients with a history of ischemic stroke under the age of 50 and age- and sex-matched healthy control subjects. Release of IL-8 was significantly higher in young stroke patients than in control subjects (Grau et al., 2001).

The question of whether aging is associated with chronic elevation of cytokine production or whether an increased capacity for cytokine production following the normal inflammatory challenges of life develops during aging is an interesting one to consider. Insight into this issue can be gained from the response to surgery where an inflammatory stimulus is applied at a defined moment in time, making it easy to follow the subsequent response. Ono, Aosasa, Tsujimoto, Ueno, and Mochizuki (2001) investigated the age-related changes in the inflammatory response in patients with gastric cancer undergoing distal gastrectomy. Patients were divided into two groups: >75 yr of age (elderly group) and ≤75 years of age (young group). Serum IL-6 concentrations, TNF-α production and CD11b/CD18 expression by monocytes, and the postoperative clinical course were compared between the two groups to assess the inflammatory response to surgery. TNF-α production by LPS-stimulated monocytes and CD11b/CD18 expression on monocytes were significantly higher in the elderly than in the young group. Moreover, serum IL-6 concentrations on the first postoperative day in the elderly group were significantly higher than those in the young group.

Paradoxically, both loss of body weight and lean tissue and obesity are found in elderly populations. Is there, therefore, a link between this phenomenon and increased levels of inflammation?

4.2. Loss of Lean Tissue During Aging

The loss of muscle mass and strength that occurs with aging is described clinically as sarcopenia (Rosenberg, 1989; Roubenoff, 2001). It is an important contributor to the development of frailty and functional impairment during aging. It is well established that aging is associated with a significant decline in muscle strength that becomes functionally important by the seventh decade of life. The relationship between chronic inflammation owing to disease during aging and the prevalence of low body mass are well illustrated in rheumatoid arthritis. In a study on patients with rheumatoid arthritis, the loss of body mass was greater for lean tissue than fat, with over 50% of the rheumatoid group falling into the lowest 10th percentile of a reference population for skeletal muscle mass assessed from the upper arm muscle area. In female patients there was a significant correlation between reduced fat-free mass and two indicators of inflammatory stress—erythrocyte sedimentation rate and plasma CRP concentration (Munro & Capell,1997). Clinical and animal studies show a relationship between raised plasma cytokine concentrations and low muscle mass. Visser et al. (2002) investigated whether markers of inflammation are associated with muscle mass and strength over a time course of several years in over 3000 healthy well-functioning black and white elderly persons (70–79 yr). Mid-thigh muscle cross-sectional area , appendicular muscle mass, and muscle strength were assessed. Plasma concentrations of IL-6 and TNF-α were also measured. Higher cytokine concentrations were associated with lower muscle mass and lower muscle strength. The most consistent relationship across the gender and race groups was observed for IL-6 and grip strength. When an overall indicator of elevated cytokine production was created by combining the concentrations of IL-6 and TNF-α, with the exception of white men, elderly persons having high concentrations of IL-6 (>1.80 pg/mL) as well as high levels of TNF-α (>3.20 pg/mL) had a smaller muscle area, less appendicular muscle mass, and lower muscle strength compared to those with low levels of both cytokines. Thus, raised plasma concentrations of IL-6 and TNF-α are associated with lower muscle mass and lower muscle strength in well-functioning older men and women as well as those suffering frank inflammatory disease.

Nutrient intake is clearly another important determinant of lean body weight and fat mass and may play a part in the decline in lean tissue with age as well as an increase in inflammatory stress. A recent survey of 40,000 subjects in 88 communities in NHANES III in the United States also included a survey of about 5000 elderly people ranging in age from 60 to 69 yr, 70 to 79 yr, and 80+ yr (Marwick, 1997). The report indicated that the median intake of total energy was in general lower than the recommended 2300 kcal for men and 1900 kcal for women (Marwick, 1997).

4.3. The Link Between Obesity, Aging, and Inflammatory Stress

Chronic inflammation is either a causative agent or a closely associated process in the pathology of obesity, insulin insensitivity, and atherosclerosis.The incidence of these conditions increases with aging. A fundamental question is which precedes the other—the general increase in inflammation or the development of diseases with overt and covert inflammatory bases? This "chicken-and-egg" question is difficult to answer. However, examination of data from studies conducted in elderly populations may throw some light on the answer to this conumdrum.

There are at least two potential mechanisms for the higher level of chronic inflammation observed in elderly than in younger subjects. The first of these is that the elderly are experiencing a higher level of asymptomatic urinary infection. This possibility was studied in 40 consecutive patients (70–91 yr) admitted to the hospital for functional disability. Patients were examined for the presence or absence of bacteria in the urine. Twenty subjects had a positive urine culture, and 20 sex- and age-matched subjects had a negative urine culture. Inclusion criteria were temperature <37.8°C, no clinical signs of infection, and no current antibiotic treatment. Patients with asymptomatic bacteriuria had significantly increased levels of TNF receptors and a higher number of neutrophils in the blood compared to the group without bacteriuria. Thus, the study provides some support for the hypothesis that asymptomatic urinary infections are associated with low-grade inflammatory activity in frail, elderly subjects (Prio, Bruunsgaard, Roge, & Pedersen, 2002).

A second potential mechanism resides in endocrine changes during aging. In aging, dysregulation of secretion of hormones that come under the regulation of the hypothalamic–pituitary–adrenal axis may occur. This may have an effect on the regulation of cortisol secretion, as mentioned earlier. Cortisol is important as an anti-inflammatory agent. The effect of aging on glucocorticoid sensitivity of pro-inflammatory cytokine production was examined in elderly men, testosterone-treated elderly men, and young controls. Stress-induced increases in cortisol did not differ significantly between experimental groups, but glucocorticoid sensitivity increased significantly in young controls and testosterone-treated elderly men, whereas a decrease was found in untreated elderly men. As the increase in glucocorticoid sensitivity after stress serves to protect the individual from detrimental increases of pro-inflammatory cytokines, the disturbed mechanism in elderly men may result in an increase in inflammatory stress (Rohleder, Kudielka, Hellhammer, Wolf, & Kirschbaum, 2002).

There is now a large body of evidence suggesting that the decline in ovarian function with menopause is associated with spontaneous increases in pro-inflammatory cytokine production. As mentioned earlier, studies in men and postmenopausal women indicate a remarkable individual constancy in the ability of PBMCs to produce TNF-α ex vivo, and genetic determinants underlie this constancy. However in premenopausal women production is highly variable at an individual level, indicating how ovarian hormones are able to override the influence of genotype (Jacob et al., 1990). The exact mechanisms by which estrogen interferes with cytokine activity are still incompletely known but may include interactions of the estrogen receptor with other transcription factors, modulation of nitric oxide activity, antioxidative effects, plasma membrane actions, and changes in immune cell function. Experimental and clinical studies also strongly support a link between the increased state of pro-inflammatory cytokine activity and postmenopausal bone loss (Pfeilschifter et al., 2002).

4.4. Influence of Genotype on Inflammation and Aging

Recent evidence indicates the presence of SNPs, associated with the strength of the inflammatory response, affects longevity. Human longevity may be directly correlated with optimal functioning of the immune system. Therefore, it is likely that one of the genetic determinants of longevity resides in polymorphisms for genes influencing the activity of the immune system.

It has been estimated that up to 7000 variations in the genome contribute to life span (Martin, 1997). Those contributing to loss of muscle and bone mass during aging are related to the inflammatory process and include pro- and anti-inflammatory cytokines and their receptors.

Studies in mice have shown that the genes controlling the major histocompatibility complex (MHC), known to control a variety of immune functions, are associated with differences in the life span of different strains of mice, but a major difference between observations in mice and humans is that the latter have a lifetime experience of exposure to pathogens, whereas for laboratory animals this exposure is kept to a minimum. Thus, although HLA studies in mice of different genotypes may be interpreted to support studies of MHC effects on longevity in humans, in mice the association may be by way of altered susceptibility to lymphomas, whereas in human beings the effect on longevity is likely to be via an altered response to pathogens and susceptibility to infectious disease.

A number of cross-sectional studies have examined the role of HLA genes on human longevity by comparing HLA antigen frequencies between groups of young and elderly persons. Conflicting findings have been obtained. When this topic was reviewed (Caruso et al., 2001), it was concluded that in humans there may be an association between longevity and some HLA-DR alleles or the HLA-B8,DR3 haplotype. These genotypes are involved in the antigen nonspecific control of immune response, in other words, the component of immune function associated with inflammation and cytokine biology.

Recent evidence indicates that presence of SNPs in certain pro- and anti-inflammatory cytokine genes influences life span. When 700 individuals between 60 and 110 yr of age were studied, it was noted that not only was plasma IL-6 concentration positively related to age but individuals with a SNP in the promoter region of the IL-6 gene, which predisposes to high levels of production of the cytokine (-174 GG), decreased in frequency with age. The effect was seen in men but not in women (Bonafè, Olivieri, & Cavallone, 2001). Although men with SNPs made up 58% of the 60- to 80-yr-old age group, the percentage fell to 38% in subjects <99 years of age. Conversely, one of three SNPs in the IL-10 gene (-1082 GG), which is closely linked to higher production of the anti-inflammatory cytokine IL-10 (Hutchinson, Pravica, Hajeer, & Sinnott, 1999; Turner et al., 1997), was found in higher proportions in male centenarians than in younger controls (58 vs 34%). In females this genotype exerted no effect upon longevity (Lio et al., 2002). Thus, it would appear that genetic characteristics that might influence the balance between pro- and anti-inflammatory cytokines influence mortality in men but not in women (Franceschi et al., 2000). A study on SNPs that influence interferon (IFN)-γ production further reinforces the concept that possession of a genotype that predisposes to a raised pro-inflammatory status is not compatible with a long life span (Lio et al., 2002). In women, possession of the A allele, which is associated with low production of IFN-γ, significantly increased the possibility of reaching old age. It might be concluded that possession of high-producing alleles of the IL-10 is universally protective against morbidity as well as mortality. Possession of a genotype that results in low levels of IL-10 production (-1082 AA) increases the risk of developing inflammatory diseases (Hajeer, Lazanes, & Turner, 1998; Huizinga, Keijsers, & Yanni, 2002; Tagore, Gonsalkorale, & Pravica, 1999). However, as already mentioned, in a large survey of hospital admission in the Netherlands, patients with raised IL-10:IL-6 ratios had higher mortality rates (Van Dissel et al., 1998).

Not all studies implicate cytokine gene SNP in longevity. Cytokine gene polymorphisms at IL-1α, IL-1β, IL-1RA, IL-6, IL-10, and TNF-α were measured in 250 Finnish nonagenarians (52 men and 198 women) and in 400 healthy blood donors (18–60 yr) used as controls. No statistically significant differences were found in the distribution of genotype, allelic frequencies, and A2+ carrier status between nonagenarians and younger controls (Wang, Hurme, Jylha, & Hervonen, 2001).

In a review on the different impact of genetic factors on the probability of reaching old age, Franceschi et al. (2000) concluded from studies conducted in Italy that emerging evidence (regarding mtDNA haplogroups, thyrosine hydroxylase, and IL-6 genes) suggests that female longevity is less dependent on genetics than male longevity and that female centenarians are more likely to have had a healthier lifestyle and more favorable environmental conditions than males. However, a recent study conducted by our group suggests that although a pro-inflammatory genotype may be disadvantageous to elderly males, it may confer a survival benefit in females. Subsequent survival was studied in 79 elderly geriatric patients (87 ± 7 yr) after a period of hospitalization for a range of conditions necessitating geriatric care. Although women possessing a pro-inflammatory genotype (TNF-α–308 A allele or IL-6–174 GG) had improved 3 yr survival rates, men possessing pro-inflammatory genotypes (IL-1β-511 T allele or LT-α +252 AA) had shortened survival rates (Grimble, Thorell, et al., 2003) (Table 3).

5. THE POTENTIAL FOR MODULATION OF THE INFLAMMATORY RESPONSE BY IMMUNONUTRITION

As outlined in the preceding sections, the inflammatory response, although essential for survival in the presence of pathogens, can exert deleterious effects on the host.The clear need to find ways of modulating cytokine production and other aspects of inflammation has fostered the research area of immunonutrition.

In a clinical context the purpose of immunonutrition is to find nutritional means of altering the patient's inflammatory response to infection and injury, from the detrimental to the beneficial side of the pivot on which an individual undergoing a response is positioned. While inflammation may be exerting deleterious effects most obviously in patients, people on the borderline of health and disease living in the general population

Table 4
Nutrients Commonly Used in Immunonutrient Supplements and Their Potential Mode of Action

- *n*-3 polyunsaturated fatty acids: act as anti-inflammatory agents and reverse immunosuppression
- Sulfur amino acids and their precursors: enhance antioxidant status via GSH synthesis
- Glutamine: nutrient for immune cells, improves gut barrier function, precursor for GSH
- Arginine: stimulates nitric oxide and growth hormone production, improves helper T-cell numbers
- Nucleotides: RNA and DNA precursors, improve T-cell function

may also require nutritional modulation of ongoing inflammatory processes. During the last 20 years the pace of evolution of immunomodulatory feeds and intravenous solutions has accelerated. These products contain combinations of a number of components to which various functional attributes are ascribed them (Table 4) (Grimble, 2001a).

Many studies have indicated that *n*-3 polyunsaturated fatty acids (PUFAs), glutamine, arginine, sulfur amino acids, and nucleotides are all potentially capable of shifting the balance from a disadvantageous to an advantageous response to infection and injury. The examples used here are illustrative rather than comprehensive. A number of studies indicate that improvement of antioxidant status is associated with an increase in cellular aspects of immune function. Meta-analyses have been conducted on the efficacy of immunonutrients that influence antioxidant status. In clinical trials, indices such as infection rates, mortality rates, and length of stay are often measured in the absence of functional and biochemical aspects of the response, such as T-cell function, cytokine production, and antioxidant status, and vice versa, giving a rather incomplete picture of the mechanisms of any observed effects of immunonutrition. However, Beale, Bryg, & Bihari (1999), in a meta-analysis of 12 studies containing more than 1400 patients receiving enteral immunonutrition, observed that although there was no effect upon mortality, there were significant reductions in infection rates, time spent on a ventilator, and length of hospital stay. While this finding indicates that immunonutrition may be useful in modulating the inflammatory process in patients experiencing severe inflammation, the consistency of the effects observed was disappointing.

There are at least three major reasons why it is difficult to demonstrate a consistent effect. First, patients used as the subjects of clinical trials of immunonutrients will constitute a diverse population—different ages, at different stages of a disease process, and undergoing complex clinical treatment in addition to nutrient therapy. Second, patients will have differing genetic backgrounds that will influence the intensity of the inflammatory and immune responses they are undergoing. This issue is dealt with below. Third, nutrients may exert paradoxical effects, as illustrated by the findings of the first observations of the effects of fish oil on cytokine production in healthy subjects. The findings of Endres et al. (1989) that a daily supplement of 18 g/d of fish oil given to nine young men for 6 wk was able to reduce ex vivo production of IL-1 and TNF-α by LPS-stimulated PBMCs aroused great interest in fish oil as an anti-inflammatory nutrient. This perception was supported by a large amount of animal data. However, Endres' data showed a wide variability in the effect of the fish oil supplements. The standard deviations of the mean for IL-1β and TNF-α production were 59 and 51%, respectively. This indicates that cytokine production could have risen or fallen as a consequence of taking the supplement.

The effects of supplementing 116 healthy young men with 6 g/d of fish oil for 12 wk, on TNF-α production by PBMCs stimulated with endotoxin have been studied in the author's laboratory. It was found that 51% of subjects experienced a fall in production and 49% a rise. Although the ability of fish oil to increase TNF-α production is at first sight paradoxical, earlier work of Dinarello, Bishai, Rosenwasser, and Coceani (1984) and Kunkel, Remick, Spengler, and Chensue (1987) indicated that fish oil could potentially change cytokine production in either direction. What mechanisms could result in this divergent effect? Inflammation will result in activation of phospholipase A_2, which releases arachidonic acid (AA) (C20:4 *n*-6) from the cell membrane for prostaglandin E_2 (PGE2) or leukotriene B_4 (LT B4) synthesis. The in vitro studies (Kunkel et al., 1987) showed that PGE2 suppressed TNF-α production, whereas LTB4 had the opposite effect (Dinarello et al., 1984). Fish oil is rich in eicosapentaenoic acid (C20:5 *n*-3), which will replace AA in the cell membrane and results in the production of PGE3 and LT B5. PGE3 and LT B5 are considerably less potent than the corresponding compounds produced from AA, and thus dietary fish oil may lessen the inhibitory influence of PGE2 or the stimulatory influence of LTB4 on TNF-α production, resulting in a potential increase or decrease, respectively, in production of the cytokine. Fish oil could thus result in an inflammatory cytokine response, which could fall on either side of the pivot.

5.1. Immunomodulation by Enhancement of Antioxidant Defenses

The response to bacterial invasion of the body, or injury, contains a paradox. Although the inflammatory response and the T-cell response both play a part in defeating the invader, the inflammatory response may in some clinical circumstances exert an inhibitory influence on T-cell function. In severely infected or traumatized patients, an enhanced inflammatory state occurs, which is associated with immunosuppression. In vitro studies support this inverse relationship. PBMCs taken from healthy young subjects and incubated with GSH show decreased PGE2 and LTB4 production (reduced inflammation) and an increase in mitogenic index and IL-2 production (enhanced immune function) (Wu, Meydani, Sastre, Hayek, & Meydani, 1994).

Thus, enhancement of antioxidant defenses reduces the likelihood of the inflammatory response suppressing T-cell function (Grimble, 1997, 2001b). Although all antioxidants are important owing to the linked nature of antioxidant defense (Fig. 8), GSH plays a pivotal role as it acts directly as an antioxidant and maintains other components of defense in a reduced state through enzymic conversion between the oxidized and reduced states. Various compounds can be used to increase GSH synthesis (Fig. 9). *N*-Acetyl cysteine (NAC) and the GSH prodrug oxothiazalidine-4-carboxylate (procysteine) have been used in a number of clinical studies. Tissue GSH content is also influenced by protein and sulfur amino acid intake. Unfortunately, surgery, a wide range of diseases that have an inflammatory component, and aging and protein energy malnutrition decrease GSH concentration in blood and other tissues (Boya et al., 1999; Loguercio et al., 1999; Luo, Hammarqvist, Anderson, & Wernerman, 1996; Micke, Beeh, Schlaak, & Buhl, 2001; Nuttal et al., 1999; Reid et al., 2000) (Table 5). Within 24 h of elective abdominal surgery, muscle GSH content falls by >30%. Values return to normal 72 h postoperatively. A smaller perturbation in blood GSH occurs over a shorter time course.

Modification of the GSH content of liver, lung, spleen, and thymus in young rats by feeding diets containing a range of casein (a protein with a low sulfur amino acid content) concentrations changed immune cell numbers in lung (Hunter & Grimble, 1994). It was

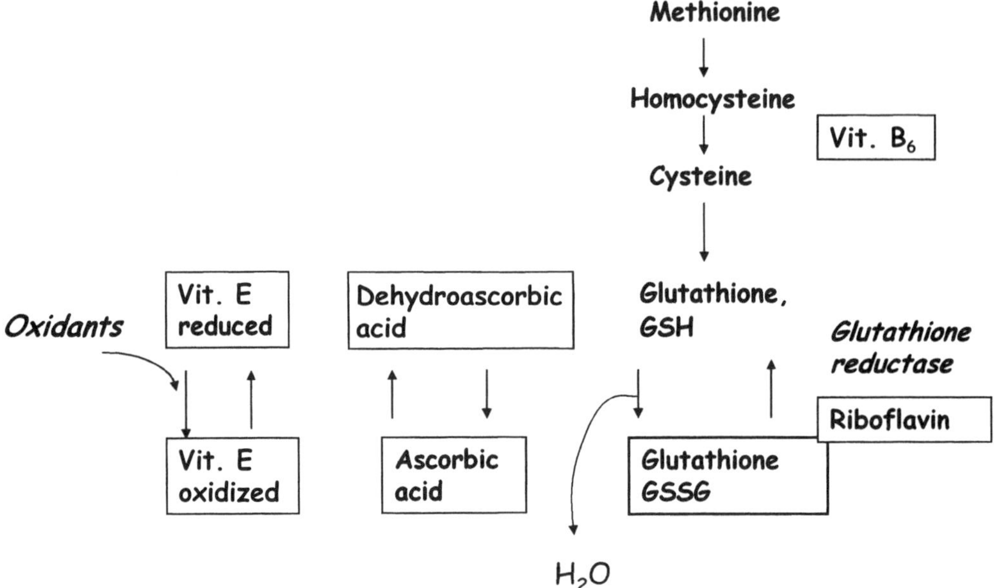

Fig. 8. The interlinked nature of the antioxidant defenses.

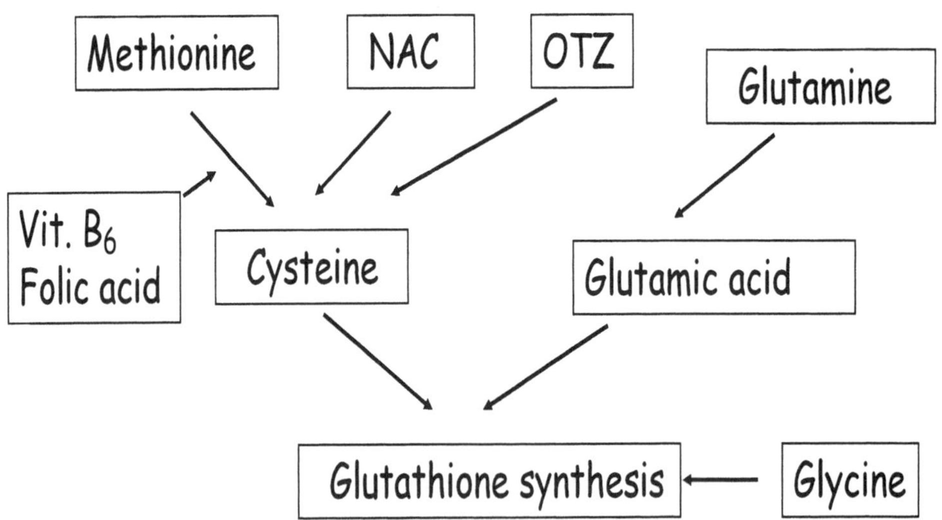

Fig. 9. Potential means of enhancing GSH synthesis by immunonutrients. NAC, *N*-acetyl cysteine; OTZ, l-2-oxothiazolidine-4-carboxylate.

found that in unstressed animals the number of lung neutrophils decreased as dietary protein intake and tissue GSH content fell. However, in animals given an inflammatory challenge (endotoxin), liver and lung GSH concentrations increased directly in relation to dietary protein intake. Lung neutrophils, however, became related inversely with tissue GSH content. Addition of methionine to the protein-deficient diets normalized tissue GSH content and restored lung neutrophil numbers to those seen in unstressed animals fed a diet with adequate protein content (Fig. 10).

Table 5
Conditions Associated With Decreases in Glutathione Content of Tissues

Condition or disease	*Tissue, fluid, or cell showing decrease in GSH content*
Surgical stress	Skeletal muscle, plasma
HIV infection	PBMCs, lung lavage fluid
Sepsis	PBMCs, lung lavage fluid
Cirrhosis	Plasma, red blood cells
Ulcerative colitis	Colonic cells, red blood cells
Type 2 diabetes	Whole blood, red blood cells
Protein–energy malnutrition	Plasma, red blood cells
Old age	Plasma

GSH, glutathione; PBMCs, peripheral blood mononuclear cells; HIV, human immunodeficiency virus.

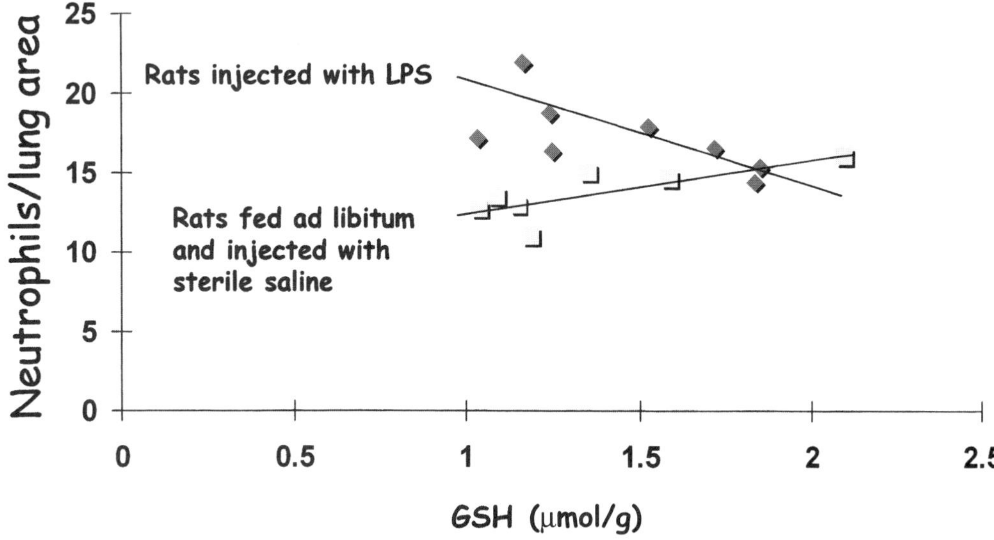

Fig. 10. The effect of dietary sulfur amino acid intake on lung neutrophil content in unstressed rats and stressed rats receiving an intraperitoneal injection of *E. coli* endotoxin.

Why does tissue GSH content have differing effects on immune cell populations depending on whether or not an inflammatory response is occurring? A partial explanation may come from an in vitro study using HeLa cells and cells from human embryonic kidney. In the study, both TNF-α and hydrogen peroxide resulted in activation of NF-κB and AP1 (Wesselborg, Bauer, Vogt, Schmitz, & Schulze-Osthoff, 1997). Addition of the antioxidant sorbitol to the medium suppressed NF-κB activation as expected, but unexpectedly activated AP1. Thus, the antioxidant environment of the cell might exert opposite effects upon transcription factors closely associated with inflammation (e.g., NF-κB) and cellular proliferation (e.g., AP1). Evidence for this biphasic effect was seen when GSH was incubated with immune cells from young adults (Wu et al., 1994). A rise in cellular GSH content was accompanied by an increase in IL-2 production and lymphocyte proliferation (enhancement of T-cell function) and a decrease in production of the inflammatory mediators PGE2 and LTB4 (anti-inflammatory influence). Without doubt, a decline in antioxidant status in the presence of oxidant stress will increase inflammatory stress. The interaction between oxidant stress and an impaired ability to synthesize GSH, a situation that stimulates inflammation, is clearly seen in cirrhosis, a disease that results in high levels of oxidative stress and an impaired ability to synthesize GSH (Pena, 1999). In Pena an inverse relationship between GSH concentration and the ability of monocytes to produce IL-1, IL-8, and TNF-α was observed. Treatment of cirrhotic patients with the procysteine increased monocyte GSH content and reduced IL-1, IL-8, and TNF-α production. Septic patients given an infusion of NAC (150 mg/kg bolus followed by infusion of 50 mg/kg over 4-h) showed a decrease in plasma IL-8 and soluble TNF receptor p55, had a reduced requirement for ventilator support, and spent 19 fewer days in intensive care than patients not receiving NAC (Spapen et al., 1998). De Rosa et al. (2000) showed that NAC was able to restore tissue GSH concentrations in individuals with HIV infection. In a study on HIV-positive patients, Brietkreutz et al. (2000) showed that a dose of 600 mg/d of NAC for 7 mo resulted in a decrease in plasma IL-6 (decreased inflammation), an increase in natural killer cell activity, and increased responsiveness of T lymphocytes to tetanus toxin stimulation (improved lymphocyte function).

Antioxidants might act to prevent NF-κB activation by quenching oxidants. However, NF-κB and AP1 may not respond to changes in cell redox state in the same way. When rats were subjected to depletion of effective tissue GSH pools by administration of diethyl maleate, there was a significant reduction in lymphocyte proliferation in spleen and mesenteric lymph nodes (Robinson et al., 1993). An increase in inflammatory stress would be expected in this study. Thus, it can be hypothesized that antioxidants exert an immunoenhancing effect by activating transcription factors that are strongly associated with cell proliferation (e.g., AP1) and an anti-inflammatory effect by preventing activation of NF-κB by oxidants produced during the inflammatory response (Dröge et al., 1994).Thus, inclusion of antioxidants or substances that increase GSH synthesis in immunonutrient mixes would seem to be beneficial.

Improvement of antioxidant defenses is also possible by feeding other components of antioxidant defenses. Supplementation of the diet of healthy subjects and smokers with 600 IU/d α-tocopherol for 4 wk suppressed the ability of PBMCs to produce TNF-α (Mol, de Rijke, Demacher, & Stalenhoef, 1997). The same dose given to healthy elderly subjects for 235 d increased delayed-type hypersensitivity and raised antibody titers to hepatitis B (Meydani et al., 1997). An enteral feed enriched with vitamin E, vitamin C, and taurine given to intensive-care patients decreased total lymphocyte and neutrophil content in bronchioalveolar lavage fluid (decreased inflammation) and resulted in a reduction in organ failure rate, a reduced requirement for artificial ventilation, and a reduction of 5 d in intensive-care stay (Gadek et al., 1999).

5.2. Influence of Glutamine on Inflammation and Immune Function

A number of roles have been ascribed to glutamine as an immunonutrient: (a) as an essential nutrient for immune cells, (b) as an important modulator of gut barrier function, and (c) as a substrate for GSH synthesis. A number of reviews have been written about the first two of these roles (Newsholme, Crabtree, Salleh, & Ardawi, 1985; Elia, 1992); we will consider the last one here. Could glutamine be exerting an anti-inflammatory influence via an effect on GSH that enhances immune function? In a study in rats, glutamine supplementation resulted in an increased production of GSH by the gut (Cao, Feng, Hoos, & Klimberg, 1998), and total parenteral nutrition (TPN) with glutamine raised plasma GSH concentrations in these animals (Denno, Rounds, Faris, Halejko, & Wilmore, 1996).

In randomized controlled trials the administration of glutamine, either as a dipeptide during TPN to surgical patients or as a glutamine-enriched enteral feed to trauma patients, resulted, respectively, in improved nitrogen retention (less tissue protein depletion) and a 6.2-d reduction in hospital stay, a concomitant suppression of the rise in plasma-soluble TNF receptors (reduced inflammation), and a lower incidence of bacteremia, pneumonia, and sepsis (improved immune function) (Houdijk et al., 1998; Morlion et al., 1998)

5.3. Dietary Intervention to Moderate Chronic Low-Grade Inflammation in the Elderly

In the previous section the influence of antioxidants on severe inflammation was considered. Do the general findings from this type of study also apply to modulation of low-grade chronic inflammation, such as has been observed in the elderly and obese?

Because aging is so closely associated with increased oxidative stress, which might both result from and contribute to a stimulation in the level of inflammation in the elderly, antioxidant therapy could produce beneficial effects. The effects would be seen in a decrease in oxidant damage, downregulation of inflammation, and, because of the inverse link between inflammation and immune function, an improvement in T-lymphocyte function. Meydani, Meydani, & Verdon (1986) reported that supplementation of aged mice (24 mo old) with dietary vitamin E (500 ppm) improved several indices of the immune system to levels comparable to those seen in young animals. Supplementation of aged mice with this vitamin also increased clearance of influenza virus from the lung to that observed in animals supplemented with other antioxidants such as melathonine, GSH, or strawberry extract, which contains a high level of flavonoids with antioxidant activity (Han et al., 2000). In a double-blind, placebo-controlled study, Meydani and colleagues (Meydani, Barklund, & Lui, 1990; Meydani et al., 1997) also reported that supplementation of elderly subjects with vitamin E for a short (1 mo) or long (4.5 mo) period of time also improved several in vitro and in vivo indices of immune response. The optimal immune response was observed with 200 IU of vitamin E per day in the long-term study. It is worth noting that this level of vitamin E has also been reported to be the optimal level for reducing plasma F_2-isoprostane, a reliable index of lipid peroxidation (Dillon, Vita, & Leeuwenburgh, 1998). Improving the immune response in the elderly may result in a lower incidence of infections, which are prevalent among the elderly, and thus may contribute to a longer and healthier life. Many observational and clinical trials have also indicated that a high intake or high plasma level of this vitamin is associated with a low risk of cardiovascular disease. The vitamin may be operating at two levels; first, by protecting LDL from peroxidation, thereby reducing its atherogenicity, and second, by lowering the level of chronic inflammation by downregulation of NF-κB. A reduction in platelet aggregability may also arise out of this action (Huang et al., 2001; Tanus-Santos et al., 2002). Indeed, several lines of evidence indicated that supplements of vitamin E may prevent cardiovascular disease by reducing the susceptibility of LDLs to oxidation (Jailal, Fuller, & Huet, 1995), reducing the expression of chemokines, adhesion molecule expression, and monocyte adhesion (Wu, Koga, Martin, & Meydani, 1999), decreasing smooth muscle proliferation (Azzi, Boscoboinik, & Marilley, 1995), and decreasing platelet aggregation (Steiner 1999).

Another anti-inflammatory approach using nutrients would be to supplement diets of the elderly with *n*-3 PUFAs. Supplementation with *n*-3 PUFAs from fish oil, however, has been reported to suppress the immune response (Meydani, Endres, & Woods, 1991; Meydani, 1993), which hampers enthusiasm for the use of *n*-3 PUFAs for their benefits in CVD. However, the latter concern could be addressed by including a vitamin E supplement along with fish oil supplements. In a recent study it was found that supplementing elderly persons with (*n*-3) fatty acids of fish oil in combination with vitamin E while maintaining the anti-inflammatory properties of (*n*-3) PUFAs did not reduce immune indices in the elderly (Wu, Meydani, & Han, 2000).

6. INFLUENCE OF GENOTYPE ON RESPONSE TO NUTRIENTS

6.1. Fish Oil

Fish oil supplementation is not universally efficacious in the treatment of inflammatory disease (Grimble, 1998). Rheumatoid arthritis and inflammatory bowel disease have been the most successfully treated of all inflammatory diseases (Calder, 1997). The anti-inflammatory mechanism may be through suppression of TNF-α production. Endres et al. (1989) reported that large doses (15 g/d for 6 wk) of oil in nine healthy volunteers resulted in a small but statistically significant reduction in TNF-α and IL-1β production from PBMCs. Subsequently, fewer than half of 11 similar small intervention studies were able to demonstrate a statistically significant reduction in cytokine production. To understand the differences in response more closely, the author's laboratory conducted a study on 111 young men fed 6 g fish oil daily for 12 wk and measured TNF-α production by PBMCs before and after supplementation in relation to the SNP at −308 in the TNF-α and at +252 in the LT-α genes. No significant effect of fish oil on cytokine production was noted in the group as a whole. However, when data were examined according to tertile of TNF-α production prior to supplementation, homozygosity for TNFB2 (LT-α+252 A) was 2.5 times more frequent in the highest than in the lowest tertile of production. The percentage of individuals in whom fish oil suppressed production was lowest (22%) in the lowest tertile and doubled with each ascending tertile. In the highest tertile, mean values were decreased by 43% ($p < 0.05$). In the lowest tertile, mean values were increased by 62% ($p < 0.05$). TNFB2 (LT-α+252 AA) homozygotes were strongly represented among unresponsive individuals in the lowest tertile of TNF-α production prior to supplementation. In this lowest tertile, only TNFB1/B2 (LT-α+252 GA) heterozygous subjects were responsive to the suppressive effects of fish oil. In the medium tertile, this genotype was six times more frequent than other LT-α genotypes among responsive individuals. No relationship between possession of TNF1 or 2 (TNF-α−308 G or A) alleles and responsiveness to fish oil was found. Clearly, although the level of inflammation determines whether fish oil will exert an anti-inflammatory influence or not and is influenced by the TNFB2 (LT-α+252 A) allele, the precise genomic mechanism for an anti-inflammatory effect is unclear at present (Grimble et al., 2002).

6.2. Vitamin E

Antioxidant intake also modifies cytokine production. In a study on healthy men and women and smokers, dietary supplementation with 600 IU/d α-tocopherol for 1 mo suppressed the ability of PBMCs to produce TNF-α. Production was reduced by 22 and

33% in nonsmokers and smokers, respectively (Mol et al., 1997). In a similar dietary intervention study on normolipaemic and hypertriglyceridaemic subjects given 600 IU/d of α-tocopherol for 6 wk, reduced TNF-α, IL-1β, and IL-8 production by LPS-stimulated blood mononuclear cells occurred (Mol et al., 1997; van Tits, Demacker, de Graaf, Hak-Lemmers, & Stalenhoef, 2000). A similar effect of α-tocopherol was noted in a study on normal subjects and type 2 diabetics (Devaraj & Jialal, 2000). However, there were large standard deviations in the data from these studies, indicating major intraindividual variability in the ability of vitamin E to suppress production of the cytokine. Although a number of studies have shown that α-tocopherol suppresses superoxide production, the situation with regard to nitric oxide is less clear (Mol et al., 1997; van Tits et al., 2000)κ The α-tocopherol derivative pentamethyl-hydroxychromane inhibited LPS-stimulated NF-κB and iNOS activation in cultured J774 macrophages (Hattori, 1995). At present it is not known whether antioxidants interact differently with SNPs in the genes associated with oxidant stress and inflammation than they do with the other anti-inflammatory nutrient, *n*-3 PUFA. This topic is currently an area of active research at the author's laboratory.

Proteomic studies have shown that iNOS and SOD are both influenced by the NRAMP1 gene (Kovorova, Necasova, Porkertova, Radzoich, & Macela, 2001). The production of oxidant molecules enhancing pro-inflammatory cytokine production via high levels of NF-kB activation may thus be under a genomic influence owing to the aforementioned variations in the NRAMP1 gene (Formica, Roach, & Blackwell, 1994). A better understanding of this interaction and of the interaction of *n*-3 PUFAs and antioxidants with genotype may allow the better design of nutrient products for the treatment of inflammatory disease.

7. CONCLUSIONS

It is clear from the current understanding about the purpose and functioning of the immune system throughout the life cycle that it is a powerful biological entity that profoundly alters body function while it is carrying out its prime purpose of defending the body against invasion by pathogens. However, within the response lie the seeds of disaster at an individual level, for the inflammatory component of the response can turn against the body, particularly as the body ages or becomes obese. The response, which can be devastating when directed against microbes entering the body, also sows the seeds of atherosclerosis, degradation of brain function, and insulin insensitivity and hastens the passage of HIV-infected individuals towards full-blown AIDS. Along with the insights arising from the unraveling of the human genome has come evidence that the inflammatory response is able to protect the human species from invasion by pathogens but not all individuals within the species from ill health. The differing ability of humans, particularly the male of the species, at an individual level to mount an inflammatory response of different levels of intensity owing to genotype can result in widely contrasting outcomes of invasion of the body by pathogens. On the one hand, individuals may effectively fight off invasion provided the immune response follows a normal pathway, whereas other individuals within the same community encoutering the same pathogens will die from the strength and nature of the response rather than from the direct effects of the invader. Insights gained from the genomic influences on cytokine production and the response to malaria suggest that the retention of alleles in pro-inflammatory cytokine genes that resulted in enhanced cytokine production within the human gene pool over generations could be a result of the heterozygotes' better capacity for fighting pathogens, whereas homozygotes of the high-producing genotype run an increased risk of a strong adverse inflammatory response. In the case of sickle cell anemia, where heterozygotic individuals reap an advantage in resistance to malaria by possession of only one copy of the anemia allele, homozygous individuals for the sickle cell trait pay the price for possession of two copies of the allele and die young. Because of the overall advantage of this situation to the species, the potentially disadvantageous allele will be retained within the human gene pool over generations.

With the twin discoveries that nutrients can modulate the inflammatory response and that cytokine genotype can modulate the effectiveness of nutrients in controlling inflammation, nutritional science sits at an exciting moment in its development. The mapping of how pro- and anti-inflammatory cytokine genotypes interact with responsiveness to immunonutrients at an indivividual level will allow tailor-made nutritional treatments of all diseases that have an underlying inflammatory basis. Furthermore, a better understanding of how nutritonal therapies and genetics interact will allow the twin adverse biological factors increasing the level of inflammatory stress in populations—obesity and aging—to be tackled by targeted nutritional therapy.

ACKNOWLEDGMENTS

The author is grateful to the BBSRC for funding much of the work reported in this chapter. The author is also grateful to collegues in the United Kingdom, Sweden, and Switzerland for scientific collaboration and advice.

REFERENCES

Ables, G. P., Takamatsu, D., Noma, H., El-Shazly, S., Jin, H. K., Taniguchi, T., Sekikawa, K., & Watanabe, T. (2001). The roles of Nramp1 and Tnfα genes in nitric oxide production and their effect on the growth of Salmonella typhimurium in macrophages from Nramp1 congenic and tumor necrosis factor-alpha-/- mice. *Journal of Interferon Cytokine Research, 21*, 53–62.

Allen, R. D. (1999). Polymorphism of the human TNF-α promoter—random variation or functional diversity? *Molecular Immunolology, 36*, 1017–1027.

Armitage, G. C. (2000). Periodontal infections and cardiovascular disease—how strong is the association? *Oral Disease, 6*, 335–350.

Arnalich, F., Garcia-Palomero, E., Lopez, J., Jiminez, M., Madero, R., Renart, J., Vazquez, J. J., & Montiel, C. (2000). Predictive value of nuclear factor kappaB activity and plasma cytokine levels in patients with sepsis. *Infection and Immununity, 68*, 1942–1945.

Azzi, A., Boscoboinik, D., & Marilley, D. (1995). Vitamin E: A sensor and an information transducer of the cell oxidation state. *American Journal of Clinical Nutrition, 62* (6 Suppl.), 1337S–1346S.

Baggio, G., Donnazzan, S., Monti, D., & Mari, D. (1998). Lipoprotein(a) and lipoprotein profile in healthy centenarians: A reappraisal of vascular risk factors. *FASEB Journal, 12*, 433–437.

Beale, R. J., Bryg, D. J., & Bihari, D. J. (1999). Immunonutrition in the critically ill: A systematic review of clinical outcome. *Critical Care Medicine, 27*, 2799–2805.

Bell, D. S. (2000). Inflammation, insulin resistance, infection, diabetes, and atherosclerosis. *Endocrinological Practice, 6*, 272–276.

Bethin, K. E., Vogt, S. K., & Muglia, L. J. (2000). Interleukin-6 is an essential, corticotropin-releasing hormone-independent stimula-torof the adrenal axis during immune system activation. *Proceedings of the National Academy of Science USA, 97*, 9317–9322.

Bidwell, J., Keen, L., Gallagher, G., Kimberly, R., Huizinga, T., McDermott, M. F., Oksenberg, J., McNicholl, J., Pociot, F., Hardt, C., & D'Alfonso, S. (2001). Cytokine gene polymorphism in human disease: On-line databases, supplement 1. *Genes and Immunology, 2*, 61–70.

Bonafè, M., Olivieri, F., & Cavallone, L. (2001). A gender-dependent genetic predisposition to produce high levels of IL-6 is detrimental to longevity. *European Journal of Immunology, 31*, 2357–2361.

Bonora, E., Kiechl, S., & Oberhollenzer, E. (2000). Impaired glucose tolerance, type 2 diabetes mellitus and carotid atherosclerosis: Prospective results of the Bruneck Study. *Diabetologia, 43*, 156–164.

Boya, P., de la Pena, A., Beloqui, O., Larrea, E., Conchillo, M., Castelruiz, Y., Civeira, M. P., & Prieto, J. (1999). Antioxidant status and glutathione metabolism in peripheral blood mononuclear cells from patients with chronic hepatitis C. *Journal of Hepatology, 31*, 808–814.

Breitkreutz, R., Pittack, N., Nebe, C. T., Schuster, D., Brust, J., Beichert, M., Hack, V., Daniel, V., Edler, L., & Droge, W. (2000). Improvement of immune functions in HIV infection by sulfur supplementation: Two randomized trials. *Journal of Molecular Medicine, 78*, 55–62.

Bryson, B. (2003). In *A short history of nearly everything*. New York: Doubleday.

Calder, P. C. (1997). *n*-3 Polyunsaturated fatty acids and cytokine production in health and disease. *Annals of Nutrition and Metabolism, 41*, 203–234.

Cao, Y., Feng, Z., Hoos, A., & Klimberg, V. S. (1998). Glutamine enhances gut glutathione production. *Journal of Parenteral and Enteral Nutrition, 22*, 224–227.

Caruso, C., Candore, G., Romano, G. C., Lio, D., Bonafe, M., Valensin, S., & Franceschi, C. (2001). Immunogenetics of longevity. Is major histocompatibility complex polymorphism relevant to the control of human longevity? A review of literature data . *Mechanisms of Ageing and Development, 122*, 445–462.

Chambers, J. C., Eda, S., & Bassett, P. (2001). C-reactive protein, insulin resistance, central obesity, and coronary heart disease risk in Indian Asians from the United Kingdom compared with European whites. *Circulation, 104*, 145–150.

Chernoff, A. E., Granowitz, E. V., Shapiro, L., Vannier, E., Lonnemann, G., Angel, J. B., Kennedy, J. S., Rabson, A. R., Wolff, S. M., & Dinarello, C. A. (1995). A randomized, controlled trial of IL-10 in humans. Inhibition of inflammatory cytokine production and immune responses. *Journal of Immunology, 154*, 5492–5499.

Chorazy, P. A., Schumacher, H. R., Jr., & Edlind, T. D. (1992). Glutathione peroxidase in rheumatoid arthritis: Analysis of enzyme activity and DNA polymorphism. *DNA Cell Biology, 11*, 221–225.

Choi, S. S., Gatanaga, M., Granger, G. A., & Gatanaga, T. (1996). Prostaglandin-E2 regulation of tumor necrosis factor receptor release in human monocytic THP-1 cells. *Cellular Immunology, 170*, 178–184.

Chu, N. F., Spiegelman, D., & Hotamisligil, G. S. (2001). Plasma insulin, leptin, and soluble TNF receptors levels in relation to obesity-related atherogenic and thrombogenic cardiovascular disease risk factors among men. *Atherosclerosis, 157*, 495–503.

Cnop, M., Landchild, M. J., & Vidal, J. (2002).The concurrent accumulation of intra-abdominal and subcutaneous fat explains the association between insulin resistance and plasma leptin concentrations : Distinct metabolic effects of two fat compartments. *Diabetes, 51*, 1005–1015.

Corry, D. B., & Tuck, M. L. (2001). Selective aspects of the insulin resistance syndrome. *Current Opinion in Nephrology and Hypertension, 10*, 507–514.

Debril, M. B., Renaud, J. P., Fajas, L., & Auwerx, J. (2001). The pleiotropic functions of peroxisome proliferator-activated receptor gamma. *Journal of Molecular Medicine, 79*, 30–47.

Denno, R., Rounds, J. D., Faris, R., Halejko, L. B., & Wilmore, D. W. (1996). Glutamine enriched TPN enhances plasma glutathione in resting state. *Journal of Surgical Research, 61*, 35–38.

De Rosa, S. C., Zaretsky, M. D., Dubs, J. D., Roederer, M., Anderson, M., Green, A., Mitra, D., Watanabe, N., Nakamura, H., Tjioe, I., Deresinski, S. C., Moore, W. A., Ela, S. W., Parks, D., Herzenberg, L. A., & Herzenberg, L. A. (2000). *N*-Acetylcysteine replenishes glutathione in HIV infection. *European Journal of Clinical Investigation, 30*, 915–929.

Devaraj, S., & Jialal, I. (2000). Low-density lipoprotein postsecretory modification, monocyte function, and circulating adhesion molecules in type 2 diabetic patients with and without macrovascular complications: The effect of alpha-tocopherol supplementation. *Circulation, 102*, 191–196.

Diamond J. (1999). In *Guns, germs and steel: The fate of human societies*. New York: W. W. Norton & Co.

Dillon, G., Vita, J. A., & Leeuwenburgh, C. (1998). α-Tocopherol supplementation reduces systemic markers of oxidative damage in healthy adults. *Circulation, 17S*, 671I.

Dinarello, C. A., Bishai, I., Rosenwasser, L. J., & Coceani, F. (1984). The influence of lipoxygenase inhibitors on the in vitro production of human leukocytic pyrogen and lymphocyte activating factor (interleukin-1). *International Journal of Immunopharmacology, 6*, 43–50.

Dröge, W., Schulze-Osthoff, K., Mihm, S., Galter, D., Schenk, H., Eck, H. P., Roth, S., & Gmünder, H. (1994). Functions of glutathione and glutathione disulphide in immunology and immunopathology. *FASEB Journal, 8*, 1131–1138.

Duncan, B. B., & Schmidt, M. I. (2001). Chronic activation of the innate immune system may underlie the metabolic syndrome. *Sao Paulo Medical Journal, 119*, 122–127.

Elia, M. (1992). Glutamine in parenteral nutrition. International Journal of Food Science and *Nutrition, 43*, 47–49.

Emanuelli, B., Peraldi, P., & Filloux, C. (2001). SOCS-3 inhibits insulin signaling and is up-regulated in response to tumor necrosis factor-alpha in the adipose tissue of obese mice. *Journal of Biological Chemistry, 276*, 47,944–47,949.

Endres, S., Ghorbani, R., Kelley, V. E., Georgilis, K., Lonnemann, G., van der Meer, J. W. M., Cannon, J. G., Rogers, T. S., Klempner, M. S., Weber, P. C., Schaefer, E. J., Wolff, S. M., & Dinarello, C. A. (1989). The effect of dietary supplementation with n-3 polyunsaturated fatty acids on the synthesis of interleukin-1 and tumor necrosis factor by mononuclear cells. *New England Journal of Medicine, 320*, 265–271.

Ershler, W. B., & Kerller, E. T. (2000). Age-associated increased interleukin-6 gene expression, late diseases, and frailty. *Annual Reviews of Medicine, 51*, 245–270.

Espevik, T., Figari, I. S., Shalaby, M. R., Lackides, G. A., Lewis, G. D., Shepard, H. M., & Palladino, M. A., Jr. (1987). Inhibition of cytokine production by cyclosporin A and transforming growth factor beta. *Journal of Experimental Medicine, 166*, 571–576.

Faggioni, R., Feingold, K. R., & Grunfeld, C. (2001). Leptin regulation of the immune response and the immunodeficiency of malnutrition. *FASEB Journal, 15*, 2565–2571.

Fagiolo, U., Cossarizza, A., Scala, E., Fanales-Belasio, E., Ortolani, C., Cozzi, E., Monti, D., Franceschi, C., & Paganelli, R. (1993). Increased cytokine production in mononuclear cells of healthy elderly people. *European Journal of Immunology, 23*, 2375–2378.

Ferrucci, L, Harris, T. B., Guralnik, J. M., & Tracy, R. P. (1999). Serum IL-6 level and the development of disability in older persons. *Journal of the American Geriatric Society, 47*, 639–646.

Festa, A., D'Agostino, R., Jr., & Williams, K. (2001). The relation of body fat mass and distribution to markers of chronic inflammation. *International Journal of Obesity and Related Metabolic Disorders, 25*, 1407–1415.

Folsom, A. R., Pankow, J. S., & Tracy, R. P. (2001). The Investigators of the NHBLI Family Heart Study. Association of C-reactive protein with markers of prevalent atherosclerotic disease. *American Journal of Cardiology, 88*, 112–117.

Formica, S., Roach, T. I., & Blackwell, J. M. (1994). Interaction with extracellular matrix proteins influences Lsh/Ity/Bcg (candidate Nramp) gene regulation of macrophage priming/activation for tumour necrosis factor-alpha and nitrite release. *Immunology, 82*, 42–50.

Forsberg, L., Lyrenas, L., de Faire, U., & Morgenstern, R. (2001). A common functional C-T substitution polymorphism in the promoter region of the human catalase gene influences transcription factor binding, reporter gene transcription and is correlated to blood catalase levels. *Free Radical Biology and Medicine, 30*, 500–505.

Franceschi, C., Motta, L., Valensin, S., Rapisarda, R., Franzone, A., Berardelli, M., Motta, M., Monti, D., Bonafe, M., Ferrucci, L., Deiana, L., Pes, G. M., Carru, C., Desole, M. S., Barbi, C., Sartoni, G., Gemelli, C., Lescai, F., Olivieri, F., Marchegiani, F., et al. (2000). Do men and women follow different trajectories to reach extreme longevity? Italian Multicenter Study on Centenarians (IMUSCE). *Aging (Milano), 12*, 77–84.

Fruchart, J. C., Staels, B., & Duriez, P. (2001). PPARS, metabolic disease and atherosclerosis. *Pharmacological Research, 44*, 345–352.

Gadek, J. E., De Michele, S. J., Karlstad, M. D., Pacht, E. R., Donahoe, M., Albertson, T. E., Van Hoozen, C., Wennberg, A. K., Nelson, J. L., Nourselehi, M., & The Enteral Nutrition in ARDS Study Group. (1999). Effect of enteral feeding with eicosapentaenoic acid, γ-linolenic acid, and antioxidants in patients with acute respiratory distress syndrome. *Critical Care Medicine, 27*, 1409–1420.

Grau, A. J., Aulmann, M., Lichy, C., Meiser, H., Buggle, F., Brandt, T., & Grond-Ginsbach, C. (2001). Increased cytokine release by leucocytes in survivors of stroke at young age. *European Journal of Clinical Investigation, 31*, 999–1006.

Grimble, R. (1990). Serum albumin and mortality. *Lancet, 1*, 348.

Grimble, R. F. (1996). Theory and efficacy of antioxidant therapy. *Current Opinion in Critical Care, 2*, 260–266.

Grimble, R. F. (1997). Effect of antioxidative vitamins on immune function with clinical applications. *International Journal of Vitamin Nutrition Research, 67*, 312–320.

Grimble, R. F. (1998). Dietary lipids and the inflammatory response. *Proceedings of the Nutrition Society, 57*, 535–542.

Grimble, R. F. (2001a). Nutritional modulation of immune function. *Proceedings of the Nutrition Society, 60*, 389–397.

Grimble, R. (2001b). Stress proteins in disease: Metabolism on a knife edge. *Clinical Nutrition, 20*, 469–476.

Grimble, R. F. (2002). Inflammatory status and insulin resistance. *Current Opinion in Clinical Nutrition and Metabolic Care, 5*, 551–559.

Grimble, R. F. (2003). Inflammatory response in the elderly. *Current Opinion in Clinical Nutrition and Metabolic Care, 6*, 21–29.

Grimble, R. F., Andersson, P., Madden, J., Palmblad, J., Persson, M., Vedin, I., & Cederholm, T. (2003). Gene:gene interactions influence the outcome in elderly patients. *Clinical Nutrition, 22*, S39.

Grimble, R. F., Howell, W. M., O'Reilly, G., Turner, S. J., Markovic, O., Hirrell, S., East, J. M., & Calder, P. C. (2002).The ability of fish oil to suppress tumor necrosis factor-alpha production by peripheral blood mononuclear cells in healthy men is associated with polymorphisms in genes which influence TNF-alpha production. *American Journal of Clinical Nutrition, 76*, 454–459.

Grimble, R. F., Thorell, A., Nygren, J., Ljungqvist, O., Barber, N., Grant, S., & Madden, J. (2003). Cytokine genotype and gender influence the inflammatory response to surgery. *Clinical Nutrition, 22*, S45.

Hajeer, A. H., Lazarus, M., & Turner, D. (1998). IL-10 gene promoter polymorphisms in rheumatoid arthritis. *Scandinavian Journal of Rheumatology, 27*, 142–145.

Hak, A. E., Pols, H. A., & Stehouwer, C. D. (2001). Markers of inflammation and cellular adhesion molecules in relation to insulin resistance in nondiabetic elderly: The Rotterdam study. *Journal of Clinical Endocrinology and Metabolism, 86*, 4398–4405.

Han, S. N., Meydani, M., Wu, D., Bender, B. S., Smith, D. E., Vina, J., Cao, G. P., & Meydani, S. N. (2000). Effect of long-term dietary antioxidant supplementation on influenza virous infection. *Journal of Gerontology Biological Sciences and Medical Sciences, 55*, B496–503.

Harris, T. B., Ferrucci, T., Tracy, R. P., & Corti, M. (1999). Associations between elevated interleukin-6 and C-reactive protein levels with mortality in the elderly. *American Journal of Medicine, 106*, 506–512.

Hattori, S., Hattori, Y., Banba, N., Kasai, K., & Shimoda S. (1995). Pentamethyl-hydroxychromane, vitamin E derivative, inhibits induction of nitric oxide synthase by bacterial lipopolysaccharide. *Biochemistry and Molecular Biology International, 35*, 177–183.

Hegazy, D. M., O'Reilly, D. A., & Yang, B. M. (2001). NFkappaB polymorphisms and susceptibility to type 1 diabetes. *Genes and Immunology, 2*, 304–308.

Hotamisligil, G. S., Budavari, A., Murray, D., & Spiegelman, B. M. I. (1994). Reduced tyrosine kinase activity of the insulin receptor in obesity-diabetes. *Journal of Clinical Investigation, 94*, 1543–1549.

Hotamisligil, G. S., Peraldi. P., Budavari. A., Ellis, R., White, M. F., & Spiegelman, B. M. I. (1996). IRS-1-mediated inhibition of insulin receptor tyrosine kinase activity in TNF-alpha- and obesity-induced insulin resistance. *Science, 271*, 665–668.

Hotamisligil, G. S., & Spiegelman, B. M. I. (1994). Tumor necrosis factor a: A key component of the obesity-diabetes link. *Diabetes, 43*, 1271–1278.

Houdijk, A. P. J., Rijnsburger, E. R., Jansen, J., Wesdorp, R. I. C., Weiss, J. K., McCamish, M. A., Teerlink, T., Meuwissen, S. G. M., Haarman, H. J. ThM., Thijs, L. G., & Van Leeuwen, P. A. M. (1998). Randomised trial of glutamine-enriched enteral nutrition on infectious morbidity in patients with multiple trauma. *Lancet, 352*, 772–776.

Huang, Y. C., Guh, J. H., Cheng, Z. J., Chang, Y. L., Hwang, T. L., Liao, C. H., Tzeng, C. H., & Teng, C. M. (2001). Inhibition of the expression of inducible nitric oxide synthase and cyclooxygenase-2 in macrophages in macrophages by & HQ derivatives: Involvement of IkappaB-alpha stabilisation. *European Journal of Pharmacology, 418*, 133–139.

Huizinga, T. W., Keijsers, V., & Yanni, G. (2002). Are differences in interleukin 10 production associated with joint damage? *Rheumatology, 39*, 1180–1188.

Hunter, E. A. L., & Grimble, R. F. (1994). Cysteine and methionine supplementation modulate the effect of tumor necrosis factor α on protein synthesis, glutathione and zinc content of tissues in rats fed a low-protein diet. *Journal of Nutrition, 124*, 2319–2328.

Hutchinson, I. V., Pravica, V., Hajeer, A., & Sinnott, P. J. (1999). Identification of high and low responders to allographs. *Review in Immunogenetics, 1*, 323–333.

Iwamoto, Y., Nishimura, F., & Nakagawa, M. (2001). The effect of antimicrobial periodontal treatment on circulating tumor necrosis factor-alpha and glycated hemoglobin level in patients with type 2 diabetes. *Journal of Periodontolology, 72*, 774–778.

Jacob, C. O., Franek, Z., Lewis, G. D., Koo, M., Hansen, J. A., & McDevitt, H. O. (1990). Heritable major histocompatibility complex class II-associated differences in production of tumor necrosis factor-α: Relevance to genetic predisposition to systemic lupus erythematosus. *Proceedings of the National Academy of Science, 87*, 1233–1237.

Jacob, R. A., Kelley, D. S., Pianalto, F. S., Swendseid, M. E., Henning, S. M., Zhang, J. Z., Ames, B. N. Fraga, C. G., & Peters, J. H. (1991). Immunocompetence and oxidant defense during ascorbate depletion of healthy men. *American Journal of Clinical Nutrition, 54*, 1302S–1309S.

Jersmann, H. P., Hii, C. S., Ferrante, J. V., & Ferrante, A. (2001). Bacterial lipopolysaccharide and tumor necrosis factor alpha synergistically increase expression of human endothelial adhesion molecules through activation of NF-kappaB and p38 mitogen-activated protein kinase signaling pathways. *Infection and Immunology, 69*, 1273–1279.

Jialal, I., Fuller, C. J., & Huet, B. A. (1995). The effect of alpha-tocopherol supplementation on LDL oxidation. *Arteriosclerosis, Thrombosis and Vascular Biology, 15*, 190–198.

Jonkers, I. J., Mohrschladt, M. F., & Westendorp. R. G. (2002). Severe hypertriglyceridemia with insulin resistance is associated with systemic inflammation: Reversal with bezafibrate therapy in a randomized controlled trial. *American Journal of Medicine, 112*, 275–280.

Kol, A., Sukhova, G. K., Lichtman, A. H., & Libby, P. (1998). Chlamydial heat shock protein 60 localizes in human atheroma and regulates macrophage tumor necrosis factor-a andmatrix metalloproteinase expression. *Circulation, 98*, 300–307.

Kovarova, H., Necasova, R., Porkertova, S., Radzioch, D., & Macela, A. (2001). A Natural resistance to intracellular pathogens: Modulation of macrophage signal transduction related to the expression of the Bcg locus. *Proteomics, 1*, 587–596.

Kudoh, A., Katagai, H., Takazawa, T., & Matsuki, A. (2001). Plasma proinflammatory cytokine response to surgical stress in elderly patients. *Cytokine, 15*, 270–273.

Kunkel, S. L., Remick, D. G., Spengler, M., & Chensue, S. W. (1987). Modulation of macrophage-derived interleukin-1 and tumour necrosis factor by prostaglandin E_2. *Advances in Prostaglandin, Leukotriene and Thromboxane Research, 17A*, 155–156.

Lio, D., Scola, L., Crivello, A., Bonafe, M., Franceschi, C., Olivieri, F., Colonna Romano, G., Candore, G., & Caruso, C. (2002). Allele frequencies of +874TgA single nucleotide polymorphism at the first intron of interferon-gamma gene in a group of Italian centenarians. *Experimental Gerontolology, 37*, 315–319.

Loguercio, C., Blanco, F. D., De Girolamo, V., Disalvo, D., Nardi, G., Parente, A., & Blanco, C. D. (1999). Ethanol consumption, amino acid and glutathione blood levels in patients with and without chronic liver disease. *Alcohol Clinical and Experimental Research, 23*, 1780–1784.

Luo, J. L., Hammarqvist, F., Andersson, K., & Wernerman, J. (1996). Skeletal muscle glutathione after surgical trauma. *Annals of Surgery, 223*, 420–427.

Martin, G. M. (1997). Genetics and the pathobiology of ageing. *Philosophical Transactions of the Royal Society of London. Series B, Biological Sciences, 352*, 1773–1780.

Marwick, C. (1997). NHANES III health data relevant for aging nation. *Journal of the American Medical Association, 277*, 100–102.

McGuire, W., Hill, A. V., Allsopp, C. E., Greenwood, B. M. & Kwiatkowski, D. (1994). Variation in the TNF-alpha promoter region associated with susceptibility to cerebral malaria. *Nature, 371*, 508–510.

Messer, G., Spengler, U., Jung, M. C., Honold, G., Blomer, K., Pape, G. R., Riethmuller, G., & Weiss, E. H. (1991). Polymorphic structure of the tumour necrosis factor (TNF) locus: An Nco I polymorphism in the first intron of the human TNF-β gene correlates with a variant amino acid in position 26 and a reduced level of TNFα production. *Journal of Experimental Medicine, 173*, 209–219.

Meydani, S. N., Barklund, P. M., & Liu, S. (1990). Vitamin E supplementation enhances cell-mediated immunity in healthy elderly subjects. *American Journal of Clinical Nutrition, 52*, 557–563.

Meydani, S. N., Endres, S., & Woods, M. N. (1991). Oral (n-3) fatty acid supplementation supresses cytokine production and lymphocyte proliferation: Comparison between young and older women. *Journal of Nutrition, 121*, 547–555.

Meydani, S. N., Lichenstein, A. H., & Cornwall, S. (1993). Immunological effects of national cholesterol education panel (NCEP) step-2 diets with and without fish-derived (n-3) fatty acid enrichment. *Journal of Clinical Investigation, 92*, 105–113.

Meydani, S. N., Meydani, M., Blumberg, J. B., Leka, L. S., Silber, G., Loszewski, R., Thompson, C., Pedrosa, R. D., Diamond, D., & Stoller, D. (1997). Vitamin E supplementation and in vivo immune response in healthy subjects. A randomized controlled trial. *Journal of the American Medical Association, 277*, 1370–1386.

Meydani, S. N., Meydani, M., & Verdon, C. P. (1986). Vitamin E supplementation suppresses prostaglandin E2 synthesis and enhances the immune response of aged mice. *Mechanisms of Ageing and Development, 34*, 191–201.

Micke, P., Beeh, K. M., Schlaak, J. F., & Buhl, R. (2001). Oral supplementation with whey proteins increases plasma glutathione levels in HIV-infected patients. *European Journal of Clinical Investigation, 31*, 171–178.

Mira, J. P., Cariou, A., Grall, F., Delclaux, C., Losser, M. R., Heshmati, F., Cheval, C., Monchi, M., Teboul, J. L., Riche, F., Leleu, G., Arbibe, L., Mignon, A., Delpech, M., & Dhainaut, J. F. (1999). Association of TNF2, a TNF-alpha promoter polymorphism, with septic shock susceptibility and mortality: A multicenter study. *Journal of the American Medical Association, 282*, 561–568.

Mitrunen, K., Sillanpaa, P., Kataja, V., Eskelinen, M., Kosma, V. M., Benhamou, S., Uusitupa, M., & Hirvonen, A. (2001). Association between manganese superoxide dismutase (MnSOD) gene polymorphism and breast cancer risk. *Carcinogenesis, 22*, 827–829.

Mol, J. T. M., de Rijke, Y. B., Demacher, P. M. N., & Stalenhoef, A. F. H. (1997). Plasma levels of lipid and cholesterol oxidation products and cytokines in diabetes mellitus and smokers: Effect of vitamin E treatment. *Atherosclerosis, 129*, 169–176.

Moller, D. E. (2000). Potential role of TNF-alpha in the pathogenesis of insulin resistance and type 2 diabetes. *Trends Endocrinology Metabolism, 11*, 212–217.

Momoi, A., Murao, K., & Imachi, H. (2001). Inhibition of monocyte chemoattractant protein-1 expression in cytokine-treated human lung epithelial cells by thiazolidinedione. *Chest, 120*, 1293–1300.

Morlion, B. J., Stehle, P., Wachtler, P., Siedhoff, H-P., Koller, M., Konig, W., Furst, P., & Puchstein, C. (1998). Total parenteral nutrition with glutamine dipeptide after major surgery. A double blind controlled study. *Annals of Surgery, 227*, 302–308.

Munro, R., & Capell, H. (1997). Prevalence of low body mass in rheumatoid arthritis: Association with the acute phase response. *Annals of Rheumatic Disease, 56*, 326–369.

Mysliwska, J., Bryl, E., Foerster, A., & Mysliwski, A. (1998). Increase in IL-6 and decrease of interleukin 2 production during the ageing process are influenced by health status. *Mechanisms of Ageing and Development, 100*, 313–328.

Newsholme, E. A., Crabtree, B., Salleh, M., & Ardawi, M. (1985). Glutamine metabolism in lymphocytes. Its biochemistry, physiology and clinical importance. *Quarterly Journal of Experimental Physiology, 70*, 473–489.

Nilsson, J., Jovinge, S., Niemann, A., Reneland, R., & Lithell, H. (1998). Relation between plasma tumor necrosis factor-alpha and insulin sensitivity in elderly men with non-insulin-dependent diabetes mellitus. *Arteriosclerosis, Thrombosis and Vascular Biology, 18*, 1199–1202.

Nishimura, F., & Murayama, Y. (2001). Periodontal inflammation and insulin resistance—lessons from obesity. *Journal of Dental Research, 80*, 1690–1694.

Nuttall, S. L., Dunne, F., Kendall, M. J., & Martin, U. (1999). Age-dependent oxidative stress in elderly patients with non-insulin-dependent diabetes mellitus. *Quarterly Journal of Medicine, 92*, 33–38.

Onat, A., Sansoy, V., & Yildirim, B. (2001). C-reactive protein and coronary heart disease in western Turkey. *American Journal of Cardiology, 88*, 601–607.

Ono, S., Aosasa, S., Tsujimoto, H., Ueno, C., & Mochizuki, H. (2001). Increased monocyte activation in elderly patients after surgical stress. *European Journal of Surgical Research, 33*, 33–38.

Pannacciulli, N., Cantatore, F. P., & Minenna, A. (2001). C-reactive protein is independently associated with total body fat, central fat, and insulin resistance in adult women. *International Journal of Obesity and Related Metabolic Disorders, 25*, 1416–1420.

Paolini-Giacobino, A. A., Grimble, R., & Pichard, C. (2003). Genomic interactions with disease and nutrition. *Clinical Nutrition, 22*, 507–514.

Pena, L. R., Hill, D. B., & McClain, C. J. (1999). Treatment with glutathione precursor decreases cytokine activity. *Journal of Parenteral and Enteral Nutrition, 23*, 1–6.

Perrey, C., Pravica, V., Sinnott, P. J., & Hutchinson, I. V. (1998). Genotyping for polymorphisms in interferon-gamma, interleukin-10, transforming growth factor-beta 1 and tumour necrosis factor-alpha genes: a technical report. *Transplantation Immunology, 6*, 193–197.

Pfeilschifter, J., Koditz, R., Pfohl, M., & Schatz, H. (2002). Changes in proinflammatory cytokine activity after menopause. *Endocrinological Reviews, 23*, 90–119.

Pradhan, A. D., Manson, J. E., Rifai, N. (2001). C-reactive protein, interleukin 6, and risk of developing type 2 diabetes mellitus. *Journal of the American Medical Association, 286*, 327–334.

Prio, T. K., Bruunsgaard, H., Roge, B., & Pedersen, B. K. (2002). Asymptomatic bacteriuria in elderly humans is associated with increased levels of circulating TNF receptors and elevated numbers of neutrophils. *Experimental Gerontology, 37*, 693–699.

Reid, C. L., Hutchinson, I. V., Campbell, I. T., & Little, R. A. (1999). Genetic variation in cytokine production may be protective of ICU admission and may influence mortality. *Clinical Nutrition, 18*, 45.

Reid. M., Badaloo, A., Forrester, T., Morlese, J. F., Frazer, M., Heird, W. C., & Jahoor, F. (2000). In vivo rates of erythrocyte glutathione synthesis in children with severe protein-energy malnutrition. *American Journal of Physiology, 278*, E405–412.

Rink, L., Cakman, I., & Kirchner, H. (1998). Altered cytokine production in the elderly. *Mechanisms of Ageing and Development, 102*, 199–209.

Robinson, M. K., Rodrick, M. L., Jacobs, D. O., Rounds, J. D., Collins, K. H., Saporoschetz, I. B., Mannick, J. A., & Wilmore, D. W. (1993). Glutathione depletion in rats impairs T-cell and macrophage immune function. *Archives of Surgery, 128*, 29–34.

Rohleder, N., Kudielka, B. M., Hellhammer, D. H., Wolf, J. M., & Kirschbaum, C. (2002). Age and sex steroid-related changes in glucocorticoid sensitivity of proinflammatory cytokine production after psychosocial stress. *Journal of Neuroimmunology, 126*, 69–77.

Romano, M., Pomilio, M., & Vigneri, S. (2001). Endothelial perturbation in children and adolescents with type 1 diabetes: Association with markers of the inflammatory reaction. *Diabetes Care, 24*, 1674–1678.

Rosenberg, I. H. (1989). Epidemiologic and methodologic problems in determining nutritional status of older persons. *American Journal of Clinical Nutrition, 50* (Suppl.), 1231–1233.

Ross, R. (1993). The pathogenesis of atherosclerosis: A perspective for the 1990s. *Nature, 362*, 801–809.

Roubenoff, R. (2001). Origins and clinical relevance of sarcopenia. *Canadian Journal of Applied Physiology, 26*, 78–89.

Sakao, S., Tatsumi, K., Igari, H., Shino, Y., Shirasawa, H., & Kuriyama, T. (2001). Association of tumor necrosis factor alpha gene promoter polymorphism with the presence of chronic obstructive pulmonary disease. *American Journal of Respiratory and Critical Care Medicine, 163*, 420–422.

Saldeen, T. G., & Rand, K. (1998). Interactive role of infection, inflammation and traditional risk factors in atherosclerosis and coronary artery disease. *Journal of the American College of Cardiology, 31*, 1217–1225.

Schreck, R., Rieber, P., & Baeurerle, P. A. (1991). Reactive oxygen intermediates as apparently widely used messengers in the activation of nuclear transcription factor-κB and HIV-1. *EMBO Journal, 10*, 2247–2256.

Schaaf, B. M., Seitzer, U., Pravica, V., Aries, S. P., & Zabel, P. (2001). Tumor necrosis factor-alpha −308 promoter gene polymorphism and increased tumor necrosis factor serum bioactivity in farmer's lung patients. *American Journal of Respiratory and Critical Care Medicine, 163*, 379–382.

Schroder, J., Kahlke, V., Book, M., & Stuber, F. (2000). Gender differences in sepsis: Genetically determined? *Shock, 14*, 307–310.

Searle, S., & Blackwell, J. M. (1999). Evidence for a functional repeat polymorphism in the promoter of the human NRAMP1 gene that correlates with autoimmune versus infectious disease susceptibility. *Journal of Medical Genetics, 36*, 295–299.

Shurtz-Swirski, R., Sela, S., & Herskovits, A. T. (2001). Involvement of peripheral polymorphonuclear leukocytes in oxidative stress and inflammation in type 2 diabetic patients. *Diabetes Care, 24*, 104–110.

Spapen, H., Zhang, H., Demanet, C., Vleminckx, W., Vincent, J.L., & Huyghens, L. (1998). Does *N*-acetyl cysteine inflkuence cytokine response during early human septic shock? *Chest, 113*, 1616–1624.

Spitzer, J. J., Bagby, G. J., Meszaros, K., & Lang, C. H. (1988). Alterations in lipid and carbohydrate metabolism in sepsis. *Journal of Parenteral and Enteral Nutrition, 12* (Suppl.), 53S–58S.

Spitzer, J. J., Bagby, G. J., Meszaros, K., & Lang, C. H. (1989). Altered control of carbohydrate metabolism in endotoxemia. *Progress in Clinical and Biological Research, 286*, 145–165.

Staal, F. J. T., Ela, S. W., & Roederer, M. (1992). Glutathione deficiency in human immunodeficiency virus infection. *Lancet, i*, 909–912.

Steiner, M. (1999). Vitamin E, a modifier of platelet function: Rationale and use in cardiovascular and cerebrovascular disease. *Nutrition Reviews, 57*, 306–309.

Stuber, F., Petersen, M., Bokelmann, F., & Schade, U. (1996). A genomic polymorphism within the tumor necrosis factor locus influences plasma tumor necrosis factor-alpha concentrations and outcome of patients with severe sepsis. *Critical Care Medicine, 24*, 381–384.

Tagore, A., Gonsalkorale, W. W., & Pravica, V. (1999). Interleukin 10 (IL-10) genotypes in inflammatory bowel disease. *Tissues Antigens, 54*, 386–390.

Taniguchi, T., Koido, Y., Aiboshi, J., Yamashita, T., Suzaki, S., & Kurokawa, A. (1999). Change in the ratio of interleukin-6 to interleukin-10 predicts a poor outcome in patients with systemic inflammatory response syndrome. *Critical Care Medicine, 27,* 1262–1264.

Tanus-Santos, J. E., Desai, M., Deak, L. R., Pezzullo, J. C., Abernethy, D. R., Flockhart, D. A., & Freedman, J. E. (2002). Effects of endothelial nitric oxide synthase gene polymorphisms on platelet function, nitric oxide release, and interactions with estradiol. *Pharmacogenetics, 12*, 407–413.

Turner, D. M., Williams, D. M., & Sankaran, D. (1997). An investigation of polymorphisms in the interleukin-10 gene promoter. *European Journal of Immunogenetics, 24*, 108–116.

van Dissel, J. T., van Langevelde, P., Westendorp, R. G., Kwappenberg, K., & Frolich, M. (1998). Anti-inflammatory cytokine profile and mortality in febrile patients. *Lancet, 351*, 950–955.

van Tits, L. J., Demacker, P. N., de Graaf, J., Hak-Lemmers, H. L., & Stalenhoef, A. F. (2000). Alpha-tocopherol supplementation decreases production of superoxide and cytokines by leukocytes ex vivo in both normolipidemic and hypertriglyceridemic individuals. *American Journal of Clinical Nutrition, 71*, 458–464.

Visser, M., Pahor, M., Taaffe, D. R., Goodpaster, B. H., Simonsick, E. M., Newman, A. B., Nevitt, M., & Harris, T. B. (2002). Relationship of interleukin-6 and tumor necrosis factor-alpha with muscle mass and muscle strength in elderly men and women: The Health ABC Study. *Journal of Gerontolology Biological Science and Medical Science, 57*, M326–332.

Vozarova, B., Weyer, C., & Hanson, K. (2001). Circulating interleukin-6 in relation to adiposity, insulin action, and insulin secretion. *Obesity Research, 9*, 414–417.

Vozarova, B., Weyer, C., & Lindsay, R. S. (2002). High white blood cell count is associated with a worsening of insulin sensitivity and predicts the development of type 2 diabetes. *Diabetes, 51*, 455–461.

Wada, K., Nakajima, A., & Blumberg, R. S. (2001). PPAR-gamma and inflammatory bowel disease: a new therapeutic target for ulcerative colitis and Crohn's disease. *Trends in Molecular Medicine, 7*, 329–331.

Wang, X. Y., Hurme, M., Jylha, M., & Hervonen, A. (2001). Lack of association between human longevity and polymorphisms of IL-1 cluster, IL-6, IL-10 and TNF-alpha genes in Finnish nonagenarians. *Mechanisms of Ageing and Development, 123*, 29–38.

Warzocha, K., Ribeiro, P., Bienvenu, J., Roy, P., Charlot, C., Rigal, D., Coiffier, B., & Salles, G. (1998). Genetic polymorphisms in the tumor necrosis factor locus influence non-Hodgkin's lymphoma outcome. *Blood, 91*, 3574–3581.

Wesselborg, S., Bauer, M. K. A., Vogt, M., Schmitz, M. L., & Schulze-Osthoff, K. (1997). Activation of transcription factor NF-kappa B and p38 mitogen-activated protein kinase is mediated by distinct and separate stress effector pathways. *Journal of Biological Chemistry, 272*, 12,422–12,429.

Weyer, C., Yudkin, J. S., & Stehouwer, C. D. (2002). Humoral markers of inflammation and endothelial dysfunction in relation to adiposity and in vivo insulin action in Pima Indians. *Atherosclerosis, 161*, 233–242.

Willeit, J., & Kiechl, S. (2000). Biology of arterial atheroma. *Cerebrovascular Disease. 10* (Suppl. 5), 1–8.

Wilson, A. G., Clay, F. E., & Crane, A. M. (1995). Comparative genetic association of human leukocyte antigen class II and tumor necrosis factor-alpha with dermatitis herpetiformis. *Journal of Investigative Dermatology, 104*, 856–858.

Wilson, A. G., de Vries, N., Pociot, F., di Giovine, F. S., van der Putte, L. B., & Duff, G.W. (1993). An allelic polymorphism within the human tumor necrosis factor alpha promoter region is strongly associated with HLA-A1, B8, and DR3 alleles. *Journal of Experimental Medicine, 177*, 557–560.

Wilson, A. G., Gordon, C., & di Giovine, F. S. (1994). A genetic association between systemic lupus erythematosus and tumor necrosis factor alpha. *European Journal of Immunology, 24*, 191–195.

Wu, D., Koga, T., Martin, K. R., & Meydani, M. (1999). Effect of vitamin E on human aortic endothelial cell production of chemokines and adhesion to monocytes. *Atherosclerosis, 147*, 297–307.

Wu, D., Meydani, S. N., & Han, S. N. (2000). Effect of dietary supplementation with fish oil in combination with different levels of vitamin E on immune response in healthy elderly human subjects. *FASEB. Journal, 14*, A238.

Wu, D., Meydani, S. N., Sastre, J., Hayek, M., & Meydani, M. (1994). In vitro glutathione supplementation enhances interleukin-2 production and mitogenic responses in peripheral blood mononuclear cells from young and old subjects. *Journal of Nutrition, 124*, 655–663.

Wu, T., Dorn, J. P., & Donahue, R. P. (2002). Associations of serum C-reactive protein with fasting insulin, glucose, and glycosylated hemoglobin: The Third National Health and Nutrition Examination Survey, 1988—1994. *American Journal of Epidemiology, 155*, 65–71.

Yaqoob, P., Newsholme, E. A., & Calder, P.C. (1999). Production of tumour necrosis factor—alpha increases with age and BMI in healthy women. *Proceedings of the Nutrition Society, 58*, 129A.

Young, D. G., Skibinski, G., Mason, J. I., & James, K. (1999). The influence of age and gender on serum dehydroepiaandrosterone sulphate (DHEA-S), IL-6, IL-6 soluble receptor (IL-6 sR) and transforming growth factor beta 1 (TGF-beta 1) levels in normal healthy blood donors. *Clinical and Experimental Immunology, 117*, 476–481.

Zhai, R., Jetten, M., Schins, R. P., Franssen, H., & Borm, P. J. (1998). Polymorphisms in the promoter of the tumor necrosis factor-alpha gene in coal miners. *American Journal of Industrial Medicine, 34*, 318–324.

Ziccardi, P., Nappo, F., & Giugliano, G. (2002). Reduction of inflammatory cytokine concentrations and improvement of endothelial functions in obese women after weight loss over one year. *Circulation, 105*, 804–809.

Index

L

M

N

About the Editors

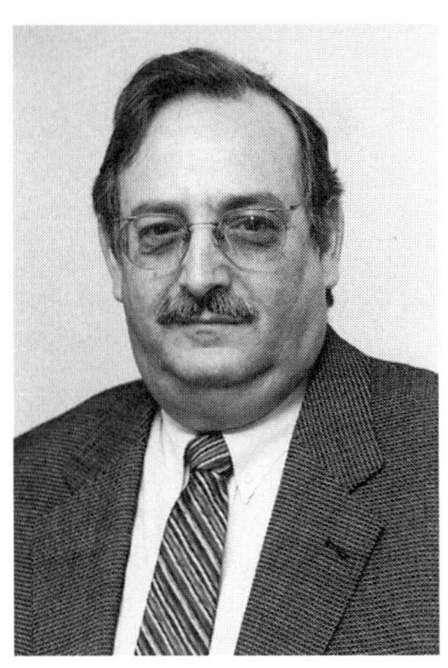

Shlomo Yehuda has a PhD in Psychology and Brain Science from M.I.T. He is a Professor in the Department of Psychology and is the Director of the Psychopharmacology Laboratory at Bar Ilan University. He currently holds the Ginsburg Chair for Alzheimer research and is active at the Farber Center. He was a research associate in Professor Wurtman's Lab at M.I.T., a visiting professor at Professor Kastin's Peptide Laboratory (Tulane Medical School, New Orleans, LA), and Rosenstadt Professor at Toronto Medical School–Nutrition Department. He has published over 150 scientific papers and 4 books in the following fields: Brain Biochemistry, Effects of Nutrients on Brain and Behavior (mainly brain iron and essential fatty acids), and Aging of the Brain and Animal Models of Neurological Disorders.

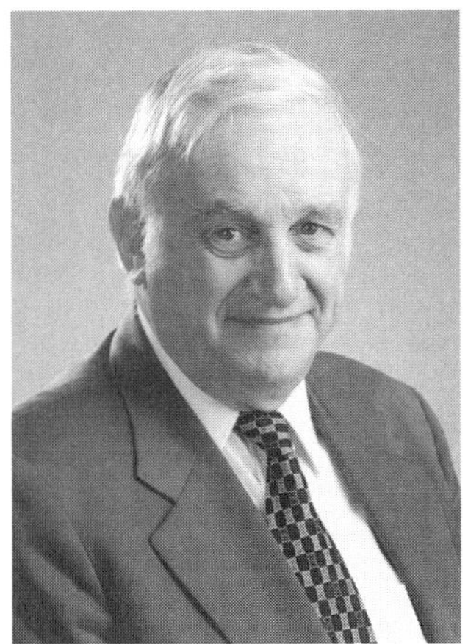

David I. Mostofsky is Professor of Experimental Psychology at Boston University, and holds associate appointments at several major medical institutions in the Boston area. A Charter Fellow of the Academy for Behavioral Medicine Research, he has been active in Behavioral Medicine and Psychopharmacology for many years, and has published numerous articles and books on a variety of topics in this area, especially with regard to epilepsy, pain, essential fatty acids, and psychoneuroimmunology. He has been the recipient of many awards including a Marshal Fund Award, Einstein Award, NIH/ Fogarty Fellowship, and a Fulbright Fellowship.

About the Series Editor

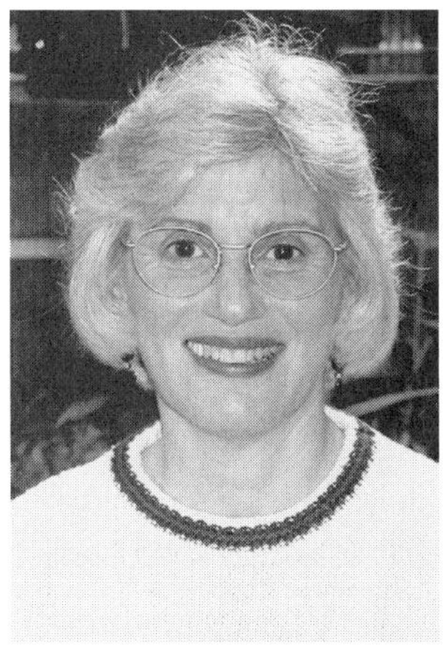

Dr. Adrianne Bendich is Clinical Director of Calcium Research at GlaxoSmithKline Consumer Healthcare, where she is responsible for leading the innovation and medical programs in support of several leading consumer brands including TUMS and Os-Cal. Dr. Bendich has primary responsibility for the coordination of GSK's support for the Women's Health Initiative (WHI) intervention study. Prior to joining GlaxoSmithKline, Dr. Bendich was at Roche Vitamins Inc., and was involved with the groundbreaking clinical studies proving that folic acid-containing multivitamins significantly reduce major classes of birth defects. Dr. Bendich has co-authored more than 100 major clinical research studies in the area of preventive nutrition. Dr. Bendich is recognized as a leading authority on antioxidants, nutrition and bone health, immunity, and pregnancy outcomes, vitamin safety, and the cost-effectiveness of vitamin/mineral supplementation.

In addition to serving as Series Editor for Humana Press and initiating the development of the 20 currently published books in the *Nutrition and Health*™ series, Dr. Bendich is the editor of 11 books, including *Preventive Nutrition: The Comprehensive Guide for Health Professionals.* She also serves as Associate Editor for *Nutrition: The International Journal of Applied and Basic Nutritional Sciences,* and Dr. Bendich is on the Editorial Board of the *Journal of Women's Health and Gender-Based Medicine,* as well as a past member of the Board of Directors of the American College of Nutrition. Dr. Bendich also serves on the Program Advisory Committee for Helen Keller International.

Dr. Bendich was the recipient of the Roche Research Award, was a Tribute to Women and Industry Awardee, and a recipient of the Burroughs Wellcome Visiting Professorship in Basic Medical Sciences, 2000–2001. Dr. Bendich holds academic appointments as Adjunct Professor in the Department of Preventive Medicine and Community Health at UMDNJ, Institute of Nutrition, Columbia University P&S, and Adjunct Research Professor, Rutgers University, Newark Campus. She is listed in *Who's Who in American Women.*